# The DIABETES Carbohydrate & Fat Gram Guide

**4TH EDITION**

Quick, Easy Meal Planning Using Carbohydrate and Fat Gram Counts

LEA ANN HOLZMEISTER, RD, CDE

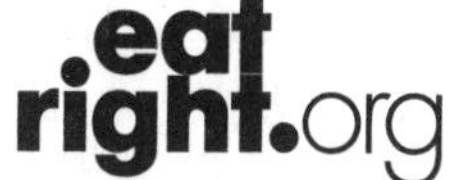


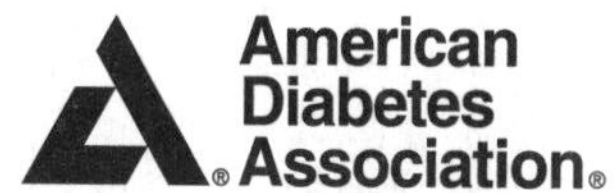

*Director, Book Publishing,* Robert Anthony; *Managing Editor,* Abe Ogden; *Acquisitions Editor,* Victor Van Beuren; *Editor,* Rebekah Renshaw; *Production Manager,* Melissa Sprott; *Composition,* ADA; *Cover Design,* pixiedesign, llc; *Printer,* Transcontinental Printing.



Printed in Canada
3 5 7 9 10 8 6 4

The suggestions and information contained in this publication are generally consistent with the Clinical Practice Recommendations and other policies of the American Diabetes Association, but they do not represent the policy or position of the Association or any of its boards or committees. Reasonable steps have been taken to ensure the accuracy of the information presented. However, the American Diabetes Association cannot ensure the safety or efficacy of any product or service described in this publication. Individuals are advised to consult a physician or other appropriate health care professional before undertaking any diet or exercise program or taking any medication referred to in this publication. Professionals must use and apply their own professional judgment, experience, and training and should not rely solely on the information contained in this publication before prescribing any diet, exercise, or medication. The American Diabetes Association—its officers, directors, employees, volunteers, and members—assumes no responsibility or liability for personal or other injury, loss, or damage that may result from the suggestions or information in this publication.

∞ The paper in this publication meets the requirements of the ANSI Standard Z39.48-1992 (permanence of paper).

ADA titles may be purchased for business or promotional use or for special sales. To purchase more than 50 copies of this book at a discount, or for custom editions of this book with your logo, contact the American Diabetes Association at the address below, at booksales@diabetes.org, or by calling 703-299-2046.

American Diabetes Association
1701 North Beauregard Street
Alexandria, Virginia 22311

DOI: 10.2337/9781580403405

**Library of Congress Cataloging-in-Publication Data**

Holzmeister, Lea Ann.
ADA diabetes carb & fat gram guide / Lea Ann Holzmeister. — 4th ed.
p. cm.
Rev. ed. of: The diabetes carbohydrate & fat gram guide. 3rd ed. c2005.
Includes bibliographical references and index.
ISBN 978-1-58040-340-5 (alk. paper)
1. Diabetes—Diet therapy. 2. Food exchange lists. 3. Food—Carbohydrate content—Tables. 4. Food—Fat content—Tables. I. Holzmeister, Lea Ann. Diabetes carbohydrate & fat gram guide. II. Title. III. Title: ADA diabetes carb and fat gram guide.
RC662.H66 2010
641.5'6314—dc22

2010018330

# *Dedication*

*To Jeff, Erin, Adam, and Emily, who I always count on.*

# *Table of Contents*

# *Preface to the Fourth Edition*

Since the third edition of the *Diabetes Carbohydrate and Fat Gram Guide* was first published, many new food products have been introduced, and fast-food restaurants have revised their menus. This fourth edition includes over 1,000 new listings, as well as one additional nutrient category. Because of new research about the effect of trans fat on health, this nutrient factor has been added for each food. In addition to saturated fat grams, this nutrient fact will help you evaluate the type of fat in foods.

Celiac disease is a lifelong digestive disease, affecting children and adults. People with type 1 diabetes have an increased risk of developing celiac disease. Celiac disease damages the small intestine and interferes with the digestion of food. People with celiac disease cannot tolerate gluten, a protein in wheat, rye, and barley. Consequently, all gluten must be eliminated from the diet. To help those affected, a chapter on gluten-free foods has been added in this new edition.

To prepare this new edition, we contacted food companies and fast-food franchises to obtain current nutrition information and product listings, and scanned grocery store shelves for the newest foods and most up-to-date nutrition facts. The result is a more complete resource for anyone who is concerned about nutrition.

# *Introduction*

Since its discovery hundreds of years ago, diabetes has been linked with what people eat. What people with diabetes are advised to eat, and how they plan their meals has changed over the years, however. The latest American Diabetes Association (ADA) Nutrition Principles and Recommendations in Diabetes (published each January in Supplement 1 of the journal *Diabetes Care*) emphasizes attaining and maintaining the best metabolic outcomes, including:

- Blood glucose in the normal range or as close to normal as is safely possible to prevent or reduce the risk for complications of diabetes;
- A lipid profile that reduces the risk for vascular disease;
- Blood pressure levels in the normal range or as close to normal as is safely possible.

The goals also recommend prevention and treatment of chronic complications of diabetes, which may require changes in eating patterns and lifestyle. People with diabetes should always consider improving health through healthy food choices and physical activity while considering personal and cultural preferences.

Many people with diabetes use some type of meal-planning system to help them meet their individual nutrition goals. Just as there is no one diet that is right for everyone with diabetes, there is also no one meal-planning approach that meets everyone's needs. It is important to know your own nutrition goals. A registered dietitian (RD) can help you determine your individual nutrition goals and develop a meal plan based on your food preferences, lifestyle, blood glucose and blood lipid (fat) levels, overall health, and abilities. If you're not currently seeing a dietitian, your doctor may be able to recommend one. Or visit the American Dietetic Association's web site at www.eatright.org.

## Types of Meal-Planning Approaches

Four types of meal-planning approaches are described in this book:

- Carbohydrate counting
- Fat gram counting
- Food exchange system
- Calorie counting

The advantages and disadvantages of each are discussed, and information about where to learn more is provided.

It is important to select a meal-planning approach that you are comfortable using and that will work toward achieving your goals. You do not have to use the same approach your entire life. As your individual nutrition goals change, so may your meal-planning approach. Before switching, though, it is a good idea to consult with your dietitian.

### *Carbohydrate Counting*

Carbohydrate counting has been used for many years in Europe and in the United States. The three main nutrients in the foods we eat are carbohydrate, protein, and fat. The carbohydrate in foods affects your blood glucose level more than protein or fat. In carbohydrate counting, you count only carbohydrate.

To use carbohydrate counting, you must know your total carbohydrate allotment for the day. A dietitian can help you determine this. Together, you and your dietitian will make a carbohydrate-counting meal plan based on your usual food intake, lifestyle, diabetes medications, and physical activity. Once you have your carbohydrate-counting meal plan, you'll need to become familiar with the carbohydrate content in foods. Carbohydrate is found in many foods, such as grains, vegetables, fruits, milk, and table sugar. It is important to count all carbohydrate regardless of its source.

The two main types of carbohydrate are sugars and starches. According to ADA's nutrition recommendations, both the amount (grams) of carbohydrate and the type of carbohydrate in a food influence blood glucose level. However, monitoring total grams of carbohydrate and eating the same amount of carbohydrate at meals and snacks each day remains a key strategy in achieving good blood glucose control.

Carbohydrate counting can provide some advantages over other meal-planning approaches. Some people feel that focusing on only one nutrient makes this system easier. With the focus on carbohydrate, food and insulin can be matched more precisely. Matching food and insulin increases flexibility in meal and snack times. This can be particularly helpful when your appetite varies or your schedule changes. Also, insulin can be matched to carbohydrate eaten at specific times during the day. For example, some people need more insulin at breakfast for each gram of carbohydrate eaten. Thus, carbohydrate counting may be most appropriate for people who take insulin.

One disadvantage of carbohydrate counting is that when you focus only on carbohydrate, it is easy to lose sight of the overall nutritional quality of foods. For example, counting the carbohydrate in foods like fried chicken or a regular hotdog, but ignoring their fat content, may lead you to eat these fatty foods more often. Too much fat in the diet increases your risk of heart disease, cancer, and weight gain. If you pay no attention to the overall nutritional quality of foods, you may end up eating a diet that is too high in fat or protein.

To learn more about carbohydrate counting, contact your dietitian. The American Diabetes Association and the American Dietetic Association have jointly published two instructional booklets on carbohydrate counting: *Count Your Carbs, Getting Started* and *Advanced Carbohydrate Counting*. You can obtain these booklets from your dietitian or by ordering them online at http://store.diabetes.org or www.eatright.org.

### *Fat-Gram Counting*

Fat-gram counting has been around since the 1980s, when it was introduced as a tool to teach low-fat eating to reduce the risk of cancer. Since that time, it has also been used for heart-healthy eating for heart disease and reduced-calorie eating for weight reduction. Fat-gram counting may be particularly useful for people with type 2 diabetes who are overweight. Fat provides two and a half times as many calories per gram as carbohydrate or protein.

The first step in using fat gram counting is to establish a daily calorie requirement based on your height, weight, activity level, and weight goal. Your dietitian can help you determine this. Then, based on your nutrition goals, a daily fat-gram goal will be determined. In fat-gram counting, you keep a record of the foods you eat and their fat content.

There are some advantages to fat-gram counting. It is simple, and it allows a considerable amount of flexibility and control over your food choices. With fat-gram counting, you will usually improve the overall quality of your food choices, because you will tend to select low-fat foods, such as fruits, vegetables, grains, and low-fat dairy products. Like carbohydrate counting, you are focusing on only one nutrient. This can be especially appealing when weight loss is the primary goal and other approaches have not worked.

One disadvantage of fat-gram counting is that it does not take into consideration foods that may affect your blood glucose. Therefore, your blood glucose values may be inconsistent.

To learn more about fat-gram counting, contact your dietitian. Your local American Heart Association may also have additional information on fat gram counting programs.

### *Exchange System*

For many years, the exchange system has been used as a meal-planning approach for people with diabetes, regardless of the type of diabetes and how it is treated. This system groups foods with similar nutritional value into lists, with the goal of helping people with diabetes eat consistent amounts of nutrients. Each food has approximately the same number of calories, carbohydrate, protein, and fat as the other foods on the same list. Any food on a list can be traded or "exchanged" for any other food on the same list.

To use the exchange system, you need an individualized meal plan that tells you how many exchanges from each list to select for meals and snacks. Your dietitian can help you design your individualized meal plan and teach you how to use this system.

The American Diabetes Association and The American Dietetic Association's *Choose Your Foods: Exchange Lists for Diabetes* booklet groups food into four broad groups: the carbohydrate group, the meat and meat substitutes group, the fat group, and the alcohol group. The carbohydrate group includes five lists: the starch list; the fruit list; the milk list; the sweets, desserts and other carbohydrates list; and the nonstarchy vegetable list. The meat and meat substitutes group includes four lists: the lean list, the medium-fat list, the high-fat list, and plant-based proteins list. The fat group includes a monounsaturated fats (unsaturated) list, a polyunsaturated fats list, and a saturated fats list. In addition to these lists, there are a free foods list, a combination foods list, a fast foods list, and an alcohol list.

One advantage of the exchange system is its emphasis on more than one nutrient and the importance of the overall nutritional content of foods. This system also encourages consistency in the timing and amount of your meals and snacks. People wanting to lose weight might find this approach useful for learning the caloric and fat values of foods. Food exchanges can also be used as a reference for those using carbohydrate counting. Each serving of a food in the carbohydrate group counts as 15 grams of carbohydrate.

One disadvantage of this system is the level of understanding needed to grasp the concept of grouping or "exchanging" foods.

It also requires learning where a food that is not listed fits. To learn more about the exchange system for meal planning, contact your dietitian.

### *Calorie Counting*

Calorie counting has been used for many years as a way to achieve weight loss, weight gain, or weight maintenance. This approach is most appropriate for people who are overweight and do not take insulin. Even modest weight loss improves blood glucose levels.

To use calorie counting, you and your dietitian establish a calorie goal that will help you achieve your weight goal. Your weight goal will be based on your current weight, height, and activity level. If you desire to lose weight, your calorie goal will be set lower than your usual intake of calories. If you wish to maintain your current weight, your calorie goal will be set at a calorie level similar to your current intake of calories. You keep records of the foods you eat and their calorie content. A periodic comparison of your food records and weekly weight can give you feedback on how you are progressing toward your weight goal. These records can also help you identify problem areas. For example, you might realize, after reviewing your records, that you tend to overeat when away from home. Knowing this information will help you and your dietitian develop strategies for changing this behavior.

The main advantage of calorie counting is the expanded choice of foods, which gives you more flexibility in what you eat. You decide whether and how a food might fit into your meal plan. For example, say your daily calorie goal is 1,500 calories, and a food you want to eat contains 600 calories. You can eat that food as long as you plan what other foods you'll eat that day to add up to the remaining 900 calories. Your serving size, too, is based on how you want to "spend" your calories. You might decide you can work in only half a serving of pasta salad, or you might choose to have a double serving of pasta salad.

One disadvantage of calorie counting might be the amount of time involved in keeping records and calculating the calorie content of foods. Also, because this approach does not guide you toward making nutritionally balanced choices, you may end up with a high-fat diet or one low in essential vitamins and minerals. Your dietitian can provide you with basic nutrition guidelines by which to select your foods to ensure that you meet your nutrition goals as well.

## Estimating Serving Sizes

The success of any meal-planning approach depends on how accurately you estimate your serving sizes. Therefore, it is essential to train your eyes to do this. Equip your kitchen with measuring spoons, measuring cups, and a food scale. Use these tools to measure and weigh foods consistently for two weeks or until you have trained your eyes to recognize what a cup of pasta looks like on your plate or how much one cup of milk fills your favorite glass.

Without some practice, it is surprisingly easy to mistakenly pour yourself one cup instead of a half cup of juice. A cup of juice has twice the carbohydrate and calories of a half cup of juice. This might tip you over your calorie or carbohydrate goal. If you do this with two to three foods each day, it could spoil your efforts at weight loss and blood glucose control.

Of course, it is not practical to measure servings when you eat out in a restaurant, but training your eyes will help. Fortunately, the serving sizes of fast foods are fairly standardized among restaurants, (e.g., a taco at any Taco Bell restaurant is likely to be the same size).

## How Food Counts Can Work For You

The meal-planning approach you select will determine what you will "count" in your diet. But using a meal-planning approach to guide your food choices is only a starting point. To reach your individual goals (such as blood glucose, blood lipids, weight, and general health), you need to respond every day to blood glucose changes and periodically to other indicators of your progress (such as blood lipid levels, weight gain, or weight loss).

### *Food Counts and Blood Glucose*

Making the connection between what you eat and how it affects your blood glucose level can be a very powerful step toward achieving your blood glucose goals. Once you have recorded your food intake and blood glucose values, you can learn to analyze the data to see how individual foods and meals affect your blood glucose. You can then try adjusting food intake, physical activity, and diabetes medications.

### *Food Counts and Blood Lipids*

Counting total fat, saturated fat, and trans fat in your diet while keeping tabs on your blood lipid levels (total cholesterol, HDL cholesterol, LDL cholesterol, and triglycerides) allows you to determine whether your meal plan is helping you to achieve your blood lipid goals. Suppose you have been advised to follow a diet with less than 70 grams of fat, minimal trans fat, and less than 25 grams of saturated fat per day in an attempt to reduce your total cholesterol from 250 to 200 mg/dl. By comparing your food records of total fat, saturated fat, and trans fat intake to your blood lipid levels over time, you can determine how close you are coming to your blood lipid goals.

## Using This Book of Food Counts

This book is intended to be a comprehensive listing of both generic and brand-name foods that are available nationally. The nutrition information in this fourth edition comes from several sources, including:

- The U.S. Department of Agriculture
- The Agricultural Research Service
- The USDA National Nutrient Database for Standard Reference, Release 21
- The American Diabetes Association and the American Dietetic Association's *Choose Your Foods: Exchange Lists for Diabetes* nutrient database
- A variety of food-processing companies and fast-food franchises
- Nutrition Facts from food labels

Foods are listed alphabetically throughout by food category and manufacturer. Nutrient information for foods from mixes (for example, puddings and cakes) reflect values after the food has been prepared according to package directions.

This book lists the calories, carbohydrate, fat, calories from fat, saturated fat, trans fat, cholesterol, sodium, fiber, and protein of many foods. These particular nutrients were selected because they are the most commonly monitored by people with diabetes (See Table 1.)

The nutrient values you use will depend on your meal-planning approach. You may need one, two, or even more of the values to figure out how a food fits in your plan. Values have been rounded to the nearest calorie, gram (g), or milligram (mg) per serving. (A gram is a unit of mass and weight in the metric system; an ounce is about 30 grams.) The serving sizes listed in this book are those most commonly used. Similar foods will have the same serving sizes. The serving size may be very different from the amount you serve yourself or eat. If your serving size is different, ask your dietitian to help you recalculate the numbers.

The exchange values of foods have been calculated using the "rounding-off method" (Wheeler ML, Franz M, Barrier PH, Holler H, Cronmiller N, Delahanty LM: Macronutrient and energy database for the 1995 Exchange Lists for Meal Planning: A rationale for clinical practice decisions. *J Am Diet Assoc* 96:1167–1170, 1996). Table 2 shows the amount of nutrients in one serving from each list.

Some of the foods in this book have a nutrient claim, such as "reduced-fat" or "low-calorie," as part of their name. These claims have standard meanings set by the Food and Drug Administration (FDA). Some of these terms and their meanings are listed in Table 3.

## TABLE 1. American Diabetes Association Nutrient Recommendations

Weight loss is recommended for overweight and obese individuals. Most healthy, normal-weight adults require 1,800 to 2,500 calories per day. However, your calorie needs are best determined by your dietitian.

**Carbohydrate:** Carbohydrates raise your blood glucose level, therefore, monitoring carbohydrate intake is recommended. A healthy diet includes carbohydrate from fruits, vegetables, whole grains, legumes, and low-fat milk. Your dietitian can help you determine how much carbohydrate you need in a day.

**Fat:** Fat may contribute to weight gain. People who are overweight should consider reducing their intake of fat. Your dietitian can help you determine what percentage of your daily calories should come from fat.

**Saturated Fat/Trans Fat:** Saturated fat and trans fat can raise your blood cholesterol level. Most people should get no more than 7% of their daily calories from saturated fat. Intake of trans fat should be minimized.

**Cholesterol:** Cholesterol, which is found in foods from animal sources, can raise your blood cholesterol level. Limit cholesterol in your diet to 200 milligrams or less daily.

**Sodium:** Sodium has been linked to high blood pressure (hypertension) and cardiovascular health risks. People with normal blood pressure should get no more than 2,300 milligrams of sodium per day. People with diabetes, heart failure, and high blood pressure are advised to get 2,000 milligrams or less of sodium per day.

*(Table 1 continues on next page.)*

## TABLE 1. American Diabetes Association Nutrient Recommendations (*Continued*)

**Fiber:** For most adults, including people with diabetes, daily consumption of 25–38 grams of dietary fiber from both soluble and insoluble fibers from a wide variety of food sources is recommended. Dietary fiber may be helpful in the treatment and prevention of constipation and several gastrointestinal disorders. Soluble fiber has a beneficial effect on serum lipids and provides satiety value to your diet.

**Protein:** Most adults, including people with diabetes, require approximately 15–20% of their calories from protein. Individuals with diabetes and kidney disease may require a reduction of protein intake.

**Alcohol:** If adults choose to use alcohol, daily intake should be limited to a moderate amount, one drink per day or less for women and two drinks per day or less for men. For individuals with diabetes who take diabetes medication, alcohol should be consumed only with food.

TABLE 2. Nutrient Content of Exchange Lists

| Food List | Carbohydrate (g) | Protein (g) | Fat (g) | Calories |
|---|---|---|---|---|
| **Carbohydrates** | | | | |
| Starch | 15 | 0–3 | 0–1 | 80 |
| Fruit | 15 | 0 | 0 | 60 |
| Milk | | | | |
| Fat-free, Low-Fat | 12 | 8 | 0–3 | 100 |
| Reduced-Fat, 2% | 12 | 8 | 5 | 120 |
| Whole | 12 | 8 | 8 | 160 |
| Sweets, Desserts, and Other Carbohydrate | 15 | Varies | Varies | Varies |
| Nonstarchy Vegetables | 5 | 2 | 0 | 25 |
| **Meat and Meat Substitutes** | | | | |
| Lean | 0 | 7 | 0-3 | 45 |
| Medium-Fat | 0 | 7 | 4-7 | 75 |
| High-Fat | 0 | 7 | 8+ | 100 |
| Plant-Based Proteins | Varies | 7 | Varies | Varies |

*(Table 2 continues on next page.)*

## TABLE 2. Nutrient Content of Exchange Lists (Continued)

| Food List | Carbohydrate (g) | Protein (g) | Fat (g) | Calories |
|---|---|---|---|---|
| **Fats** | | | | |
| Monounsaturated Fats | 0 | 0 | 5 | 45 |
| Polyunsaturated Fats | 0 | 0 | 5 | 45 |
| Saturated Fats | 0 | 0 | 5 | 45 |
| **Free Foods** | 5 or less | Varies | Varies | Less than 20 |
| **Combination Foods** | Varies | Varies | Varies | Varies |
| **Fast Foods** | Varies | Varies | Varies | Varies |
| **Alcohol** | Varies | 0 | 0 | ~100 |

Adapted from the American Diabetes Association and the American Dietetic Association: *Choose Your Foods: Exchange Lists for Diabetes*. Alexandria, VA, 2008, p. 4.

## TABLE 3. Nutrient Claims on Food Labels

| Term | Meaning |
|---|---|
| **Calorie-Free** | Less than 5 calories per serving |
| **Cholesterol-Free** | Less than 2 mg of cholesterol per serving and 2 g or less of saturated fat per serving |
| **Extra Lean** | Less than 5 g of fat, 2 g of saturated fat, and 95 mg of cholesterol per serving |
| **Fat-Free** | Less than 0.5 g of fat per serving |
| **Lean** | Less than 10 g of fat, 4 g of saturated fat, and 95 mg of cholesterol per serving |
| **Light or Lite** | 33.3% fewer calories or 50% less fat per serving than comparison food |
| **Low-Calorie** | 40 calories or less per serving |
| **Low-Cholesterol** | 20 mg or less of cholesterol per serving and 2 g or less of saturated fat per serving |
| **Low-Fat** | 3 g or less of fat per serving |
| **Low-Saturated Fat** | 1 g or less of saturated fat per serving and 15% or less of calories from saturated fat |
| **Low-Sodium** | 140 mg or less of sodium per serving |
| **Reduced** | 25% less per serving than comparison food |
| **Saturated Fat-Free** | Less than 0.5 g of saturated fat and 0.5 g of trans fatty acids per serving |
| **Sodium-Free** | Less than 5 mg of sodium per serving |
| **Sugar-Free** | Less than 0.5 g of sugar per serving |

# ALCOHOL, BEER, SPIRITS, WINE

| | Serving | Calories | Fat (g) | Cal. from Fat | Sat. Fat (g) | Trans Fat (g) | Chol. (mg) | Sod. (mg) | Carb. (g) | Fiber (g) | Prot. (g) | Servings/Exchanges |
|---|---|---|---|---|---|---|---|---|---|---|---|---|
| **BEER** | | | | | | | | | | | | |
| Beer, Light | 12 oz | 103 | 0 | 0 | 0 | 0 | 0 | 14 | 6 | 0 | <1 | 1 alcohol, 1/2 carb |
| Beer, Non-alcoholic | 12 oz | 70 | 0 | 0 | 0 | 0 | 0 | 8 | 13 | 0 | 1 | 1 alcohol |
| Beer, Regular | 12 oz | 153 | 0 | 0 | 0 | 0 | 0 | 14 | 13 | 0 | 1 | 1 alcohol, 1 carb |
| **Brands** | | | | | | | | | | | | |
| Bud Light | 12 oz | 110 | 0 | 0 | 0 | 0 | 0 | 11 | 7 | 0 | 1 | 1 alcohol, 1/2 carb |
| Budweiser | 12 oz | 145 | 0 | 0 | 0 | 0 | 0 | 11 | 11 | 0 | 1 | 1 alcohol, 1/2 carb |
| Budweiser Select | 12 oz | 95 | 0 | 0 | 0 | 0 | 0 | NA | 3 | 0 | <1 | 1 alcohol |
| Coors Light | 12 oz | 102 | 0 | 0 | 0 | 0 | 0 | NA | 5 | 0 | 0 | 1 alcohol |
| Michelob Amber | 12 oz | 114 | 0 | 0 | 0 | 0 | 0 | NA | 4 | 0 | 1 | 1 alcohol |
| Michelob Light | 12 oz | 123 | 0 | 0 | 0 | 0 | 0 | NA | 9 | 0 | 1 | 1 alcohol, 1/2 carb |
| Michelob Ultra | 12 oz | 95 | 0 | 0 | 0 | 0 | 0 | 9 | 3 | 0 | <1 | 1 alcohol |

ALCOHOL, BEER, SPIRITS, WINE

| | Serving | Calories | Fat (g) | Cal. from Fat | Sat. Fat (g) | Trans Fat (g) | Chol. (mg) | Sod. (mg) | Carb. (g) | Fiber (g) | Prot. (g) | Servings/Exchanges |
|---|---|---|---|---|---|---|---|---|---|---|---|---|
| Miller Genuine Draft Light | 12 oz | 110 | 0 | 0 | 0 | 0 | 0 | NA | 7 | 0 | 0 | 1 alcohol, 1/2 carb |
| Miller Light | 12 oz | 95 | 0 | 0 | 0 | 0 | 0 | NA | 3 | 0 | <1 | 1 alcohol |
| O'Doul's Brew | 12 oz | 65 | 0 | 0 | 0 | 0 | 0 | NA | 13 | 0 | <1 | 1 carb |
| O'Doul's Amber | 12 oz | 90 | 0 | 0 | 0 | 0 | 0 | NA | 18 | 0 | 2 | 1 carb |
| **COCKTAILS** | | | | | | | | | | | | |
| Daiquiri, Canned | 4 oz | 152 | 0 | 0 | 0 | 0 | 0 | 49 | 19 | 0 | 0 | 1 carb |
| Piña Colada, Canned | 4 oz | 309 | 10 | 90 | 9 | 0 | 0 | 93 | 36 | 0 | <1 | 2 1/2 carb, 2 fat |
| Piña Colada, from Mix | 4 oz | 219 | 2 | 18 | 2 | 0 | 0 | 8 | 29 | 0 | 0 | 2 carb |
| Tequila Sunrise, Canned | 4 oz | 137 | 0 | 0 | 0 | 0 | 0 | 71 | 14 | 0 | <1 | 1 carb |
| Whiskey Sour, Canned | 4 oz | 147 | 0 | 0 | 0 | 0 | 0 | 54 | 17 | 0 | 0 | 1 carb |
| **LIQUEURS** | | | | | | | | | | | | |
| Coffee Liqueur, 53 Proof | 1.5 oz | 170 | 0 | 0 | 0 | 0 | 0 | 4 | 24 | 0 | 0 | 1 1/2 carb |

| | | | | | | | | | | | | |
|---|---|---|---|---|---|---|---|---|---|---|---|---|
| Crème de Menthe | 1.5 oz | 186 | 0 | 0 | 0 | 0 | 0 | 2 | 21 | 0 | 0 | 1 1/2 carb |
| **MIXERS (NON-ALCOHOLIC)** | | | | | | | | | | | | |
| ***Finest Call*** | | | | | | | | | | | | |
| Margarita Mix | 4 oz | 160 | 0 | 0 | 0 | 0 | 0 | 0 | 40 | 0 | 0 | 2 1/2 carb |
| Sweet & Sour Mix | 4 oz | 110 | 0 | 0 | 0 | 0 | 0 | 80 | 24 | 0 | 0 | 2 carb |
| ***Jose Cuervo*** | | | | | | | | | | | | |
| Margarita Mix | 4 oz | 110 | 0 | 0 | 0 | 0 | 0 | 55 | 28 | 0 | 0 | 2 carb |
| Strawberry Margarita Mix | 4 oz | 100 | 0 | 0 | 0 | 0 | 0 | 80 | 24 | 0 | 0 | 1 1/2 carb |
| ***Master of Mixes*** | | | | | | | | | | | | |
| Margarita Mixer | 4 oz | 140 | 0 | 0 | 0 | 0 | 0 | 25 | 34 | 0 | 0 | 2 carb |
| Piña Colada Mixer | 4 oz | 230 | 1.5 | 14 | 0 | 0 | 0 | 45 | 53 | 0 | 0 | 3 1/2 carb |
| Strawberry Daiquiri | 4 oz | 140 | 0 | 0 | 0 | 0 | 0 | 25 | 34 | 0 | 0 | 2 carb |
| Sweet 'N Sour Mixer | 4 oz | 110 | 0 | 0 | 0 | 0 | 0 | 55 | 26 | 0 | 0 | 2 carb |
| ***On the House*** | | | | | | | | | | | | |
| Bloody Mary Mix | 4 oz | 25 | 0 | 0 | 0 | 0 | 0 | 630 | 6 | 0 | 0 | 1 vegetable |

ALCOHOL, BEER, SPIRITS, WINE

| | Serving | Calories | Fat (g) | Cal. from Fat | Sat. Fat (g) | Trans Fat (g) | Chol. (mg) | Sod. (mg) | Carb. (g) | Fiber (g) | Prot. (g) | Servings/Exchanges |
|---|---|---|---|---|---|---|---|---|---|---|---|---|
| Mai Tai Cocktail Mix | 4 oz | 150 | 0 | 0 | 0 | 0 | 0 | 75 | 38 | 0 | 0 | 2 1/2 carb |
| Margarita Mix | 4 oz | 100 | 0 | 0 | 0 | 0 | 0 | 75 | 25 | 0 | 0 | 1 1/2 carb |
| Piña Colada Mix | 4 oz | 160 | 0 | 0 | 0 | 0 | 0 | 100 | 38 | 0 | 0 | 2 1/2 carb |
| Strawberry Daiquiri Mix | 4 oz | 200 | 0 | 0 | 0 | 0 | 0 | 75 | 50 | 0 | 0 | 3 carb |
| Sweet & Sour Cocktail Mix | 4 oz | 110 | 0 | 0 | 0 | 0 | 0 | 75 | 26 | 0 | 0 | 2 carb |
| Tom Collins Mix | 3 oz | 160 | 0 | 0 | 0 | 0 | 0 | 90 | 39 | 0 | 0 | 2 1/2 carb |
| ***Rose's*** | | | | | | | | | | | | |
| Grenadine | 2 Tbsp | 90 | 0 | 0 | 0 | 0 | 0 | 10 | 22 | 0 | 0 | 1 1/2 carb |
| Sweetened Lime Juice | 1 tsp | 10 | 0 | 0 | 0 | 0 | 0 | 0 | 2 | 0 | 0 | free |
| ***Sauza*** | | | | | | | | | | | | |
| Blue Raspberry Margarita Mix | 3 oz | 80 | 0 | 0 | 0 | 0 | 0 | 45 | 19 | 0 | 0 | 1 carb |

| | | | | | | | | | | | | |
|---|---|---|---|---|---|---|---|---|---|---|---|---|
| Margarita Mix | 3 oz | 70 | 0 | 0 | 0 | 0 | 0 | 65 | 18 | 0 | 0 | 1 carb |
| Strawberry Margarita Mix | 3 oz | 80 | 0 | 0 | 0 | 0 | 0 | 45 | 19 | 0 | 0 | 1 carb |
| ***Stirrings*** | | | | | | | | | | | | |
| Bloody Mary Mix | 4 oz | 40 | 0 | 0 | 0 | 0 | 0 | 750 | 10 | 0 | 0 | 1/2 carb |
| Cosmopolitan | 3 oz | 60 | 0 | 0 | 0 | 0 | 0 | 0 | 16 | 0 | 0 | 1 carb |
| Pomegranate Martini | 3 oz | 60 | 0 | 0 | 0 | 0 | 0 | 0 | 15 | 0 | 0 | 1 carb |
| **SPIRITS (GIN, RUM, VODKA, WHISKEY)** | | | | | | | | | | | | |
| 100 Proof | 1.5 oz | 124 | 0 | 0 | 0 | 0 | 0 | 0 | 0 | 0 | 0 | 1 alcohol |
| 86 Proof | 1.5 oz | 105 | 0 | 0 | 0 | 0 | 0 | 0 | 0 | 0 | 0 | 1 alcohol |
| 80 Proof | 1.5 oz | 97 | 0 | 0 | 0 | 0 | 0 | 0 | 0 | 0 | 0 | 1 alcohol |
| **WINE** | | | | | | | | | | | | |
| Cooking Wine | 5 oz | 72 | 0 | 0 | 0 | 0 | 0 | 908 | 9 | 0 | <1 | 1 alcohol, 1/2 carb |
| Dry Dessert Wine | 5 oz | 224 | 0 | 0 | 0 | 0 | 0 | 13 | 17 | 0 | 0 | 1 alcohol, 1 carb |
| Light Wine | 5 oz | 72 | 0 | 0 | 0 | 0 | 0 | 10 | 2 | 0 | 0 | 1 alcohol |
| Non-alcoholic | 5 oz | 9 | 0 | 0 | 0 | 0 | 0 | 10 | 2 | 0 | <1 | 1 alcohol |

ALCOHOL, BEER, SPIRITS, WINE

| | Serving | Calories | Fat (g) | Cal. from Fat | Sat. Fat (g) | Trans Fat (g) | Chol. (mg) | Sod. (mg) | Carb. (g) | Fiber (g) | Prot. (g) | Servings/Exchanges |
|---|---|---|---|---|---|---|---|---|---|---|---|---|
| Sake | 1 oz | 39 | 0 | 0 | 0 | 0 | 0 | 1 | 1.5 | 0 | 0 | 1/2 alcohol |
| Sweet Dessert wine | 5 oz | 236 | 0 | 0 | 0 | 0 | 0 | 13 | 20 | 0 | 0 | 1 alcohol, 1 carb |
| Wine Cooler | 12 oz | 20 | 0 | 0 | 0 | 0 | 0 | 5 | 35 | 0 | 0 | 1 alcohol, 2 carb |
| ***Red Table Wine*** | | | | | | | | | | | | |
| Barbera | 5 oz | 125 | 0 | 0 | 0 | 0 | 0 | NA | 4 | 0 | 0 | 1 alcohol |
| Burgundy | 5 oz | 127 | 0 | 0 | 0 | 0 | 0 | NA | 6 | 0 | 0 | 1 alcohol |
| Cabernet Franc | 5 oz | 122 | 0 | 0 | 0 | 0 | 0 | NA | 4 | 0 | 0 | 1 alcohol |
| Cabernet Sauvignon | 5 oz | 120 | 0 | 0 | 0 | 0 | 0 | NA | 4 | 0 | 0 | 1 alcohol |
| Carignane | 5 oz | 109 | 0 | 0 | 0 | 0 | 0 | NA | 4 | 0 | 0 | 1 alcohol |
| Claret | 5 oz | 122 | 0 | 0 | 0 | 0 | 0 | NA | 5 | 0 | 0 | 1 alcohol |
| Gamay | 5 oz | 115 | 0 | 0 | 0 | 0 | 0 | NA | 4 | 0 | 0 | 1 alcohol |
| Lemberger | 5 oz | 118 | 0 | 0 | 0 | 0 | 0 | NA | 4 | 0 | 0 | 1 alcohol |
| Merlot | 5 oz | 122 | 0 | 0 | 0 | 0 | 0 | 6 | 4 | 0 | 0 | 1 alcohol |
| Mouvedre | 5 oz | 129 | 0 | 0 | 0 | 0 | 0 | NA | 4 | 0 | 0 | 1 alcohol |

| | | | | | | | | | | | | |
|---|---|---|---|---|---|---|---|---|---|---|---|---|
| Petite Sirah | 5 oz | 125 | 0 | 0 | 0 | 0 | 0 | NA | 4 | 0 | 0 | 1 alcohol |
| Pinot Noir | 5 oz | 121 | 0 | 0 | 0 | 0 | 0 | NA | 3 | 0 | 0 | 1 alcohol |
| Sangiovese | 5 oz | 126 | 0 | 0 | 0 | 0 | 0 | NA | 4 | 0 | 0 | 1 alcohol |
| Syrah | 5 oz | 122 | 0 | 0 | 0 | 0 | 0 | NA | 4 | 0 | 0 | 1 alcohol |
| Zinfandel | 5 oz | 129 | 0 | 0 | 0 | 0 | 0 | NA | 4 | 0 | 0 | 1 alcohol |
| ***White Table Wine*** | | | | | | | | | | | | |
| Chenin Blanc | 5 oz | 118 | 0 | 0 | 0 | 0 | 0 | NA | 4 | 0 | 0 | 1 alcohol |
| Fune Blanc | 5 oz | 121 | 0 | 0 | 0 | 0 | 0 | NA | 3 | 0 | 0 | 1 alcohol |
| Gewurztraminer | 5 oz | 119 | 0 | 0 | 0 | 0 | 0 | NA | 4 | 0 | 0 | 1 alcohol |
| Muller Thurgau | 5 oz | 112 | 0 | 0 | 0 | 0 | 0 | NA | 5 | 0 | 0 | 1 alcohol |
| Muscat | 5 oz | 123 | 0 | 0 | 0 | 0 | 0 | NA | 8 | 0 | 0 | 1 alcohol |
| Pinot Blanc | 5 oz | 119 | 0 | 0 | 0 | 0 | 0 | NA | 3 | 0 | 0 | 1 alcohol |
| Pinot Gris (Grigio) | 5 oz | 122 | 0 | 0 | 0 | 0 | 0 | NA | 3 | 0 | 0 | 1 alcohol |
| Reisling | 5 oz | 118 | 0 | 0 | 0 | 0 | 0 | NA | 6 | 0 | 0 | 1 alcohol |
| Sauvignon Blanc | 5 oz | 119 | 0 | 0 | 0 | 0 | 0 | NA | 3 | 0 | 0 | 1 alcohol |

| | Serving | Calories | Fat (g) | Cal. from Fat | Sat. Fat (g) | Trans Fat (g) | Chol. (mg) | Sod. (mg) | Carb. (g) | Fiber (g) | Prot. (g) | Servings/Exchanges |
|---|---|---|---|---|---|---|---|---|---|---|---|---|
| **BEANS, PEAS, LENTILS** | | | | | | | | | | | | |
| Baked Beans with Beef, Canned | 1/2 cup | 161 | 5 | 45 | 2 | 0 | 29 | 632 | 23 | 7 | 9 | 1 1/2 starch, 1 med-fat meat |
| Baked Beans, No Pork | 1/2 cup | 78 | <1 | 0 | 0 | 0 | 0 | 333 | 17 | 4 | 4 | 1 starch |
| Baked Beans, Vegetarian, Canned | 1/2 cup | 119 | <1 | 0 | <1 | 0 | 0 | 436 | 27 | 5 | 6 | 2 starch |
| Black Beans, Cooked | 1/2 cup | 114 | 0.5 | 5 | 0 | 0 | 0 | 1 | 21 | 8 | 8 | 1 1/2 starch, 1 lean meat |
| Black-Eyed Peas, Cooked | 1/2 cup | 100 | 0.5 | 5 | 0 | 0 | 0 | 3 | 18 | 6 | 7 | 1 starch, 1 lean meat |
| Black Turtle Soup Beans, Cooked | 1/2 cup | 120 | <1 | 0 | <1 | 0 | 0 | 3 | 23 | 5 | 8 | 1 1/2 starch, 1 lean meat |
| Fava/Broadbeans, Canned | 1/2 cup | 91 | <1 | 0 | <1 | 0 | 0 | 580 | 16 | 5 | 7 | 1 starch, 1 lean meat |

| | | | | | | | | | | | | |
|---|---|---|---|---|---|---|---|---|---|---|---|---|
| French Beans, Cooked | 1/2 cup | 114 | <1 | 0 | <1 | 0 | 0 | 5 | 21 | 8 | 6 | 1 1/2 starch |
| Garbanzo Beans/ Chickpeas, Cooked | 1/2 cup | 134 | 2 | 20 | 0 | 0 | 0 | 6 | 23 | 6 | 7 | 1 1/2 starch |
| Great Northern Beans, Cooked | 1/2 cup | 104 | <1 | 0 | <1 | 0 | 0 | 2 | 19 | 6 | 7 | 1 starch, 1 lean meat |
| Hummus | 1/2 cup | 210 | 11 | 100 | 2 | 0 | 0 | 300 | 25 | 6 | 6 | 1 1/2 starch, 2 fat |
| Kidney Beans, California Red, | 1/2 cup | 110 | <1 | 0 | <1 | 0 | 0 | 4 | 20 | 8 | 8 | 1 starch, 1 lean meat |
| Kidney Beans, Red, Cooked | 1/2 cup | 112 | <1 | 0 | 0 | 0 | 0 | 2 | 20 | 6 | 8 | 1 starch, 1 lean meat |
| Kidney Beans, Royal Red, Cooked | 1/2 cup | 109 | <1 | 0 | <1 | 0 | 0 | 4 | 19 | 8 | 8 | 1 starch, 1 lean meat |
| Lentils, Cooked | 1/2 cup | 115 | <1 | 0 | <1 | 0 | 0 | 2 | 20 | 8 | 9 | 1 starch, 1 lean meat |
| Lima Beans, Canned | 1/2 cup | 99 | <1 | 0 | 0 | 0 | 0 | 280 | 18 | 6 | 7 | 1 starch, 1 lean meat |
| Lima Beans, Frozen | 1/2 cup | 76 | <1 | 0 | 0 | 0 | 0 | 40 | 14 | 4 | 5 | 1 starch, 1 lean meat |
| Navy Beans, Cooked | 1/2 cup | 129 | 0.5 | 5 | 0 | 0 | 0 | 1 | 24 | 6 | 8 | 1 1/2 starch, 1 lean meat |
| Pink Beans, Cooked | 1/2 cup | 126 | <1 | 0 | <1 | 0 | 0 | 2 | 24 | 5 | 8 | 1 1/2 starch, 1 lean meat |

BEANS, PEAS, LENTILS

| | Serving | Calories | Fat (g) | Cal. from Fat | Sat. Fat (g) | Trans Fat (g) | Chol. (mg) | Sod. (mg) | Carb. (g) | Fiber (g) | Prot. (g) | Servings/Exchanges |
|---|---|---|---|---|---|---|---|---|---|---|---|---|
| Pinto Beans, Cooked | 1/2 cup | 122 | 0.5 | 5 | 0 | 0 | 0 | 1 | 22 | 8 | 8 | 1 1/2 starch, 1 lean meat |
| Pork & Beans in Sweet Sauce, Canned | 1/2 cup | 142 | 2 | 20 | <1 | 0 | 9 | 423 | 27 | 5 | 7 | 2 starch |
| Pork & Beans in Tomato Sauce | 1/2 cup | 116 | 1 | 10 | 0 | 0 | 9 | 538 | 23 | 5 | 6 | 1 1/2 starch |
| Refried Beans/Frijoles | 1/2 cup | 100 | 0.5 | 5 | 0 | 0 | 10 | 570 | 17 | 6 | 6 | 1 starch, 1 lean meat |
| Split Peas, Cooked | 1/2 cup | 116 | <1 | 0 | 0 | 0 | 0 | 2 | 21 | 8 | 8 | 1 1/2 starch, 1 lean meat |
| White Beans, Cooked | 1/2 cup | 125 | <1 | 0 | 0 | 0 | 0 | 5 | 23 | 6 | 9 | 1 1/2 starch, 1 lean meat |
| White Beans, Small, Cooked | 1/2 cup | 127 | 0 | 0 | 0 | 0 | 0 | 2 | 23 | 9 | 8 | 1 1/2 starch, 1 lean meat |
| Yellow Beans, Cooked | 1/2 cup | 127 | <1 | 0 | <1 | 0 | 0 | 4 | 22 | 9 | 8 | 1 1/2 starch, 1 lean meat |
| **Brands (Canned Beans)** | | | | | | | | | | | | |
| ***Allens*** | | | | | | | | | | | | |

| | | | | | | | | | | | | |
|---|---|---|---|---|---|---|---|---|---|---|---|---|
| Baby Butter Beans | 1/2 cup | 120 | 0.5 | 5 | 0 | 0 | 0 | 460 | 22 | 6 | 7 | 1 1/2 starch, 1 lean meat |
| Black Beans | 1/2 cup | 100 | 0.5 | 5 | 0 | 0 | 0 | 400 | 19 | 8 | 6 | 1 starch, 1 lean meat |
| Black-Eyed Peas | 1/2 cup | 120 | 1 | 10 | 0 | 0 | 0 | 420 | 20 | 5 | 7 | 1 starch, 1 lean meat |
| Dark Red Kidney Beans | 1/2 cup | 130 | 0.5 | 5 | 0 | 0 | 0 | 310 | 22 | 8 | 8 | 1 1/2 starch, 1 lean meat |
| Garbanzo Beans | 1/2 cup | 120 | 2.5 | 25 | 0 | 0 | 0 | 330 | 19 | 8 | 5 | 1 starch |
| Great Northern Beans | 1/2 cup | 100 | 0.5 | 5 | 0 | 0 | 0 | 310 | 19 | 7 | 6 | 1 starch, 1 lean meat |
| Lima Beans | 1/2 cup | 120 | 0 | 0 | 0 | 0 | 0 | 370 | 23 | 8 | 7 | 1 1/2 starch, 1 lean meat |
| Navy Beans | 1/2 cup | 110 | 1 | 10 | 0 | 0 | 0 | 380 | 19 | 6 | 6 | 1 starch, 1 lean meat |
| Pinto Beans | 1/2 cup | 110 | 1 | 10 | 0 | 0 | 0 | 290 | 20 | 7 | 5 | 1 starch |
| Red Beans | 1/2 cup | 100 | 0.5 | 5 | 0 | 0 | 0 | 310 | 19 | 9 | 6 | 1 starch, 1 lean meat |
| Refried Beans | 1/2 cup | 150 | 2.5 | 25 | 1 | 0 | 0 | 260 | 24 | 11 | 7 | 1 1/2 starch, 1 lean meat |
| Refried Black Beans, No Fat Added | 1/2 cup | 120 | 0 | 0 | 0 | 0 | 0 | 500 | 23 | 8 | 7 | 1 1/2 starch, 1 lean meat |
| ***B & M*** | | | | | | | | | | | | |
| Baked Beans, Bacon, Onion & Brown Sugar | 1/2 cup | 190 | 2 | 20 | 0.5 | 0 | <5 | 450 | 36 | 8 | 8 | 2 1/2 starch |

| | Serving | Calories | Fat (g) | Cal. from Fat | Sat. Fat (g) | Trans Fat (g) | Chol. (mg) | Sod. (mg) | Carb. (g) | Fiber (g) | Prot. (g) | Servings/Exchanges |
|---|---|---|---|---|---|---|---|---|---|---|---|---|
| Baked Beans, Barbeque | 1/2 cup | 190 | 0.5 | 5 | 0 | 0 | 0 | 570 | 39 | 9 | 8 | 2 1/2 starch |
| Baked Beans, Country Style | 1/2 cup | 170 | 1.5 | 15 | 0.5 | 0 | <5 | 710 | 35 | 7 | 7 | 2 starch |
| Baked Beans, Maple Flavor | 1/2 cup | 180 | 1 | 10 | 0 | 0 | 0 | 340 | 31 | 8 | 7 | 2 starch |
| Baked Beans, Original | 1/2 cup | 170 | 2 | 20 | 0.5 | 0 | <5 | 400 | 31 | 8 | 7 | 2 starch |
| Baked Beans, Red Kidney | 1/2 cup | 200 | 3 | 25 | 1 | 0 | <5 | 460 | 36 | 6 | 8 | 2 1/2 starch |
| Baked Beans, Vegetarian | 1/2 cup | 160 | 1 | 10 | 0 | 0 | 0 | 380 | 28 | 8 | 7 | 2 starch |
| ***Bush's*** | | | | | | | | | | | | |
| Baked Beans, Bold & Spicy | 1/2 cup | 110 | 1 | 10 | 0 | 0 | 0 | 560 | 24 | 5 | 6 | 1 1/2 starch |

| | | | | | | | | | | | | |
|---|---|---|---|---|---|---|---|---|---|---|---|---|
| Baked Beans, Boston Style | 1/2 cup | 150 | 1 | 10 | 0 | 0 | 0 | 440 | 31 | 5 | 6 | 2 starch |
| Baked Beans, Country Style | 1/2 cup | 160 | 1 | 10 | 0 | 0 | 0 | 680 | 33 | 5 | 6 | 2 starch |
| Baked Beans | 1/2 cup | 140 | 1 | 10 | 0 | 0 | 0 | 550 | 29 | 5 | 6 | 2 starch |
| Baked Beans, Honey Baked | 1/2 cup | 160 | 1 | 10 | 0 | 0 | 0 | 540 | 32 | 6 | 6 | 2 starch |
| Baked Beans, Maple Cured Bacon | 1/2 cup | 140 | 1 | 10 | 0 | 0 | 0 | 620 | 28 | 5 | 6 | 2 starch |
| Baked Beans, Onion | 1/2 cup | 140 | 1 | 10 | 0 | 0 | 0 | 550 | 29 | 5 | 6 | 2 starch |
| Baked Beans, Original | 1/2 cup | 140 | 1 | 10 | 0 | 0 | 0 | 550 | 29 | 5 | 6 | 2 starch |
| Baked Beans, Vegetarian | 1/2 cup | 130 | 0 | 0 | 0 | 0 | 0 | 550 | 29 | 5 | 6 | 2 starch |
| Black Beans | 1/2 cup | 110 | 0.5 | 5 | 0 | 0 | 0 | 450 | 23 | 7 | 8 | 1 1/2 starch |
| Black Beans, Frijoles Negros Condimentados | 1/2 cup | 110 | 0.5 | 5 | 0 | 0 | 0 | 450 | 23 | 7 | 8 | 1 1/2 starch, 1 lean meat |

## BEANS, PEAS, LENTILS

| | Serving | Calories | Fat (g) | Cal. from Fat | Sat. Fat (g) | Trans Fat (g) | Chol. (mg) | Sod. (mg) | Carb. (g) | Fiber (g) | Prot. (g) | Servings/Exchanges |
|---|---|---|---|---|---|---|---|---|---|---|---|---|
| Black-Eyed Peas | 1/2 cup | 100 | 0 | 0 | 0 | 0 | 0 | 480 | 15 | 3 | 5 | 1 starch |
| Black-Eyed Peas with Bacon | 1/2 cup | 95 | 1.5 | 15 | 0 | 0 | 0 | 370 | 17 | 3 | 6 | 1 starch, 1 lean meat |
| Black-Eyed Peas with Snaps | 1/2 cup | 110 | 0.5 | 5 | 0 | 0 | 0 | 550 | 17 | 5 | 7 | 1 starch, 1 lean meat |
| Butter Beans, Baby | 1/2 cup | 120 | 0.5 | 5 | 0 | 0 | 0 | 510 | 19 | 5 | 7 | 1 starch, 1 lean meat |
| Cannellini Beans | 1/2 cup | 110 | 0.5 | 0 | 0 | 0 | 0 | 300 | 18 | 6 | 7 | 1 starch, 1 lean meat |
| Chili Beans | 1/2 cup | 120 | 1 | 10 | 0.5 | 0 | 0 | 480 | 20 | 6 | 6 | 1 starch, 1 lean meat |
| Chili Beans, Red Beans in Chili Sauce | 1/2 cup | 100 | 0.5 | 5 | 0 | 0 | 0 | 480 | 22 | 7 | 6 | 1 1/2 starch |
| Crowder Peas | 1/2 cup | 110 | 1 | 10 | 0 | 0 | 0 | 500 | 18 | 5 | 7 | 1 starch, 1 lean meat |
| Field Peas with Snaps | 1/2 cup | 80 | 0 | 0 | 0 | 0 | 0 | 430 | 16 | 2 | 5 | 1 starch |
| Garbanzo Beans | 1/2 cup | 105 | 2 | 15 | 0 | 0 | 0 | 470 | 20 | 5 | 6 | 1 starch, 1 lean meat |
| Great Northern Beans | 1/2 cup | 80 | 0 | 0 | 0 | 0 | 0 | 460 | 17 | 6 | 6 | 1 starch, 1 lean meat |

| | | | | | | | | | | | | |
|---|---|---|---|---|---|---|---|---|---|---|---|---|
| Grillin' Beans, Bourbon & Brown Sugar | 1/2 cup | 170 | 0.5 | 5 | 0 | 0 | 0 | 480 | 35 | 6 | 7 | 1 starch, 1 lean meat |
| Grillin' Beans, Smoke-house Tradition | 1/2 cup | 170 | 1 | 10 | 0 | 0 | 0 | 570 | 34 | 5 | 7 | 2 starch |
| Grillin' Beans, Southern Pit BBQ | 1/2 cup | 170 | 0.5 | 5 | 0 | 0 | 0 | 550 | 35 | 6 | 6 | 2 starch |
| Grillin' Beans, Steakhouse Recipe | 1/2 cup | 180 | 0.5 | 5 | 0 | 0 | 0 | 510 | 39 | 5 | 6 | 2 1/2 starch |
| Kidney Beans, Dark Red | 1/2 cup | 105 | 0 | 0 | 0 | 0 | 0 | 260 | 22 | 8 | 7 | 1 1/2 starch, 1 lean meat |
| Kidney Beans, Light Red | 1/2 cup | 100 | 0 | 0 | 0 | 0 | 0 | 260 | 22 | 7 | 7 | 1 1/2 starch, 1 lean meat |
| Mixed Beans | 1/2 cup | 110 | 0 | 0 | 0 | 0 | 0 | 500 | 19 | 6 | 7 | 1 starch, 1 lean meat |
| Navy Beans | 1/2 cup | 80 | 0 | 0 | 0 | 0 | 0 | 470 | 17 | 7 | 6 | 1 starch, 1 lean meat |
| Pinto Beans | 1/2 cup | 110 | 0 | 0 | 0 | 0 | 0 | 390 | 19 | 6 | 6 | 1 starch, 1 lean meat |
| Pinto Beans with Pork | 1/2 cup | 120 | 2.5 | 25 | 1 | 0 | 5 | 530 | 17 | 6 | 6 | 1 starch, 1 lean meat |
| Pinto Beans, Frijoles Pintos | 1/2 cup | 80 | 0 | 0 | 0 | 0 | 0 | 450 | 18 | 7 | 6 | 1 starch, 1 lean meat |

| | Serving | Calories | Fat (g) | Cal. from Fat | Sat. Fat (g) | Trans Fat (g) | Chol. (mg) | Sod. (mg) | Carb. (g) | Fiber (g) | Prot. (g) | Servings/Exchanges |
|---|---|---|---|---|---|---|---|---|---|---|---|---|
| Purple Hull Peas | 1/2 cup | 90 | 0 | 0 | 0 | 0 | 0 | 460 | 19 | 5 | 6 | 1 starch, 1 lean meat |
| Red Beans | 1/2 cup | 110 | 0.5 | 5 | 0 | 0 | 0 | 460 | 19 | 6 | 6 | 1 starch, 1 lean meat |
| Refried Beans, Fat Free | 1/2 cup | 130 | 0 | 0 | 0 | 0 | 0 | 490 | 24 | 7 | 9 | 1 1/2 starch, 1 lean meat |
| Refried Beans, Traditional | 1/2 cup | 150 | 3 | 25 | 1 | 0 | 0 | 490 | 24 | 7 | 9 | 1 1/2 starch, 1 lean meat |
| ***Eden Organic*** | | | | | | | | | | | | |
| Aduki Beans | 1/2 cup | 110 | 0 | 0 | 0 | 0 | 0 | 10 | 19 | 5 | 7 | 1 starch, 1 lean meat |
| Baked Beans with Sorghum & Mustard | 1/2 cup | 150 | 0 | 0 | 0 | 0 | 0 | 130 | 27 | 7 | 8 | 2 starch |
| Black Beans | 1/2 cup | 110 | 1 | 10 | 0 | 0 | 0 | 15 | 18 | 6 | 7 | 1 starch, 1 lean meat |
| Black Soy Beans | 1/2 cup | 120 | 6 | 50 | 1 | 0 | 0 | 30 | 8 | 7 | 11 | 1/2 starch, 1 lean meat |
| Black-Eyed Peas | 1/2 cup | 90 | 1 | 10 | 0 | 0 | 0 | 25 | 16 | 4 | 6 | 1 starch, 1 lean meat |
| Butter Beans | 1/2 cup | 100 | 1 | 10 | 0 | 0 | 0 | 35 | 17 | 4 | 5 | 1 starch |
| Cannellini | 1/2 cup | 100 | 1 | 10 | 0 | 0 | 0 | 40 | 17 | 4 | 5 | 1 starch |

| | | | | | | | | | | | | |
|---|---|---|---|---|---|---|---|---|---|---|---|---|
| Caribbean Black Beans | 1/2 cup | 90 | 0.5 | 0 | 0 | 0 | 0 | 135 | 20 | 7 | 7 | 1 starch, 1 lean meat |
| Garbanzo Beans | 1/2 cup | 130 | 1 | 10 | 0 | 0 | 0 | 30 | 23 | 5 | 7 | 1 1/2 starch, 1 lean meat |
| Lentils with Onions & Bay Leaf | 1/2 cup | 90 | 0 | 0 | 0 | 0 | 0 | 210 | 13 | 4 | 8 | 1 starch, 1 lean meat |
| Pinto Beans | 1/2 cup | 110 | 1 | 0 | 0 | 0 | 0 | 15 | 18 | 6 | 6 | 1 starch, 1 lean meat |
| Refried Beans | 1/2 cup | 110 | 1.5 | 15 | 0 | 0 | 0 | 180 | 18 | 7 | 6 | 1 starch, 1 lean meat |
| ***Gebhardt*** | | | | | | | | | | | | |
| Fat Free Refried Beans | 1/2 cup | 80 | 0 | 0 | 0 | 0 | 0 | 500 | 17 | 5 | 6 | 1 starch, 1 lean meat |
| Jalapeño Refried Beans | 1/2 cup | 100 | 2 | 20 | 1 | 0 | 0 | 400 | 17 | 5 | 6 | 1 starch, 1 lean meat |
| Refried Beans | 1/2 cup | 90 | 2 | 20 | 0.5 | 0 | 0 | 490 | 16 | 4 | 6 | 1 starch, 1 lean meat |
| ***Old El Paso*** | | | | | | | | | | | | |
| Refried Beans, Fat-Free | 1/2 cup | 100 | 0 | 0 | 0 | 0 | 0 | 580 | 18 | 6 | 6 | 1 starch, 1 lean meat |
| Refried Beans, Fat-Free, Spicy | 1/2 cup | 90 | 0 | 0 | 0 | 0 | 0 | 510 | 16 | 5 | 5 | 1 starch |
| Refried Beans, Traditional | 1/2 cup | 90 | 0.5 | 5 | 0 | 0 | 0 | 580 | 16 | 5 | 5 | 1 starch |

## BEANS, PEAS, LENTILS

| | Serving | Calories | Fat (g) | Cal. from Fat | Sat. Fat (g) | Trans Fat (g) | Chol. (mg) | Sod. (mg) | Carb. (g) | Fiber (g) | Prot. (g) | Servings/Exchanges |
|---|---|---|---|---|---|---|---|---|---|---|---|---|
| Refried Beans, Vegetarian | 1/2 cup | 90 | 0.5 | 5 | 0 | 0 | 0 | 570 | 16 | 5 | 5 | 1 starch |
| ***Progresso*** | | | | | | | | | | | | |
| Black Beans | 1/2 cup | 100 | 0.5 | 5 | 0 | 0 | 0 | 400 | 17 | 5 | 6 | 1 starch, 1 lean meat |
| Chick Peas | 1/2 cup | 120 | 2.5 | 25 | 0 | 0 | 0 | 280 | 20 | 5 | 5 | 1 starch |
| Dark Red Kidney Beans | 1/2 cup | 110 | 0 | 0 | 0 | 0 | 0 | 340 | 20 | 6 | 8 | 1 starch, 1 lean meat |
| Fava Beans | 1/2 cup | 110 | 0.5 | 5 | 0 | 0 | 0 | 250 | 20 | 5 | 6 | 1 starch, 1 lean meat |
| ***Ranch Style*** | | | | | | | | | | | | |
| Beans, Original | 1/2 cup | 130 | 3 | 25 | 0 | 0 | 0 | 600 | 19 | 5 | 5 | 1 starch |
| Beans with Sweet Onions | 1/2 cup | 130 | 3 | 25 | 0 | 0 | <5 | 590 | 19 | 6 | 5 | 1 starch |
| Black Beans | 1/2 cup | 100 | 0.5 | 5 | 0 | 0 | 0 | 420 | 19 | 5 | 6 | 1 starch, 1 lean meat |
| Pinto Beans | 1/2 cup | 100 | 0 | 0 | 0 | 0 | 0 | 580 | 20 | 6 | 6 | 1 starch, 1 lean meat |

| | | | | | | | | | | | | |
|---|---|---|---|---|---|---|---|---|---|---|---|---|
| Beans with Jalapeño Peppers | 1/2 cup | 120 | 2.5 | 25 | 0.5 | 0 | 0 | 740 | 19 | 6 | 5 | 1 starch |
| ***Rosarita*** | | | | | | | | | | | | |
| No Fat Refried Beans | 1/2 cup | 100 | 0 | 0 | 0 | 0 | 0 | 510 | 19 | 6 | 7 | 1 starch, 1 lean meat |
| No Fat Refried Beans with Green Chili | 1/2 cup | 100 | 0 | 0 | 0 | 0 | 0 | 310 | 18 | 7 | 7 | 1 starch, 1 lean meat |
| No Fat Refried Beans with Spicy Jalapeño | 1/2 cup | 120 | 2 | 15 | 0.5 | 0 | 0 | 320 | 19 | 7 | 7 | 1 starch, 1 lean meat |
| No Fat Refried Black Beans | 1/2 cup | 110 | 0 | 0 | 0 | 0 | 0 | 320 | 19 | 8 | 7 | 1 starch, 1 lean meat |
| Refried Beans, Traditional | 1/2 cup | 120 | 2 | 20 | 0 | 0 | 0 | 310 | 18 | 6 | 7 | 1 starch, 1 lean meat |
| Refried Beans, Vegetarian | 1/2 cup | 120 | 2 | 20 | 0 | 0 | 0 | 540 | 19 | 7 | 7 | 1 starch, 1 lean meat |
| ***S & W*** | | | | | | | | | | | | |
| Baked Beans | 1/2 cup | 160 | 1 | 5 | 0 | 0 | 0 | 510 | 32 | 8 | 8 | 2 starch |

BEANS, PEAS, LENTILS

| | Serving | Calories | Fat (g) | Cal. from Fat | Sat. Fat (g) | Trans Fat (g) | Chol. (mg) | Sod. (mg) | Carb. (g) | Fiber (g) | Prot. (g) | Servings/Exchanges |
|---|---|---|---|---|---|---|---|---|---|---|---|---|
| Baked Beans, Maple | 1/2 cup | 140 | 0.5 | 5 | 0 | 0 | 5 | 440 | 28 | 4 | 6 | 2 starch |
| Black Beans | 1/2 cup | 100 | 1 | 10 | 0 | 0 | 0 | 380 | 17 | 6 | 6 | 1 starch, 1 lean meat |
| Black Beans, 50% Less Sodium | 1/2 cup | 120 | 0.5 | 5 | 0 | 0 | 0 | 180 | 22 | 5 | 8 | 1 1/2 starch, 1 lean meat |
| Chili Beans, Pinto Beans & Chipotle | 1/2 cup | 110 | 1 | 10 | 0 | 0 | 0 | 530 | 23 | 6 | 7 | 1 1/2 starch, 1 lean meat |
| Garbanzo Beans | 1/2 cup | 110 | 2.5 | 20 | 0 | 0 | 0 | 460 | 15 | 3 | 7 | 1 starch, 1 lean meat |
| Garbanzo Beans, 50% Less Sodium | 1/2 cup | 110 | 2.5 | 20 | 0 | 0 | 0 | 220 | 15 | 3 | 7 | 1 starch, 1 lean meat |
| Kidney Beans | 1/2 cup | 120 | 1 | 10 | 0 | 0 | 0 | 380 | 20 | 6 | 7 | 1 starch, 1 lean meat |
| Kidney Beans, 50% Less Sodium | 1/2 cup | 110 | 1 | 5 | 0 | 0 | 0 | 180 | 21 | 5 | 7 | 1 1/2 starch, 1 lean meat |
| Pinquitos | 1/2 cup | 110 | 0.5 | 5 | 0 | 0 | 0 | 490 | 20 | 6 | 6 | 1 starch, 1 lean meat |
| Pinto Beans | 1/2 cup | 120 | 1 | 10 | 0 | 0 | 0 | 530 | 22 | 7 | 6 | 1 1/2 starch |

| | | | | | | | | | | | | |
|---|---|---|---|---|---|---|---|---|---|---|---|---|
| Red Beans, Louisiana Style | 1/2 cup | 110 | 0.5 | 5 | 0 | 0 | 0 | 340 | 20 | 5 | 6 | 1 starch, 1 lean meat |
| White Beans | 1/2 cup | 110 | 0.5 | 5 | 0 | 0 | 0 | 480 | 19 | 6 | 7 | 1 starch, 1 lean meat |
| ***Trader Joe's*** | | | | | | | | | | | | |
| Black Beans | 1/2 cup | 110 | 0 | 0 | 0 | 0 | 0 | 430 | 19 | 6 | 6 | 1 starch, 1 lean meat |
| Cannellini White Kidney Beans | 1/2 cup | 120 | 0 | 0 | 0 | 0 | 0 | 200 | 21 | 10 | 8 | 1 1/2 starch, 1 lean meat |
| Cuban Style Black Beans | 1/2 cup | 100 | 0.5 | 5 | 0 | 0 | 0 | 370 | 19 | 6 | 6 | 1 starch, 1 lean meat |
| Garbanzo Beans | 1/2 cup | 120 | 1 | 10 | 0 | 0 | 0 | 380 | 22 | 6 | 6 | 1 1/2 starch, 1 lean meat |
| Low Fat Vegetarian Refried Pinto Beans | 1/2 cup | 110 | 0.5 | 5 | 0 | 0 | 0 | 410 | 20 | 6 | 6 | 1 starch, 1 lean meat |
| Marinated Bean Salad | 1/2 cup | 140 | 2 | 15 | 0 | 0 | 0 | 410 | 24 | 6 | 6 | 1 1/2 starch, 1 lean meat |
| Organic Baked Beans | 1/2 cup | 140 | 0 | 0 | 0 | 0 | 0 | 450 | 29 | 7 | 7 | 2 starch |
| Organic Black Beans | 1/2 cup | 110 | 0 | 0 | 0 | 0 | 0 | 440 | 20 | 6 | 6 | 1 starch, 1 lean meat |
| Organic Pinto Beans | 1/2 cup | 110 | 0 | 0 | 0 | 0 | 0 | 220 | 22 | 7 | 6 | 1 1/2 starch, 1 lean meat |

BEANS, PEAS, LENTILS

| | Serving | Calories | Fat (g) | Cal. from Fat | Sat. Fat (g) | Trans Fat (g) | Chol. (mg) | Sod. (mg) | Carb. (g) | Fiber (g) | Prot. (g) | Servings/Exchanges |
|---|---|---|---|---|---|---|---|---|---|---|---|---|
| Refried Black Beans with Jalapeño Peppers | 1/2 cup | 120 | 0.5 | 5 | 0 | 0 | 0 | 440 | 22 | 7 | 8 | 1 1/2 starch, 1 lean meat |
| ***Van Camp's*** | | | | | | | | | | | | |
| Baked Beans, Homestyle | 1/2 cup | 170 | 1 | 5 | 0 | 0 | 0 | 680 | 33 | 6 | 7 | 2 starch |
| Baked Beans, Original | 1/2 cup | 140 | 1 | 10 | 0 | 0 | 0 | 540 | 30 | 6 | 7 | 2 starch |
| Kidney Beans, Dark Red | 1/2 cup | 90 | 0 | 0 | 0 | 0 | 0 | 730 | 19 | 6 | 7 | 1 starch, 1 lean meat |
| New Orleans Red Kidney Beans | 1/2 cup | 90 | 0 | 0 | 0 | 0 | 0 | 450 | 19 | 6 | 6 | 1 starch, 1 lean meat |

# BEVERAGES, SODA, SPORTS/ENERGY DRINKS, MEAL-REPLACEMENT DRINKS, COCOA, COFFEE/CREAMER, TEA

| | Serving | Calories | Fat (g) | Cal. from Fat | Sat. Fat (g) | Trans Fat (g) | Chol. (mg) | Sod. (mg) | Carb. (g) | Fiber (g) | Prot. (g) | Servings/Exchanges |
|---|---|---|---|---|---|---|---|---|---|---|---|---|
| **COCOA, HOT CHOCOLATE, CHOCOLATE MILK** | | | | | | | | | | | | |
| Hot Chocolate (Cocoa) | 1 envelope | 80 | 3 | 30 | 2 | 0 | 0 | 170 | 15 | <1 | <1 | 1 carb, 1 fat |
| Hot Chocolate (Cocoa), Sugar Free | 1 envelope | 50 | <1 | 0 | 0 | 0 | 1 | 180 | 10 | <1 | 2 | 1/2 carb |
| Hot Cocoa Mix, Lite | 1 envelope | 80 | 1 | 0 | 0 | 0 | 0 | 0 | 17 | 1 | 2 | 1 carb |
| ***Carnation*** | | | | | | | | | | | | |
| Malted Milk | 3 Tbsp | 90 | 2 | 20 | 1 | 0 | 10 | 100 | 15 | 0 | 2 | 1 carb |
| ***Hershey's*** | | | | | | | | | | | | |
| Chocolate Goodnight Kisses Hot Cocoa | 1 envelope | 140 | 2.5 | 20 | 1.5 | 0 | <5 | 190 | 27 | 1 | 3 | 2 carb, 1 fat |

| | Serving | Calories | Fat (g) | Cal. from Fat | Sat. Fat (g) | Trans Fat (g) | Chol. (mg) | Sod. (mg) | Carb. (g) | Fiber (g) | Prot. (g) | Servings/Exchanges |
|---|---|---|---|---|---|---|---|---|---|---|---|---|
| ***Nestlé*** | | | | | | | | | | | | |
| Chocolate Caramel Hot Cocoa | 1 envelope | 100 | 3 | 25 | 2 | 0 | 0 | 190 | 19 | <1 | 1 | 1 carb, 1 fat |
| Fat Free Hot Cocoa | 1 envelope | 25 | 0 | 0 | 0 | 0 | 0 | 150 | 5 | <1 | 1 | free |
| Hot Cocoa with Mini Marshmallows | 1 envelope | 80 | 2.5 | 25 | 2 | 0 | 0 | 160 | 14 | <1 | 1 | 1 carb, 1 fat |
| Nesquik Chocolate | 2 Tbsp | 60 | 0.5 | 5 | 0 | 0 | 0 | 30 | 14 | <1 | <1 | 1 carb |
| Nesquik No Sugar Added Chocolate | 2 Tbsp | 35 | 1 | 10 | 0.5 | 0 | 0 | 70 | 7 | 1 | 1 | 1/2 carb |
| No Sugar Added Hot Cocoa | 1 envelope | 50 | 0 | 0 | 0 | 0 | 0 | 180 | 10 | <1 | 2 | 1/2 carb |
| Rich Milk Chocolate Hot Cocoa | 1 envelope | 80 | 3 | 25 | 2 | 0 | 0 | 180 | 14 | <1 | 1 | 1 carb, 1 fat |

| | | | | | | | | | | | | |
|---|---|---|---|---|---|---|---|---|---|---|---|---|
| ***Ovaltine*** | | | | | | | | | | | | |
| Malted Milk Drink, Chocolate Malt | 4 Tbsp | 80 | 0 | 0 | 0 | 0 | 0 | 115 | 18 | <1 | 1 | 1 carb |
| Malted Milk Drink, Rich Chocolate | 4 Tbsp | 80 | 0 | 0 | 0 | 0 | 0 | 140 | 19 | 0 | <1 | 1 carb |
| ***Swiss Miss*** | | | | | | | | | | | | |
| Dark Chocolate Hot Cocoa | 1 envelope | 150 | 3.5 | 30 | 0 | 0 | 0 | 170 | 28 | 1 | 1 | 2 carb, 1 fat |
| Milk Chocolate Hot Cocoa | 1 envelope | 120 | 2 | 20 | 2 | 0 | 0 | 160 | 23 | <1 | 1 | 1 1/2 carb |
| **COFFEE** | | | | | | | | | | | | |
| Coffee, Brewed | 8 oz | 2 | 0 | 0 | 0 | 0 | 0 | 5 | 0 | 0 | 0 | free |
| Coffee, Instant | 8 oz | 5 | 0 | 0 | 0 | 0 | 0 | 10 | <1 | 0 | 0 | free |
| ***General Foods*** | | | | | | | | | | | | |
| Chai Latte | 1 1/3 Tbsp | 70 | 2 | 20 | 2 | 0 | 0 | 60 | 12 | 0 | 0 | 1 carb |

BEVERAGES, SODA, SPORTS/ENERGY DRINKS

| | Serving | Calories | Fat (g) | Cal. from Fat | Sat. Fat (g) | Trans Fat (g) | Chol. (mg) | Sod. (mg) | Carb. (g) | Fiber (g) | Prot. (g) | Servings/Exchanges |
|---|---|---|---|---|---|---|---|---|---|---|---|---|
| International Coffees, All Varieties | 1 1/3 Tbsp | 50–70 | 1.5–3 | 15–30 | 0.5–2.5 | 0 | 0 | 30–110 | 10–12 | 0 | 0–1 | 1 carb |
| International Coffees, Sugar-Free, Mocha | 1 1/3 Tbsp | 30 | 2 | 20 | 2 | 0 | 0 | 30 | 2 | 0 | 0 | free |
| ***Hills Brothers*** | | | | | | | | | | | | |
| Cappuccino, French Vanilla | 3 Tbsp | 120 | 4.5 | 40 | 3.5 | 0 | 0 | 105 | 19 | 0 | 2 | 1 carb, 1 fat |
| ***Starbucks*** | | | | | | | | | | | | |
| Coffee Frappuccino Coffee Drink | 9.5-oz bottle | 200 | 3 | 30 | 2 | 0 | 15 | 100 | 37 | 0 | 6 | 2 1/2 carb, 1 fat |
| Doubleshot Coffee Drink | 6.5-oz can | 140 | 6 | 50 | 3.5 | 0 | 20 | 70 | 18 | 0 | 4 | 1 carb, 1 fat |
| Mocha Frappuccino Coffee Drink | 9.5-oz bottle | 180 | 3 | 30 | 2 | 0 | 15 | 95 | 33 | 0 | 7 | 2 carb, 1 fat |

| | | | | | | | | | | | | |
|---|---|---|---|---|---|---|---|---|---|---|---|---|
| Mocha Lite Frappuccino Coffee Drink | 9.5-oz bottle | 100 | 3 | 30 | 2 | 0 | 15 | 95 | 12 | 0 | 6 | 1 carb, 1 fat |
| Vanilla Frappuccino Coffee Drink | 9.5-oz bottle | 200 | 3 | 30 | 2 | 0 | 15 | 100 | 37 | 0 | 6 | 2 1/2 carb, 1 fat |
| **COFFEE CREAMER** | | | | | | | | | | | | |
| ***Cremora*** | | | | | | | | | | | | |
| Lite & Creamy | 1 tsp | 10 | 0 | 0 | 0 | 0 | 0 | 5 | 1 | 0 | 0 | free |
| Original | 1 tsp | 10 | 0.5 | 5 | 0.5 | 0 | 0 | 10 | 0 | 0 | 0 | free |
| ***International Delight Coffee House*** | | | | | | | | | | | | |
| Caramel Macchiato | 1 Tbsp | 40 | 1.5 | 15 | 1 | 0 | 0 | 5 | 7 | 0 | 0 | 1/2 carb |
| Vanilla Latte | 1 Tbsp | 40 | 1.5 | 15 | 1 | 0 | 0 | 5 | 7 | 0 | 0 | 1/2 carb |
| ***Nestlé Coffee-Mate (Liquid)*** | | | | | | | | | | | | |
| Cinnamon Vanilla Crème, Fat Free | 1 Tbsp | 25 | 0 | 0 | 0 | 0 | 0 | 25 | 5 | 0 | 0 | free |
| French Vanilla | 1 Tbsp | 35 | 1.5 | 15 | 0 | 0 | 0 | 30 | 5 | 0 | 0 | 1 fat |
| Hazelnut | 1 Tbsp | 35 | 1.5 | 15 | 0 | 0 | 0 | 30 | 2 | 0 | 0 | free |

| | Serving | Calories | Fat (g) | Cal. from Fat | Sat. Fat (g) | Trans Fat (g) | Chol. (mg) | Sod. (mg) | Carb. (g) | Fiber (g) | Prot. (g) | Servings/Exchanges |
|---|---|---|---|---|---|---|---|---|---|---|---|---|
| Original | 1 Tbsp | 15 | 1 | 10 | 0 | 0 | 0 | 0 | 2 | 0 | 0 | free |
| Vanilla Caramel | 1 Tbsp | 35 | 1.5 | 15 | 0 | 0 | 0 | 30 | 5 | 0 | 0 | 1 fat |
| ***Nestlé Coffee-Mate (Powder)*** | | | | | | | | | | | | |
| Fat Free | 1 tsp | 10 | 0 | 0 | 0 | 0 | 0 | 0 | 2 | 0 | 0 | free |
| French Vanilla | 4 tsp | 60 | 2.5 | 25 | 2 | 0 | 0 | 15 | 9 | 0 | 0 | 1/2 carb, 1 fat |
| Hazelnut | 4 tsp | 60 | 3 | 25 | 2.5 | 0 | 0 | 15 | 9 | 0 | 0 | 1/2 carb, 1 fat |
| Original | 1 tsp | 10 | 0.5 | 5 | 0.5 | 0 | 0 | 0 | 1 | 0 | 0 | free |
| Vanilla Caramel | 4 tsp | 60 | 3 | 25 | 2.5 | 0 | 0 | 15 | 9 | 0 | 0 | 1/2 carb, 1 fat |
| **FRUIT PUNCH & LEMONADE** | | | | | | | | | | | | |
| Fruit Punch Mix | 8 oz | 97 | 0 | 0 | 0 | 0 | 0 | 8 | 25 | 0 | 0 | 1 1/2 carb |
| Lemonade, Prepared | 8 oz | 112 | 0 | 0 | 0 | 0 | 0 | 19 | 29 | 0 | 0 | 2 carb |
| ***Country Time*** | | | | | | | | | | | | |
| Lemonade, Powder | 8 oz | 60 | 0 | 0 | 0 | 0 | 0 | 25 | 16 | 0 | 0 | 1 carb |
| Lite Lemonade | 8 oz | 35 | 0 | 0 | 0 | 0 | 0 | 10 | 8 | 0 | 0 | 1/2 carb |

| | | | | | | | | | | | | |
|---|---|---|---|---|---|---|---|---|---|---|---|---|
| Pink Lemonade | 8 oz | 60 | 0 | 0 | 0 | 0 | 0 | 0 | 16 | 0 | 0 | 1 carb |
| ***Crystal Light*** | | | | | | | | | | | | |
| Crystal Light Bottles | 8 oz | 5 | 0 | 0 | 0 | 0 | 0 | 10 | 0 | 0 | 0 | free |
| Crystal Light Drinks, Lemonades, or Teas | 8 oz | 5 | 0 | 0 | 0 | 0 | 0 | 0–35 | 0 | 0 | 0 | free |
| ***Kool-Aid*** | | | | | | | | | | | | |
| Drink Mix from Powder, All Varieties | 8 oz | 60 | 0 | 0 | 0 | 0 | 0 | 0 | 16 | 0 | 0 | 1 carb |
| ***Tang*** | | | | | | | | | | | | |
| Orange Drink Mix, Powder | 8 oz | 40 | 0 | 0 | 0 | 0 | 0 | 0 | 9 | 0 | 0 | 1/2 carb |
| Orange Drink Mix, Sugar-Free, Powder | 8 oz | 5 | 0 | 0 | 0 | 0 | 0 | 0 | 0 | 0 | 0 | free |
| ***Tropicana*** | | | | | | | | | | | | |
| Lemonade | 12-oz can | 150 | 0 | 0 | 0 | 0 | 0 | 90 | 40 | 0 | 0 | 2 1/2 carb |

BEVERAGES, SODAS SPORTS/ENERGY DRINKS

| | Serving | Calories | Fat (g) | Cal. from Fat | Sat. Fat (g) | Trans Fat (g) | Chol. (mg) | Sod. (mg) | Carb. (g) | Fiber (g) | Prot. (g) | Servings/Exchanges |
|---|---|---|---|---|---|---|---|---|---|---|---|---|
| **SODA DRINKS** | | | | | | | | | | | | |
| **Average (All Brands)** | | | | | | | | | | | | |
| Soda Drink, Small | 16 oz | 207 | 0 | 0 | 0 | 0 | 0 | 20 | 53 | 0 | 0 | 2 1/2 carb |
| Soda Drink, Medium | 22 oz | 284 | 0 | 0 | 0 | 0 | 0 | 27 | 73 | 0 | 0 | 5 carb |
| Soda Drink, Large | 32 oz | 413 | 0 | 0 | 0 | 0 | 0 | 39 | 106 | 0 | 0 | 7 carb |
| Club Soda | 12 oz | 0 | 0 | 0 | 0 | 0 | 0 | 75 | 0 | 0 | 0 | free |
| Cream Soda | 12 oz | 189 | 0 | 0 | 0 | 0 | 0 | 45 | 49 | 0 | 0 | 3 carb |
| Diet Cola/Coke with Aspartame | 12 oz | 4 | 0 | 0 | 0 | 0 | 0 | 21 | <1 | 0 | 0 | free |
| Ginger Ale | 12 oz | 124 | 0 | 0 | 0 | 0 | 0 | 26 | 32 | 0 | 0 | 3 carb |
| Grape Soda | 12 oz | 160 | 0 | 0 | 0 | 0 | 0 | 56 | 42 | 0 | 0 | 3 carb |
| Lemon-Lime Soda | 12 oz | 147 | 0 | 0 | 0 | 0 | 0 | 40 | 38 | 0 | 0 | 2 1/2 carb |
| Orange Soda | 12 oz | 179 | 0 | 0 | 0 | 0 | 0 | 45 | 46 | 0 | 0 | 3 carb |
| Root Beer | 12 oz | 152 | 0 | 0 | 0 | 0 | 0 | 48 | 39 | 0 | 0 | 2 1/2 carb |

| **Brands** | | | | | | | | | | | | |
|---|---|---|---|---|---|---|---|---|---|---|---|---|
| 7-Up | 12 oz | 140 | 0 | 0 | 0 | 0 | 0 | 40 | 39 | 0 | 0 | 2 1/2 carb |
| 7-Up, Cherry | 12 oz | 140 | 0 | 0 | 0 | 0 | 0 | 40 | 39 | 0 | 0 | 2 1/2 carb |
| 7-Up, Diet | 12 oz | 170 | 0 | 0 | 0 | 0 | 0 | 45 | 46 | 0 | 0 | 3 carb |
| A&W Root Beer | 12 oz | 170 | 0 | 0 | 0 | 0 | 0 | 47 | 65 | 0 | 0 | 3 carb |
| A&W Cream Soda | 12 oz | 190 | 0 | 0 | 0 | 0 | 0 | 70 | 47 | 0 | 0 | 3 carb |
| Barq's Root Beer | 12 oz | 160 | 0 | 0 | 0 | 0 | 0 | 70 | 45 | 0 | 0 | 3 carb |
| Canada Dry Ginger Ale | 12 oz | 140 | 0 | 0 | 0 | 0 | 0 | 50 | 36 | 0 | 0 | 2 1/2 carb |
| ***Coca-Cola*** | | | | | | | | | | | | |
| Coca-Cola Classic | 12 oz | 140 | 0 | 0 | 0 | 0 | 0 | 50 | 39 | 0 | 0 | 2 1/2 carb |
| Coca-Cola Zero | 12 oz | 0 | 0 | 0 | 0 | 0 | 0 | 40 | 0 | 0 | 0 | free |
| Cherry Coke | 12 oz | 150 | 0 | 0 | 0 | 0 | 0 | 35 | 42 | 0 | 0 | 3 carb |
| Diet Coke | 12 oz | 0 | 0 | 0 | 0 | 0 | 0 | 40 | 0 | 0 | 0 | free |
| Diet Coke with Lime | 12 oz | 0 | 0 | 0 | 0 | 0 | 0 | 40 | 0 | 0 | 0 | free |
| Vanilla Coke | 12 oz | 150 | 0 | 0 | 0 | 0 | 0 | 35 | 42 | 0 | 0 | 3 carb |
| Diet Rite | 12 oz | 0 | 0 | 0 | 0 | 0 | 0 | 0 | 0 | 0 | 0 | free |

| | Serving | Calories | Fat (g) | Cal. from Fat | Sat. Fat (g) | Trans Fat (g) | Chol. (mg) | Sod. (mg) | Carb. (g) | Fiber (g) | Prot. (g) | Servings/Exchanges |
|---|---|---|---|---|---|---|---|---|---|---|---|---|
| Dr. Pepper | 12 oz | 150 | 0 | 0 | 0 | 0 | 0 | 55 | 40 | 0 | 0 | 2 1/2 carb |
| Fanta Orange | 12 oz | 160 | 0 | 0 | 0 | 0 | 0 | 55 | 44 | 0 | 0 | 3 carb |
| Fresca | 12 oz | 0 | 0 | 0 | 0 | 0 | 0 | 35 | 0 | 0 | 0 | free |
| ***Hansen's Natural Cane Soda*** | | | | | | | | | | | | |
| Club Soda | 8 oz | 0 | 0 | 0 | 0 | 0 | 0 | 0 | 40 | 0 | 0 | free |
| Creamy Root Beer | 12 oz | 160 | 0 | 0 | 0 | 0 | 0 | 0 | 43 | 0 | 0 | 3 carb |
| Diet Black Cherry | 12 oz | 0 | 0 | 0 | 0 | 0 | 0 | 0 | 0 | 0 | 0 | free |
| Diet Green Tea Soda, Tangerine | 8 oz | 0 | 0 | 0 | 0 | 0 | 0 | 0 | 0 | 0 | 0 | free |
| Ginger Ale | 8 oz | 90 | 0 | 0 | 0 | 0 | 0 | 0 | 24 | 0 | 0 | 1 1/2 carb |
| Mango Orange | 12 oz | 170 | 0 | 0 | 0 | 0 | 0 | 0 | 44 | 0 | 0 | 3 carb |
| Natural Green Tea Soda, Pomegranate | 8 oz | 90 | 0 | 0 | 0 | 0 | 0 | 0 | 22 | 0 | 0 | 1 1/2 carb |
| Natural Soda Tonic | 8 oz | 90 | 0 | 0 | 0 | 0 | 0 | 0 | 24 | 0 | 0 | 1 1/2 carb |

| | | | | | | | | | | | | |
|---|---|---|---|---|---|---|---|---|---|---|---|---|
| Raspberry | 12 oz | 140 | 0 | 0 | 0 | 0 | 0 | 0 | 37 | 0 | 0 | 2 1/2 carb |
| Mountain Dew | 12 oz | 170 | 0 | 0 | 0 | 0 | 0 | 65 | 46 | 0 | 0 | 3 carb |
| Mountain Dew Code Red | 12 oz | 170 | 0 | 0 | 0 | 0 | 0 | 105 | 46 | 0 | 0 | 3 carb |
| Mountain Dew–Diet | 12 oz | 0 | 0 | 0 | 0 | 0 | 0 | 50 | 0 | 0 | 0 | free |
| MUG Root Beer | 12 oz | 160 | 0 | 0 | 0 | 0 | 0 | 65 | 43 | 0 | 0 | 3 carb |
| ***Pepsi*** | | | | | | | | | | | | |
| Diet Pepsi | 12 oz | 0 | 0 | 0 | 0 | 0 | 0 | 35 | 0 | 0 | 0 | free |
| Pepsi | 12 oz | 150 | 0 | 0 | 0 | 0 | 0 | 30 | 41 | 0 | 0 | 3 carb |
| Pepsi Max | 12 oz | 0 | 0 | 0 | 0 | 0 | 0 | 35 | 0 | 0 | 0 | 2 carb |
| Pepsi Natural | 12 oz | 150 | 0 | 0 | 0 | 0 | 0 | 35 | 39 | 0 | 0 | 2 1/2 carb |
| Wild Cherry Pepsi | 12 oz | 160 | 0 | 0 | 0 | 0 | 0 | 30 | 42 | 0 | 0 | 3 carb |
| Sierra Mist | 12 oz | 140 | 0 | 0 | 0 | 0 | 0 | 35 | 39 | 0 | 0 | 2 1/2 carb |
| Slice Orange | 12 oz | 180 | 0 | 0 | 0 | 0 | 0 | 35 | 48 | 0 | 0 | 3 carb |
| ***Sprite*** | | | | | | | | | | | | |
| Sprite Zero | 12 oz | 0 | 0 | 0 | 0 | 0 | 0 | 35 | 0 | 0 | 0 | free |
| Sprite | 12 oz | 140 | 0 | 0 | 0 | 0 | 0 | 65 | 38 | 0 | 0 | 2 1/2 carb |

BEVERAGES, SODA, SPORTS/ENERGY DRINKS

| | Serving | Calories | Fat (g) | Cal. from Fat | Sat. Fat (g) | Trans Fat (g) | Chol. (mg) | Sod. (mg) | Carb. (g) | Fiber (g) | Prot. (g) | Servings/Exchanges |
|---|---|---|---|---|---|---|---|---|---|---|---|---|
| Squirt | 12 oz | 140 | 0 | 0 | 0 | 0 | 0 | 50 | 39 | 0 | 0 | 2 1/2 carb |
| Sunkist Orange | 12 oz | 190 | 0 | 0 | 0 | 0 | 0 | 65 | 52 | 0 | 0 | 3 carb |
| TAB | 12 oz | 0 | 0 | 0 | 0 | 0 | 0 | 40 | 0 | 0 | 0 | free |
| **SPORTS/NUTRITION/ENERGY DRINKS** | | | | | | | | | | | | |
| Accelerade | 1 scoop (12 oz) | 120 | 1 | 10 | 0 | 0 | 0 | 190 | 21 | 0 | 5 | 1 1/2 carb |
| Accelerade, Citrus Grapefruit | 8 oz | 80 | 0 | 0 | 0 | 0 | 0 | 120 | 15 | 0 | 4 | 1 carb |
| All Sport Body Quencher | 8 oz | 60 | 0 | 0 | 0 | 0 | 0 | 55 | 16 | 0 | 0 | 1 carb |
| All Sport Naturally Zero | 8 oz | 0 | 0 | 0 | 0 | 0 | 0 | 55 | 0 | 0 | 0 | free |
| AMP Energy Drink | 8 oz | 110 | 0 | 0 | 0 | 0 | 0 | 65 | 29 | 0 | 0 | 2 carb |
| AMP Energy Drink, Sugar Free | 8 oz | 5 | 0 | 0 | 0 | 0 | 0 | 75 | <1 | 0 | 0 | free |
| Boost | 8 oz | 240 | 4 | 35 | 0.5 | 0 | 5 | 130 | 41 | 0 | 10 | 3 carb |

| | | | | | | | | | | | | |
|---|---|---|---|---|---|---|---|---|---|---|---|---|
| Boost Glucose Control | 8 oz | 190 | 7 | 60 | 1 | 0 | 10 | 180 | 16 | 3 | 16 | 1 carb, 2 lean meat |
| Boost High Protein | 8 oz | 240 | 6 | 50 | 0.5 | 0 | 10 | 170 | 33 | 0 | 15 | 2 carb, 1 med-fat meat |
| Boost Plus | 8 oz | 360 | 14 | 130 | 1.5 | 0 | 10 | 170 | 45 | 0 | 14 | 3 carb, 1 med-fat meat, 2 fat |
| Carnation Instant Breakfast Essentials, Powder Mix | 1 packet | 130 | 0–1 | 0–10 | 0.5 | 0 | <5 | 80–160 | 26–27 | 0–1 | 5 | 2 carb |
| Carnation Instant Breakfast Essentials, Ready-to-Drink | 10.8-oz bottle | 250–260 | 5 | 50 | 1.5 | 0 | 10 | 180 | 34–41 | 0–1 | 14 | 2 carb, 1 med-fat meat |
| Carnation Instant Breakfast Essentials, Sugar-Free | 1 packet | 60–70 | 0–1 | 0–10 | 0 | 0 | <5 | 60–70 | 12 | 3–4 | 5 | 1 carb |
| Carnation Instant Breakfast, Sugar-Free, Ready-to-Drink | 10.8-oz bottle | 150 | 5 | 50 | 1.5 | 0 | 10 | 240 | 16 | 2 | 13 | 1 carb, 1 med-fat meat |

BEVERAGES, SODA, SPORTS/ENERGY DRINKS

| | Serving | Calories | Fat (g) | Cal. from Fat | Sat. Fat (g) | Trans Fat (g) | Chol. (mg) | Sod. (mg) | Carb. (g) | Fiber (g) | Prot. (g) | Servings/Exchanges |
|---|---|---|---|---|---|---|---|---|---|---|---|---|
| Clif Quench Sport Drink, All Varieties | 8 oz | 45 | 0 | 0 | 0 | 0 | 0 | 130 | 11 | 0 | 0 | 1 carb |
| CytoSport Cytomax Performance Ready-to-Drink | 8 oz | 50 | 0 | 0 | 0 | 0 | 0 | 55 | 13 | 0 | 0 | 1 carb |
| CytoSport Cytomax Powder | 1 scoop | 90 | 0 | 0 | 0 | 0 | 0 | 120 | 22 | 0 | 0 | 1 1/2 carb |
| CytoSport Muscle Milk Light Ready-to-Drink | 14 oz | 160 | 4.5 | 40 | 1 | 0 | 10 | 340 | 10 | 5 | 20 | 1/2 carb, 3 lean meat |
| CytoSport Muscle Milk Powder | 1 scoop | 150 | 6 | 55 | 3 | 0 | 8 | 115 | 8 | 2.5 | 16 | 1/2 carb, 2 lean meat |
| CytoSport Muscle Milk Ready-to-Drink | 14 oz | 230 | 9 | 80 | 1.5 | 0 | 10 | 350 | 12 | 2 | 25 | 1 carb, 3 lean meat |
| Gatorade (All Varieties) | 8 oz | 50 | 0 | 0 | 0 | 0 | 0 | 110 | 14 | 0 | 0 | 1 carb |

| | | | | | | | | | | | | |
|---|---|---|---|---|---|---|---|---|---|---|---|---|
| Gatorade G2 | 8 oz | 25 | 0 | 0 | 0 | 0 | 0 | 110 | 7 | 0 | 0 | 1/2 carb |
| Glaceau Vitamin Water (All Varieties) | 8 oz | 50 | 0 | 0 | 0 | 0 | 0 | 0 | 13 | 0 | 0 | 1 carb |
| KMX Energy Drink (All Varieties) | 8.4 oz | 120 | 0 | 0 | 0 | 0 | 0 | 75 | 31 | 0 | 0 | 2 carb |
| Monster Energy Drink | 8 oz | 100 | 0 | 0 | 0 | 0 | 0 | 180 | 27 | 0 | 0 | 2 carb |
| Monster Energy Drink, Lo-Carb | 8 oz | 10 | 0 | 0 | 0 | 0 | 0 | 180 | 3 | 0 | 0 | free |
| No Fear | 8 oz | 130 | 0 | 0 | 0 | 0 | 0 | 115 | 36 | 0 | 0 | 2 1/2 carb |
| No Fear Blood Shot | 8 oz | 100 | 0 | 0 | 0 | 0 | 0 | 160 | 24 | 0 | 0 | 1 1/2 carb |
| No Fear Motherload | 8 oz | 130 | 0 | 0 | 0 | 0 | 0 | 100 | 34 | 0 | 0 | 2 carb |
| No Fear Sugar Free | 8 oz | 10 | 0 | 0 | 0 | 0 | 0 | 100 | 1 | 0 | 0 | free |
| Powerade (All Varieties) | 8 oz | 50 | 0 | 0 | 0 | 0 | 0 | 100 | 14 | 0 | 0 | 1 carb |
| Powerade Zero | 8 oz | 0 | 0 | 0 | 0 | 0 | 0 | 55 | 0 | 0 | 0 | free |
| Propel Fitness Water | 8 oz | 10 | 0 | 0 | 0 | 0 | 0 | 75 | 2 | 0 | 0 | free |
| Red Bull Energy Drink | 8.4 oz | 110 | 0 | 0 | 0 | 0 | 0 | 100 | 28 | 0 | <1 | 2 carb |

| | Serving | Calories | Fat (g) | Cal. from Fat | Sat. Fat (g) | Trans Fat (g) | Chol. (mg) | Sod. (mg) | Carb. (g) | Fiber (g) | Prot. (g) | Servings/Exchanges |
|---|---|---|---|---|---|---|---|---|---|---|---|---|
| Rockstar Energy Drink | 8 oz | 140 | 0 | 0 | 0 | 0 | 0 | 40 | 31 | 0 | 0 | 2 carb |
| ***R.W. Knudsen*** | | | | | | | | | | | | |
| Recharge Sports | 8 oz | 70 | 0 | 0 | 0 | 0 | 0 | 25 | 18 | 0 | 0 | 1 carb |
| Simply Nutritious Mega Green | 8 oz | 130 | 0 | 0 | 0 | 0 | 0 | 35 | 31 | 0 | 1 | 2 carb |
| Simply Nutritious Plum Boost | 8 oz | 120 | 0 | 0 | 0 | 0 | 0 | 10 | 33 | 0 | 0 | 2 carb |
| Simply Nutritious VitaJuice | 8 oz | 120 | 0 | 0 | 0 | 0 | 0 | 40 | 31 | 0 | 0 | 2 carb |
| Sparkling Essence Organic Blueberry | 8 oz | 0 | 0 | 0 | 0 | 0 | 0 | 0 | 0 | 0 | 0 | free |
| ***Ross Products*** | | | | | | | | | | | | |
| Ensure | 8 oz | 250 | 6 | 55 | 1 | 0 | 5 | 190 | 41 | 0 | 9 | 2 1/2 carb, 1 fat |
| Ensure High Calcium | 8 oz | 220 | 6 | 50 | 1 | 0 | <5 | 290 | 31 | 0 | 10 | 2 carb, 1 med-fat meat |

| | | | | | | | | | | | | |
|---|---|---|---|---|---|---|---|---|---|---|---|---|
| Ensure High Protein | 8 oz | 230 | 6 | 50 | 1 | 0 | <5 | 290 | 31 | 0 | 12 | 2 carb, 1 med-fat meat |
| Ensure Plus | 8 oz | 350 | 11 | 100 | 1.5 | 0 | 10 | 220 | 50 | 0 | 13 | 3 carb, 2 fat |
| Glucerna, Chocolate | 8 oz | 200 | 7 | 60 | 0.5 | 0 | <5 | 210 | 27 | 5 | 10 | 2 carb, 2 fat |
| ***Slim-Fast*** | | | | | | | | | | | | |
| Easy to Digest | 10.8-oz can | 180 | 5 | 45 | 1 | 0 | <5 | 240 | 26 | 3 | 10 | 1 med-fat meat, 1 1/2 carb |
| High Protein Extra Creamy Chocolate | 10.8-oz can | 190 | 5 | 45 | 2 | 0 | 10 | 220 | 24 | 5 | 15 | 1 1/2 carb, 2 lean meat |
| Lower Carb Creamy Chocolate | 10.8-oz can | 190 | 9 | 80 | 1.5 | 0 | 15 | 260 | 6 | 4 | 20 | 1/2 carb, 3 lean meat |
| Optima Creamy Milk Chocolate | 10.8-oz can | 190 | 6 | 25 | 2.5 | 0 | 5 | 200 | 25 | 5 | 10 | 1 1/2 carb, 1 med-fat meat |
| Original Creamy Milk Chocolate | 10.8-oz can | 220 | 3 | 25 | 1 | 0 | 5 | 220 | 40 | 5 | 10 | 2 1/2 carb, 1 lean meat |
| ***Snapple Elements*** | | | | | | | | | | | | |
| Diet Ice Drinks | 8 oz | 10 | 0 | 0 | 0 | 0 | 0 | 10 | 2 | 0 | 0 | free |

| | Serving | Calories | Fat (g) | Cal. from Fat | Sat. Fat (g) | Trans Fat (g) | Chol. (mg) | Sod. (mg) | Carb. (g) | Fiber (g) | Prot. (g) | Servings/Exchanges |
|---|---|---|---|---|---|---|---|---|---|---|---|---|
| Juice Drinks (Spark) | 8 oz | 110–130 | 0 | 0 | 0 | 0 | 0 | 10–35 | 28–29 | 0 | 0 | 2 carb |
| ***SoBe*** | | | | | | | | | | | | |
| Adrenaline Rush Energy | 8 oz | 130 | 0 | 0 | 0 | 0 | 0 | 95 | 34 | 0 | 0 | 2 carb |
| Energy | 8 oz | 110 | 0 | 0 | 0 | 0 | 0 | 15 | 27 | 0 | 0 | 2 carb |
| Lean Diet Energy | 8 oz | 5 | 0 | 0 | 0 | 0 | 0 | 15 | 1 | 0 | 0 | free |
| Lifewater | 8 oz | 40 | 0 | 0 | 0 | 0 | 0 | 20 | 17 | 0 | 0 | 1 carb |
| Nirvana | 8 oz | 120 | 0 | 0 | 0 | 0 | 0 | 15 | 29 | 0 | 0 | 2 carb |
| Power | 8 oz | 110 | 0 | 0 | 0 | 0 | 0 | 15 | 27 | 0 | 0 | 2 carb |
| ***Starbucks*** | | | | | | | | | | | | |
| DoubleShot Coffee Drink | 8 oz | 170 | 7 | 60 | 4.5 | 0 | 25 | 85 | 22 | 0 | 5 | 1 low-fat milk, 1/2 carb |
| Frappuccino-Vanilla | 8 oz | 170 | 2.5 | 25 | 1.5 | 0 | 10 | 85 | 31 | 0 | 5 | 1 low-fat milk, 1 carb |

| | Serving | Calories | Fat (g) | Cal. from Fat | Sat. Fat (g) | Trans Fat (g) | Chol. (mg) | Sod. (mg) | Carb. (g) | Fiber (g) | Prot. (g) | Servings/Exchanges |
|---|---|---|---|---|---|---|---|---|---|---|---|---|
| **BREAD, BAGELS, ROLLS, BISCUITS, TORTILLAS, PANCAKES, WAFFLES, STUFFING, CROUTONS** | | | | | | | | | | | | |
| Bagel, Cinnamon Raisin | 1, 2–3 inches | 97 | 1 | 10 | 0 | 0 | 0 | 114 | 20 | <1 | 4 | 1 starch |
| Bagel, Plain | 1, 2–3 inches | 95 | <1 | 0 | 0 | 0 | 0 | 184 | 18 | <1 | 4 | 1 starch |
| Biscuit | 1, 2 1/2 inches | 127 | 6 | 55 | <1 | 0 | 0 | 368 | 17 | <1 | 2 | 1 starch, 1 fat |
| Bread Sticks, Plain | 2, 4-inch | 42 | 1 | 10 | 0 | 0 | 0 | 66 | 7 | 0 | 1 | 1/2 starch |
| Bread, Butter Croissant | 1, small | 171 | 9 | 80 | 5 | 0 | 28 | 312 | 19 | 1 | 3 | 1 starch, 2 fat |
| Bread, Corn | 1.5-oz piece | 113 | 3 | 30 | 1 | 0 | 17 | 280 | 19 | 1 | 3 | 1 starch, 1 fat |
| Bread, Cracked Wheat | 1 slice | 65 | 1 | 10 | 0 | 0 | 0 | 134 | 12 | 1 | 2 | 1 starch |

## BREAD, BAGELS, ROLLS, BISCUITS, TORTILLAS

| | Serving | Calories | Fat (g) | Cal. from Fat | Sat. Fat (g) | Trans Fat (g) | Chol. (mg) | Sod. (mg) | Carb. (g) | Fiber (g) | Prot. (g) | Servings/Exchanges |
|---|---|---|---|---|---|---|---|---|---|---|---|---|
| Bread, French, Vienna, or Sourdough | 1 small slice | 92 | 1 | 10 | <1 | 0 | 0 | 208 | 18 | <1 | 4 | 1 starch |
| Bread, Italian | 1 slice | 81 | 1 | 10 | <1 | 0 | 0 | 175 | 15 | <1 | 3 | 1 starch |
| Bread, Multi Grain | 1 slice | 69 | 1 | 10 | 0 | 0 | 0 | 109 | 11 | 2 | 3 | 1 starch |
| Bread, Oatmeal | 1 slice | 73 | 1 | 10 | 0 | 0 | 0 | 162 | 13 | 1 | 2 | 1 starch |
| Bread, Pita | 1/2 | 82 | <1 | 0 | 0 | 0 | 0 | 161 | 17 | 1 | 3 | 1 starch |
| Bread, Pita, Whole Wheat | 1, large | 170 | 2 | 20 | 0 | 0 | 0 | 340 | 35 | 5 | 6 | 2 starch |
| Bread, Pumpernickel | 1 slice | 80 | 1 | 10 | 0 | 0 | 0 | 215 | 15 | 2 | 3 | 1 starch |
| Bread, Raisin | 1 slice | 71 | 1 | 10 | 0 | 0 | 0 | 101 | 14 | 1 | 2 | 1 starch |
| Bread, Rye | 1 slice | 83 | 1 | 10 | 0 | 0 | 0 | 211 | 16 | 2 | 3 | 1 starch |
| Bread, Wheat Bran | 1 slice | 89 | 1 | 10 | 0 | 0 | 0 | 175 | 17 | 1 | 3 | 1 starch |
| Bread, Wheat, Reduced Calorie | 2 slices | 91 | 1 | 10 | 0 | 0 | 0 | 235 | 20 | 6 | 4 | 1 starch |
| Bread, White | 1 slice | 67 | 1 | 10 | 0 | 0 | 0 | 134 | 12 | 1 | 2 | 1 starch |

| | | | | | | | | | | | | |
|---|---|---|---|---|---|---|---|---|---|---|---|---|
| Bread, White, Reduced Calorie | 2 slices | 95 | 1 | 10 | 0 | 0 | 0 | 208 | 20 | 5 | 4 | 1 starch |
| Bread, Whole Wheat | 1 slice | 69 | 1 | 10 | 0 | 0 | 0 | 148 | 13 | 2 | 3 | 1 starch |
| Bun, Hamburger | 1/2 | 60 | 1 | 10 | 0 | 0 | 0 | 103 | 11 | <1 | 2 | 1 starch |
| Bun, Hot Dog | 1/2 | 61 | 1 | 10 | 0 | 0 | 0 | 120 | 11 | <1 | 2 | 1 starch |
| Chapati | 1, 6-inch | 71 | <1 | 0 | 0 | 0 | 0 | 131 | 15 | 2 | 3 | 1 starch |
| Croutons | 1 cup | 122 | 2 | 20 | <1 | 0 | 0 | 209 | 22 | 2 | 4 | 1 1/2 starch |
| Egg Bread/Challah | 1 slice | 113 | 2 | 20 | <1 | 0 | 20 | 197 | 19 | <1 | 4 | 1 starch |
| English Muffin | 1/2 | 67 | 0.5 | 5 | 0 | 0 | 0 | 132 | 13 | 1 | 2 | 1 starch |
| French Toast, Frozen | 1 slice | 126 | 4 | 35 | 1 | 0 | 48 | 292 | 19 | <1 | 4 | 1 starch, 1 fat |
| French Toast, Homemade with 2% Milk | 1 slice | 149 | 7 | 65 | 2 | 0 | 75 | 311 | 16 | NA | 5 | 1 starch, 1 fat |
| Naan | 1/4, large | 75 | 2 | 20 | 0 | 0 | 9 | 90 | 13 | <1 | 2 | 1 starch |
| Pancakes, Plain, Frozen | 1, 4-inch | 82 | 1 | 10 | 0 | 0 | 3 | 183 | 16 | <1 | 2 | 1 starch |
| Roll, Plain | 1 | 85 | 2 | 20 | 0.5 | 0 | 0 | 148 | 14 | 1 | 2 | 1 starch |
| Roll, Whole Wheat | 1 | 74 | 1 | 10 | 0 | 0 | 0 | 134 | 14 | 2 | 2 | 1 starch |

BREAD, BAGELS, ROLLS, BISCUITS, TORTILLAS

| | Serving | Calories | Fat (g) | Cal. from Fat | Sat. Fat (g) | Trans Fat (g) | Chol. (mg) | Sod. (mg) | Carb. (g) | Fiber (g) | Prot. (g) | Servings/Exchanges |
|---|---|---|---|---|---|---|---|---|---|---|---|---|
| Taco Shells | 2 | 124 | 6 | 55 | 1 | 0 | 0 | 98 | 17 | 2 | 2 | 1 starch, 1 fat |
| Tortilla, Corn | 1, 6-inch | 52 | 0.5 | 5 | 0 | 0 | 0 | 11 | 11 | 2 | 1 | 1 starch |
| Tortilla, Flour | 1, 6-inch | 112 | 3 | 30 | <1 | 0 | 0 | 229 | 19 | 1 | 3 | 1 starch |
| Tortilla, Flour | 1/3 of 10 1/2-inch | 185 | 4 | 40 | 1 | 0 | 0 | 272 | 32 | 2 | 5 | 2 starch, 1 fat |
| Waffles, Toaster Style | 1, 4-inch | 96 | 3 | 30 | <1 | 0 | 3 | 217 | 15 | 1 | 2 | 1 starch, 1 fat |
| **Brands** | | | | | | | | | | | | |
| ***Aunt Hattie's*** | | | | | | | | | | | | |
| All Natural 100% Whole Grain | 1 slice | 100 | 1.5 | 10 | 0 | 0 | 0 | 240 | 19 | 3 | 4 | 1 starch |
| All Natural Dark 12 Grain | 1 slice | 120 | 2 | 20 | 0 | 0 | 0 | 200 | 20 | 1 | 4 | 1 starch |
| All Natural Double Fiber | 1 slice | 100 | 1.5 | 10 | 0 | 0 | 0 | 190 | 22 | 6 | 4 | 1 1/2 starch |
| Homestyle Potato | 1 slice | 80 | 1 | 5 | 0 | 0 | 0 | 180 | 15 | 0 | 3 | 1 starch |

| | | | | | | | | | | | | |
|---|---|---|---|---|---|---|---|---|---|---|---|---|
| Homestyle Wheat | 1 slice | 70 | 1 | 10 | 0 | 0 | 0 | 140 | 13 | 1 | 2 | 1 starch |
| Homestyle White | 1 slice | 70 | 1 | 10 | 0 | 0 | 0 | 160 | 13 | 0 | 2 | 1 starch |
| Light 9 Grain | 2 slices | 90 | 0.5 | 5 | 0 | 0 | 0 | 260 | 16 | 4 | 4 | 1 starch |
| Low Carb | 1 slice | 45 | 0.5 | 5 | 0 | 0 | 0 | 120 | 7 | 2 | 4 | 1/2 starch |
| Potato Hamburger Buns | 1 | 140 | 2 | 20 | 0 | 0 | 0 | 220 | 25 | 1 | 4 | 1 1/2 starch |
| Potato Hot Dog Buns | 1 | 140 | 2 | 20 | 0 | 0 | 0 | 250 | 25 | 1 | 5 | 1 1/2 starch |
| Soft Wheat with Buttermilk | 1 slice | 70 | 1 | 10 | 0 | 0 | 0 | 150 | 13 | 1 | 3 | 1 starch |
| Wheat Berry | 1 slice | 110 | 1.5 | 10 | 0 | 0 | 0 | 230 | 20 | 2 | 4 | 1 starch |
| ***Aunt Jemima*** | | | | | | | | | | | | |
| Pancake/Waffle Mix, Buttermilk | 1/3 cup | 110 | 0.5 | 5 | 0 | 0 | 0 | 480 | 23 | 1 | 4 | 1 1/2 starch |
| Pancake/Waffle Mix, Original | 1/3 cup | 150 | 0 | 0 | 0 | 0 | 0 | 740 | 33 | 1 | 4 | 2 starch |
| Pancake/Waffle Mix, Whole Wheat | 1/4 cup | 120 | 0.5 | 5 | 0 | 0 | 0 | 620 | 26 | 3 | 4 | 2 starch |

BREAD, BAGELS, ROLLS, BISCUITS, TORTILLAS

| | Serving | Calories | Fat (g) | Cal. from Fat | Sat. Fat (g) | Trans Fat (g) | Chol. (mg) | Sod. (mg) | Carb. (g) | Fiber (g) | Prot. (g) | Servings/Exchanges |
|---|---|---|---|---|---|---|---|---|---|---|---|---|
| ***Betty Crocker*** | | | | | | | | | | | | |
| Bisquick, Original | 1/3 cup | 160 | 5 | 45 | 1.5 | 1.5 | 0 | 490 | 26 | 1 | 3 | 2 starch, 1 fat |
| Heart Smart | 1/3 cup | 140 | 2.5 | 25 | 0 | 0 | 0 | 340 | 27 | <1 | 3 | 2 starch, 1 fat |
| ***Food for Life*** | | | | | | | | | | | | |
| Ezekial 4:9 100% Whole Wheat Sprouted | 1 slice | 80 | 0.5 | 5 | 0 | 0 | 0 | 75 | 15 | 3 | 4 | 1 starch |
| Ezekiel 4:9 Low Sodium | 1 slice | 80 | 0.5 | 5 | 0 | 0 | 0 | 0 | 15 | 3 | 4 | 1 starch |
| ***Healthy Choice*** | | | | | | | | | | | | |
| Hearty 100% Whole Grain | 1 slice | 80 | 1 | 10 | 0 | 0 | 0 | 170 | 18 | 3 | 3 | 1 starch |
| Hearty 7 Grain | 1 slice | 80 | 1 | 10 | 0 | 0 | 0 | 170 | 18 | 3 | 4 | 1 starch |
| ***Holsum*** | | | | | | | | | | | | |
| Hamburger Buns | 1 | 110 | 1.5 | 15 | 0 | 0 | 0 | 220 | 20 | 1 | 4 | 1 starch |
| Hot Dog Buns | 1 | 110 | 1.5 | 15 | 0 | 0 | 0 | 220 | 20 | 1 | 4 | 1 starch |

| | | | | | | | | | | | | |
|---|---|---|---|---|---|---|---|---|---|---|---|---|
| Thin White Sandwich | 1 slice | 70 | 1 | 10 | 0 | 0 | 0 | 160 | 14 | 0 | 2 | 1 starch |
| ***Home Pride*** | | | | | | | | | | | | |
| Butter Top White | 1 slice | 70 | 1 | 10 | 0 | 0 | 0 | 140 | 14 | 0 | 2 | 1 starch |
| ***Jiffy*** | | | | | | | | | | | | |
| Buttermilk Biscuit Mix | 1/3 cup | 160 | 5 | 45 | 2 | 0 | <5 | 420 | 27 | <1 | 3 | 2 starch, 1 fat |
| Corn Muffin Mix | 1/4 cup | 150 | 4.5 | 40 | 2 | 0 | <5 | 340 | 27 | <1 | 2 | 1 starch, 1 fat |
| ***Kellogg's Eggo*** | | | | | | | | | | | | |
| French Toast Sticks | 2 slices | 220 | 6 | 60 | 1.5 | 0 | 25 | 540 | 35 | <1 | 5 | 2 starch, 1 fat |
| Pancakes, Blueberry | 3 | 260 | 8 | 70 | 1.5 | 0 | 15 | 500 | 42 | 1 | 6 | 3 starch, 2 fat |
| Pancakes, Buttermilk | 3 | 280 | 9 | 80 | 1.5 | 0 | 15 | 580 | 44 | 1 | 6 | 2 starch, 2 fat |
| Waffles, Apple Cinnamon | 2 | 190 | 6 | 60 | 1.5 | 0 | 15 | 370 | 29 | 1 | 4 | 2 starch, 1 fat |
| Waffles, Blueberry | 2 | 190 | 6 | 60 | 1.5 | 0 | 15 | 370 | 29 | <1 | 4 | 2 starch, 1 fat |
| Waffles, Buttermilk | 2 | 180 | 6 | 60 | 2 | 0 | 15 | 420 | 26 | 1 | 5 | 2 starch, 1 fat |
| Waffles, Chocolate Chip | 2 | 210 | 7 | 60 | 2.5 | 0 | 15 | 380 | 32 | 1 | 4 | 2 starch, 1 fat |
| Waffles, Cinnamon Toast | 3 | 300 | 11 | 100 | 3 | 0 | 20 | 490 | 45 | 1 | 5 | 3 starch, 2 fat |

| | Serving | Calories | Fat (g) | Cal. from Fat | Sat. Fat (g) | Trans Fat (g) | Chol. (mg) | Sod. (mg) | Carb. (g) | Fiber (g) | Prot. (g) | Servings/Exchanges |
|---|---|---|---|---|---|---|---|---|---|---|---|---|
| Waffles, French Toast | 1 | 140 | 6 | 50 | 2 | 0 | 10 | 240 | 19 | <1 | 3 | 1 starch, 1 fat |
| Waffles, Homestyle | 2 | 190 | 7 | 70 | 2 | 0 | 20 | 430 | 27 | <1 | 4 | 2 starch, 1 fat |
| Waffles, Minis Homestyle | 3 | 260 | 10 | 90 | 2.5 | 0 | 25 | 610 | 38 | 1 | 6 | 2 1/2 starch, 2 fat |
| Waffles, Nutri-Grain Whole Wheat | 2 | 170 | 6 | 50 | 1.5 | 0 | 0 | 400 | 26 | 3 | 4 | 2 starch, 1 fat |
| Waffles, Special K | 3 | 160 | 2.5 | 20 | 0.5 | 0 | 20 | 440 | 29 | <1 | 5 | 2 starch, 1 fat |
| Waffles, Waf-Fulls, Strawberry | 1 | 170 | 5 | 45 | 1.5 | 0 | 10 | 300 | 27 | <1 | 3 | 2 starch, 1 fat |
| ***Krusteaz*** | | | | | | | | | | | | |
| Buttermilk Pancakes | 3 | 280 | 4 | 35 | 0.5 | 0 | 10 | 710 | 52 | 3 | 8 | 3 1/2 starch, 1 fat |
| Homestyle French Toast | 2 | 230 | 5 | 50 | 1 | 0 | 95 | 540 | 36 | 2 | 9 | 2 1/2 starch, 1 fat |
| Mini Pancakes | 12 | 220 | 2.5 | 20 | 0.5 | 0 | 0 | 580 | 43 | 2 | 6 | 3 starch, 1 fat |
| ***Marshall's*** | | | | | | | | | | | | |

| | | | | | | | | | | | | |
|---|---|---|---|---|---|---|---|---|---|---|---|---|
| Biscuits, Buttermilk | 3 | 240 | 12 | 110 | 3 | 3.5 | 0 | 600 | 29 | 1 | 4 | 2 starch, 2 fat |
| Biscuits, Homestyle | 1 | 120 | 6 | 50 | 3 | 1.5 | 0 | 330 | 15 | 0 | 2 | 1 starch, 1 fat |
| ***Milton's*** | | | | | | | | | | | | |
| Gourmet White | 1 slice | 110 | 0.5 | 5 | 0 | 0 | 0 | 110 | 23 | 1 | 4 | 1 1/2 starch |
| Multi-Grain 100% Whole Wheat Bread | 1 slice | 110 | 0.5 | 5 | 0 | 0 | 0 | 220 | 22 | 5 | 5 | 1 1/2 starch |
| Whole Grain Plus | 1 slice | 90 | 0.5 | 5 | 0 | 0 | 0 | 125 | 16 | 5 | 4 | 1 starch |
| ***Mission*** | | | | | | | | | | | | |
| 96% Fat Free Flour Tortilla, Large Burrito Size | 1 | 180 | 2.5 | 20 | 0.5 | 0 | 0 | 450 | 35 | 5 | 5 | 2 starch, 1 fat |
| 96% Fat Free Flour Tortilla, Medium Soft Taco Size | 1 | 130 | 1.5 | 15 | 0 | 0 | 0 | 330 | 26 | 3 | 4 | 2 starch |
| 96% Fat Free Whole Wheat Flour Tortilla, Soft Taco Size | 1 | 130 | 2 | 15 | 0 | 0 | 0 | 340 | 25 | 3 | 4 | 1 1/2 starch |

BREAD, BAGELS, ROLLS, BISCUITS, TORTILLAS

| | Serving | Calories | Carb. (g) | Fat (g) | Cal. from Fat | Sat. Fat (g) | Trans Fat (g) | Chol. (mg) | Sod. (mg) | Fiber (g) | Prot. (g) | Servings/Exchanges |
|---|---|---|---|---|---|---|---|---|---|---|---|---|
| Carb Balance Flour Tortilla, Fajita Size | 1 | 80 | 2 | 15 | 0 | 0 | 0 | 220 | 12 | 7 | 3 | 1 starch |
| Carb Balance Flour Tortilla, Medium Soft Taco Size | 1 | 120 | 3.5 | 25 | 1.5 | 0 | 0 | 330 | 18 | 11 | 5 | 1 starch, 1 fat |
| Carb Balance Whole Wheat Flour Tortilla, Small Fajita Size | 1 | 80 | 2 | 10 | 0 | 0 | 0 | 220 | 12 | 8 | 3 | 1 starch |
| Life Balance Flour Tortilla, Medium Soft Taco Size | 1 | 130 | 3 | 30 | 1.5 | 0 | 0 | 290 | 20 | 3 | 4 | 1 starch, 1 fat |
| Life Balance Whole Wheat Tortilla, Soft Taco Size | 1 | 130 | 3 | 30 | 1.5 | 0 | 0 | 310 | 19 | 4 | 4 | 1 starch, 1 fat |
| Multi-Grain Flour Tortilla, Soft Taco Size | 1 | 150 | 4.5 | 35 | 1.5 | 0 | 0 | 460 | 23 | 5 | 5 | 1 1/2 starch, 1 fat |

| | | | | | | | | | | | | |
|---|---|---|---|---|---|---|---|---|---|---|---|---|
| Tortilla Wraps, Jalapeño Cheddar | 1 | 210 | 4.5 | 40 | 2 | 0 | 0 | 850 | 35 | 1 | 5 | 2 starch, 1 fat |
| Tortilla Wraps, Multi-Grain | 1 | 210 | 6 | 50 | 2.5 | 0 | 0 | 660 | 32 | 7 | 6 | 2 starch, 1 fat |
| Tortilla Wraps, Sun Dried Tomato Basil | 1 | 210 | 4.5 | 40 | 2 | 0 | 0 | 570 | 35 | 2 | 6 | 2 starch, 1 fat |
| Tortilla, Large Burrito Size | 1 | 210 | 5 | 45 | 2 | 0 | 0 | 630 | 36 | 1 | 6 | 2 1/2 starch, 1 fat |
| Tortilla, Medium Soft Taco | 1 | 150 | 3.5 | 35 | 1.5 | 0 | 0 | 440 | 25 | 1 | 4 | 1 1/2 starch, 1 fat |
| Tortilla, Small Fajita | 1 | 110 | 3 | 25 | 1 | 0 | 0 | 320 | 18 | 1 | 3 | 1 starch, 1 fat |
| White Corn Tortilla | 2 | 90 | 1 | 10 | 0 | 0 | 0 | 10 | 17 | 3 | 2 | 1 starch |
| Yellow Corn Tortilla | 2 | 110 | 1.5 | 15 | 0 | 0 | 0 | 10 | 22 | 3 | 2 | 1 1/2 starch |
| ***Mrs. Cubbinson's*** | | | | | | | | | | | | |
| Caesar Salad | 5 | 35 | 0 | 0 | 0 | 0 | 0 | 65 | 4 | 0 | <1 | 1/2 starch |
| Fat Free Herb Seasoned | 5 | 30 | 0 | 0 | 0 | 0 | 0 | 105 | 5 | 0 | 1 | 1/2 starch |

BREAD, BAGELS, ROLLS, BISCUITS, TORTILLAS

| | Serving | Calories | Fat (g) | Cal. from Fat | Sat. Fat (g) | Trans Fat (g) | Chol. (mg) | Sod. (mg) | Carb. (g) | Fiber (g) | Prot. (g) | Servings/Exchanges |
|---|---|---|---|---|---|---|---|---|---|---|---|---|
| ***Nature's Own*** | | | | | | | | | | | | |
| 100% Whole Wheat | 1 slice | 60 | 1 | 10 | 0 | 0 | 0 | 125 | 11 | 2 | 4 | 1 starch |
| Double Fiber Wheat | 1 slice | 50 | 0.5 | 5 | 0 | 0 | 0 | 135 | 13 | 5 | 3 | 1 starch |
| Honey Wheat | 1 slice | 70 | 0.5 | 5 | 0 | 0 | 0 | 120 | 14 | <1 | 2 | 1 starch |
| White Wheat | 2 slices | 100 | 2 | 15 | 0 | 0 | 0 | 230 | 22 | 5 | 6 | 1 1/2 starch |
| ***Old El Paso*** | | | | | | | | | | | | |
| Taco Shells, Corn | 3 | 150 | 7 | 60 | 3 | 0 | 0 | 135 | 19 | 1 | 2 | 1 starch, 1 fat |
| Tostada Shells, Corn | 3 | 150 | 7 | 60 | 3 | 0 | 0 | 135 | 19 | 1 | 2 | 1 starch, 1 fat |
| ***Oroweatx*** | | | | | | | | | | | | |
| 100% Whole Wheat English Muffin | 1 | 130 | 1.5 | 15 | 0 | 0 | 0 | 240 | 25 | 4 | 5 | 1 1/2 starch |
| 100% Whole Wheat Hamburger Buns | 1 | 180 | 3 | 25 | 0.5 | 0 | 0 | 370 | 32 | 6 | 9 | 2 starch, 1 fat |
| Country Buttermilk | 1 slice | 100 | 1 | 10 | 0 | 0 | 0 | 180 | 19 | <1 | 3 | 1 starch |

| | | | | | | | | | | | | |
|---|---|---|---|---|---|---|---|---|---|---|---|---|
| Country Potato | 1 slice | 100 | 1 | 10 | 0 | 0 | 0 | 190 | 20 | <1 | 3 | 1 starch |
| Country White | 1 slice | 110 | 1.5 | 15 | 0 | 0 | 0 | 240 | 20 | <1 | 3 | 1 starch |
| Double Fiber | 1 slice | 70 | 1 | 10 | 0 | 0 | 0 | 160 | 16 | 6 | 3 | 1 starch |
| Health Nut | 1 slice | 100 | 2 | 20 | 0 | 0 | 0 | 190 | 18 | 2 | 4 | 1 starch |
| Jewish Rye | 1 slice | 80 | 1 | 10 | 0 | 0 | 0 | 170 | 15 | 1 | 3 | 1 starch |
| Oatnut | 1 slice | 100 | 1.5 | 15 | 0 | 0 | 0 | 190 | 19 | 1 | 4 | 1 starch |
| Russian Rye | 1 slice | 70 | 1 | 10 | 0 | 0 | 0 | 200 | 13 | <1 | 2 | 1 starch |
| Seven Grain | 1 slice | 100 | 1 | 10 | 0 | 0 | 0 | 180 | 20 | 2 | 3 | 1 starch |
| Whole Grain & Flax Seed | 1 slice | 100 | 1.5 | 15 | 0 | 0 | 0 | 160 | 17 | 3 | 4 | 1 starch |
| ***Ortega*** | | | | | | | | | | | | |
| Taco Shells, Corn | 2 | 120 | 6 | 50 | 1 | 0 | 0 | 170 | 16 | 2 | 2 | 1 starch, 1 fat |
| Tostada Shells | 2 | 120 | 6 | 50 | 1 | 0 | 0 | 170 | 19 | 2 | 2 | 1 starch, 1 fat |
| ***Pepperidge Farm*** | | | | | | | | | | | | |
| 9 Grain | 1 slice | 100 | 2 | 15 | 0 | 0 | 0 | 130 | 20 | 3 | 4 | 1 starch |
| German Dark Wheat | 1 slice | 100 | 1.5 | 15 | 0 | 0 | 0 | 150 | 20 | 3 | 4 | 1 starch |

BREAD, BAGELS, ROLLS, BISCUITS, TORTILLAS

| | Serving | Calories | Fat (g) | Cal. from Fat | Sat. Fat (g) | Trans Fat (g) | Chol. (mg) | Sod. (mg) | Carb. (g) | Fiber (g) | Prot. (g) | Servings/Exchanges |
|---|---|---|---|---|---|---|---|---|---|---|---|---|
| Honey Flax | 1 slice | 100 | 2 | 15 | 0 | 0 | 0 | 120 | 19 | 3 | 5 | 1 starch |
| ***Bagels and Rolls*** | | | | | | | | | | | | |
| Bagel, Cinnamon and Raisin | 1 | 270 | 1 | 10 | 0 | 0 | 0 | 450 | 57 | 3 | 8 | 4 starch |
| Bagel, Everything | 1 | 260 | 1.5 | 15 | 0.5 | 0 | 0 | 480 | 53 | 2 | 9 | 3 1/2 starch |
| Bagel, Mini Plain | 1 | 110 | 0.5 | 5 | 0 | 0 | 0 | 200 | 22 | 1 | 4 | 1 1/2 starch |
| Bagel, Plain | 1 | 260 | 1 | 10 | 0 | 0 | 0 | 500 | 54 | 3 | 9 | 3 1/2 starch |
| Buns, Sandwich with Sesame Seeds | 1 | 130 | 3 | 30 | 0.5 | 0 | 0 | 220 | 22 | 1 | 5 | 1 1/2 starch, 1 fat |
| Buns, Classic 100% Whole Wheat Hamburger | 1 | 120 | 2 | 20 | 0 | 0 | 0 | 190 | 18 | 2 | 6 | 1 starch |
| English Muffin, 100% Whole Wheat | 1 | 140 | 1.5 | 15 | 0.5 | 0 | 0 | 210 | 26 | 3 | 6 | 2 starch |

| | | | | | | | | | | | | |
|---|---|---|---|---|---|---|---|---|---|---|---|---|
| English Muffin, Original | 1 | 130 | 1.5 | 15 | 0.5 | 0 | 0 | 170 | 25 | 1 | 5 | 1 1/2 starch |
| Mini Bagel, Brown Sugar Cinnamon | 1 | 120 | 0.5 | 5 | 0 | 0 | 0 | 150 | 24 | 2 | 4 | 1 1/2 starch |
| Rolls, Hamburger Classic | 1 | 120 | 2 | 20 | 0.5 | 0 | 0 | 180 | 22 | 1 | 5 | 1 1/2 starch |
| Rolls, Soft Country Dinner | 1 | 90 | 1.5 | 15 | 0 | 0 | 0 | 150 | 17 | 1 | 3 | 1 starch |
| Rolls, Soft Hoagie with Sesame Seeds | 1 | 210 | 6 | 55 | 1.5 | 0 | 0 | 350 | 35 | 2 | 7 | 2 starch, 1 fat |
| ***Croutons*** | | | | | | | | | | | | |
| Seasoned | 6 | 30 | 1 | 10 | 0 | 0 | 0 | 75 | 5 | 0 | <1 | 1/2 starch |
| Whole Grain | 6 | 30 | 1 | 10 | 0 | 0 | 0 | 70 | 5 | <1 | 1 | 1/2 starch |
| ***Farm House Hearty Sliced Bread*** | | | | | | | | | | | | |
| 12 Grain | 1 slice | 120 | 2 | 15 | 0 | 0 | 0 | 180 | 21 | 3 | 4 | 1 starch |
| 7 Grain | 1 slice | 110 | 1.5 | 15 | 0.5 | 0 | 0 | 170 | 21 | 2 | 4 | 1 starch |
| Crunchy Oat | 1 slice | 120 | 1.5 | 15 | 0.5 | 0 | 0 | 160 | 21 | 2 | 5 | 1 starch |
| Hearty White | 1 slice | 120 | 1.5 | 15 | 0.5 | 0 | 0 | 250 | 22 | 1 | 4 | 1 starch |

BREAD, BAGELS, ROLLS, BISCUITS, TORTILLAS

| | Serving | Calories | Fat (g) | Cal. from Fat | Sat. Fat (g) | Trans Fat (g) | Chol. (mg) | Sod. (mg) | Carb. (g) | Fiber (g) | Prot. (g) | Servings/Exchanges |
|---|---|---|---|---|---|---|---|---|---|---|---|---|
| Soft 100% Whole Wheat | 1 slice | 110 | 2 | 15 | 0.5 | 0 | 0 | 150 | 19 | 3 | 5 | 1 starch |
| Soft Oatmeal | 1 slice | 120 | 1.5 | 15 | 0.5 | 0 | 0 | 200 | 21 | 1 | 4 | 1 starch |
| Sourdough | 1 slice | 120 | 1.5 | 15 | 0.5 | 0 | 0 | 220 | 22 | 1 | 4 | 1 starch |
| Sweet Buttermilk | 1 slice | 120 | 1.5 | 15 | 0.5 | 0 | 0 | 190 | 23 | 1 | 4 | 1 starch |
| ***Hot & Crusty Breads*** | | | | | | | | | | | | |
| Twin French | 4-inch slice | 150 | 1.5 | 15 | 0 | 0 | 0 | 260 | 29 | 1 | 5 | 1 starch |
| ***Light Style Breads*** | | | | | | | | | | | | |
| Extra Fiber | 3 slices | 120 | 1 | 10 | 0 | 0 | 0 | 250 | 26 | 6 | 6 | 1 1/2 starch |
| Oatmeal | 3 slices | 140 | 1 | 10 | 0 | 0 | 0 | 260 | 27 | 2 | 7 | 2 starch |
| Seven Grain | 3 slices | 130 | 1 | 10 | 0 | 0 | 0 | 270 | 26 | 4 | 7 | |
| Soft Wheat | 3 slices | 130 | 1.5 | 15 | 0 | 0 | 0 | 270 | 25 | 4 | 8 | 1 1/2 starch |
| ***Party Breads*** | | | | | | | | | | | | |
| Dark Pumpernickel | 5 slices | 130 | 1.5 | 15 | 0 | 0 | 0 | 320 | 23 | 3 | 5 | 1 1/2 starch |

| | | | | | | | | | | | | |
|---|---|---|---|---|---|---|---|---|---|---|---|---|
| Jewish Rye | 5 slices | 130 | 2 | 18 | 0 | 0 | 0 | 460 | 25 | 2 | 4 | 1 1/2 starch |
| ***Rye & Pumpernickel*** | | | | | | | | | | | | |
| Deli Swirl | 1 slice | 80 | 1 | 10 | 0 | 0 | 0 | 180 | 14 | 1 | 3 | 1 starch |
| Pumpernickel | 1 slice | 80 | 1 | 10 | 0 | 0 | 0 | 190 | 15 | 1 | 3 | 1 starch |
| Seedless Rye | 1 slice | 80 | 1 | 10 | 0 | 0 | 0 | 180 | 14 | 1 | 3 | 1 starch |
| ***Variety Breads*** | | | | | | | | | | | | |
| 100% Whole Wheat Thin Sliced | 1 slice | 70 | 1 | 10 | 0 | 0 | 0 | 65 | 12 | 2 | 2 | 1 starch |
| Oatmeal | 1 slice | 70 | 1 | 10 | 0 | 0 | 0 | 85 | 12 | 1 | 2 | 1 starch |
| ***Very Thin Breads*** | | | | | | | | | | | | |
| 100% Whole Wheat | 3 slices | 110 | 2 | 20 | 0.5 | 0 | 0 | 230 | 20 | 3 | 4 | 1 starch |
| White | 3 slices | 120 | 1 | 10 | 0 | 0 | 0 | 250 | 24 | 1 | 4 | 1 1/2 starch |
| ***White Breads*** | | | | | | | | | | | | |
| Italian Bread | 1 slice | 90 | 1 | 10 | 0 | 0 | 0 | 190 | 17 | <1 | 3 | 1 starch |
| Original Whole Grain White | 2 slices | 110 | 2 | 20 | 0.5 | 0 | 0 | 200 | 22 | 3 | 4 | 1 1/2 starch |

BREAD, BAGELS, ROLLS, BISCUITS, TORTILLAS

| | Serving | Calories | Fat (g) | Cal. from Fat | Sat. Fat (g) | Trans Fat (g) | Chol. (mg) | Sod. (mg) | Carb. (g) | Fiber (g) | Prot. (g) | Servings/Exchanges |
|---|---|---|---|---|---|---|---|---|---|---|---|---|
| Sandwich | 2 slices | 130 | 2.5 | 25 | 0.5 | 0 | 0 | 250 | 23 | <1 | 4 | 1 1/2 starch, 1 fat |
| ***Pillsbury*** | | | | | | | | | | | | |
| Bread, Crusty French | 1/6 batch | 120 | 1.5 | 15 | 0.5 | 0 | 0 | 300 | 24 | <1 | 4 | 1 1/2 starch |
| Crescent Rolls, Original | 1 | 110 | 6 | 60 | 2 | 1.5 | 0 | 220 | 11 | 0 | 2 | 1 starch, 1 fat |
| Crescent Rolls, Reduced Fat | 1 | 90 | 4.5 | 35 | 0.5 | 0 | 0 | 220 | 12 | 0 | 2 | 1 starch, 1 fat |
| Crescent Rounds | 1 | 110 | 6 | 60 | 2 | 1.5 | 0 | 220 | 11 | 0 | 2 | 1 starch, 1 fat |
| Pizza Crust, Thin | 1/5 can | 180 | 5 | 45 | 1 | 0 | 0 | 360 | 29 | 1 | 5 | 2 starch, 1 fat |
| ***Pillsbury Grands*** | | | | | | | | | | | | |
| Big Biscuits, Butter Tastin | 1 | 180 | 8 | 70 | 2 | 3.5 | 0 | 580 | 25 | <1 | 3 | 1 1/2 starch, 2 fat |
| Big Biscuits, Buttermilk | 1 | 180 | 8 | 70 | 2 | 2 | 0 | 540 | 25 | <1 | 3 | 1 1/2 starch, 2 fat |
| Big Biscuits, Flaky Layers | 1 | 180 | 8 | 70 | 2 | 2 | 0 | 540 | 25 | <1 | 4 | 1 1/2 starch, 2 fat |

| | | | | | | | | | | | | |
|---|---|---|---|---|---|---|---|---|---|---|---|---|
| Big Biscuits, Reduced Fat Flaky Layers | 1 | 160 | 6 | 50 | 2 | 0 | 0 | 570 | 26 | <1 | 4 | 2 starch, 1 fat |
| Biscuits, Buttermilk | 1 | 100 | 4 | 40 | 1 | 1 | 0 | 360 | 14 | <1 | 2 | 1 starch, 1 fat |
| Biscuits, Honey Butter | 1 | 110 | 4 | 35 | 1 | 1 | 0 | 290 | 15 | 0 | 2 | 1 starch, 1 fat |
| ***Progresso*** | | | | | | | | | | | | |
| Bread Crumbs, Italian Style | 1/4 cup | 110 | 1.5 | 15 | 0.5 | 0 | 0 | 470 | 20 | 1 | 4 | 1 starch |
| Bread Crumbs, Parmesan | 1/4 cup | 110 | 1.5 | 15 | 0.5 | 0 | 0 | 870 | 19 | 1 | 4 | 1 starch |
| Bread Crumbs, Plain | 1/4 cup | 110 | 1.5 | 15 | 0.5 | 0 | 0 | 220 | 19 | 1 | 4 | 1 starch |
| ***Roman Meal*** | | | | | | | | | | | | |
| Sandwich Bread | 1 slice | 60 | 1 | 5 | 0 | 0 | 0 | 140 | 12 | 1 | 3 | 1 starch |
| Whole Grain Bread | 2 slices | 130 | 2 | 15 | 0 | 0 | 0 | 240 | 24 | 2 | 5 | 1 1/2 starch |
| ***Rudi's Organic*** | | | | | | | | | | | | |
| 100% Whole Wheat bread | 1 slice | 100 | 1 | 10 | 0 | 0 | 0 | 140 | 19 | 3 | 4 | 1 starch |

| | Serving | Calories | Fat (g) | Cal. from Fat | Sat. Fat (g) | Trans Fat (g) | Chol. (mg) | Sod. (mg) | Carb. (g) | Fiber (g) | Prot. (g) | Servings/Exchanges |
|---|---|---|---|---|---|---|---|---|---|---|---|---|
| 7 Grain Flax | 1 slice | 100 | 1.5 | 15 | 0 | 0 | 0 | 150 | 18 | 4 | 4 | 1 starch |
| Honey Whole Wheat | 1 slice | 100 | 1 | 10 | 0 | 0 | 0 | 170 | 19 | 3 | 5 | 1 starch |
| Multigrain Oat | 1 slice | 110 | 1 | 10 | 0 | 0 | 0 | 180 | 21 | 2 | 4 | 1 starch |
| Spelt | 1 slice | 100 | 1 | 10 | 0 | 0 | 0 | 210 | 22 | 2 | 3 | 1 starch |
| Spelt Ancient Grain | 1 slice | 120 | 2.5 | 25 | 0 | 0 | 0 | 170 | 20 | 2 | 4 | 1 starch, 1 fat |
| Wheat & Oat | 1 slice | 90 | 1 | 10 | 0 | 0 | 0 | 190 | 18 | 4 | 3 | 1 starch |
| ***Sara Lee*** | | | | | | | | | | | | |
| Classic White | 2 slices | 160 | 2 | 20 | 0.5 | 0 | 0 | 270 | 30 | 1 | 5 | 2 starch |
| Whole Grain White | 2 slices | 150 | 2 | 20 | 0.5 | 0 | 0 | 220 | 28 | 2 | 5 | 2 starch |
| ***Shake 'N Bake*** | | | | | | | | | | | | |
| Coating Mix, Classic Italian | 1/8 pkt | 35 | 0.5 | 5 | 0 | 0 | 0 | 280 | 7 | 0 | <1 | 1/2 starch |
| Coating Mix, Original Chicken | 1/8 pkt | 40 | 1 | 10 | 0 | 0 | 0 | 220 | 7 | 0 | <1 | 1/2 starch |

| | | | | | | | | | | | | |
|---|---|---|---|---|---|---|---|---|---|---|---|---|
| Coating Mix, Original Pork | 1/8 pkt | 40 | 0 | 0 | 0 | 0 | 0 | 240 | 8 | 0 | 1 | 1/2 starch |
| Coating Mix, Parmesan | 1/8 pkt | 35 | 0.5 | 5 | 0 | 0 | 0 | 290 | 7 | 0 | 1 | 1/2 starch |
| ***Stove Top*** | | | | | | | | | | | | |
| Stuffing Mix for Pork | 1/2 cup | 160 | 7 | 60 | 1.5 | 1.5 | 0 | 510 | 21 | 1 | 3 | 1 starch, 2 fat |
| Stuffing Mix for Turkey | 1/2 cup | 160 | 7 | 60 | 1.5 | 0 | 1.5 | 520 | 21 | 1 | 3 | 1 starch, 2 fat |
| Stuffing Mix, Chicken Flavor | 1/2 cup | 150 | 7 | 60 | 1 | 1.5 | 0 | 520 | 20 | <1 | 3 | 1 starch, 2 fat |
| Stuffing Mix, Corn Bread | 1/2 cup | 160 | 7 | 60 | 1.5 | 1.5 | 0 | 570 | 22 | <1 | 3 | 1 1/2 starch, 2 fat |
| Stuffing Mix, Herbs | 1/2 cup | 160 | 7 | 60 | 1.5 | 1.5 | 0 | 530 | 21 | 1 | 3 | 1 starch, 2 fat |
| ***Trader Joe's*** | | | | | | | | | | | | |
| 100% Stone Ground Whole Grain | 1 slice | 100 | 0.5 | 5 | 0 | 0 | 0 | 200 | 22 | 3 | 4 | 1 1/2 starch |
| 100% Whole Grain Fiber Bread | 1 slice | 90 | 1 | 10 | 0 | 0 | 0 | 160 | 20 | 5 | 4 | 1 starch |

BREAD, BAGELS, ROLLS, BISCUITS, TORTILLAS

| | Serving | Calories | Fat (g) | Cal. from Fat | Sat. Fat (g) | Trans Fat (g) | Chol. (mg) | Sod. (mg) | Carb. (g) | Fiber (g) | Prot. (g) | Servings/Exchanges |
|---|---|---|---|---|---|---|---|---|---|---|---|---|
| California Style Complete Protein | 1 slice | 90 | 0.5 | 5 | 0 | 0 | 0 | 160 | 15 | 2 | 5 | 1 starch |
| Gourmet White | 1 slice | 120 | 3.5 | 35 | 0 | 0 | 0 | 260 | 19 | 1 | 3 | 1 starch, 1 fat |
| Harvest Whole Wheat | 1 slice | 90 | 1 | 10 | 0 | 0 | 0 | 180 | 19 | 3 | 3 | 1 1/2 starch |
| Multi-Grain | 1 slice | 120 | 1 | 10 | 0 | 0 | 0 | 170 | 24 | 1 | 3 | 1 1/2 starch |
| Omega Seed Bread | 1 slice | 140 | 4 | 35 | 0.5 | 0 | 0 | 140 | 22 | 3 | 4 | 1 1/2 starch, 1 fat |
| Organic Flourless Sprouted 7 Grain | 1 slice | 80 | 0.5 | 5 | 0 | 0 | 0 | 65 | 16 | 3 | 4 | 1 starch |
| Potato | 1 slice | 110 | 1.5 | 10 | 0 | 0 | 0 | 180 | 20 | 1 | 4 | 1 starch |
| Seeded Harvest | 2 oz | 130 | 2 | 20 | 0 | 0 | 0 | 250 | 25 | 2 | 5 | 1 1/2 starch |
| Sprouted Multigrain | 1 slice | 90 | 0.5 | 5 | 0 | 0 | 0 | 170 | 15 | 2 | 5 | 1 starch |
| Sprouted Wheat Berry | 1 slice | 90 | 1 | 10 | 0 | 0 | 0 | 140 | 18 | 2 | 4 | 1 starch |
| Whole Grain | 1 slice | 90 | 0.5 | 5 | 0 | 0 | 0 | 200 | 19 | 3 | 3 | 1 starch |
| Whole Wheat | 1 slice | 100 | 1.5 | 15 | 0 | 0 | 0 | 190 | 20 | 3 | 5 | 1 starch |

***Wonder***

| | | | | | | | | | | | | |
|---|---|---|---|---|---|---|---|---|---|---|---|---|
| Classic White | 1 slice | 70 | 1 | 10 | 0 | 0 | 0 | 150 | 14 | 0 | 2 | 1 starch |
| Made with Whole Grain White | 2 slices | 130 | 2 | 20 | 0.5 | 0 | 0 | 300 | 25 | 4 | 6 | 1 1/2 starch |
| Texas Toast | 1 slice | 100 | 1 | 10 | 0 | 0 | 0 | 200 | 19 | <1 | 3 | 1 starch |

| | Serving | Calories | Fat (g) | Cal. from Fat | Sat. Fat (g) | Trans Fat (g) | Chol. (mg) | Sod. (mg) | Carb. (g) | Fiber (g) | Prot. (g) | Servings/Exchanges |
|---|---|---|---|---|---|---|---|---|---|---|---|---|
| **BREAKFAST CEREAL, READY-TO-EAT CEREAL, HOT CEREAL** | | | | | | | | | | | | |
| Bran, 100%, Wheat, | 1/2 cup | 63 | 1 | 10 | 0 | 0 | 0 | 1 | 19 | 12 | 5 | 1 starch |
| Bran, Oat, Uncooked | 1/4 cup | 58 | 2 | 20 | 0 | 0 | 0 | 1 | 16 | 4 | 4 | 1 starch |
| Bulgur, Cooked | 1/2 cup | 76 | 0 | 0 | 0 | 0 | 0 | 5 | 17 | 4 | 3 | 1 starch |
| Corn Grits, White or Yellow, Cooked | 1/2 cup | 71 | 0 | 0 | 0 | 0 | 0 | 2 | 16 | <1 | 2 | 1 starch |
| Cream of Rice, Cooked | 1/2 cup | 63 | 0 | 0 | 0 | 0 | 0 | 1 | 14 | <1 | 1 | 1 starch |
| Cream of Wheat, Cooked | 1/2 cup | 65 | 0 | 0 | 0 | 0 | 0 | 69 | 13 | <1 | 2 | 1 starch |
| Farina, Cooked | 1/2 cup | 56 | 0 | 0 | 0 | 0 | 0 | 2 | 12 | <1 | 2 | 1 starch |
| Granola, Homemade | 1/2 cup | 298 | 15 | 135 | 2.5 | 0 | 0 | 15 | 33 | 6 | 9 | 2 starch, 3 fat |
| Kasha or Buckwheat Groats, Cooked | 1/2 cup | 77 | 0.5 | 5 | 0 | 0 | 0 | 3 | 17 | 2 | 3 | 1 starch |
| Millet, Cooked | 1/4 cup | 52 | 0.5 | 5 | 0 | 0 | 0 | 1 | 10 | <1 | 2 | 1/2 starch |

| | | | | | | | | | | | | |
|---|---|---|---|---|---|---|---|---|---|---|---|---|
| Muesli | 1/4 cup | 74 | 1 | 10 | 0 | 0 | 0 | 64 | 15 | 2 | 2 | 1 starch |
| Oatmeal Cereal, Cooked | 1/2 cup | 73 | 1 | 10 | <1 | 0 | 0 | 1 | 13 | 2 | 3 | 1 starch |
| Puffed Rice | 1 1/2 cup | 80 | 0 | 0 | 0 | 0 | 0 | 1 | 18 | <1 | 2 | 1 starch |
| Puffed Wheat | 1 1/2 cup | 66 | 0.5 | 5 | 0 | 0 | 0 | 1 | 14 | 2 | 3 | 1 starch |
| Shredded Wheat, Plain | 1/2 cup | 83 | 0 | 0 | 0 | 0 | 0 | 2 | 20 | 3 | 3 | 1 starch |
| Wheatena, Cooked | 1/2 cup | 68 | 0.5 | 5 | 0 | 0 | 0 | 2 | 14 | 3 | 2 | 1 starch |
| **Brands** | | | | | | | | | | | | |
| ***Active Lifestyle*** | | | | | | | | | | | | |
| Original | 1 cup | 110 | 0 | 0 | 0 | 0 | 0 | 220 | 22 | <1 | 7 | 1 1/2 starch |
| Strawberry | 1 cup | 110 | 0 | 0 | 0 | 0 | 0 | 220 | 25 | 1 | 3 | 1 1/2 starch |
| ***General Mills*** | | | | | | | | | | | | |
| Basic 4 | 1 cup | 200 | 2 | 20 | 1 | 0 | 0 | 320 | 43 | 3 | 4 | 3 starch |
| Boo Berry | 1 cup | 130 | 1 | 10 | 0 | 0 | 0 | 190 | 28 | 1 | 1 | 2 starch |
| Cheerios | 1 cup | 100 | 2 | 15 | 0 | 0 | 0 | 190 | 20 | 3 | 3 | 1 starch |
| Cheerios Plus, Multi-Grain | 1 cup | 110 | 1 | 10 | 0 | 0 | 0 | 200 | 24 | 3 | 2 | 1 1/2 starch |

BREAKFAST CEREAL, READY-TO-EAT CEREAL, HOT CEREAL

| | Serving | Calories | Fat (g) | Cal. from Fat | Sat. Fat (g) | Trans Fat (g) | Chol. (mg) | Sod. (mg) | Carb. (g) | Fiber (g) | Prot. (g) | Servings/Exchanges |
|---|---|---|---|---|---|---|---|---|---|---|---|---|
| Cheerios, Apple Cinnamon | 3/4 cup | 120 | 1.5 | 15 | 0 | 0 | 0 | 120 | 25 | 1 | 2 | 1 1/2 starch |
| Cheerios, Banana Nut | 3/4 cup | 100 | 1 | 10 | 0 | 0 | 0 | 160 | 23 | 1 | 1 | 1 1/2 starch |
| Cheerios, Berry Burst Triple Berry | 1 cup | 100 | 1 | 10 | 0 | 0 | 0 | 170 | 22 | 2 | 2 | 1 1/2 starch |
| Cheerios, Frosted | 3/4 cup | 110 | 1 | 10 | 0 | 0 | 0 | 170 | 23 | 2 | 2 | 1 1/2 starch |
| Cheerios, Fruity | 3/4 cup | 100 | 1.5 | 15 | 0 | 0 | 0 | 135 | 23 | 2 | 1 | 1 1/2 starch |
| Cheerios, Honey Nut | 3/4 cup | 110 | 1.5 | 15 | 0 | 0 | 0 | 190 | 22 | 2 | 2 | 1 1/2 starch |
| Cheerios, Oat Cluster Crunch | 3/4 cup | 100 | 1 | 10 | 0 | 0 | 0 | 135 | 22 | 2 | 2 | 1 1/2 starch |
| Cheerios, Yogurt Burst Strawberries | 3/4 cup | 120 | 1.5 | 15 | 0.5 | 0 | 0 | 180 | 24 | 2 | 2 | 1 1/2 starch |
| Chex, Chocolate | 3/4 cup | 130 | 2.5 | 25 | 0.5 | 0 | 0 | 240 | 26 | <1 | 2 | 2 starch, 1 fat |
| Chex, Cinnamon | 3/4 cup | 120 | 2 | 20 | 0 | 0 | 0 | 190 | 25 | 0 | 2 | 1 1/2 starch |

| | | | | | | | | | | | | |
|---|---|---|---|---|---|---|---|---|---|---|---|---|
| Chex, Corn | 1 cup | 120 | 0.5 | 5 | 0 | 0 | 0 | 290 | 26 | 1 | 2 | 2 starch |
| Chex, Honey Nut | 3/4 cup | 120 | 0.5 | 5 | 0 | 0 | 0 | 230 | 28 | 1 | 2 | 2 starch |
| Chex, Multi-Bran | 1 cup | 160 | 1.5 | 10 | 0 | 0 | 0 | 310 | 39 | 6 | 3 | 2 1/2 starch |
| Chex, Rice | 1 cup | 100 | 0 | 0 | 0 | 0 | 0 | 250 | 23 | 0 | 2 | 1 1/2 starch |
| Chex, Strawberry | 3/4 cup | 130 | 2 | 15 | 0 | 0 | 0 | 200 | 26 | <1 | 1 | 2 starch |
| Chex, Wheat | 1 cup | 160 | 1 | 10 | 0 | 0 | 0 | 340 | 38 | 5 | 5 | 2 1/2 starch |
| Cinnamon Toast Crunch | 3/4 cup | 130 | 3 | 30 | 0.5 | 0 | 0 | 220 | 25 | 1 | 1 | 1 1/2 starch, 1 fat |
| Cinnamon Toast Crunch, Reduced Sugar | 3/4 cup | 110 | 2.5 | 20 | 0 | 0 | 0 | 170 | 23 | 3 | 2 | 1 1/2 starch, 1 fat |
| Cocoa Puffs | 1 cup | 110 | 1.5 | 10 | 0 | 0 | 0 | 150 | 23 | 1 | 1 | 1 1/2 starch |
| Cookie Crisp | 1 cup | 100 | 1 | 10 | 0 | 0 | 0 | 150 | 22 | 1 | 1 | 1 1/2 starch |
| Cookie Crisp, Sprinkles | 3/4 cup | 100 | 1 | 10 | 0 | 0 | 0 | 150 | 23 | 1 | 1 | 1 1/2 starch |
| Count Chocula | 3/4 cup | 110 | 1 | 10 | 0 | 0 | 0 | 160 | 23 | 1 | 1 | 1 1/2 starch |
| Country Corn Flakes | 1 cup | 120 | 0.5 | 5 | 0 | 0 | 0 | 300 | 28 | 1 | 2 | 2 starch |
| Dora the Explorer | 3/4 cup | 100 | 1.5 | 15 | 0 | 0 | 0 | 180 | 23 | 3 | 1 | 1 1/2 starch |
| Fiber One | 1/2 cup | 60 | 1 | 10 | 0 | 0 | 0 | 105 | 25 | 14 | 2 | 1 1/2 starch |

## BREAKFAST CEREAL, READY-TO-EAT CEREAL, HOT CEREAL

| | Serving | Calories | Fat (g) | Cal. from Fat | Sat. Fat (g) | Trans Fat (g) | Chol. (mg) | Sod. (mg) | Carb. (g) | Fiber (g) | Prot. (g) | Servings/Exchanges |
|---|---|---|---|---|---|---|---|---|---|---|---|---|
| Fiber One, Caramel Delight | 1 cup | 180 | 3 | 25 | 0 | 0 | 0 | 260 | 41 | 9 | 3 | 2 1/2 starch, 1 fat |
| Fiber One, Frosted Shredded Wheat | 1 cup | 200 | 1 | 10 | 0 | 0 | 0 | 0 | 50 | 9 | 5 | 3 starch |
| Fiber One, Honey Clusters | 1 cup | 160 | 1.5 | 15 | 0 | 0 | 0 | 290 | 42 | 13 | 5 | 3 starch |
| Fiber One, Raisin Bran Clusters | 1 cup | 170 | 1 | 10 | 0 | 0 | 0 | 260 | 45 | 11 | 4 | 3 starch |
| Frankenberry | 1 cup | 130 | 1.5 | 10 | 0 | 0 | 0 | 190 | 28 | 1 | 1 | 2 starch |
| Golden Grahams | 3/4 cup | 120 | 1 | 10 | 0 | 0 | 0 | 270 | 26 | 1 | 2 | 2 starch |
| Honey Kix | 1 1/4 cup | 120 | 1 | 10 | 0 | 0 | 0 | 230 | 28 | 3 | 2 | 2 starch |
| Honey Nut Clusters | 1 cup | 210 | 1 | 10 | 0 | 0 | 0 | 290 | 49 | 3 | 4 | 3 starch |
| Kaboom | 1 1/4 cup | 110 | 1 | 10 | 0 | 0 | 0 | 210 | 28 | 4 | 1 | 2 starch |
| Kix | 1 1/4 cup | 110 | 1 | 5 | 0 | 0 | 0 | 210 | 26 | 3 | 2 | 1 1/2 starch |

| | | | | | | | | | | | | |
|---|---|---|---|---|---|---|---|---|---|---|---|---|
| Kix, Berry Berry | 3/4 cup | 100 | 1 | 10 | 0 | 0 | 0 | 180 | 22 | 1 | 1 | 1 1/2 starch |
| Lucky Charms | 1 cup | 110 | 1 | 10 | 0 | 0 | 0 | 190 | 22 | 1 | 2 | 1 1/2 starch |
| Lucky Charms, Chocolate | 1 cup | 110 | 1 | 10 | 0 | 0 | 0 | 160 | 24 | 1 | 1 | 1 1/2 starch |
| Oatmeal Crisp, Almond | 1 cup | 240 | 5 | 45 | 0 | 0 | 0 | 250 | 47 | 4 | 5 | 3 starch, 1 fat |
| Oatmeal Crisp, HeartyRaisin | 1 cup | 230 | 2.5 | 20 | 0.5 | 0 | 0 | 135 | 51 | 4 | 5 | 3 1/2 starch, 1 fat |
| Para Su Familia Raisin Bran | 1 1/4 cup | 170 | 1 | 10 | 0 | 0 | 0 | 300 | 41 | 6 | 4 | 2 1/2 starch |
| Raisin Nut Bran | 3/4 cup | 180 | 3 | 30 | 0.5 | 0 | 0 | 230 | 38 | 5 | 4 | 2 1/2 starch, 1 fat |
| Reese's Puffs | 3/4 cup | 120 | 3 | 30 | 0.5 | 0 | 0 | 180 | 22 | 1 | 2 | 1 1/2 starch, 1 fat |
| Total Blueberry Pomegranate | 1 cup | 170 | 2 | 15 | 0 | 0 | 0 | 95 | 38 | 4 | 5 | 2 1/2 starch |
| Total Cinnamon Crunch | 1 cup | 190 | 2.5 | 25 | 0 | 0 | 0 | 200 | 40 | 4 | 4 | 2 1/2 starch, 1 fat |
| Total Cranberry Crunch | 1 1/4 cup | 190 | 1.5 | 15 | 0 | 0 | 0 | 230 | 44 | 4 | 4 | 3 starch |
| Total Raisin Bran | 1 cup | 160 | 1 | 5 | 0 | 0 | 0 | 230 | 40 | 5 | 3 | 2 1/2 starch |

BREAKFAST CEREAL, READY-TO-EAT CEREAL, HOT CEREAL

| | Serving | Calories | Fat (g) | Cal. from Fat | Sat. Fat (g) | Trans Fat (g) | Chol. (mg) | Sod. (mg) | Carb. (g) | Fiber (g) | Prot. (g) | Servings/Exchanges |
|---|---|---|---|---|---|---|---|---|---|---|---|---|
| Total Whole-Grain | 3/4 cup | 100 | 0.5 | 5 | 0 | 0 | 0 | 190 | 23 | 3 | 2 | 1 1/2 starch |
| Trix | 1 cup | 120 | 1 | 10 | 0 | 0 | 0 | 190 | 28 | 1 | 1 | 2 starch |
| Wheaties | 3/4 cup | 100 | 0.5 | 5 | 0 | 0 | 0 | 190 | 22 | 3 | 3 | 1 1/2 starch |
| ***Health Valley Organic*** | | | | | | | | | | | | |
| Cranberry Crunch | 3/4 cup | 190 | 4 | 35 | 0 | 0 | 0 | 100 | 38 | 3 | 4 | 2 1/2 starch, 1 fat |
| Heart Wise | 1 cup | 200 | 3 | 25 | 0 | 0 | 0 | 140 | 37 | 5 | 11 | 2 1/2 starch, 1 fat |
| Low Fat Date Almond Flavor Granola | 2/3 cup | 180 | 1 | 10 | 0 | 0 | 0 | 90 | 43 | 6 | 5 | 3 starch |
| Low Fat Raisin Cinnamon Fruit Granola | 2/3 cup | 180 | 1 | 10 | 0 | 0 | 0 | 90 | 43 | 6 | 5 | 3 starch |
| Organic Amaranth Flakes | 1 cup | 100 | 1 | 10 | 0 | 0 | 0 | 90 | 23 | 3 | 3 | 1 1/2 starch |
| Organic Blue Corn Flakes | 3/4 cup | 100 | 0 | 0 | 0 | 0 | 0 | 10 | 24 | 3 | 3 | 1 1/2 starch |

| | | | | | | | | | | | | |
|---|---|---|---|---|---|---|---|---|---|---|---|---|
| Organic Chocolate Blast-Ems | 3/4 cup | 120 | 1.5 | 15 | 0 | 0 | 0 | 90 | 25 | 3 | 3 | 1 1/2 starch |
| Organic Fiber 7 | 1 cup | 160 | 1 | 10 | 0 | 0 | 0 | 100 | 37 | 7 | 6 | 2 1/2 starch |
| Organic Golden Flax Cereal | 1 cup | 180 | 3.5 | 30 | 0 | 0 | 0 | 65 | 37 | 6 | 6 | 2 1/2 starch, 1 fat |
| Organic Multi-Grain Apple Cinnamon Square-Ems | 1 1/4 cup | 210 | 3 | 30 | 0 | 0 | 0 | 125 | 44 | 8 | 5 | 3 starch, 1 fat |
| Organic Oat Bran Flakes | 1 cup | 190 | 1.5 | 15 | 0.5 | 0 | 0 | 190 | 39 | 4 | 5 | 2 1/2 starch |
| ***Kashi*** | | | | | | | | | | | | |
| 7 Grain Puffs | 1 cup | 70 | 0.5 | 5 | 0 | 0 | 0 | 0 | 15 | 1 | 2 | 1 starch |
| 7 Whole Grain Flakes | 1 cup | 180 | 1 | 10 | 0 | 0 | 0 | 150 | 41 | 6 | 6 | 2 1/2 starch |
| Cinnamon Harvest | 1 cup | 190 | 1 | 10 | 0 | 0 | 0 | 0 | 44 | 5 | 4 | 3 starch |
| GoLean | 1 cup | 140 | 1 | 10 | 0 | 0 | 0 | 85 | 30 | 10 | 13 | 2 starch |
| GoLean Crunch | 1 cup | 190 | 3 | 25 | 0 | 0 | 0 | 100 | 37 | 8 | 9 | 2 1/2 starch, 1 fat |
| GoLean Crunch Honey Almond Flax | 1 cup | 200 | 4.5 | 40 | 0 | 0 | 0 | 140 | 36 | 8 | 9 | 2 1/2 starch, 1 fat |

BREAKFAST CEREAL, READY-TO-EAT CEREAL, HOT CEREAL

| | Serving | Calories | Fat (g) | Cal. from Fat | Sat. Fat (g) | Trans Fat (g) | Chol. (mg) | Sod. (mg) | Carb. (g) | Fiber (g) | Prot. (g) | Servings/Exchanges |
|---|---|---|---|---|---|---|---|---|---|---|---|---|
| Good Friends | 1 cup | 160 | 1.5 | 15 | 0 | 0 | 0 | 110 | 42 | 12 | 5 | 3 starch |
| Good Friends Cinna-Raisin Crunch | 1 cup | 170 | 1.5 | 15 | 0 | 0 | 0 | 105 | 41 | 8 | 4 | 3 starch |
| Heart to Heart Honey Toasted | 3/4 cup | 110 | 1.5 | 15 | 0 | 0 | 0 | 90 | 25 | 5 | 4 | 1 1/2 starch |
| Heart to Heart Oat Flakes & Wild Blueberry Clusters | 1 cup | 200 | 2 | 15 | 0 | 0 | 0 | 135 | 44 | 4 | 6 | 3 starch |
| Heart to Heart Warm Cinnamon | 3/4 cup | 110 | 1.5 | 15 | 0 | 0 | 0 | 80 | 24 | 5 | 4 | 1 1/2 starch |
| Honey Sunshine | 3/4 cup | 100 | 1.5 | 10 | 0 | 0 | 0 | 135 | 25 | 6 | 2 | 1 1/2 starch |
| Island Vanilla | 27 biscuits | 180 | 1 | 5 | 0 | 0 | 0 | 0 | 44 | 6 | 6 | 3 starch |
| Organic Promise Autumn Wheat | 29 biscuits | 180 | 1 | 10 | 0 | 0 | 0 | 0 | 43 | 6 | 6 | 3 starch |

| | | | | | | | | | | | | |
|---|---|---|---|---|---|---|---|---|---|---|---|---|
| Organic Promise Strawberry Fields | 1 cup | 120 | 0 | 0 | 0 | 0 | 0 | 200 | 28 | 1 | 2 | 2 starch |
| Vive Toasted Graham & Vanilla | 1 1/4 cup | 170 | 2.5 | 25 | 1 | 0 | 0 | 100 | 43 | 12 | 4 | 3 starch, 2 fat |
| ***Kellogg's*** | | | | | | | | | | | | |
| All-Bran | 1/2 cup | 80 | 1 | 10 | 0 | 0 | 0 | 80 | 23 | 10 | 4 | 1 1/2 starch |
| All-Bran Bran Buds | 1/3 cup | 70 | 1 | 10 | 0 | 0 | 0 | 200 | 24 | 13 | 2 | 1 1/2 starch |
| All-Bran Complete Wheat Flakes | 3/4 cup | 90 | 0.5 | 5 | 0 | 0 | 0 | 210 | 23 | 5 | 3 | 1 1/2 starch |
| All-Bran Yogurt Bites | 1 1/4 cup | 190 | 3 | 30 | 0 | 0 | 0 | 240 | 44 | 10 | 6 | 3 starch, 1 fat |
| Apple Jacks | 1 cup | 100 | 0.5 | 5 | 0 | 0 | 0 | 130 | 25 | 3 | 1 | 1 1/2 starch |
| Cocoa Krispies | 3/4 cup | 120 | 1 | 10 | 0.5 | 0 | 0 | 150 | 27 | 1 | 1 | 2 starch |
| Corn Flakes | 1 cup | 100 | 0 | 0 | 0 | 0 | 0 | 200 | 24 | 1 | 2 | 1 1/2 starch |
| Corn Flakes Touch of Honey | 1 cup | 120 | 0 | 0 | 0 | 0 | 0 | 220 | 27 | <1 | 2 | 2 starch |
| Corn Pops | 110 | 120 | 0 | 0 | 0 | 0 | 0 | 110 | 26 | 0 | 1 | 2 starch |

BREAKFAST CEREAL, READY-TO-EAT CEREAL, HOT CEREAL

| | Serving | Calories | Fat (g) | Cal. from Fat | Sat. Fat (g) | Trans Fat (g) | Chol. (mg) | Sod. (mg) | Carb. (g) | Fiber (g) | Prot. (g) | Servings/Exchanges |
|---|---|---|---|---|---|---|---|---|---|---|---|---|
| Cracklin' Oat Bran | 3/4 cup | 200 | 7 | 60 | 3 | 0 | 0 | 150 | 35 | 6 | 4 | 2 starch, 1 fat |
| Crispix | 1 cup | 110 | 0 | 0 | 0 | 0 | 0 | 220 | 25 | <1 | 2 | 2 starch |
| Eggo Cinnamon Toast | 1 cup | 130 | 3 | 30 | 0 | 0 | 0 | 130 | 26 | 2 | 2 | 2 starch, 1 fat |
| Froot Loops | 1 cup | 110 | 1 | 10 | 0.5 | 0 | 0 | 135 | 25 | 3 | 1 | 1 1/2 starch |
| Frosted Flakes | 3/4 cup | 110 | 0 | 0 | 0 | 0 | 0 | 140 | 27 | 1 | 1 | 2 starch |
| Frosted Flakes, 1/3 Less Sugar | 1 cup | 120 | 0 | 0 | 0 | 0 | 0 | 180 | 28 | <1 | 1 | 2 starch |
| Frosted Mini-Wheats Little Bites Chocolate | 52 biscuits | 200 | 2 | 15 | 1 | 0 | 0 | 200 | 45 | 6 | 5 | 3 starch |
| Frosted Mini-Wheats Little Bites Honey Nut | 46 biscuits | 190 | 1 | 10 | 0 | 0 | 0 | 120 | 47 | 6 | 5 | 3 starch |
| Frosted Mini-Wheats Strawberry Delight | 24 biscuits | 180 | 1 | 10 | 0 | 0 | 0 | 0 | 43 | 5 | 4 | 3 starch |
| Honey Smacks | 3/4 cup | 100 | 0.5 | 5 | 0 | 0 | 0 | 50 | 24 | 1 | 2 | 1 1/2 starch |

| | | | | | | | | | | | | |
|---|---|---|---|---|---|---|---|---|---|---|---|---|
| Keebler Cookie Crunch | 1 cup | 110 | 1 | 10 | 0 | 0 | 0 | 170 | 26 | 1 | 2 | 2 starch |
| Mini-Wheats, Big Bite | 5 biscuits | 180 | 1 | 10 | 0 | 0 | 0 | 5 | 41 | 5 | 5 | 3 starch |
| Mini-Wheats, Blueberry | 24 biscuits | 180 | 1 | 10 | 0 | 0 | 0 | 0 | 43 | 5 | 4 | 3 starch |
| Mini-Wheats, Frosted Bite Size | 24 biscuits | 200 | 1 | 10 | 0 | 0 | 0 | 5 | 48 | 6 | 6 | 3 starch |
| Mini-Wheats, Frosted Maple & Brown Sugar | 24 biscuits | 190 | 1 | 10 | 0 | 0 | 0 | 0 | 44 | 5 | 4 | 3 starch |
| Product 19 | 1 cup | 100 | 0 | 0 | 0 | 0 | 0 | 210 | 25 | 1 | 2 | 1 1/2 starch |
| Raisin Bran | 1 cup | 190 | 1.5 | 15 | 0 | 0 | 0 | 350 | 45 | 7 | 5 | 3 starch |
| Raisin Bran Crunch | 1 cup | 190 | 1 | 9 | 0 | 0 | 0 | 210 | 45 | 4 | 3 | 3 starch |
| Raisin Bran Extra | 1 cup | 190 | 3 | 25 | 1.5 | 0 | 0 | 350 | 44 | 7 | 5 | 3 starch |
| Rice Krispies | 1 1/4 cup | 130 | 0 | 0 | 0 | 0 | 0 | 220 | 29 | <1 | 2 | 2 starch |
| Smart Start Original | 1 cup | 190 | 0.5 | 5 | 0 | 0 | 0 | 280 | 43 | 3 | 3 | 3 starch |
| Smart Start Strong Heart Strawberry Bites | 30 biscuits | 200 | 2.5 | 20 | 0.5 | 0 | 0 | 130 | 43 | 6 | 6 | 3 starch, 1 fat |

BREAKFAST CEREAL, READY-TO-EAT CEREAL, HOT CEREAL

| | Serving | Calories | Fat (g) | Cal. from Fat | Sat. Fat (g) | Trans Fat (g) | Chol. (mg) | Sod. (mg) | Carb. (g) | Fiber (g) | Prot. (g) | Servings/Exchanges |
|---|---|---|---|---|---|---|---|---|---|---|---|---|
| Smart Start Toasted Oat | 1 1/4 cup | 220 | 2.5 | 20 | 0.5 | 0 | 0 | 140 | 48 | 5 | 6 | 3 starch, 1 fat |
| Special K | 1 cup | 120 | 0.5 | 5 | 0 | 0 | 0 | 220 | 23 | 1 | 6 | 1 1/2 starch |
| Special K Chocolatey Delight | 3/4 cup | 120 | 2 | 20 | 2 | 0 | 0 | 180 | 25 | 1 | 2 | 1 1/2 starch |
| Special K Fruit & Yogurt | 3/4 cup | 120 | 1 | 10 | 0.5 | 0 | 0 | 135 | 27 | 1 | 2 | 2 starch |
| Special K Red Berries | 1 cup | 120 | 0 | 0 | 0 | 0 | 0 | 220 | 25 | 1 | 3 | 1 1/2 starch |
| Special K Vanilla Almond | 1 cup | 110 | 1.5 | 15 | 0 | 0 | 0 | 160 | 25 | 1 | 2 | 1 1/2 starch |
| ***Malt-O-Meal*** | | | | | | | | | | | | |
| Apple Zings | 1 cup | 130 | 1 | 5 | 0 | 0 | 0 | 150 | 30 | 1 | 1 | 2 starch |
| Berry Colossal Crunch | 3/4 cup | 120 | 1.5 | 15 | 0 | 0 | 0 | 230 | 26 | 0 | 1 | 2 starch |
| Blueberry Muffin Tops | 3/4 cup | 130 | 3.5 | 30 | 0.5 | 0 | 0 | 140 | 24 | 1 | 1 | 1 1/2 starch, 1 fat |
| Cinnamon Toasters | 3/4 cup | 130 | 3.5 | 30 | 0.5 | 0 | 0 | 140 | 24 | 1 | 1 | 1 1/2 starch, 1 fat |
| Cocoa Roos | 3/4 cup | 120 | 1.5 | 15 | 0 | 0 | 0 | 135 | 26 | <1 | 1 | 2 starch |

| | | | | | | | | | | | | |
|---|---|---|---|---|---|---|---|---|---|---|---|---|
| Creamy Hot Wheat | 3 Tbsp | 130 | 0 | 0 | 0 | 0 | 0 | 0 | 27 | 1 | 4 | 2 starch |
| Crispy Rice | 1 1/4 cup | 130 | 0 | 0 | 0 | 0 | 0 | 300 | 26 | 0 | 2 | 2 starch |
| Dyno Bites | 3/4 cup | 120 | 1 | 10 | 0 | 0 | 0 | 150 | 26 | 0 | 1 | 2 starch |
| Frosted Flakes | 3/4 cup | 120 | 0 | 0 | 0 | 0 | 0 | 180 | 28 | 1 | 1 | 2 starch |
| Frosted Mini Spooners | 1 cup | 190 | 1 | 10 | 0 | 0 | 0 | 10 | 45 | 6 | 5 | 3 starch |
| Golden Puffs | 3/4 cup | 110 | 0 | 0 | 0 | 0 | 0 | 65 | 24 | 0 | 2 | 2 starch |
| Honey & Oat Blenders | 3/4 cup | 120 | 1.5 | 15 | 0 | 0 | 0 | 150 | 25 | 1 | 2 | 1 1/2 starch |
| Honey Buzzers | 1 1/3 cup | 110 | 0.5 | 5 | 0 | 0 | 0 | 220 | 26 | 1 | 1 | 2 starch |
| Honey Graham Squares | 3/4 cup | 130 | 3 | 25 | 0.5 | 0 | 0 | 270 | 25 | 1 | 1 | 1 1/2 starch, 1 fat |
| Honey Nut Scooters | 1 cup | 110 | 1.5 | 10 | 0 | 0 | 0 | 210 | 24 | 2 | 2 | 1 1/2 starch |
| Hot Wheat Cereal, Chocolate | 3 Tbsp dry | 130 | 0 | 0 | 0 | 0 | 0 | 0 | 27 | 1 | 4 | 2 starch |
| Hot Wheat Cereal, Maple & Brown Sugar | 1/4 cup dry | 170 | 0 | 0 | 0 | 0 | 0 | 0 | 37 | 1 | 4 | 2 1/2 starch |
| Hot Wheat Cereal, Quick Original | 3 Tbsp dry | 130 | 0.5 | 5 | 0 | 0 | 0 | 0 | 27 | 1 | 5 | 2 starch |

BREAKFAST CEREAL, READY-TO-EAT CEREAL, HOT CEREAL

| | Serving | Calories | Fat (g) | Cal. from Fat | Sat. Fat (g) | Trans Fat (g) | Chol. (mg) | Sod. (mg) | Carb. (g) | Fiber (g) | Prot. (g) | Servings/Exchanges |
|---|---|---|---|---|---|---|---|---|---|---|---|---|
| Marshmallow Mateys | 1 cup | 120 | 1 | 10 | 0 | 0 | 0 | 200 | 25 | 1 | 2 | 1 1/2 starch |
| Raisin Bran | 1 cup | 220 | 1.5 | 10 | 0 | 0 | 0 | 340 | 49 | 6 | 5 | 3 starch |
| Tootie Fruities | 1 cup | 130 | 1 | 10 | 0 | 0 | 0 | 150 | 28 | 1 | 2 | 2 starch |
| ***Nature's Path Organic*** | | | | | | | | | | | | |
| Organic Flax Plus Multibran | 3/4 cup | 110 | 1.5 | 15 | 0 | 0 | 0 | 135 | 23 | 5 | 4 | 1 1/2 starch |
| Organic Flax Plus Raisin Bran | 3/4 cup | 190 | 2.5 | 20 | 0 | 0 | 0 | 190 | 41 | 8 | 6 | 2 1/2 starch, 1 fat |
| Organic Hemp Plus Granola | 3/4 cup | 260 | 10 | 90 | 1.5 | 0 | 0 | 35 | 36 | 5 | 6 | 2 1/2 starch, 2 fat |
| Organic Heritage Heirloom Whole Grains | 3/4 cup | 120 | 1 | 10 | 0 | 0 | 0 | 130 | 24 | 5 | 4 | 1 1/2 starch |
| Organic Optimum Blueberry Cinnamon | 1 cup | 200 | 3 | 25 | 0 | 0 | 0 | 230 | 38 | 7 | 9 | 2 1/2 starch, 1 fat |

| | | | | | | | | | | | | |
|---|---|---|---|---|---|---|---|---|---|---|---|---|
| Organic Pumpkin Flax Plus Granola | 3/4 cup | 260 | 10 | 90 | 1.5 | 0 | 0 | 45 | 37 | 5 | 6 | 2 1/2 starch, 2 fat |
| ***Post*** | | | | | | | | | | | | |
| Alpha-Bits | 1 cup | 110 | 1 | 10 | 0 | 0 | 0 | 160 | 23 | 2 | 2 | 1 1/2 starch |
| Banana Nut Crunch | 1 cup | 240 | 6 | 50 | 0.5 | 0 | 0 | 230 | 44 | 4 | 5 | 3 starch, 1 fat |
| Blueberry Morning | 1 1/4 cup | 220 | 3 | 30 | 0 | 0 | 0 | 280 | 45 | 2 | 3 | 3 starch, 1 fat |
| Bran Flakes | 3/4 cup | 100 | 0.5 | 5 | 0 | 0 | 0 | 220 | 24 | 5 | 3 | 1 1/2 starch |
| Cocoa Pebbles | 3/4 cup | 110 | 1.5 | 10 | 1 | 0 | 0 | 180 | 26 | 3 | 1 | 2 starch |
| Cranberry Almond Crunch | 3/4 cup | 200 | 2.5 | 35 | 0 | 0 | 0 | 115 | 39 | 3 | 4 | 2 1/2 starch, 1 fat |
| Fruity Pebbles | 3/4 cup | 110 | 1 | 10 | 1 | 0 | 0 | 180 | 26 | 3 | 1 | 2 starch |
| Golden Crisp | 3/4 cup | 110 | 0 | 0 | 0 | 0 | 0 | 25 | 24 | <1 | 2 | 1 1/2 starch |
| Grape Nuts | 1/2 cup | 200 | 1 | 10 | 0 | 0 | 0 | 290 | 48 | 7 | 6 | 3 starch |
| Grape Nuts Flakes | 3/4 cup | 110 | 1 | 10 | 0 | 0 | 0 | 110 | 24 | 3 | 3 | 1 1/2 starch |
| Great Grains, Crunchy Pecan | 1/2 cup | 220 | 6 | 60 | 0.5 | 0 | 0 | 150 | 38 | 4 | 5 | 2 1/2 starch, 1 fat |

BREAKFAST CEREAL, READY-TO-EAT CEREAL, HOT CEREAL

| | Serving | Calories | Fat (g) | Cal. from Fat | Sat. Fat (g) | Trans Fat (g) | Chol. (mg) | Sod. (mg) | Carb. (g) | Fiber (g) | Prot. (g) | Servings/Exchanges |
|---|---|---|---|---|---|---|---|---|---|---|---|---|
| Great Grains, Raisin/ Date/Pecan | 1/2 cup | 210 | 4.5 | 40 | 0 | 0 | 0 | 130 | 40 | 4 | 4 | 2 1/2 starch, 1 fat |
| Honey Bunches of Oats, Honey Roasted | 3/4 cup | 120 | 1.5 | 15 | 0 | 0 | 0 | 150 | 25 | 2 | 2 | 1 1/2 starch |
| Honeycombs | 1 1/3 cup | 120 | 1.5 | 10 | 0 | 0 | 0 | 180 | 27 | 2 | 2 | 2 starch |
| Raisin Bran | 1 cup | 190 | 1 | 10 | 0 | 0 | 0 | 300 | 46 | 8 | 4 | 3 starch |
| Shredded Wheat | 2 biscuits | 160 | 1 | 10 | 0 | 0 | 0 | 0 | 40 | 6 | 5 | 2 1/2 starch |
| Shredded Wheat 'n Bran | 1 1/4 cup | 200 | 1 | 10 | 0 | 0 | 0 | 0 | 49 | 8 | 6 | 3 starch |
| Shredded Wheat, Frosted | 1 cup | 180 | 1 | 10 | 0 | 0 | 0 | 0 | 43 | 5 | 4 | 3 starch |
| Shredded Wheat, Honey Nut | 1 cup | 190 | 1.5 | 15 | 0 | 0 | 0 | 70 | 44 | 5 | 4 | 3 starch |
| ***Quaker*** | | | | | | | | | | | | |
| High Fiber Oatmeal Cinnamon Swirl | 1 pkt | 160 | 2 | 20 | 0.5 | 0 | 0 | 210 | 34 | 10 | 4 | 2 starch |

| | | | | | | | | | | | | |
|---|---|---|---|---|---|---|---|---|---|---|---|---|
| Instant Hot Oatmeal | 1 pkt | 100 | 2 | 20 | 0 | 0 | 0 | 80 | 19 | 3 | 4 | 1 starch |
| Instant Hot Oatmeal Express, Baked Apple | 1 cup | 200 | 2.5 | 25 | 0.5 | 0 | 0 | 250 | 41 | 4 | 5 | 2 1/2 starch, 1 fat |
| Instant Hot Oatmeal Express, Cinnamon | 1 cup | 200 | 2.5 | 25 | 0.5 | 0 | 0 | 250 | 41 | 4 | 5 | 2 1/2 starch, 1 fat |
| Instant Hot Oatmeal, Apple & Cinnamon | 1 pkt | 130 | 1.5 | 15 | 0.5 | 0 | 0 | 170 | 27 | 3 | 3 | 2 starch |
| Instant Hot Oatmeal, Apple & Cinnamon, Lower Sugar | 1 pkt | 110 | 1.5 | 15 | 0.5 | 0 | 0 | 170 | 22 | 3 | 3 | 1 1/2 starch |
| Instant Hot Oatmeal, Cinnamon Roll | 1 pkt | 160 | 2 | 20 | 0.5 | 0 | 0 | 240 | 33 | 3 | 4 | 2 starch |
| Instant Hot Oatmeal, Cinnamon Spice | 1 pkt | 170 | 2 | 20 | 0.5 | 0 | 0 | 250 | 35 | 3 | 4 | 2 starch |
| Instant Hot Oatmeal, Maple & Brown Sugar | 1 pkt | 160 | 2 | 20 | 0 | 0 | 0 | 270 | 33 | 3 | 4 | 2 starch |

BREAKFAST CEREAL, READY-TO-EAT CEREAL, HOT CEREAL

| | Serving | Calories | Fat (g) | Cal. from Fat | Sat. Fat (g) | Trans Fat (g) | Chol. (mg) | Sod. (mg) | Carb. (g) | Fiber (g) | Prot. (g) | Servings/Exchanges |
|---|---|---|---|---|---|---|---|---|---|---|---|---|
| Instant Hot Oatmeal, Maple & Brown Sugar, Low Sugar | 1 pkt | 120 | 2 | 20 | 0 | 0 | 0 | 290 | 24 | 3 | 4 | 1 1/2 starch |
| Instant Hot Oatmeal, Peaches & Cream | 1 pkt | 130 | 2 | 20 | 0.5 | 0 | 0 | 190 | 27 | 2 | 3 | 2 starch |
| Instant Hot Oatmeal, Raisin & Spice | 1 pkt | 150 | 2 | 20 | 0 | 0 | 0 | 240 | 33 | 3 | 3 | 2 starch |
| Instant Hot Oatmeal, Raisin/Date/Walnut | 1 pkt | 140 | 2.5 | 25 | 0 | 0 | 0 | 240 | 27 | 3 | 3 | 2 starch, 1 fat |
| Instant Hot Oatmeal, Strawberries & Cream | 1 pkt | 130 | 2 | 20 | 0.5 | 0 | 0 | 180 | 27 | 2 | 3 | 2 starch |
| Life | 3/4 cup | 120 | 1.5 | 15 | 0 | 0 | 0 | 160 | 25 | 2 | 3 | 1 1/2 starch |
| Life, Cinnamon | 3/4 cup | 120 | 1.5 | 15 | 0 | 0 | 0 | 150 | 25 | 2 | 3 | 1 1/2 starch |
| Life, Maple & Brown Sugar | 3/4 cup | 120 | 1.5 | 15 | 0 | 0 | 0 | 150 | 25 | 2 | 3 | 1 1/2 starch |

| | | | | | | | | | | | | |
|---|---|---|---|---|---|---|---|---|---|---|---|---|
| Natural Granola Oats, Honey & Raisins | 1/2 cup | 210 | 6 | 50 | 3.5 | 0 | 0 | 25 | 38 | 3 | 5 | 2 1/2 starch, 1 fat |
| Natural Granola, Lowfat | 2/3 cup | 210 | 3 | 25 | 1.5 | 0 | 0 | 135 | 45 | 3 | 4 | 3 starch, 1 fat |
| Oat Bran | 1 1/4 cup | 210 | 3 | 25 | 0.5 | 0 | 0 | 210 | 43 | 6 | 7 | 3 starch |
| Old-Fashioned Hot Oats | 1/2 cup | 150 | 3 | 25 | 0.5 | 0 | 0 | 0 | 27 | 4 | 5 | 2 starch, 1 fat |
| Quick Hot Oats | 1/2 cup | 150 | 3 | 25 | 0.5 | 0 | 0 | 0 | 27 | 4 | 5 | 2 starch |
| Simple Harvest Apples & Cinnamon (Hot Cereal) | 1 pkt | 150 | 1.5 | 15 | 0 | 0 | 0 | 90 | 33 | 4 | 4 | 2 starch |
| Simple Harvest Maple Brown Sugar with Pecans (Hot Cereal) | 1 pkt | 160 | 3.5 | 30 | 0 | 0 | 0 | 75 | 30 | 4 | 4 | 2 starch, 1 fat |
| Take Heart Instant Oatmeal Blueberry | 1 pkt | 160 | 2.5 | 25 | 0.5 | 0 | 0 | 105 | 33 | 6 | 4 | 2 starch, 1 fat |
| Take Heart Instant Golden Maple | 1 pkt | 160 | 2.5 | 25 | 0.5 | 0 | 0 | 110 | 33 | 5 | 4 | 2 starch, 1 fat |

BREAKFAST CEREAL, READY-TO-EAT CEREAL, HOT CEREAL

| | Serving | Calories | Fat (g) | Cal. from Fat | Sat. Fat (g) | Trans Fat (g) | Chol. (mg) | Sod. (mg) | Carb. (g) | Fiber (g) | Prot. (g) | Servings/Exchanges |
|---|---|---|---|---|---|---|---|---|---|---|---|---|
| Toasted Oatmeal Squares, Brown Sugar | 1 cup | 210 | 2.5 | 25 | 0.5 | 0 | 0 | 250 | 44 | 5 | 6 | 3 starch, 1 fat |
| Toasted Oatmeal Squares, Cinnamon | 1 cup | 230 | 2.5 | 25 | 0.5 | 0 | 0 | 260 | 47 | 5 | 6 | 3 starch, 1 fat |
| Weight Control Instant Oatmeal Banana Bread | 1 pkt | 160 | 3 | 25 | 0.5 | 0 | 0 | 260 | 29 | 6 | 7 | 2 starch, 1 fat |
| Weight Control Instant Oatmeal Maple & Brown Sugar | 1 pkt | 160 | 3 | 25 | 0.5 | 0 | 0 | 310 | 29 | 6 | 7 | 2 starch, 1 fat |
| ***Trader Joe's*** | | | | | | | | | | | | |
| Apple & Cinnamon Instant Oatmeal | 1 pouch | 130 | 1.5 | 15 | 0 | 0 | 0 | 170 | 27 | 3 | 3 | 2 starch |
| Banana Nut Clusters | 1 cup | 240 | 8 | 70 | 0.5 | 0 | 0 | 140 | 40 | 2 | 4 | 2 1/2 starch, 2 fat |

| | | | | | | | | | | | | |
|---|---|---|---|---|---|---|---|---|---|---|---|---|
| Gluten Free Granola Loaded Fruit & Nut | 3/4 cup | 270 | 13 | 120 | 2 | 0 | 0 | 45 | 34 | 3 | 4 | 2 starch, 3 fat |
| Gourmet Flakes & Chocolate | 1 1/4 cup | 230 | 4.5 | 40 | 2.5 | 0 | 0 | 290 | 43 | 3 | 4 | 3 starch, 1 fat |
| High Fiber Cereal | 2/3 cup | 80 | 0.5 | 5 | 0 | 0 | 0 | 70 | 23 | 9 | 3 | 1 1/2 starch |
| High Fiber Fruit & Nut Medley | 2/3 cup | 90 | 1.5 | 15 | 0 | 0 | 0 | 55 | 25 | 7 | 2 | 1 1/2 starch |
| Honey Almond & Flax 9 Grain Crunch | 1 cup | 190 | 5 | 45 | 0 | 0 | 0 | 125 | 33 | 8 | 10 | 2 starch, 1 fat |
| Honey Nut O's | 3/4 cup | 120 | 1.5 | 15 | 0 | 0 | 0 | 200 | 24 | 2 | 2 | 1 1/2 starch |
| Joe's O's | 1 cup | 110 | 1.5 | 15 | 0 | 0 | 0 | 280 | 22 | 3 | 3 | 1 1/2 starch |
| Just The Clusters Maple Pecan Granola | 2/3 cup | 250 | 10 | 90 | 1 | 0 | 0 | 70 | 38 | 3 | 5 | 2 1/2 starch, 2 fat |
| Lowfat Granola Mixed Berry | 3/4 cup | 210 | 2.5 | 20 | 0 | 0 | 0 | 75 | 45 | 5 | 4 | 3 starch, 1 fat |
| Lowfat Granola with Almonds | 3/4 cup | 210 | 3 | 25 | 0 | 0 | 0 | 75 | 44 | 5 | 4 | 3 starch, 1 fat |

BREAKFAST CEREAL, READY-TO-EAT CEREAL, HOT CEREAL

| | Serving | Calories | Fat (g) | Cal. from Fat | Sat. Fat (g) | Trans Fat (g) | Chol. (mg) | Sod. (mg) | Carb. (g) | Fiber (g) | Prot. (g) | Servings/Exchanges |
|---|---|---|---|---|---|---|---|---|---|---|---|---|
| Oat 'n Wheat Bran Swirls | 1/2 cup | 200 | 7 | 60 | 0 | 0 | 0 | 135 | 34 | 4 | 4 | 2 starch, 1 fat |
| Organic Cinnamon Spice Instant Oatmeal | 1 pkt | 150 | 1.5 | 15 | 0 | 0 | 0 | 90 | 30 | 2.5 | 4 | 2 starch |
| Organic Corn Flakes | 1 cup | 110 | 0 | 0 | 0 | 0 | 0 | 280 | 26 | <1 | 2 | 2 starch |
| Organic Golden Flax | 3/4 cup | 200 | 3.5 | 30 | 0.5 | 0 | 0 | 65 | 37 | 6 | 6 | 2 1/2 starch, 1 fat |
| Organic Granny's Apple Granola | 2/3 cup | 210 | 7 | 60 | 0.5 | 0 | 0 | 45 | 31 | 4 | 5 | 2 starch, 1 fat |
| Organic High Fiber O's | 1 1/4 cup | 190 | 1 | 10 | 0 | 0 | 0 | 115 | 44 | 9 | 6 | 3 starch |
| Organic Honey Crunch 'n Oats | 3/4 cup | 120 | 1 | 10 | 0 | 0 | 0 | 135 | 25 | 2 | 2 | 1 1/2 starch |
| Organic Morning Lite | 1 cup | 170 | 2.5 | 25 | 0 | 0 | 0 | 70 | 40 | 10 | 3 | 2 1/2 starch, 1 fat |
| Organic Oats & Flax | 1 pkt | 150 | 2 | 25 | 0 | 0 | 0 | 130 | 29 | 3 | 4 | 2 starch |
| Organic Raisin Bran | 1 cup | 170 | 1 | 10 | 0 | 0 | 0 | 120 | 44 | 8 | 4 | 3 starch |

| | | | | | | | | | | | | |
|---|---|---|---|---|---|---|---|---|---|---|---|---|
| Organic Raisin Bran Clusters | 1 cup | 190 | 3 | 25 | 0 | 0 | 0 | 150 | 40 | 7 | 6 | 2 1/2 starch, 1 fat |
| Pomegranate Blueberry Flakes & Clusters | 1 cup | 210 | 2 | 20 | 0 | 0 | 0 | 110 | 46 | 4 | 4 | 3 starch |
| Quick Cook Steel Cut Oats | 1/4 cup dry | 150 | 2.5 | 25 | 0.5 | 0 | 0 | 0 | 27 | 4 | 5 | 2 starch, 1 fat |
| Shredded Bite Size Wheats | 1 cup | 180 | 1 | 10 | 0 | 0 | 0 | 0 | 38 | 5 | 5 | 2 1/2 starch |
| Soy & Flax Clusters | 1 cup | 190 | 3 | 25 | 0 | 0 | 0 | 135 | 38 | 6 | 7 | 2 1/2 starch, 1 fat |
| Strawberry Yogurt O's | 3/4 cup | 110 | 2.5 | 25 | 0 | 0 | 0 | 60 | 22 | 3 | 2 | 1 1/2 starch 1 fat |
| Super Nutty Toffee Clusters | 3/4 cup | 250 | 9 | 80 | 1.5 | 0 | 0 | 105 | 38 | 3 | 5 | 2 1/2 starch, 2 fat |
| Toasted Oatmeal Flakes | 3/4 cup | 110 | 1 | 10 | 0 | 0 | 0 | 190 | 23 | 3 | 3 | 1 1/2 starch |
| Triple Berry-O's | 3/4 cup | 110 | 1 | 10 | 0 | 0 | 0 | 180 | 25 | 3 | 2 | 1 1/2 starch |
| Triple Nut Reduced Sugar & Flakes | 1/2 cup | 130 | 4 | 35 | 0 | 0 | 0 | 55 | 21 | 2 | 3 | 1 1/2 starch, 1 fat |

BREAKFAST CEREAL, READY-TO-EAT CEREAL, HOT CEREAL

| | Serving | Calories | Fat (g) | Cal. from Fat | Sat. Fat (g) | Trans Fat (g) | Chol. (mg) | Sod. (mg) | Carb. (g) | Fiber (g) | Prot. (g) | Servings/Exchanges |
|---|---|---|---|---|---|---|---|---|---|---|---|---|
| Twigs, Flakes & Clusters | 1 cup | 170 | 1.5 | 15 | 0 | 0 | 0 | 105 | 41 | 12 | 5 | 2 1/2 starch |
| Vanilla Almond Clusters | 1 cup | 220 | 6 | 60 | 0.5 | 0 | 0 | 150 | 38 | 2 | 5 | 2 1/2 starch, 1 fat |
| Vanilla Almond Granola | 2/3 cup | 250 | 9 | 80 | 1 | 0 | 0 | 70 | 39 | 3 | 5 | 2 1/2 starch, 2 fat |
| Very Berry Clusters | 1 cup | 230 | 5 | 50 | 0.5 | 0 | 0 | 120 | 42 | 3 | 5 | 3 starch, 1 fat |

| | Serving | Calories | Fat (g) | Cal. from Fat | Sat. Fat (g) | Trans Fat (g) | Chol. (mg) | Sod. (mg) | Carb. (g) | Fiber (g) | Prot. (g) | Servings/Exchanges |
|---|---|---|---|---|---|---|---|---|---|---|---|---|
| **BUTTER, MARGARINE, SOUR CREAM** | | | | | | | | | | | | |
| Butter, Light | 1 Tbsp | 50 | 6 | 55 | 3.5 | 0 | 15 | 100 | 0 | 0 | 0 | 1 fat |
| Butter, Stick | 1 tsp | 34 | 4 | 35 | 2 | 0 | 10 | 27 | 0 | 0 | 0 | 1 fat |
| Butter, Whipped | 2 tsp | 33 | 4 | 35 | 2 | 0 | 10 | 33 | 0 | 0 | 0 | 1 fat |
| Margarine, Fat-Free | 1 Tbsp | 6 | 0 | 0 | 0 | 0 | 0 | 85 | <1 | 0 | 0 | free |
| Margarine, Liguid | 1 tsp | 34 | 4 | 35 | <1 | NA | 0 | 37 | 0 | 0 | 0 | 1 fat |
| Margarine, Stick | 1 tsp | 30 | 3 | 25 | <1 | NA | 0 | 37 | 0 | 0 | 0 | 1 fat |
| Margarine, Tub | 1 tsp | 24 | 3 | 27 | <1 | NA | 0 | 29 | 0 | 0 | 0 | 1 fat |
| Margarine-like Spread, Light or Lower Fat | 1 Tbsp | 46 | 5 | 45 | 1 | NA | 0 | 86 | 0 | 0 | 0 | 1 fat |
| Sour Cream, Fat-Free | 1 Tbsp | 30 | 0 | 0 | 0 | 0 | 5 | 20 | 3 | 0 | 1 | free |
| Sour Cream, Reduced-Fat or Light | 3 Tbsp | 45 | 4 | 35 | 3 | 0 | 18 | 38 | 3 | 0 | 3 | 1 fat |
| Sour Cream, Regular | 2 Tbsp | 62 | 5 | 45 | 3 | 0 | 19 | 14 | 1 | 0 | <1 | 1 fat |

BUTTER, MARGARINE, SOUR CREAM

| | Serving | Calories | Fat (g) | Cal. from Fat | Sat. Fat (g) | Trans Fat (g) | Chol. (mg) | Sod. (mg) | Carb. (g) | Fiber (g) | Prot. (g) | Servings/Exchanges |
|---|---|---|---|---|---|---|---|---|---|---|---|---|
| **Brands** | | | | | | | | | | | | |
| ***Benecol Spread*** | | | | | | | | | | | | |
| Light | 1 Tbsp | 50 | 5 | 50 | 0.5 | 0 | 0 | 110 | 0 | 0 | 0 | 1 fat |
| Regular | 1 Tbsp | 70 | 8 | 70 | 1 | 0 | 0 | 110 | 0 | 0 | 0 | 2 fat |
| ***Blue Bonnet Margarine*** | | | | | | | | | | | | |
| Light Stick | 1 Tbsp | 50 | 5 | 50 | 1 | 1 | 0 | 80 | <1 | 0 | 0 | 1 fat |
| Regular Stick | 1 Tbsp | 80 | 9 | 80 | 2 | 1.5 | 0 | 110 | 0 | 0 | 0 | 2 fat |
| Regular Tub | 1 Tbsp | 60 | 7 | 60 | 1.5 | 1 | 0 | 125 | 0 | 0 | 0 | 1 fat |
| ***Breakstone's/Knudsen*** | | | | | | | | | | | | |
| Sour Cream | 2 Tbsp | 60 | 5 | 50 | 3.5 | 0 | 20 | 10 | 1 | 0 | 1 | 1 fat |
| Sour Cream, Fat Free | 2 Tbsp | 30 | 0 | 0 | 0 | 0 | 5 | 25 | 6 | 0 | 1 | 1/2 carb |
| Sour Cream, Reduced Fat | 2 Tbsp | 40 | 3 | 30 | 2 | 0 | 15 | 20 | 2 | 0 | 1 | free |
| ***Brummel & Brown Margarine Spread with Yogurt*** | | | | | | | | | | | | |

| | | | | | | | | | | | | |
|---|---|---|---|---|---|---|---|---|---|---|---|---|
| Tub | 1 Tbsp | 45 | 5 | 45 | 1.5 | 0 | 0 | 90 | 0 | 0 | 0 | 1 fat |
| ***Butter Buds*** | | | | | | | | | | | | |
| Butter Replacement, Dry | 1 Tbsp | 15 | 0 | 0 | 0 | 0 | 0 | 360 | 6 | 0 | 0 | free |
| ***Canola Harvest Margarine*** | | | | | | | | | | | | |
| Baking Margarine | 2 tsp | 70 | 8 | 70 | 1.5 | 2.5 | 0 | 70 | 0 | 0 | 0 | 2 fat |
| Flaxseed Blend | 2 tsp | 70 | 8 | 70 | 1 | 0 | 0 | 70 | 0 | 0 | 0 | 2 fat |
| Olive Oil Blend | 2 tsp | 70 | 8 | 70 | 1 | 0 | 0 | 70 | 0 | 0 | 0 | 2 fat |
| Original | 2 tsp | 70 | 8 | 70 | 1 | 0 | 0 | 70 | 0 | 0 | 0 | 2 fat |
| Regular Soft Tub | 1 Tbsp | 100 | 11 | 100 | 1.5 | 0 | 0 | 100 | 0 | 0 | 0 | 2 fat |
| ***Canola*** | | | | | | | | | | | | |
| 100% Canola Margarine | 1 Tbsp | 100 | 11 | 100 | 2 | 0 | 0 | 120 | 0 | 0 | 0 | 2 fat |
| ***Daisy*** | | | | | | | | | | | | |
| Sour Cream | 2 Tbsp | 60 | 5 | 45 | 3.5 | 0 | 20 | 15 | 1 | 0 | 1 | 1 fat |
| Sour Cream, Light | 2 Tbsp | 60 | 2.5 | 25 | 2.5 | 0 | 10 | 25 | 2 | 0 | 2 | 1 fat |
| ***Fleischmann's Margarine*** | | | | | | | | | | | | |
| Original Tub | 1 Tbsp | 60 | 7 | 60 | 1 | 0 | 0 | 35 | 0 | 0 | 0 | 1 fat |

| | Serving | Calories | Fat (g) | Cal. from Fat | Sat. Fat (g) | Trans Fat (g) | Chol. (mg) | Sod. (mg) | Carb. (g) | Fiber (g) | Prot. (g) | Servings/Exchanges |
|---|---|---|---|---|---|---|---|---|---|---|---|---|
| Original Tub with Olive Oil | 1 Tbsp | 60 | 6.5 | 60 | 1 | 0 | 0 | 45 | 0 | 0 | 0 | 1 fat |
| ***Gold n Soft*** | | | | | | | | | | | | |
| Original Tub | 1 Tbsp | 100 | 10 | 90 | 2.5 | 0 | 0 | 90 | 0 | 0 | 0 | 2 fat |
| ***I Can't Believe It's Not Butter*** | | | | | | | | | | | | |
| Light Spread | 1 Tbsp | 50 | 5 | 45 | 1 | 0 | 0 | 85 | 0 | 0 | 0 | 1 fat |
| Original Spread | 1 Tbsp | 70 | 8 | 70 | 2 | 0 | 0 | 90 | 0 | 0 | 0 | 2 fat |
| Regular Stick | 1 Tbsp | 100 | 11 | 90 | 3.5 | 0 | 0 | 95 | 0 | 0 | 0 | 2 fat |
| Spray Original | 5 sprays | 0 | 0 | 0 | 0 | 0 | 0 | 15 | 0 | 0 | 0 | free |
| ***IMO*** | | | | | | | | | | | | |
| Sour Cream Substitute | 2 Tbsp | 60 | 5 | 50 | 5 | 0 | 0 | 30 | 2 | 0 | 1 | 1 fat |
| ***Imperial*** | | | | | | | | | | | | |
| Regular Stick | 1 Tbsp | 80 | 8 | 80 | 1.5 | 2 | 0 | 105 | 0 | 0 | 0 | 2 fat |
| ***Land O'Lakes*** | | | | | | | | | | | | |

| | | | | | | | | | | | | |
|---|---|---|---|---|---|---|---|---|---|---|---|---|
| Country Morning Blend Soft Spread | 1 Tbsp | 100 | 11 | 100 | 2.5 | 2 | 0 | 80 | 0 | 0 | 0 | 2 fat |
| Country Morning Blend Stick | 1 Tbsp | 100 | 11 | 100 | 2.5 | 2.5 | 0 | 90 | 0 | 0 | 0 | 2 fat |
| Fresh Buttery Taste Soft Spread | 1 Tbsp | 70 | 8 | 70 | 2 | 0 | 0 | 80 | 0 | 0 | 0 | 2 fat |
| Fresh Buttery Taste Stick Spread | 1 Tbsp | 90 | 10 | 90 | 2 | 2 | 0 | 95 | 0 | 0 | 0 | 2 fat |
| Garlic Butter Tub | 1 Tbsp | 90 | 10 | 90 | 5 | 0 | 20 | 110 | 0 | 0 | 0 | 2 fat |
| Honey Butter Tub | 1 Tbsp | 90 | 8 | 70 | 4 | 0.5 | 15 | 40 | 4 | 0 | 0 | 2 fat |
| Light Butter Stick | 1 Tbsp | 50 | 6 | 50 | 3.5 | 0 | 15 | 100 | 0 | 0 | 0 | 1 fat |
| Margarine Soft Tub | 1 Tbsp | 100 | 11 | 100 | 3 | 0 | 0 | 125 | 0 | 0 | 0 | 2 fat |
| Margarine Stick | 1 Tbsp | 100 | 11 | 100 | 2 | 2.5 | 0 | 105 | 0 | 0 | 0 | 2 fat |
| Salted Butter Stick | 1 Tbsp | 100 | 11 | 100 | 7 | 0 | 30 | 95 | 0 | 0 | 0 | 2 fat |
| Salted Whipped Light Butter | 1 Tbsp | 45 | 5 | 45 | 3 | 0 | 15 | 85 | 0 | 0 | 0 | 1 fat |

| | Serving | Calories | Fat (g) | Cal. from Fat | Sat. Fat (g) | Trans Fat (g) | Chol. (mg) | Sod. (mg) | Carb. (g) | Fiber (g) | Prot. (g) | Servings/Exchanges |
|---|---|---|---|---|---|---|---|---|---|---|---|---|
| Spreadable Butter with Canola Oil | 1 Tbsp | 100 | 11 | 100 | 4.5 | 0 | 20 | 90 | 0 | 0 | 0 | 2 fat |
| Spreadable Butter with Olive Oil | 1 Tbsp | 90 | 10 | 90 | 4 | 0 | 15 | 90 | 0 | 0 | 0 | 2 fat |
| Spreadable Light Butter with Canola Oil | 1 Tbsp | 50 | 5 | 50 | 2 | 0 | 5 | 90 | 0 | 0 | 0 | 1 fat |
| Unsalted Butter Stick | 1 Tbsp | 100 | 11 | 100 | 7 | 0 | 30 | 0 | 0 | 0 | 0 | 2 fat |
| Whipped Salted Butter | 1 Tbsp | 50 | 6 | 50 | 3.5 | 0 | 15 | 50 | 0 | 0 | 0 | 1 fat |
| ***Nucoa Margarine*** | | | | | | | | | | | | |
| Regular Stick | 1 Tbsp | 100 | 11 | 100 | 2 | 1.5 | 0 | 160 | 0 | 0 | 0 | 2 fat |
| Parkay | | | | | | | | | | | | |
| Squeeze | 1 Tbsp | 70 | 8 | 70 | 1.5 | 0 | 0 | 110 | 0 | 0 | 0 | 2 fat |
| ***Promise*** | | | | | | | | | | | | |
| Activ | 1 Tbsp | 45 | 5 | 45 | 1 | 0 | <5 | 85 | 0 | 0 | 0 | 1 fat |

| | | | | | | | | | | | | |
|---|---|---|---|---|---|---|---|---|---|---|---|---|
| Fat Free Spread | 1 Tbsp | 5 | 0 | 5 | 0 | 0 | 0 | 90 | 0 | 0 | 0 | free |
| Light Spread | 1 Tbsp | 45 | 5 | 45 | 1 | 0 | 0 | 85 | 0 | 0 | 0 | 1 fat |
| Regular Spread | 1 Tbsp | 80 | 8 | 80 | 1.5 | 0 | 0 | 85 | 0 | 0 | 0 | 2 fat |
| ***Shedd's Spread Country Crock*** | | | | | | | | | | | | |
| Calcium Plus Vitamin D Spread | 1 Tbsp | 50 | 5 | 45 | 1 | 0 | 0 | 95 | 0 | 0 | 0 | 1 fat |
| Churn Style Spread | 1 Tbsp | 80 | 8 | 80 | 1.5 | 0 | 0 | 95 | 0 | 0 | 0 | 2 fat |
| Honey Spread | 1 Tbsp | 50 | 5 | 45 | 1 | 0 | 0 | 95 | 0 | 0 | 0 | 1 fat |
| Light Spread | 1 Tbsp | 50 | 5 | 50 | 1.5 | 0 | 0 | 85 | 0 | 0 | 0 | 1 fat |
| Omega Plus Light Spread | 1 Tbsp | 50 | 5 | 45 | 1 | 0 | 0 | 80 | 0 | 0 | 0 | 1 fat |
| Omega Plus Spread | 1 Tbsp | 70 | 8 | 70 | 1.5 | 0 | 0 | 100 | 0 | 0 | 0 | 2 fat |
| Regular Tub | 1 Tbsp | 60 | 7 | 60 | 1.5 | 0 | 0 | 110 | 0 | 0 | 0 | 1 fat |
| Spreadable Butter | 1 Tbsp | 80 | 9 | 80 | 3.5 | 0 | 15 | 65 | 0 | 0 | 0 | 2 fat |
| Spreadable Sticks | 1 Tbsp | 80 | 8 | 80 | 1.5 | 0 | 0 | 90 | 0 | 0 | 0 | 2 fat |
| Whipped Easy Squeeze | 1 Tbsp | 60 | 7 | 60 | 1 | 0 | 0 | 85 | 0 | 0 | 0 | 1 fat |

BUTTER, MARGARINE, SOUR CREAM

| | Serving | Calories | Fat (g) | Cal. from Fat | Sat. Fat (g) | Trans Fat (g) | Chol. (mg) | Sod. (mg) | Carb. (g) | Fiber (g) | Prot. (g) | Servings/Exchanges |
|---|---|---|---|---|---|---|---|---|---|---|---|---|
| ***Smart Balance*** | | | | | | | | | | | | |
| 67% Buttery Spread | 1 Tbsp | 80 | 9 | 80 | 2.5 | 0 | 0 | 90 | 0 | 0 | 0 | 2 fat |
| Butter Blend Regular Stick | 1 Tbsp | 100 | 11 | 100 | 5 | 0 | 15 | 100 | 0 | 0 | 0 | 2 fat |
| Butter Blend Regular Stick with Omega-3 | 1 Tbsp | 100 | 11 | 100 | 5 | 0 | 15 | 100 | 0 | 0 | 0 | 2 fat |
| Heart Right Buttery Spread | 1 Tbsp | 80 | 8 | 80 | 2.5 | 0 | 0 | 85 | 0 | 0 | 0 | 2 fat |
| Light 32% Buttery Spread | 1 Tbsp | 45 | 5 | 45 | 1.5 | 0 | 0 | 85 | 0 | 0 | 0 | 1 fat |
| Low Sodium Buttery Spread | 1 Tbsp | 65 | 7 | 65 | 2 | 0 | 0 | 30 | 0 | 0 | 0 | 1 fat |
| Omega Plus | 1 Tbsp | 80 | 9 | 80 | 2.5 | 0 | 0 | 90 | 0 | 0 | 0 | 2 fat |
| Omega-3 Buttery Spread | 1 Tbsp | 80 | 9 | 80 | 2.5 | 0 | 0 | 85 | 0 | 0 | 0 | 2 fat |

| | | | | | | | | | | | | |
|---|---|---|---|---|---|---|---|---|---|---|---|---|
| Omega-3 Light Buttery Spread | 1 Tbsp | 50 | 5 | 50 | 1.5 | 0 | 0 | 80 | 0 | 0 | 0 | 1 fat |
| Omega-3 with Extra Virgin Olive Oil Buttery Spread | 1 Tbsp | 60 | 7 | 60 | 2 | 0 | 0 | 70 | 0 | 0 | 0 | 1 fat |
| Omega-3 with Extra Virgin Olive Oil Light Buttery Spread | 1 Tbsp | 50 | 5 | 50 | 1.5 | 0 | 0 | 70 | 0 | 0 | 0 | 1 fat |
| Organic Buttery Spread | 1 Tbsp | 80 | 9 | 80 | 2.5 | 0 | 0 | 100 | 0 | 0 | 0 | 2 fat |
| Regular Buttery Spread Light with Flax Oil | 1 Tbsp | 45 | 5 | 45 | 1.5 | 0 | 0 | 90 | 0 | 0 | 0 | 1 fat |
| Regular Buttery Spread with Flax Oil | 1 Tbsp | 80 | 9 | 80 | 2.5 | 0 | 0 | 85 | 0 | 0 | 0 | 2 fat |
| ***Smart Beat*** | | | | | | | | | | | | |
| Smart Squeeze | 1 Tbsp | 5 | 0 | 0 | 0 | 0 | 0 | 100 | 0 | 0 | 0 | free |

## CANDY, SWEETS

| | Serving | Calories | Fat. (g) | Cal. from Fat | Sat. Fat (g) | Trans Fat (g) | Chol. (mg) | Sod. (mg) | Carb. (g) | Fiber (g) | Prot. (g) | Servings/Exchanges |
|---|---|---|---|---|---|---|---|---|---|---|---|---|
| Almond Roca | 1 oz | 124 | 5 | 45 | 3 | 0 | 3 | 51 | 19 | <1 | 2 | 1 carb, 1 fat |
| Almonds, Chocolate Coated | 1/4 cup | 234 | 18 | 162 | 3 | 0 | <1 | 24 | 16 | 4 | 5 | 1 carb, 4 fat |
| Almonds, Sugar Coated | 7 | 116 | 4 | 35 | <1 | 0 | 0 | 3 | 20 | <1 | 2 | 1 carb, 1 fat |
| Butterscotch | 5 pieces | 119 | 1 | 10 | <1 | 0 | 3 | 13 | 29 | 0 | <1 | 2 carb |
| Candies, Chocolate Covered, Caramel with Nuts | 3 pieces | 197 | 9 | 80 | 2 | 0 | 0 | 10 | 26 | 2 | 4 | 2 carb, 2 fat |
| Candy Corn | 26 pieces | 140 | 0 | 0 | 0 | 0 | 0 | 80 | 36 | 0 | 0 | 2 1/2 carb |
| Caramels | 3 | 116 | 3 | 30 | 2 | 0 | 2 | 74 | 23 | <1 | 1 | 1 1/2 carb, 1 fat |
| Cherries, Chocolate Covered | 2 | 110 | 4 | 35 | 3 | 0 | 0 | 15 | 18 | 2 | <1 | 1 carb, 1 fat |
| Chewing Gum | 1 piece | 10 | <1 | 0 | 0 | 0 | 0 | <1 | 3 | 0 | 0 | free |

| | | | | | | | | | | | | |
|---|---|---|---|---|---|---|---|---|---|---|---|---|
| Chewing Gum, Sugar Free | 1 piece | 11 | <1 | 0 | 0 | 0 | 0 | <1 | 4 | 0 | 0 | free |
| Divinity, Homemade | 3 pieces | 120 | 0 | 0 | 0 | 0 | 0 | 11 | 29 | 0 | <1 | 2 carb |
| Fruit Leather | 1 oz | 102 | <1 | 0 | 0 | 0 | 0 | 114 | 24 | 0 | 0 | 1 1/2 carb |
| Fudge, Chocolate, Homemade | 3 pieces | 210 | 5 | 45 | 3 | 0 | 7 | 23 | 40 | 0 | 1 | 2 1/2 carb, 1 fat |
| Fudge, Vanilla, Homemade | 1 oz | 105 | 2 | 20 | <1 | 0 | 5 | 19 | 23 | 0 | <1 | 1 1/2 carb |
| Gumdrops, Sugar Free | 10 small | 81 | 0 | 0 | 0 | 0 | 0 | 16 | 44 | 0 | 0 | 3 carb |
| Gummy Bears | 10 small | 85 | 0 | 0 | 0 | 0 | 0 | 15 | 22 | 0 | 0 | 1 1/2 carb |
| Hard Candy, All Flavors | 1 oz | 106 | 0 | 0 | 0 | 0 | 0 | 11 | 28 | 0 | 0 | 2 carb |
| Jellybeans | 10 | 40 | <1 | 0 | 0 | 0 | 0 | 3 | 10 | 0 | 0 | 1/2 carb |
| Lollipops | 1 | 22 | 0 | 0 | 0 | 0 | 0 | 2 | 6 | 0 | 0 | 1/2 carb |
| Peanut Brittle, Homemade | 1 oz | 122 | 5 | 45 | 1 | 0 | 3 | 111 | 18 | <1 | 2 | 1 carb, 1 fat |
| Peanuts, Milk Chocolate Coated | 1/4 cup | 193 | 13 | 115 | 5 | 0 | 3 | 15 | 18 | 2 | 5 | 1 carb, 3 fat |

| | Serving | Calories | Fat (g) | Cal. from Fat | Sat. Fat (g) | Trans Fat (g) | Chol. (mg) | Sod. (mg) | Carb. (g) | Fiber (g) | Prot. (g) | Servings/Exchanges |
|---|---|---|---|---|---|---|---|---|---|---|---|---|
| Peanuts, Yogurt Covered | 1/4 cup | 194 | 13 | 115 | 3 | 0 | 1 | 15 | 16 | 2 | 4 | 1 carb, 3 fat |
| Praline, Homemade | 1 oz | 129 | 7 | 65 | <1 | 0 | 0 | 18 | 18 | <1 | <1 | 1 carb, 1 fat |
| Raisins, Milk Chocolate Covered | 1/4 cup | 185 | 7 | 65 | 4 | 0 | 1 | 17 | 33 | 2 | 2 | 2 carb, 1 fat |
| Raisins, Yogurt Covered | 1/4 cup | 176 | 7 | 65 | 5 | 0 | 1 | 16 | 31 | 1 | 2 | 2 carb, 1 fat |
| Taffy, Homemade | 1 oz | 11 | <1 | 0 | <1 | 0 | 3 | 15 | 26 | 0 | 0 | 2 carb |
| Toffee, Homemade | 1 oz | 157 | 9 | 80 | 6 | 0 | 29 | 38 | 18 | 0 | 0 | 1 carb, 2 fat |
| Truffles, Homemade | 1 oz | 143 | 10 | 90 | 5 | 0 | 15 | 19 | 13 | <1 | 2 | 1 carb, 2 fat |
| **Brands** | | | | | | | | | | | | |
| ***Concorde*** | | | | | | | | | | | | |
| Bit-O-Honey Chews | 6 | 186 | 4 | 36 | NA | 0 | <1 | 124 | 39 | NA | 1 | 2 1/2 carb, 1 fat |
| ***DeMet's*** | | | | | | | | | | | | |
| Turtles | 3 pieces | 260 | 15 | 130 | 6 | 0 | 5 | 45 | 29 | 1 | 3 | 2 carb, 3 fat |
| Turtles, Sugar Free | 3 pieces | 150 | 11 | 100 | 6 | 0 | <5 | 70 | 20 | <1 | 2 | 1 carb, 2 fat |

| ***Hershey's*** | | | | | | | | | | | | |
|---|---|---|---|---|---|---|---|---|---|---|---|---|
| 5th Avenue Bar | 2-oz bar | 260 | 12 | 110 | 4.5 | 0 | 0 | 120 | 37 | 2 | 4 | 2 1/2 carb, 2 fat |
| Almond Joy | 1.6-oz bar | 220 | 13 | 110 | 8 | 0 | 0 | 50 | 26 | 2 | 2 | 2 carb, 3 fat |
| BreathSavers Mints | 1 | 5 | 0 | 0 | 0 | 0 | 0 | 0 | 2 | 0 | 0 | free |
| Cadbury Chocolate | 7 blocks | 200 | 11 | 100 | 7 | 0 | 10 | 40 | 23 | <1 | 3 | 1 1/2 carb, 2 fat |
| Cadbury's Caramello Bar | 1.6-oz bar | 220 | 10 | 90 | 6 | 0 | 10 | 45 | 29 | <1 | 3 | 2 carb, 2 fat |
| Chocolate Candy, Sugar Free | 5 pieces | 160 | 13 | 110 | 8 | 0 | 10 | 15 | 24 | 3 | 1 | 1 1/2 carb, 3 fat |
| Chocolate Kisses | 9 | 230 | 13 | 120 | 8 | 0 | 10 | 35 | 24 | 1 | 3 | 1 1/2 carb, 3 fat |
| Cookies & Creme Bar | 1.2-oz bar | 170 | 9 | 80 | 6 | 0 | 5 | 75 | 21 | 0 | 3 | 1 1/2 carb, 2 fat |
| Good & Plenty Licorice | 1.4 oz | 140 | 0 | 0 | 0 | 0 | 0 | 120 | 35 | 0 | <1 | 2 carb |
| Heath Toffee Bar | 1.4-oz bar | 210 | 13 | 110 | 7 | 0 | 10 | 135 | 24 | <1 | 1 | 1 1/2 carb, 3 fat |

CANDY, SWEETS

| | Serving | Calories | Fat (g) | Cal. from Fat | Sat. Fat (g) | Trans Fat (g) | Chol. (mg) | Sod. (mg) | Carb. (g) | Fiber (g) | Prot. (g) | Servings/Exchanges |
|---|---|---|---|---|---|---|---|---|---|---|---|---|
| Hershey's 100 Calorie Pretzel Bar | 1 bar | 100 | 4.5 | 40 | 2.5 | 0 | 0 | 105 | 13 | 0 | 1 | 1 carb, 1 fat |
| Hershey's Bliss Milk Chocolate | 6 pieces | 210 | 14 | 120 | 9 | 0 | 5 | 40 | 24 | 1 | 3 | 1 1/2 carb, 3 fat |
| Hershey's Extra Dark Chocolate Bar | 3 blocks | 210 | 13 | 120 | 8 | 0 | <5 | 5 | 20 | 4 | 3 | 1 carb, 3 fat |
| Hershey's Miniatures | 5 pieces | 210 | 13 | 110 | 7 | 0 | 5 | 50 | 25 | 2 | 3 | 1 1/2 carb, 3 fat |
| Hershey's Nuggets | 4 pieces | 200 | 12 | 110 | 7 | 0 | 10 | 35 | 25 | 1 | 3 | 1 1/2 carb, 2 fat |
| Hershey's Sugar Free Chocolates | 5 pieces | 160 | 13 | 110 | 8 | 0 | 10 | 15 | 24 | 3 | 1 | 1 1/2 carb, 3 fat |
| Hershey's Take 5 | 1.5-oz bar | 200 | 11 | 90 | 5 | 0 | 0 | 180 | 25 | 1 | 4 | 1 1/2 carb, 2 fat |
| Jolly Rancher Candy | 3 pieces | 50 | 0 | 0 | 0 | 0 | 0 | 20 | 13 | 0 | 0 | 1 carb |
| Jolly Rancher Hard Candy, Sugar Free | 4 pieces | 35 | 0 | 0 | 0 | 0 | 0 | 0 | 13 | 0 | 0 | 1 carb |

| | | | | | | | | | | | | |
|---|---|---|---|---|---|---|---|---|---|---|---|---|
| Kit Kat Bar | 1.5-oz bar | 210 | 11 | 100 | 7 | 0 | <5 | 30 | 28 | <1 | 3 | 2 carb, 2 fat |
| Milk Chocolate Bar | 1.5-oz bar | 210 | 13 | 110 | 8 | 0 | 10 | 35 | 26 | 1 | 3 | 2 carb, 3 fat |
| Milk Chocolate Bar, Symphony | 1.5-oz bar | 220 | 14 | 130 | 8 | 0 | 10 | 65 | 23 | <1 | 3 | 1 1/2 carb, 3 fat |
| Milk Duds | 13 | 170 | 6 | 50 | 3.5 | 0 | 0 | 100 | 28 | 0 | 1 | 2 carb, 1 fat |
| Mounds | 1.75 oz | 230 | 13 | 120 | 10 | 0 | 0 | 55 | 29 | 3 | 2 | 2 carb, 3 fat |
| Mr. Goodbar | 1.75-oz bar | 250 | 17 | 140 | 7 | 0 | <5 | 65 | 26 | 2 | 5 | 2 carb, 3 fat |
| PayDay | 2.08-oz bar | 240 | 13 | 120 | 2.5 | 0 | 0 | 120 | 27 | 2 | 7 | 2 carb, 3 fat |
| Reese's Peanut Butter Cups | 1.5 oz 2 pieces | 210 | 13 | 110 | 4.5 | 0 | <5 | 150 | 24 | 1 | 5 | 1 1/2 carb, 3 fat |
| Reese's Pieces | 1.5 oz | 210 | 10 | 90 | 8 | 0 | 0 | 85 | 26 | 1 | 5 | 2 carb, 2 fat |
| Reese's Sticks | 1.5-oz bar | 210 | 13 | 110 | 5 | 0 | 0 | 130 | 23 | 1 | 4 | 1 1/2 carb, 3 fat |

CANDY, SWEETS

| | Serving | Calories | Fat (g) | Cal. from Fat | Sat. Fat (g) | Trans Fat (g) | Chol. (mg) | Sod. (mg) | Carb. (g) | Fiber (g) | Prot. (g) | Servings/Exchanges |
|---|---|---|---|---|---|---|---|---|---|---|---|---|
| Reese's 100 Calorie Peanut Butter Wafer | 1 bar | 100 | 6 | 50 | 2.5 | 0 | 0 | 50 | 11 | 0 | 2 | 1 carb, 1 fat |
| Reese's Fast Break | 2-oz bar | 260 | 12 | 100 | 4.5 | 0 | 0 | 190 | 35 | 2 | 5 | 2 carb, 2 fat |
| Reese's NutRageous | 1.82-oz bar | 260 | 16 | 140 | 5 | 0 | 0 | 100 | 28 | 2 | 6 | 2 carb, 3 fat |
| Reese's Peanut Butter Cups, Sugar Free | 5 pieces | 180 | 13 | 110 | 6 | 0 | <5 | 120 | 27 | 6 | 3 | 2 carb, 3 fat |
| Rolos Caramel | 1.7-oz pkg | 220 | 10 | 80 | 7 | 0 | 5 | 80 | 33 | 0 | 2 | 2 carb, 2 fat |
| Skor Bar | 1.4-oz bar | 200 | 12 | 110 | 7 | 0 | 20 | 130 | 25 | <1 | 1 | 1 1/2 carb, 2 fat |
| Special Dark Sweet Chocolate Bar | 1.5 oz | 180 | 12 | 110 | 8 | 0 | <5 | 15 | 25 | 3 | 2 | 1 1/2 carb, 3 fat |
| Tootsie Rolls | 6 small | 140 | 3 | 30 | 0.5 | 0 | 1 | 15 | 28 | 0 | 1 | 2 carb, 1 fat |

| | | | | | | | | | | | | |
|---|---|---|---|---|---|---|---|---|---|---|---|---|
| Twizzlers, Strawberry | 4 pieces | 160 | 1 | 5 | 0 | 0 | 0 | 95 | 36 | 0 | 1 | 2 1/2 carb |
| Twizzlers, Sugar Free | 6 pieces | 130 | 1 | 10 | 0 | 0 | 0 | 105 | 33 | 0 | 1 | 2 carb |
| Whatchamacallit Bar | 1.6 oz | 230 | 12 | 110 | 9 | 0 | <5 | 140 | 28 | <1 | 3 | 2 carb, 2 fat |
| Whoppers Chocolate Malted Milk Balls | 1.5-oz pkg | 190 | 7 | 60 | 7 | 0 | 0 | 115 | 31 | 0 | 1 | 2 carb, 1 fat |
| York 100 Calorie Bars | 1 bar | 100 | 6 | 50 | 4 | 0 | 0 | 10 | 11 | <1 | <1 | 1 carb, 1 fat |
| York Peppermint Pattie | 1 pattie | 140 | 2.5 | 25 | 1.5 | 0 | 0 | 10 | 31 | <1 | <1 | 2 carb, 1 fat |
| York Sugar Free Peppermint Patties | 3 pieces | 120 | 8 | 60 | 4.5 | 0 | 0 | 5 | 24 | 2 | 1 | 1 1/2 carb, 2 fat |
| Zagnut | 3 pieces | 200 | 8 | 70 | 3 | 0 | 0 | 90 | 31 | 1 | 3 | 2 carb, 2 fat |
| ***Just Born*** | | | | | | | | | | | | |
| Hot Tamales | 1.4 oz 20 pieces | 150 | 0 | 0 | 0 | 0 | 0 | 15 | 36 | 0 | 0 | 2 1/2 carb |
| Mike and Ike | 23 pieces | 140 | 0 | 0 | 0 | 0 | 0 | 30 | 36 | 0 | 0 | 2 1/2 carb |
| ***Kraft*** | | | | | | | | | | | | |
| Butter Mints | 7 mints | 60 | 0 | 0 | 0 | 0 | 0 | 25 | 14 | 0 | 0 | 1 carb |

| | Serving | Calories | Fat (g) | Cal. from Fat | Sat. Fat (g) | Trans Fat (g) | Chol. (mg) | Sod. (mg) | Carb. (g) | Fiber (g) | Prot. (g) | Servings/Exchanges |
|---|---|---|---|---|---|---|---|---|---|---|---|---|
| Caramels | 5 | 160 | 3.5 | 30 | 2 | 0 | 0 | 95 | 31 | 0 | 2 | 2 carb, 1 fat |
| ***M&M Mars*** | | | | | | | | | | | | |
| 3 Musketeers Bar | 1.68-oz bar | 200 | 6 | 60 | 4 | 0 | 5 | 85 | 36 | 1 | 1 | 2 1/2 carb, 1 fat |
| Dove Bar | 1 bar | 80 | 4.5 | 40 | 3 | 0 | 0 | 10 | 9 | NA | 1 | 1/2 carb, 1 fat |
| M&M's, Chocolate | 1.7 oz | 260 | 11 | 80 | 7 | 0 | 5 | 35 | 37 | 1 | 2 | 2 1/2 carb, 2 fat |
| M&M's, Peanut | 1.75 oz | 250 | 13 | 120 | 5 | 0 | 5 | 25 | 30 | 2 | 5 | 2 carb, 3 fat |
| Milky Way Bar | 2.05-oz bar | 270 | 10 | 90 | 7 | 0 | 5 | 95 | 41 | 1 | 2 | 2 1/2 carb, 2 fat |
| Munch Bar | 1 bar | 220 | 15 | 130 | 3.5 | 0 | 10 | 140 | 17 | 2 | 6 | 1 carb, 3 fat |
| Skittles | 1 bag | 230 | 2.5 | 20 | 2.5 | 0 | 0 | 10 | 51 | 0 | 0 | 3 1/2 carb, 1 fat |
| Snickers Bar | 2.07-oz bar | 280 | 14 | 130 | 5 | 0 | 5 | 140 | 36 | 1 | 4 | 2 1/2 carb, 3 fat |
| Starburst Fruit Chews | 1 pkg | 240 | 5 | 45 | 4.5 | 0 | 0 | 0 | 48 | 0 | 0 | 3 carb, 1 fat |

| | | | | | | | | | | | | |
|---|---|---|---|---|---|---|---|---|---|---|---|---|
| Twix Caramel Cookie Bar | 2-oz bar | 280 | 14 | 130 | 11 | 0 | 5 | 115 | 37 | 1 | 3 | 2 1/2 carb, 3 fat |
| ***Nestlé*** | | | | | | | | | | | | |
| 100 Grand Bar | 1.5-oz bar | 190 | 8 | 70 | 5 | 0 | 10 | 90 | 30 | 0 | 1 | 2 carb, 2 fat |
| Baby Ruth Bar | 2.1-oz bar | 280 | 14 | 120 | 8 | 0 | 0 | 130 | 39 | 1 | 4 | 2 1/2 carb, 3 fat |
| Butterfinger Bar | 2.1-oz bar | 270 | 11 | 100 | 6 | 0 | 0 | 135 | 43 | 1 | 4 | 3 carb, 2 fat |
| Chunky Bar | 1.4-oz bar | 190 | 11 | 100 | 5 | 0 | <5 | 15 | 24 | 1 | 3 | 1 1/2 carb, 2 fat |
| Crunch Bar | 1.4-oz bar | 220 | 11 | 100 | 7 | 0 | 10 | 60 | 30 | 1 | 2 | 2 carb, 2 fat |
| Goobers Chocolate-Covered Peanuts | 1.5-oz bag | 210 | 14 | 120 | 5 | 0 | 5 | 15 | 22 | 2 | 5 | 1 1/2 carb, 3 fat |
| Raisinets | 3.5-oz box | 190 | 8 | 70 | 5 | 0 | 5 | 15 | 32 | 1 | 2 | 2 carb, 2 fat |

| | Serving | Calories | Carb. (g) | Fat (g) | % Cal Fat. | Sat. Fat (g) | Trans Fat (g) | Chol (mg) | Sod. (mg) | Fiber (g) | Prot. (g) | Servings/Exchanges |
|---|---|---|---|---|---|---|---|---|---|---|---|---|
| Sno Caps | 3.1-oz box | 180 | 8 | 70 | 5 | 0 | <5 | 0 | 30 | 2 | 1 | 2 carb, 2 fat |
| ***Russell Stover*** | | | | | | | | | | | | |
| Mint Patties, Sugar Free | 3 pieces | 180 | 12 | 110 | 8 | 0 | <5 | 20 | 26 | 2 | 2 | 2 carb, 2 fat |
| Pecan Delights, Sugar Free | 3 pieces | 190 | 15 | 130 | 7 | 0 | <5 | 45 | 23 | 3 | 3 | 1 1/2 carb, 3 fat |
| Toffee Squares, Sugar Free | 3 | 190 | 15 | 130 | 7 | 0 | 0 | 45 | 23 | 2 | 3 | 1 1/2 carb, 3 fat |
| ***Storck*** | | | | | | | | | | | | |
| Swedish Fish | 7 pieces | 150 | 0 | 0 | 0 | 0 | 0 | 30 | 38 | 0 | 0 | 2 1/2 carb |
| ***Tootsie*** | | | | | | | | | | | | |
| Dots | 11 | 130 | 0 | 0 | 0 | 0 | 0 | 15 | 33 | 0 | 0 | 2 carb |
| Junior Mints | 16 (1.4 oz) | 170 | 3 | 30 | 2.5 | 0 | 0 | 30 | 35 | 1 | 1 | 2 carb, 1 fat |

| | | | | | | | | | | | | |
|---|---|---|---|---|---|---|---|---|---|---|---|---|
| Sugar Babies | 30 (1.6 oz) | 180 | 1.5 | 15 | 0 | 0 | 0 | 40 | 41 | 0 | 0 | 2 1/2 carb |
| ***Weight Watchers by Whitman's*** | | | | | | | | | | | | |
| Coconut Covered Milk Chocolate | 3 pieces | 150 | 9 | 80 | 7 | 0 | 5 | 50 | 23 | 11 | 2 | 1 1/2 carb, 2 fat |
| Pecan Crowns | 3 pieces | 160 | 10 | 90 | 6 | 0 | <5 | 20 | 24 | 9 | 2 | 1 1/2 carb, 2 fat |
| **Werther's** | | | | | | | | | | | | |
| Caramel Candies | 4 pieces | 70 | 1 | 10 | 0.5 | 0 | <5 | 30 | 15 | 0 | 0 | 1 carb |
| Caramel Candies, Sugar Free | 5 pieces | 40 | 1 | 10 | 0.5 | 0 | <5 | 55 | 15 | 0 | 0 | 1 carb |

## CHEESE, COTTAGE CHEESE, CREAM CHEESE

| | Serving | Calories | Fat (g) | Cal. from Fat | Sat. Fat (g) | Trans Fat (g) | Chol. (mg) | Sod. (mg) | Carb. (g) | Fiber (g) | Prot. (g) | Servings/Exchanges |
|---|---|---|---|---|---|---|---|---|---|---|---|---|
| American | 1 oz | 106 | 9 | 80 | 6 | 0 | 27 | 406 | <1 | 0 | 6 | 1 high-fat meat |
| American, Fat Free | 3/4-oz slice | 30 | 0 | 0 | 0 | 0 | 3 | 270 | 2 | 0 | 5 | 1 lean meat |
| American, Reduced Fat | 1 oz | 68 | 4 | 35 | 2.5 | 0 | 14 | 379 | 1 | 0 | 5 | 1 lean meat |
| Blue or Roquefort | 1 oz | 100 | 8 | 70 | 5 | 0 | 21 | 396 | <1 | 0 | 6 | 1 high-fat meat |
| Brick | 1 oz | 105 | 8 | 70 | 5 | 0 | 27 | 159 | 1 | 0 | 7 | 1 high-fat meat |
| Brie | 1 oz | 95 | 8 | 70 | 5 | 0 | 28 | 178 | 0 | 0 | 6 | 1 high-fat meat |
| Camembert | 1 oz | 85 | 7 | 65 | 4 | 0 | 20 | 239 | 0 | 0 | 6 | 1 med-fat meat |
| Cheddar | 1 oz | 114 | 9 | 80 | 6 | 0 | 30 | 176 | <1 | 0 | 7 | 1 high-fat meat |
| Cheddar/Colby, Fat Free | 1 oz | 45 | 0 | 0 | 0 | 0 | 3 | 296 | 2 | 0 | 9 | 1 lean meat |
| Cheddar/Colby, Reduced Fat | 1 oz | 80 | 5 | 45 | 4 | 0 | 15 | 230 | 1 | 0 | 7 | 1 lean meat |
| Cheese Spread | 1 oz | 82 | 6 | 55 | 4 | 0 | 16 | 381 | 3 | 0 | 5 | 1 med-fat meat |

| | | | | | | | | | | | | |
|---|---|---|---|---|---|---|---|---|---|---|---|---|
| Cheshire | 1 oz | 110 | 9 | 80 | 6 | 0 | 29 | 198 | 1 | 0 | 7 | 1 high-fat meat |
| Cottage Cheese, 1% Milkfat, Low Fat | 1/4 cup | 41 | <1 | 0 | <1 | 0 | 2 | 229 | 2 | 0 | 7 | 1 lean meat |
| Cottage Cheese, Creamed, 4.5% Milkfat | 1/4 cup | 54 | 2 | 20 | 1 | 0 | 8 | 210 | 1 | 0 | 7 | 1 lean meat |
| Cottage Cheese, Nonfat | 1/4 cup | 40 | 0 | 0 | 0 | 0 | 3 | 205 | 2.5 | 0 | 7 | 1 lean meat |
| Edam | 1 oz | 101 | 8 | 70 | 5 | 0 | 25 | 274 | 0 | 0 | 7 | 1 high-fat meat |
| Feta | 1 oz | 75 | 6 | 55 | 4 | 0 | 25 | 317 | 1 | 0 | 4 | 1 med-fat meat |
| Feta, Fat Free, Plain | 1 oz | 30 | 0 | 0 | 0 | 0 | 0 | 449 | 2 | 0 | 6 | 1 lean meat |
| Fontina | 1 oz | 110 | 9 | 80 | 5 | 0 | 33 | 227 | 0 | 0 | 7 | 1 high-fat meat |
| Gjetost | 1 oz | 132 | 8 | 70 | 5 | 0 | 27 | 170 | 12 | 0 | 3 | 1 high-fat meat |
| Goat Cheese, Hard | 1 oz | 127 | 10 | 90 | 7 | 0 | 30 | 98 | <1 | 0 | 9 | 1 high-fat meat |
| Gouda | 1 oz | 101 | 8 | 70 | 5 | 0 | 32 | 232 | 1 | 0 | 7 | 1 high-fat meat |
| Gruyere | 1 oz | 117 | 9 | 80 | 5 | 0 | 31 | 95 | 0 | 0 | 8 | 1 high-fat meat |
| Limburger | 1 oz | 93 | 8 | 70 | 5 | 0 | 26 | 227 | 0 | 0 | 6 | 1 high-fat meat |

CHEESE, COTTAGE CHEESE, CREAM CHEESE

| | Serving | Calories | Fat (g) | Cal. from Fat | Sat. Fat (g) | Trans Fat (g) | Chol. (mg) | Sod. (mg) | Carb. (g) | Fiber (g) | Prot. (g) | Servings/Exchanges |
|---|---|---|---|---|---|---|---|---|---|---|---|---|
| Mexican, Reduced Fat | 1 oz | 81 | 6 | 55 | 3 | 0 | 20 | 201 | 0 | 0 | 8 | 1 med-fat meat |
| Monterey Jack | 1 oz | 106 | 9 | 80 | 5 | 0 | 25 | 152 | 0 | 0 | 7 | 1 high-fat meat |
| Monterey Jack, Reduced Fat | 1 oz | 80 | 6 | 55 | 3.5 | 0 | 20 | 240 | 1 | 0 | 7 | 1 med-fat meat |
| Mozarella, Fat Free | 1 oz | 45 | 0 | 0 | 0 | 0 | 4 | 335 | 1 | 0 | 8 | 1 lean meat |
| Mozzarella, Part Skim | 1 oz | 72 | 5 | 45 | 3 | 0 | 18 | 175 | <1 | 0 | 7 | 1 med-fat meat |
| Mozzarella, Reduced Fat | 1 oz | 70 | 4 | 35 | 3 | 0 | 15 | 200 | <1 | 0 | 8 | 1 lean meat |
| Muenster | 1 oz | 105 | 9 | 80 | 5 | 0 | 27 | 178 | 0 | 0 | 7 | 1 high-fat meat |
| Parmesan, Grated | 2 Tbsp | 43 | 3 | 30 | 2 | 0 | 9 | 153 | 0 | 0 | 4 | 1 lean meat |
| Port du Salut | 1 oz | 100 | 8 | 70 | 5 | 0 | 35 | 151 | 0 | 0 | 7 | 1 high-fat meat |
| Provolone | 1 oz | 100 | 8 | 70 | 5 | 0 | 20 | 248 | 1 | 0 | 7 | 1 high-fat meat |
| Ricotta, Fat Free | 1/4 cup | 45 | 0 | 0 | 0 | 0 | 20 | 50 | 3 | 0 | 8 | 1 lean meat |
| Ricotta, Part Skim | 1/4 cup | 85 | 5 | 45 | 3 | 0 | 19 | 76 | 3 | 0 | 7 | 1 med-fat meat |

| | | | | | | | | | | | | |
|---|---|---|---|---|---|---|---|---|---|---|---|---|
| Romano | 1 oz | 110 | 8 | 70 | 5 | 0 | 29 | 340 | 1 | 0 | 9 | 1 high-fat meat |
| String Cheese | 1 | 83 | 5 | 45 | 3.5 | 0 | 18 | 236 | <1 | 0 | 7 | 1 med-fat meat |
| Swiss | 1 oz | 108 | 8 | 70 | 5 | 0 | 26 | 55 | 1.5 | 0 | 8 | 1 high-fat meat |
| Swiss, Fat Free | 1 oz | 41 | 0 | 0 | 0 | 0 | 7 | 352 | 3 | 0 | 7 | 1 lean meat |
| Swiss, Reduced Fat | 1 oz | 70 | 3.5 | 30 | 2 | 0 | 10 | 130 | 0 | 0 | 9 | 1 med-fat meat |
| Tilsit | 1 oz | 96 | 7 | 65 | 5 | 0 | 29 | 213 | 1 | 0 | 7 | 1 med-fat meat |
| **Brands** | | | | | | | | | | | | |
| ***Alpine Lace*** | | | | | | | | | | | | |
| American, White, Reduced Fat, Reduced Sodium | 3/4-oz slice | 70 | 5 | 45 | 3 | 0 | 15 | 310 | 1 | 0 | 5 | 1 med-fat meat |
| American, Yellow, Reduced Fat, Reduced Sodium | 3/4-oz slice | 70 | 5 | 45 | 3 | 0 | 15 | 310 | 1 | 0 | 5 | 1 med-fat meat |
| Cheddar, Reduced Fat | 3/4-oz slice | 70 | 5 | 50 | 3.5 | 0 | 15 | 135 | 0 | 0 | 6 | 1 med-fat meat |

| | Serving | Calories | Fat (g) | Cal. from Fat | Sat. Fat (g) | Trans Fat (g) | Chol. (mg) | Sod. (mg) | Carb. (g) | Fiber (g) | Prot. (g) | Servings/Exchanges |
|---|---|---|---|---|---|---|---|---|---|---|---|---|
| CO-JACK Semisoft Cheese, Reduced Fat | 3/4-oz slice | 70 | 5 | 50 | 3.5 | 0 | 15 | 150 | 0 | 0 | 5 | 1 med-fat meat |
| Mozzarella, Low Moisture, Reduced Fat | 3/4-oz slice | 60 | 4 | 35 | 2.5 | 0 | 15 | 160 | 1 | 0 | 5 | 1 med-fat meat |
| Muenster, Reduced Sodium | 3/4-oz slice | 90 | 7 | 60 | 4.5 | 0 | 15 | 110 | 1 | 0 | 6 | 1 med-fat meat |
| Provolone, Reduced Fat | 3/4-oz slice | 70 | 4.5 | 40 | 3 | 0 | 10 | 135 | 1 | 0 | 6 | 1 med-fat meat |
| Swiss, Reduced Fat | 3/4-oz slice | 70 | 4.5 | 40 | 3 | 0 | 15 | 95 | 1 | 0 | 7 | 1 med-fat meat |
| ***Athenos*** | | | | | | | | | | | | |
| Blue Cheese | 3 Tbsp | 110 | 9 | 80 | 6 | 0 | 30 | 430 | 2 | <1 | 7 | 1 high-fat meat |
| Gorgonzola | 3 Tbsp | 110 | 9 | 80 | 6 | 0 | 30 | 400 | 2 | <1 | 7 | 1 high-fat meat |
| Traditional Feta | 1/4 cup | 90 | 7 | 60 | 4 | 0 | 25 | 390 | 2 | <1 | 7 | 1 med-fat meat |

| | | | | | | | | | | | | |
|---|---|---|---|---|---|---|---|---|---|---|---|---|
| ***Breakstone's*** | | | | | | | | | | | | |
| Cottage Cheese, 2% Low Fat, Small Curd | 1/2 cup | 90 | 2.5 | 15 | 1.5 | 0 | 15 | 400 | 6 | 0 | 12 | 2 lean meat |
| Cottage Cheese, 4% Milkfat, Large Curd | 1/2 cup | 120 | 5 | 45 | 3 | 0 | 25 | 430 | 6 | 0 | 12 | 2 lean meat |
| Cottage Cheese, 4% Milkfat, Small Curd | 1/2 cup | 120 | 5 | 45 | 3 | 0 | 25 | 430 | 6 | 0 | 12 | 2 lean meat |
| Cottage Cheese, Fat Free, Small Curd | 1/2 cup | 80 | 0 | 0 | 0 | 0 | 10 | 450 | 8 | 0 | 12 | 2 lean meat |
| ***DiGiorno*** | | | | | | | | | | | | |
| Parmesan, Shredded | 1/4 cup | 110 | 8 | 70 | 4.5 | 0 | 25 | 430 | 0 | 0 | 1 | 1 high-fat meat |
| Romano, Grated | 2 tsp | 20 | 2 | 20 | 1 | 0 | 5 | 75 | 0 | 0 | 2 | free |
| ***Knudsen*** | | | | | | | | | | | | |
| Cottage Cheese, 2% Lowfat, Small Curd | 1/2 cup | 100 | 2.5 | 20 | 1.5 | 0 | 15 | 440 | 6 | 0 | 14 | 2 lean meat |
| Cottage Cheese, Nonfat | 1/2 cup | 80 | 0 | 0 | 0 | 0 | 5 | 430 | 7 | 0 | 13 | 2 lean meat |

CHEESE, COTTAGE CHEESE, CREAM CHEESE

| | Serving | Calories | Fat (g) | Cal. from Fat | Sat. Fat (g) | Trans Fat (g) | Chol. (mg) | Sod. (mg) | Carb. (g) | Fiber (g) | Prot. (g) | Servings/Exchanges |
|---|---|---|---|---|---|---|---|---|---|---|---|---|
| Cottage Doubles, Blueberry | 5.6 oz | 140 | 2.5 | 20 | 1.5 | 0 | 15 | 400 | 18 | 1 | 11 | 1 carb, 1 lean meat |
| Cottage Doubles, Peach | 5.6 oz | 140 | 2.5 | 20 | 1.5 | 0 | 15 | 390 | 17 | 0 | 11 | 1 carb, 1 lean meat |
| Creamed Cottage Cheese, Small Curd | 1/2 cup | 120 | 5 | 45 | 3 | 0 | 25 | 430 | 5 | 0 | 13 | 2 lean meat |
| LiveActive Cottage Cheese | 4 oz | 90 | 2 | 20 | 1.5 | 0 | 15 | 380 | 8 | 3 | 10 | 1/2 carb, 1 lean meat |
| ***Kraft*** | | | | | | | | | | | | |
| Cheddar & Monterey Jack, Natural 2% Reduced Fat Cubes | 7 pieces | 90 | 6 | 60 | 4 | 0 | 20 | 260 | <1 | 0 | 8 | 1 med-fat meat |
| Cheddar Cheese Sticks, Mild Cheddar | 1 oz | 120 | 10 | 90 | 6 | 0 | 30 | 180 | 0 | 0 | 6 | 1 high-fat meat |
| Cheddar, 2% Reduced Fat, Mild, Shredded | 1 oz | 90 | 7 | 60 | 4.5 | 0 | 20 | 220 | <1 | 0 | 7 | 1 med-fat meat |

| | | | | | | | | | | | | |
|---|---|---|---|---|---|---|---|---|---|---|---|---|
| Cheddar, Fat Free, Shredded | 1/4 cup | 45 | 0 | 0 | 0 | 0 | <5 | 280 | 2 | 0 | 9 | 1 lean meat |
| Cheddar, Natural | 1 oz | 120 | 10 | 90 | 6 | 0 | 30 | 180 | 0 | 0 | 6 | 1 high-fat meat |
| Cheddar, Sharp, Cheese Sticks | 1 oz | 90 | 6 | 50 | 3.5 | 0 | 20 | 240 | 1 | 0 | 7 | 1 med-fat meat |
| Cheddar, Shredded | 1 oz | 110 | 9 | 80 | 6 | 0 | 25 | 190 | 1 | 0 | 6 | 1 high-fat meat |
| Cheese Cubes, Natural, 2% Reduced Fat | 1.5 oz | 160 | 13 | 120 | 9 | 0 | 40 | 280 | 1 | 0 | 10 | 2 high-fat meat |
| Cheese Spread, Pimento | 2 Tbsp | 80 | 6 | 60 | 4 | 0 | 20 | 170 | 3 | 0 | 2 | 1 med-fat meat |
| Cheez Whiz Cheese Dip | 2 Tbsp | 90 | 7 | 60 | 4.5 | 0 | 30 | 490 | 4 | 0 | 3 | 1 med-fat meat |
| Cheez Whiz Cheese Dip, Light | 2 Tbsp | 80 | 3.5 | 30 | 2 | 0 | 20 | 500 | 6 | 0 | 6 | 1 med-fat meat |
| Classic Melts Four Cheese Shredded Cheese | 1 oz | 120 | 7 | 90 | 7 | 0 | 30 | 310 | 1 | 0 | 7 | 1 med-fat meat |

CHEESE, COTTAGE CHEESE, CREAM CHEESE

| | Serving | Calories | Fat (g) | Cal. from Fat | Sat. Fat (g) | Trans Fat (g) | Chol. (mg) | Sod. (mg) | Carb. (g) | Fiber (g) | Prot. (g) | Servings/Exchanges |
|---|---|---|---|---|---|---|---|---|---|---|---|---|
| Colby & Monterey Jack, 2% Reduced Fat, Natural | 1/4 cup | 80 | 5 | 70 | 3.5 | 0 | 15 | 220 | <1 | 0 | 7 | 1 med-fat meat |
| Colby & Monterey Jack, Shredded | 1 oz | 100 | 8 | 70 | 5 | 0 | 25 | 190 | 1 | 0 | 6 | 1 high-fat meat |
| Colby, Natural | 1 oz | 110 | 9 | 80 | 6 | 0 | 30 | 180 | 1 | 0 | 6 | 1 high-fat meat |
| Cracker Barrel, Spreadable Sharp Cheddar | 2 Tbsp | 80 | 8 | 70 | 5 | 0 | 20 | 180 | <1 | 0 | 3 | 1 high-fat meat |
| Cream Cheese, Neufchatel, Philadelphia | 1 oz | 70 | 6 | 60 | 4 | 0 | 20 | 120 | 1 | 0 | 2 | 1 med-fat meat |
| Cream Cheese, Philadelphia Brick | 1 oz | 100 | 9 | 80 | 6 | 0 | 35 | 105 | 1 | 0 | 2 | 2 fat |
| Cream Cheese, Philadelphia Brick, Fat Free | 1 oz | 30 | 0 | 0 | 0 | 0 | 5 | 200 | 2 | 0 | 4 | 1 lean meat |

| | | | | | | | | | | | | |
|---|---|---|---|---|---|---|---|---|---|---|---|---|
| Cream Cheese, Philadelphia Soft | 2 Tbsp | 90 | 9 | 80 | 5 | 0 | 35 | 125 | 2 | 0 | 2 | 2 fat |
| Cream Cheese, Philadelphia Soft, Cheesecake | 2 Tbsp | 100 | 8 | 70 | 5 | 0 | 30 | 115 | 5 | 0 | 1 | 2 fat |
| Cream Cheese, Philadelphia Soft, Fat Free | 2 Tbsp | 30 | 0 | 0 | 0 | 0 | 5 | 200 | 1 | 0 | 5 | 1 lean meat |
| Cream Cheese, Philadelphia Soft, Honey Nut | 2 Tbsp | 90 | 8 | 70 | 4.5 | 0 | 30 | 110 | 4 | 0 | 1 | 2 fat |
| Cream Cheese, Philadelphia Soft, Light | 2 Tbsp | 70 | 5 | 45 | 3 | 0 | 20 | 140 | 2 | 0 | 2 | 1 fat |
| Cream Cheese, Philadelphia Soft, Pineapple | 2 Tbsp | 90 | 7 | 70 | 4.5 | 0 | 30 | 110 | 4 | 0 | 1 | 1 fat |

| | Serving | Calories | Fat (g) | Cal. from Fat | Sat. Fat (g) | Trans Fat (g) | Chol. (mg) | Sod. (mg) | Carb. (g) | Fiber (g) | Prot. (g) | Servings/Exchanges |
|---|---|---|---|---|---|---|---|---|---|---|---|---|
| Cream Cheese, Philadelphia Soft, Salmon | 2 Tbsp | 90 | 8 | 70 | 5 | 0 | 30 | 210 | 2 | 0 | 2 | 2 fat |
| Cream Cheese, Philadelphia Soft, Strawberry | 2 Tbsp | 90 | 8 | 70 | 4.5 | 0 | 30 | 110 | 5 | 0 | 1 | 2 fat |
| Cream Cheese, Philadelphia Whipped | 2 Tbsp | 60 | 6 | 50 | 3.5 | 0 | 20 | 90 | 1 | 0 | 1 | 1 fat |
| Easy Cheese Cheddar Cheese Snack | 2 Tbsp | 90 | 6 | 60 | 3 | 0 | 20 | 410 | 2 | 0 | 5 | 1 med-fat meat |
| Easy Cheese Cheddar 'n Bacon Cheese Snack | 2 Tbsp | 90 | 7 | 60 | 4.5 | 0 | 25 | 400 | 2 | 0 | 5 | 1 med-fat meat |
| Mexican Four Cheese, Shredded, Natural | 1 oz | 100 | 8 | 70 | 5 | 0 | 25 | 180 | 1 | 0 | 6 | 1 high-fat meat |

| | | | | | | | | | | | | |
|---|---|---|---|---|---|---|---|---|---|---|---|---|
| Mexican Style, 2% Milk Reduced Fat, Natural Crumbles | 1/4 cup | 80 | 5 | 50 | 3 | 0 | 15 | 220 | <1 | 0 | 7 | 1 med-fat meat |
| Monterey Jack & Jalapeño Pepper, Natural | 1 oz | 110 | 9 | 80 | 5 | 0 | 25 | 190 | 1 | 0 | 6 | 1 high-fat meat |
| Monterey Jack, Natural | 1 oz | 110 | 9 | 80 | 6 | 0 | 30 | 190 | 0 | 0 | 6 | 1 high-fat meat |
| Mozzarella, Part-Skim, Natural | 1 oz | 80 | 6 | 50 | 3.5 | 0 | 20 | 220 | 1 | 0 | 7 | 1 med-fat meat |
| Mozzarella, Part-Skim, Shredded | 1 oz | 80 | 4 | 50 | 3.5 | 0 | 20 | 200 | 1 | 0 | 7 | 1 med-fat meat |
| Parmesan, Grated | 2 tsp | 20 | 1.5 | 15 | 1 | 0 | 5 | 85 | 0 | 0 | 2 | free |
| Romano, Grated | 2 tsp | 20 | 1.5 | 15 | 1 | 0 | 5 | 85 | 0 | 0 | 2 | free |
| Singles American, Fat Free | 2/3-oz slice | 45 | 0 | 0 | 0 | 0 | <5 | 250 | 2 | 0 | 4 | 1 lean meat |
| Singles, American | 2/3-oz slice | 60 | 4.5 | 40 | 2.5 | 0 | 15 | 250 | 1 | 0 | 3 | 1 med-fat meat |

## CHEESE, COTTAGE CHEESE, CREAM CHEESE

| | Serving | Calories | Carb. (g) | Fat (g) | % Cal Fat. | Sat. Fat (g) | Trans Fat (g) | Chol (mg) | Sod. (mg) | Fiber (g) | Prot. (g) | Servings/Exchanges |
|---|---|---|---|---|---|---|---|---|---|---|---|---|
| Singles, American, 2% Milk | 2/3-oz slice | 45 | 2.5 | 20 | 1.5 | 0 | 10 | 280 | 2 | 0 | 4 | 1 lean meat |
| Singles, Sharp Cheddar, Fat Free | 2/3-oz slice | 25 | 0 | 0 | 0 | 0 | <5 | 280 | 2 | 0 | 5 | 1 lean meat |
| Singles, Swiss | 2/3-oz slice | 45 | 2.5 | 20 | 1.5 | 0 | 10 | 270 | 2 | 0 | 4 | 1 lean meat |
| Singles, White American | 3/4-oz slice | 60 | 5 | 40 | 2.5 | 0 | 15 | 260 | 2 | 0 | 4 | 1 med-fat meat |
| Smoky Swiss & Cheddar, Natural | 1 oz | 100 | 8 | 70 | 5 | 0 | 25 | 380 | 1 | 0 | 5 | 1 high-fat meat |
| String-Ums 2% Milk String Cheese | 1 oz | 80 | 6 | 50 | 3.5 | 0 | 20 | 220 | 1 | 0 | 7 | 1 med-fat meat |
| Swiss Cheese, Shredded | 1 oz | 110 | 8 | 70 | 5 | 0 | 25 | 60 | 1 | 0 | 7 | 1 high-fat meat |

| | | | | | | | | | | | | |
|---|---|---|---|---|---|---|---|---|---|---|---|---|
| Velveeta Cheese Spread | 1 oz | 80 | 6 | 50 | 4 | 0 | 25 | 410 | 3 | 0 | 5 | 1 med-fat meat |
| Velveeta Cheese Spread, 2% Milk | 1 oz | 60 | 3 | 25 | 1.5 | 0 | 10 | 410 | 4 | 0 | 5 | 1 lean meat |
| Velveeta Cheese Spread, Mexican, Mild or Hot | 1 oz | 90 | 6 | 60 | 4 | 0 | 25 | 430 | 3 | 0 | 5 | 1 med-fat meat |
| ***Lifetime*** | | | | | | | | | | | | |
| Cheddar, Fat Free, Shredded | 1/3 cup | 45 | 0 | 0 | 0 | 0 | <5 | 310 | 2 | 0 | 8 | 1 lean meat |
| Cheddar, Low Fat | 1 oz | 40 | 0 | 0 | 0 | 0 | <5 | 220 | 1 | 1 | 8 | 1 lean meat |
| Sargento Blends | | | | | | | | | | | | |
| Cheddar, Medium, Reduced Fat Slices | 1 slice | 60 | 4 | 35 | 2.5 | 0 | 15 | 135 | 0 | 0 | 6 | 1 med-fat meat |
| Cheddar, Mild, Reduced Fat Shredded | 1/4 cup | 80 | 6 | 50 | 4 | 0 | 20 | 180 | <1 | 0 | 7 | 1 med-fat meat |
| Four Cheese Italian, Reduced Fat Shredded | 1/4 cup | 80 | 4.5 | 40 | 3 | 0 | 15 | 220 | 1 | 0 | 8 | 1 med-fat meat |

CHEESE, COTTAGE CHEESE, CREAM CHEESE

| | Serving | Calories | Fat (g) | Cal. from Fat | Sat. Fat (g) | Trans Fat (g) | Chol. (mg) | Sod. (mg) | Carb. (g) | Fiber (g) | Prot. (g) | Servings/Exchanges |
|---|---|---|---|---|---|---|---|---|---|---|---|---|
| Mozzarella, Light String | 1 piece | 50 | 2.5 | 25 | 1.5 | 0 | 10 | 160 | 1 | 0 | 6 | 1 med-fat meat |
| Swiss, Reduced Fat Slices | 1 slice | 60 | 4 | 35 | 2 | 0 | 10 | 30 | 1 | 0 | 7 | 1 med-fat meat |
| ***Shamrock*** | | | | | | | | | | | | |
| Cottage Cheese, 2% Lowfat | 1/2 cup | 100 | 2 | 20 | 1.5 | 0 | 15 | 440 | 5 | 0 | 13 | 2 lean meat |
| Cottage Cheese, 4% Original | 1/2 cup | 110 | 5 | 45 | 4.5 | 0 | 40 | 370 | 5 | 0 | 13 | 2 lean meat |
| ***Smart Balance*** | | | | | | | | | | | | |
| Cheese Product Shreds | 1 oz | 80 | 5 | 50 | 1.5 | 0 | 5 | 260 | <1 | 0 | 7 | 1 med-fat meat |
| Creamy Cheddar-Flavor Slices | 2/3-oz slice | 40 | 2 | 20 | 0.5 | 0 | <5 | 290 | 2 | 0 | 4 | 1 lean meat |
| Smart Beat Fat Free Slices | 1 slice | 25 | 0 | 0 | 0 | 0 | 0 | 170 | 3 | 0 | 3 | 1 lean meat |

| | Serving | Calories | Fat (g) | Cal. from Fat | Sat. Fat (g) | Trans Fat (g) | Chol. (mg) | Sod. (mg) | Carb. (g) | Fiber (g) | Prot. (g) | Servings/Exchanges |
|---|---|---|---|---|---|---|---|---|---|---|---|---|

# COMBINATION FOODS, ENTRÉES, SALADS

| | Serving | Calories | Fat (g) | Cal. from Fat | Sat. Fat (g) | Trans Fat (g) | Chol. (mg) | Sod. (mg) | Carb. (g) | Fiber (g) | Prot. (g) | Servings/Exchanges |
|---|---|---|---|---|---|---|---|---|---|---|---|---|
| Beef Burgundy | 1 cup | 285 | 11 | 100 | 3 | NA | 91 | 110 | 10 | 2 | 34 | 1/2 carb, 5 lean meat |
| Beef Stroganoff & Noodles | 1 cup | 342 | 20 | 180 | 8 | NA | 73 | 454 | 21 | 2 | 20 | 1 1/2 carb, 2 med-fat meat,2 fat |
| Beef with Macaroni & Tomato Sauce, Homemade | 1 cup | 254 | 10 | 90 | 4 | NA | 39 | 862 | 26 | 3 | 16 | 2 carb, 2 med-fat meat |
| Burrito, Bean | 1 | 224 | 7 | 65 | 4 | NA | 2 | 493 | 36 | 4 | 7 | 2 1/2 carb, 1 fat |
| Burrito, Beef | 1 | 262 | 11 | 100 | 6 | NA | 32 | 746 | 30 | <1 | 13 | 2 carb, 1 med-fat meat, 1 fat |
| Cabbage Rolls, Stuffed | 8 oz | 179 | 6 | 55 | 1 | NA | 11 | 551 | 23 | 4 | 8 | 1 1/2 carb, 1 med-fat meat, 1 fat |
| Chicken & Noodles, Homemade | 1 cup | 367 | 19 | 170 | 6 | NA | 96 | 600 | 26 | 2 | 22 | 2 carb, 2 med-fat meat, 2 fat |

COMBINATION FOODS, ENTRÉES, SALADS

| | Serving | Calories | Fat (g) | Cal. from Fat | Sat. Fat (g) | Trans Fat (g) | Chol. (mg) | Sod. (mg) | Carb. (g) | Fiber (g) | Prot. (g) | Servings/Exchanges |
|---|---|---|---|---|---|---|---|---|---|---|---|---|
| Chicken à la King, Homemade | 1 cup | 468 | 34 | 310 | 13 | NA | 186 | 760 | 12 | 1 | 27 | 1 carb, 3 med-fat meat, 4 fat |
| Chicken Tetrazzini | 1 cup | 372 | 20 | 180 | 7 | NA | 50 | 813 | 28 | 2 | 19 | 2 carb, 2 med-fat meat, 2 fat |
| Chiles Rellenos | 1 | 425 | 35 | 315 | 17 | NA | 165 | 620 | 7 | 1 | 23 | 1/2 carb, 3 med-fat meat, 4 fat |
| Chili Con Carne with Beans & Rice | 1 cup | 297 | 8 | 70 | 4 | NA | 25 | 1162 | 46 | 6 | 11 | 3 carb, 2 fat |
| Chili Con Carne, No Beans | 1 cup | 350 | 19 | 170 | 7 | NA | 81 | 1407 | 21 | 4 | 25 | 1 1/2 carb, 3 med-fat meat, 1 fat |
| Chimichanga, Beef & Bean | 1 | 249 | 12 | 110 | 3 | NA | 24 | 242 | 26 | 3 | 11 | 2 carb, 1 med-fat meat, 1 fat |
| Chop Suey, Beef, with Noodles | 1 cup | 425 | 25 | 225 | 5 | NA | 46 | 818 | 31 | 3 | 22 | 2 carb, 2 med-fat meat, 3 fat |

| | | | | | | | | | | | | |
|---|---|---|---|---|---|---|---|---|---|---|---|---|
| Chop Suey, Shrimp, with Noodles | 1 cup | 277 | 12 | 110 | 2 | NA | 122 | 937 | 22 | 2 | 21 | 1 1/2 carb, 2 med-fat meat |
| Chow Mein, Beef, No Noodles | 1 cup | 275 | 16 | 145 | 4 | NA | 54 | 774 | 12 | 2 | 22 | 1 carb, 3 med-fat meat |
| Chow Mein, Shrimp, with Noodles | 1 cup | 277 | 12 | 110 | 2 | NA | 122 | 937 | 22 | 2 | 21 | 1 1/2 carb, 2 med-fat meat |
| Corndog | 1 | 460 | 19 | 170 | 5 | NA | 79 | 973 | 56 | NA | 17 | 4 carb, 1 med-fat meat, 3 fat |
| Corned Beef Hash, Canned | 1 cup | 398 | 25 | 225 | 12 | NA | 73 | 1188 | 24 | 1 | 19 | 1 1/2 carb, 2 med-fat meat, 3 fat |
| Curry, Beef | 1 cup | 437 | 32 | 290 | 7 | NA | 70 | 1323 | 13 | 3 | 27 | 1 carb, 3 med-fat meat, 3 fat |
| Eggplant Parmesan | 1 cup | 320 | 22 | 200 | 10 | NA | 57 | 683 | 17 | 3 | 15 | 1 carb, 2 med-fat meat, 2 fat |
| Enchilada, Beef & Cheese | 1 | 323 | 18 | 160 | 9 | NA | 40 | 1319 | 31 | NA | 12 | 2 carb, 1 med-fat meat, 3 fat |

COMBINATION FOODS, ENTRÉES, SALADS

| | Serving | Calories | Fat (g) | Cal. from Fat | Sat. Fat (g) | Trans Fat (g) | Chol. (mg) | Sod. (mg) | Carb. (g) | Fiber (g) | Prot. (g) | Servings/Exchanges |
|---|---|---|---|---|---|---|---|---|---|---|---|---|
| Enchilada, Chicken | 1 | 195 | 9 | 80 | 4 | NA | 36 | 312 | 16 | 2 | 13 | 1 carb, 2 med-fat meat |
| Fajita, Chicken | 1 | 405 | 13 | 120 | 3 | NA | 41 | 439 | 50 | 4 | 22 | 3 carb, 2 med-fat meat, 1 fat |
| Goulash, Beef, with Noodles | 1 cup | 341 | 14 | 125 | 4 | NA | 88 | 457 | 23 | 2 | 30 | 1 1/2 carb, 3 med-fat meat |
| Lasagna | 8 oz | 302 | 12 | 110 | NA | NA | 34 | 885 | 27 | NA | 22 | 2 carb, 2 med-fat meat |
| Macaroni & Cheese | 1 cup | 228 | 10 | 90 | 4 | NA | NA | 730 | 26 | NA | 9 | 2 carb, 2 med-fat meat |
| Meat Loaf, Beef & 1/3 Pork | 1 slice | 205 | 14 | 125 | 5 | NA | 84 | 381 | 5 | <1 | 15 | 2 med-fat meat, 1 fat |
| Meat Tamale | 1 | 183 | 10 | 90 | 4 | NA | 24 | 229 | 16 | 3 | 7 | 1 carb, 1 med-fat meat, 1 fat |
| Meat Tortellini | 1 cup | 372 | 15 | 135 | 5 | NA | 238 | 797 | 33 | 1 | 25 | 2 carb, 3 med-fat meat |
| Moo Goo Gai Pan | 1 cup | 281 | 20 | 180 | 5 | NA | 39 | 327 | 12 | 3 | 15 | 2 vegetable, 2 med-fat meat, 2 fat |

| | | | | | | | | | | | | |
|---|---|---|---|---|---|---|---|---|---|---|---|---|
| Pepper, Stuffed Green Bell | 1 | 229 | 12 | 110 | 5 | NA | 34 | 201 | 20 | 2 | 11 | 1 carb, 1 vegetable, 2 med-fat meat, 2 fat |
| Pizza, Cheese, Thin Crust | 1/4 of 10-inch | 317 | 17 | 155 | 7 | NA | 20 | 770 | 28 | NA | 14 | 2 carb, 2 med-fat meat, 1 fat |
| Pizza, Meat, Thin Crust | 1/4 of 10-inch | 368 | 21 | 190 | 7 | NA | 29 | 1000 | 29 | NA | 15 | 2 carb, 2 med-fat meat, 2 fat |
| Pot Pie | 7 oz | 450 | 28 | 250 | NA | NA | 34 | 778 | 35 | NA | 13 | 2 carb, 2 med-fat meat, 4 fat |
| Quesadilla | 1 | 199 | 10 | 90 | 4 | NA | 14 | 255 | 21 | 1 | 6 | 1 1/2 carb, 2 fat |
| Quiche Lorraine | 1/8 pie | 508 | 39 | 350 | 18 | NA | 205 | 549 | 20 | <1 | 20 | 1 carb, 3 med-fat meat, 5 fat |
| Ravioli, Cheese with Tomato Sauce | 1 | 336 | 14 | 125 | 6 | NA | 160 | 1541 | 38 | 2 | 14 | 2 1/2 carb, 1 med-fat meat, 2 fat |
| Salad, Carrot Raisin | 1/2 cup | 202 | 14 | 125 | 2 | NA | 10 | 117 | 21 | 2 | 1 | 1/2 fruit, 2 vegetable, 3 fat |
| Salad, Chef Style | 1 1/2 cup | 267 | 16 | 145 | 8 | NA | 140 | 743 | 5 | NA | 26 | 1 vegetable, 3 med-fat meat |

COMBINATION FOODS, ENTRÉES, SALADS

| | Serving | Calories | Fat (g) | Cal. from Fat | Sat. Fat (g) | Trans Fat (g) | Chol. (mg) | Sod. (mg) | Carb. (g) | Fiber (g) | Prot. (g) | Servings/Exchanges |
|---|---|---|---|---|---|---|---|---|---|---|---|---|
| Salad, Egg | 1/2 cup | 293 | 28 | 250 | 6 | NA | 287 | 333 | 2 | 0 | 8 | 1 med-fat meat, 5 fat |
| Salad, Potato, No Egg | 1/2 cup | 134 | 7 | 65 | 1 | NA | 5 | 345 | 16 | 2 | 2 | 1 carb, 1 fat |
| Salad, Seafood | 1/2 cup | 166 | 12 | 110 | 2 | NA | 64 | 274 | 3 | <1 | 13 | 2 med-fat meat |
| Salad, Shrimp | 1/2 cup | 141 | 9 | 80 | 2 | NA | 103 | 196 | 3 | <1 | 13 | 2 med-fat meat |
| Salad, Three Bean | 1/2 cup | 70 | 4 | 35 | <1 | NA | 0 | 257 | 7 | 2 | 2 | 1/2 carb, 1 fat |
| Salad, Tuna | 1/2 cup | 192 | 10 | 90 | 2 | NA | 13 | 412 | 10 | 0 | 16 | 1/2 carb, 2 med-fat meat |
| Salad, Waldorf | 1/2 cup | 201 | 20 | 180 | 2 | NA | 10 | 118 | 6 | 1 | 2 | 1/2 fruit, 4 fat |
| Salmon Patty or Cake | 4.5 oz | 261 | 16 | 145 | 4 | NA | 57 | 657 | 14 | 1 | 16 | 1 carb, 2 med-fat meat, 1 fat |
| Shepherd's Pie, Beef | 1 cup | 287 | 10 | 90 | 3 | NA | 41 | 702 | 31 | 3 | 18 | 2 carb, 2 med-fat meat |
| Shrimp with Noodles & Cheese Sauce | 1 cup | 350 | 15 | 135 | 6 | NA | 220 | 698 | 24 | 2 | 28 | 1 1/2 carb, 3 med-fat meat |
| Shrimp, Stuffed | 1 cup | 276 | 14 | 125 | 3 | NA | 221 | 694 | 9 | <1 | 28 | 1/2 carb, 4 lean meat |

| | | | | | | | | | | | | |
|---|---|---|---|---|---|---|---|---|---|---|---|---|
| Sloppy Joe Gravy/ Sauce, Beef | 1 cup | 380 | 23 | 205 | 9 | NA | 81 | 1246 | 24 | 3 | 21 | 1 1/2 carb, 2 med-fat meat, 3 fat |
| Soufflé, Cheese, Homemade | 1 cup | 197 | 14 | 125 | 6 | NA | 194 | 299 | 6 | <1 | 12 | 2 med-fat meat, 1 fat |
| Soufflé, Spinach | 1 cup | 219 | 18 | 160 | 7 | NA | 184 | 763 | 3 | 3 | 12 | 2 med-fat meat, 2 fat |
| Spaghetti with Meatballs | 1 cup | 258 | 10 | 90 | 2 | NA | NA | 1220 | 29 | NA | 12 | 2 carb, 2 med-fat meat |
| Sukiyaki | 1 cup | 175 | 8 | 70 | 3 | NA | 154 | 762 | 6 | 1 | 19 | 1/2 carb, 3 lean meat |
| Swedish Meatballs with Cream Sauce | 1 cup | 404 | 23 | 205 | 10 | NA | 162 | 1157 | 17 | <1 | 31 | 1 carb, 4 med-fat meat, 1 fat |
| Sweet & Sour Pork with Rice | 1 cup | 269 | 6 | 55 | 2 | NA | 29 | 906 | 40 | 1 | 13 | 2 1/2 carb, 1 med-fat meat |
| Taco, Chicken | 1 | 173 | 8 | 70 | 3 | NA | 45 | 106 | 9 | 1 | 15 | 1/2 carb, 2 med-fat meat |
| Tostada, Bean & Cheese | 1 | 223 | 10 | 90 | 5 | NA | 30 | 543 | 27 | 7 | 10 | 2 carb, 1 med-fat meat, 1 fat |
| Tostada, Bean & Chicken | 1 | 248 | 11 | 100 | 5 | NA | 53 | 434 | 18 | 3 | 20 | 1 carb, 2 med-fat meat |

COMBINATION FOODS, ENTREES, SALADS

| | Serving | Calories | Fat (g) | Cal. from Fat | Sat. Fat (g) | Trans Fat (g) | Chol. (mg) | Sod. (mg) | Carb. (g) | Fiber (g) | Prot. (g) | Servings/Exchanges |
|---|---|---|---|---|---|---|---|---|---|---|---|---|
| Tuna-Noodle Casserole | 9 oz | 259 | 8 | 70 | NA | NA | NA | 1043 | 34 | NA | 13 | 2 carb, 2 med-fat meat |
| Turkey-Noodle Casserole | 1 cup | 326 | 13 | 115 | 4 | NA | 84 | 732 | 29 | 2 | 23 | 2 carb, 2 med-fat meat, 2 fat |
| Veal Parmigiana | 1 cup | 350 | 20 | 180 | 8 | NA | 138 | 755 | 15 | 1 | 27 | 1 strch, 3 med-fat meat |
| ***Armour LunchMakers*** | | | | | | | | | | | | |
| Cracker Crunchers, Bologna | 1 | 250 | 16 | 140 | 7 | 0 | 35 | 740 | 22 | 1 | 9 | 1 1/2 carb, 1 med-fat meat, 2 fat |
| Loco Nachos | 1 | 400 | 14 | 130 | 3 | 1.5 | 10 | 760 | 69 | 4 | 4 | 4 1/2 carb, 3 fat |
| Pepperoni Pizza | 1 | 370 | 9 | 80 | 5 | 0 | 15 | 530 | 65 | 5 | 8 | 4 carb, 2 fat |
| ***Betty Crocker*** | | | | | | | | | | | | |
| Bowl Appetit! Cheddar Broccoli Pasta | 1 bowl | 310 | 7 | 60 | 2.5 | 1.5 | 10 | 960 | 52 | 2 | 10 | 3 1/2 carb, 1 fat |
| Bowl Appetit! Parmesan Pasta | 1 bowl | 310 | 8 | 70 | 2.5 | 2.5 | <5 | 1010 | 51 | 1 | 9 | 3 1/2 carb, 2 fat |

| | | | | | | | | | | | | |
|---|---|---|---|---|---|---|---|---|---|---|---|---|
| Bowl Appetit! Teriyaki Rice | 1 bowl | 250 | 1 | 5 | 0 | 0 | 0 | 940 | 57 | 2 | 5 | 4 carb |
| Chicken Helper, Cheesy Chicken Enchilada | 1 cup | 330 | 7 | 65 | 2 | 0.5 | 60 | 820 | 42 | <1 | 25 | 3 carb, 2 lean meat |
| Chicken Helper, Chicken Fried Rice | 1 cup | 250 | 9 | 80 | 2 | 0 | 115 | 550 | 22 | 1 | 22 | 1 1/2 carb, 3 lean meat |
| Chicken Helper, Creamy Chicken & Noodles | 1 cup | 280 | 9 | 80 | 2.5 | 1 | 60 | 750 | 24 | <1 | 25 | 1 1/2 carb, 3 lean meat |
| Chicken Helper, Fettuccine Alfredo | 1 cup | 330 | 11 | 100 | 3.5 | 1.5 | 60 | 810 | 31 | 1 | 26 | 2 carb, 3 lean meat |
| Hamburger Helper, Beef Pasta | 1 cup | 280 | 11 | 100 | 4.5 | 0.5 | 55 | 760 | 23 | 1 | 21 | 1 1/2 carb, 2 med-fat meat |
| Hamburger Helper, Cheeseburger Macaroni | 1 cup | 310 | 12 | 110 | 5 | 0 | 60 | 910 | 27 | <1 | 22 | 2 carb, 2 med-fat meat |
| Hamburger Helper, Cheesy Hashbrowns | 1 cup | 400 | 19 | 170 | 6 | 0 | 55 | 990 | 38 | 2 | 20 | 2 1/2 carb, 2 med-fat meat, 2 fat |

COMBINATION FOODS, ENTREES, SALADS

| | Serving | Calories | Fat (g) | Cal. from Fat | Sat. Fat (g) | Trans Fat (g) | Chol. (mg) | Sod. (mg) | Carb. (g) | Fiber (g) | Prot. (g) | Servings/Exchanges |
|---|---|---|---|---|---|---|---|---|---|---|---|---|
| Hamburger Helper, Crunchy Taco | 1 cup | 340 | 14 | 125 | 5 | 1 | 55 | 870 | 33 | 1 | 20 | 2 carb, 2 med-fat meat, 1 fat |
| Hamburger Helper, Double Cheese Enchilada | 1 cup | 350 | 13 | 115 | 5 | 1 | 55 | 840 | 40 | <1 | 21 | 2 1/2 carb, 2 med-fat meat, 1 fat |
| Hamburger Helper, Italian Sausage | 1 cup | 290 | 11 | 100 | 4 | 0.5 | 55 | 860 | 29 | 1 | 20 | 2 carb, 2 med-fat meat |
| Hamburger Helper, Lasagna | 1 cup | 280 | 11 | 100 | 4 | 0.5 | 55 | 900 | 27 | <1 | 19 | 2 carb, 2 med-fat meat |
| Hamburger Helper, Philly Cheesesteak | 1 cup | 320 | 13 | 115 | 5 | 1 | 55 | 750 | 28 | 1 | 22 | 2 carb, 2 med-fat meat, 1 fat |
| Hamburger Helper, Potato Stroganoff | 1 cup | 290 | 14 | 125 | 5 | 1 | 60 | 790 | 26 | 1 | 21 | 2 carb, 2 med-fat meat, 1 fat |
| Hamburger Helper, Tomato Basil Penne | 1 cup | 300 | 11 | 100 | 4 | 1 | 55 | 710 | 26 | 1 | 23 | 2 carb, 3 lean meat |

| | | | | | | | | | | | | |
|---|---|---|---|---|---|---|---|---|---|---|---|---|
| Suddenly Salad, Caesar | 1 cup | 310 | 14 | 130 | 2 | 0 | 0 | 640 | 38 | 1 | 6 | 2 1/2 carb, 3 fat |
| Suddenly Salad, Chipotle Ranch | 1 cup | 290 | 16 | 140 | 2 | 0 | 15 | 450 | 32 | 2 | 6 | 2 carb, 3 fat |
| Suddenly Salad, Ranch & Bacon | 3/4 cup | 290 | 16 | 140 | 2 | 0 | 15 | 450 | 32 | 1 | 6 | 2 carb, 3 fat |
| Tuna Helper, Creamy Broccoli | 1 cup | 290 | 12 | 110 | 3 | 1.5 | 20 | 870 | 34 | 2 | 14 | 2 carb, 1 med-fat meat, 1 fat |
| Tuna Helper, Fettuccine Alfredo | 1 cup | 280 | 12 | 110 | 3.5 | 1.5 | 20 | 970 | 31 | 1 | 13 | 2 carb, 1 med-fat meat, 1 fat |
| Tuna Helper, Tetrazzini | 1 cup | 280 | 11 | 100 | 3 | 0 | 10 | 910 | 31 | 1 | 15 | 2 carb, 2 med-fat meat |
| Tuna Helper, Tuna Melt | 1 cup | 300 | 10 | 90 | 3 | 1.5 | 20 | 1050 | 39 | <1 | 14 | 2 1/2 carb, 1 med-fat meat, 1 fat |
| ***Campbell's SpaghettiOs*** | | | | | | | | | | | | |
| RavioliOs, Beef in Meat Sauce | 1 cup | 270 | 8 | 70 | 3.5 | 0 | 20 | 1090 | 38 | <1 | 11 | 2 1/2 carb, 1 med-fat meat, 1 fat |
| SpaghettiOs Meatballs | 1 cup | 240 | 8 | 70 | 3.5 | 0 | 15 | 600 | 32 | 4 | 11 | 2 carb, 2 fat |

COMBINATION FOODS, ENTREES, SALADS

| | Serving | Calories | Fat (g) | Cal. from Fat | Sat. Fat (g) | Trans Fat (g) | Chol. (mg) | Sod. (mg) | Carb. (g) | Fiber (g) | Prot. (g) | Servings/Exchanges |
|---|---|---|---|---|---|---|---|---|---|---|---|---|
| SpaghettiOs Original | 1 cup | 200 | 1.5 | 15 | 0.5 | 0 | 5 | 950 | 40 | 3 | 7 | 2 1/2 carb |
| SpaghettiOs with Meat Sauce | 1 cup | 180 | 2 | 20 | 1 | 0 | 10 | 890 | 32 | 3 | 8 | 2 carb |
| ***Chef Boyardee*** | | | | | | | | | | | | |
| Beef Ravioli | 1 cup | 240 | 8 | 70 | 3 | 0 | 15 | 900 | 35 | 3 | 8 | 2 carb, 2 fat |
| Beefaroni | 1 cup | 260 | 10 | 90 | 4.5 | 0 | 25 | 990 | 33 | 3 | 10 | 2 carb, 1 med-fat meat, 1 fat |
| Cheese Nacho Twistaroni | 1 cup | 220 | 7 | 60 | 3.5 | 0 | 15 | 950 | 32 | 2 | 8 | 2 carb, 1 fat |
| Lasagna | 1 cup | 270 | 10 | 90 | 5 | 0 | 25 | 830 | 36 | 2 | 9 | 2 1/2 carb, 2 fat |
| Healthy Choice Fresh Mixers | | | | | | | | | | | | |
| Chicken Cacciatore | 1 pkg | 310 | 4 | 35 | 1 | 0 | 30 | 600 | 49 | 6 | 20 | 3 carb, 2 lean meat |
| Sesame Teriyaki Chicken | 1 pkg | 380 | 6 | 50 | 1.5 | 0 | 20 | 600 | 69 | 3 | 13 | 4 1/2 carb, 1 fat |

| | | | | | | | | | | | | |
|---|---|---|---|---|---|---|---|---|---|---|---|---|
| Steak Portobello | 1 pkg | 290 | 6 | 50 | 1.5 | 0 | 15 | 600 | 42 | 5 | 16 | 3 carb, 1 med-fat meat |
| Sweet & Sour Chicken | 1 pkg | 390 | 3 | 25 | 1 | 0 | 25 | 400 | 78 | 5 | 12 | 5 carb, 1 fat |
| Sweet Hickory BBQ Chicken | 1 pkg | 370 | 3 | 25 | 1 | 0 | 35 | 600 | 70 | 5 | 16 | 4 1/2 carb, 1 med-fat meat |
| Tuscan Style Chicken | 1 pkg | 320 | 5 | 45 | 1.5 | 0 | 25 | 540 | 50 | 6 | 18 | 3 carb, 1 med-fat meat |
| ***Hormel*** | | | | | | | | | | | | |
| Hormel Compleats, Beef Pot Roast | 10 oz | 270 | 6 | 55 | 3 | 0 | 50 | 1470 | 29 | 3 | 24 | 2 carb, 3 lean meat |
| Hormel Compleats, Beef Steak Tips | 10 oz | 270 | 9 | 80 | 4 | 0 | 45 | 800 | 29 | 2 | 17 | 2 carb, 2 med-fat meat |
| Hormel Compleats, Chicken & Dumplings | 10 oz | 260 | 8 | 70 | 2 | 0 | 40 | 990 | 34 | 1 | 13 | 2 carb, 1 med-fat meat, 1 fat |
| Hormel Compleats, Chicken & Noodles | 10 oz | 240 | 8 | 70 | 4 | 0 | 60 | 990 | 27 | 2 | 15 | 2 carb, 1 med-fat meat, 1 fat |
| Hormel Compleats, Lasagna | 10 oz | 280 | 7 | 65 | 2 | 0 | 50 | 1100 | 42 | 3 | 13 | 3 carb, 1 med-fat meat |

| | Serving | Calories | Fat (g) | Cal. from Fat | Sat. Fat (g) | Trans Fat (g) | Chol. (mg) | Sod. (mg) | Carb. (g) | Fiber (g) | Prot. (g) | Servings/Exchanges |
|---|---|---|---|---|---|---|---|---|---|---|---|---|
| Microcup Beef Stew | 7.5 oz | 150 | 6 | 55 | 3 | 0 | 25 | 890 | 15 | 2 | 10 | 1 carb, 1 med-fat meat |
| Microcup Spaghetti with Meat Sauce | 7.5 oz | 210 | 5 | 45 | 2.5 | 0 | 15 | 750 | 31 | 3 | 10 | 2 carb, 1 med-fat meat |
| ***Marie Callender's Home-Style Creations*** | | | | | | | | | | | | |
| Classic Stroganoff | 1 pkg | 310 | 10 | 90 | 3.5 | 0 | 35 | 860 | 39 | 3 | 17 | 2 1/2 carb, 1 med-fat meat, 1 fat |
| Creamy Parmesan Chicken | 1 pkg | 490 | 23 | 210 | 10 | 0.5 | 65 | 980 | 43 | 4 | 27 | 3 carb, 3 med-fat meat, 2 fat |
| Garlic Herb Chicken | 1 pkg | 340 | 10 | 90 | 3.5 | 0 | 30 | 960 | 47 | 4 | 16 | 3 carb, 1 med-fat meat, 1 fat |
| Meatball Lasagna | 1 pkg | 310 | 9 | 80 | 3 | 0 | 20 | 760 | 43 | 6 | 14 | 3 carb, 1 med-fat meat, 1 fat |
| ***Oscar Mayer Deli Creations*** | | | | | | | | | | | | |
| Flatbread Sandwich, Chicken Bacon Ranch | 1 pkg | 320 | 13 | 120 | 4.5 | 0 | 55 | 600 | 29 | <1 | 22 | 2 carb, 2 med-fat meat, 1 fat |

| | | | | | | | | | | | | |
|---|---|---|---|---|---|---|---|---|---|---|---|---|
| Hot Sandwich Melts, Ham & Cheddar | 1 pkg | 430 | 16 | 140 | 6 | 0 | 55 | 1540 | 47 | 5 | 28 | 3 carb, 3 med-fat meat |
| Hot Sandwich Melts, Steakhouse Cheddar | 1 pkg | 450 | 16 | 140 | 6 | 0.5 | 60 | 1410 | 51 | 3 | 28 | 3 1/2 carb, 3 med-fat meat |
| Hot Sandwich Melts, Turkey Monterey | 1 pkg | 450 | 17 | 160 | 6 | 0.5 | 55 | 1170 | 51 | 4 | 25 | 3 1/2 carb, 2 med-fat meat, 1 fat |
| ***Oscar Mayer Lunchables*** | | | | | | | | | | | | |
| Lunchables, Chicken Dunks | 1 | 320 | 6 | 50 | 1.5 | 0 | 30 | 550 | 55 | 0 | 12 | 3 1/2 carb, 1 med-fat meat |
| Lunchables, Deep Dish Cheese Pizza | 1 | 370 | 11 | 90 | 3.5 | 0 | 15 | 500 | 60 | 5 | 10 | 4 carb, 2 fat |
| Lunchables, Ham & American Cracker Stackers | 1 | 370 | 16 | 140 | 8 | 0.5 | 35 | 850 | 40 | <1 | 15 | 2 1/2 carb, 1 med-fat meat, 2 fat |
| Lunchables, Mini Hot Dogs | 1 | 380 | 11 | 100 | 3.5 | 0 | 20 | 690 | 62 | 1 | 10 | 4 carb, 2 fat |

COMBINATION FOODS, ENTREES, SALADS

| | Serving | Calories | Fat (g) | Cal. from Fat | Sat. Fat (g) | Trans Fat (g) | Chol. (mg) | Sod. (mg) | Carb. (g) | Fiber (g) | Prot. (g) | Servings/Exchanges |
|---|---|---|---|---|---|---|---|---|---|---|---|---|
| Lunchables, Nachos, Cheese Dip & Salsa | 1 | 380 | 21 | 190 | 6 | 0 | 15 | 880 | 41 | <1 | 7 | 2 1/2 carb, 4 fat |
| Lunchables, Pepperoni Pizza | 1 | 410 | 11 | 100 | 5 | 0 | 30 | 630 | 64 | 3 | 16 | 4 carb, 1 med-fat meat, 1 ft |
| Lunchables, Turkey & Cheddar Cracker Stackers | 1 | 380 | 13 | 110 | 5 | 0.5 | 30 | 780 | 53 | 3 | 13 | 3 1/2 carb, 3 fat |

# COOKING OILS, FATS

| | Serving | Calories | Fat (g) | Cal. from Fat | Sat. Fat (g) | Trans Fat (g) | Chol (mg) | Sod. (mg) | Carb. (g) | Fiber (g) | Prot. (g) | Servings/Exchanges |
|---|---|---|---|---|---|---|---|---|---|---|---|---|
| **Oils** | | | | | | | | | | | | |
| Avocado Oil | 1 tsp | 41 | 4.5 | 40 | <1 | 0 | 0 | 0 | 0 | 0 | 0 | 1 fat |
| Canola Oil | 1 tsp | 40 | 4.5 | 40 | <1 | 0 | 0 | 0 | 0 | 0 | 0 | 1 fat |
| Cocoa Butter Oil | 1 tsp | 40 | 4.5 | 40 | 3 | 0 | 0 | 0 | 0 | 0 | 0 | 1 fat |
| Coconut Oil | 1 tsp | 39 | 4.5 | 40 | 4 | 0 | 0 | 0 | 0 | 0 | 0 | 1 fat |
| Cod Liver/Fish Oil | 1 tsp | 41 | 4.5 | 40 | 1 | 0 | 0 | 0 | 0 | 0 | 0 | 1 fat |
| Corn Oil | 1 tsp | 40 | 4.5 | 40 | <1 | 0 | 0 | 0 | 0 | 0 | 0 | 1 fat |
| Cottonseed Oil | 1 tsp | 40 | 4.5 | 40 | 1 | 0 | 0 | 0 | 0 | 0 | 0 | 1 fat |
| Flaxseed Oil | 1 tsp | 40 | 4.5 | 40 | <1 | 0 | 0 | 0 | 0 | 0 | 0 | 1 fat |
| Grapeseed Oil | 1 tsp | 40 | 4.5 | 40 | <1 | 0 | 0 | 0 | 0 | 0 | 0 | 1 fat |
| Hazelnut Oil | 1 tsp | 40 | 4.5 | 40 | <1 | 0 | 0 | 0 | 0 | 0 | 0 | 1 fat |
| Olive Oil | 1 tsp | 40 | 4.5 | 40 | 0.5 | 0 | 0 | 0 | 0 | 0 | 0 | 1 fat |

| | Serving | Calories | Fat (g) | Cal. from Fat | Sat. Fat (g) | Trans Fat (g) | Chol (mg) | Sod. (mg) | Carb. (g) | Fiber (g) | Prot. (g) | Servings/Exchanges |
|---|---|---|---|---|---|---|---|---|---|---|---|---|
| Palm Kernel Oil | 1 tsp | 39 | 4.5 | 40 | 3.5 | 0 | 0 | 0 | 0 | 0 | 0 | 1 fat |
| Palm Oil | 1 tsp | 40 | 4.5 | 40 | 2 | 0 | 0 | 0 | 0 | 0 | 0 | 1 fat |
| Peanut Oil | 1 tsp | 40 | 4.5 | 40 | 1 | 0 | 0 | 0 | 0 | 0 | 0 | 1 fat |
| Safflower Oil | 1 tsp | 44 | 4.5 | 40 | <1 | 0 | 0 | 0 | 0 | 0 | 0 | 1 fat |
| Sardine/Fish Oil | 1 tsp | 41 | 4.5 | 40 | 1 | 0 | 0 | 32 | 0 | 0 | 0 | 1 fat |
| Sesame Oil | 1 tsp | 40 | 4.5 | 40 | <1 | 0 | 0 | 0 | 0 | 0 | 0 | 1 fat |
| Soybean & Canola Oil | 1 tsp | 40 | 4.5 | 40 | <1 | 0 | 0 | 0 | 0 | 0 | 0 | 1 fat |
| Soybean Oil | 1 tsp | 44 | 4.5 | 40 | <1 | 0 | 0 | 0 | 0 | 0 | 0 | 1 fat |
| Sunflower Oil | 1 tsp | 40 | 4.5 | 40 | <1 | 0 | 0 | 0 | 0 | 0 | 0 | 1 fat |
| **Fats** | | | | | | | | | | | | |
| Chitterlings, Boiled | 2 Tbsp | 38 | 3 | 25 | 1.5 | 0 | 44 | 3 | 0 | 0 | 2 | 1 fat |
| Lard | 1 tsp | 39 | 4 | 35 | 2 | 0 | 4 | 0 | 0 | 0 | 0 | 1 fat |
| Salt Pork, Raw, Cured | .25 oz | 51 | 5 | 45 | 2 | 0 | 6 | 91 | 0 | 0 | <1 | 1 fat |
| Shortening | 1 tsp | 38 | 4 | 35 | 1 | 0 | 0 | 0 | 0 | 0 | 0 | 1 fat |

| | Serving | Calories | Fat (g) | Cal. from Fat | Sat. Fat (g) | Trans Fat (g) | Chol. (mg) | Sod. (mg) | Carb. (g) | Fiber (g) | Prot. (g) | Servings/Exchanges |
|---|---|---|---|---|---|---|---|---|---|---|---|---|

## DESSERTS, CAKE, PIE, CHEESECAKE, COOKIES, BROWNIES

| | Serving | Calories | Fat (g) | Cal. from Fat | Sat. Fat (g) | Trans Fat (g) | Chol. (mg) | Sod. (mg) | Carb. (g) | Fiber (g) | Prot. (g) | Servings/Exchanges |
|---|---|---|---|---|---|---|---|---|---|---|---|---|
| Angel Food Cake | 1 piece | 128 | 0 | 0 | 0 | 0 | 0 | 254 | 29 | <1 | 3 | 2 carb |
| Apple Turnover | 1 | 284 | 16 | 145 | 4 | 0 | 0 | 176 | 31 | 2 | 4 | 2 carb, 3 fat |
| Brownie | 1 small | 115 | 5 | 45 | 1 | 5 | 15 | 88 | 18 | <1 | 1 | 1 carb, 1 fat |
| Cake, Chocolate with Chocolate Icing | 1 piece | 352 | 14 | 125 | 5 | 0 | 55 | 299 | 51 | 2 | 5 | 3 1/2 carb, 3 fat |
| Cake, Frosted | 2-inch square | 175 | 6 | 55 | 2 | 0 | 18 | 194 | 29 | 1 | 2 | 2 carb, 1 fat |
| Cake, Pound with Butter | 1 piece | 109 | 6 | 55 | 3 | 0 | 62 | 111 | 14 | 0 | 2 | 1 carb, 1 fat |
| Cake, Unfrosted | 2-inch square | 97 | 3 | 30 | 1 | 0 | 18 | 168 | 17 | <1 | 2 | 1 carb, 1 fat |
| Cake, White with Vanilla Icing | 1 piece | 239 | 9 | 90 | 2 | 0 | 35 | 220 | 38 | 0 | 2 | 2 1/2 carb, 2 fat |
| Cake, Yellow with Chocolate Icing | 1 piece | 243 | 11 | 100 | 3 | 0 | 35 | 216 | 36 | 1 | 2 | 2 1/2 carb, 2 fat |

DESSERTS, CAKE, PIE, CHEESECAKE, COOKIES, BROWNIES

| | Serving | Calories | Fat (g) | Cal. from Fat | Sat. Fat (g) | Trans Fat (g) | Chol. (mg) | Sod. (mg) | Carb. (g) | Fiber (g) | Prot. (g) | Servings/Exchanges |
|---|---|---|---|---|---|---|---|---|---|---|---|---|
| Cheesecake | 1/12 cake | 271 | 13 | 117 | 7 | 0 | 29 | 376 | 35 | 2 | 5 | 2 carb, 3 fat |
| Cobbler, Apple | 1/2 cup | 225 | 6 | 55 | 1 | 0 | 2 | 109 | 42 | 1 | 3 | 3 carb, 1 fat |
| Cookies, Chocolate Chip | 1 | 78 | 5 | 45 | 1 | 0 | 5 | 58 | 9 | <1 | <1 | 1/2 carb, 1 fat |
| Cookies, Fortune | 2 | 60 | <1 | 0 | <1 | 0 | 2 | 44 | 13 | <1 | <1 | 1 carb |
| Cookies, Gingersnaps | 3 | 87 | 2 | 20 | 0.5 | 0 | 0 | 137 | 16 | <1 | 2 | 1 carb |
| Cookies, Lady Fingers | 4 | 161 | 4 | 35 | 1 | 0 | 161 | 65 | 26 | <1 | 5 | 2 carb, 1 fat |
| Cookies, Macaroons | 1 | 97 | 3 | 30 | 3 | 0 | 0 | 59 | 17 | <1 | 1 | 1 carb, 1 fat |
| Cookies, Oatmeal | 1 | 67 | 3 | 30 | <1 | 0 | 5 | 90 | 10 | NA | 1 | 1/2 carb, 1 fat |
| Cookies, Peanut Butter | 1 | 95 | 5 | 45 | <1 | 0 | 6 | 104 | 12 | NA | 2 | 1 carb, 1 fat |
| Cookies, Sandwich with Creme Filling | 2 | 93 | 4 | 45 | <1 | 1 | 0 | 97 | 14 | <1 | 1 | 1 carb, 1 fat |
| Cookies, Shortbread | 4 | 161 | 8 | 70 | 2 | 0 | 6 | 146 | 21 | <1 | 2 | 1 1/2 carb, 2 fat |
| Cookies, Soft Raisin | 1 | 60 | 2 | 20 | <1 | 0 | <1 | 51 | 10 | <1 | <1 | 1/2 carb |

| | | | | | | | | | | | | |
|---|---|---|---|---|---|---|---|---|---|---|---|---|
| Cookies, Sugar | 1 | 72 | 3 | 30 | 2 | 0 | 8 | 54 | 10 | <1 | <1 | 1/2 carb, 1 fat |
| Cookies, Sugar-free | 3 | 141 | 7 | 65 | 2 | 0 | 0 | 1 | 20 | 2 | 2 | 1 carb, 1 fat |
| Cookies, Vanilla Wafers | 5 | 88 | 3 | 30 | <1 | 0 | 10 | 70 | 15 | <1 | 1 | 1 carb, 1 fat |
| Crisp, Apple | 1/2 cup | 227 | 5 | 45 | 1 | 0 | 0 | 495 | 44 | 2 | 2 | 3 carb, 1 fat |
| Cupcake, Frosted | 1 | 174 | 6 | 65 | 1 | 0 | 8 | 186 | 29 | 0 | 2 | 2 carb, 1 fat |
| Pie, Fruit, 2-Crust | 1/6 | 284 | 13 | 115 | 2 | 0 | 0 | 300 | 42 | 2 | 2 | 3 carb, 3 fat |
| Pie, Pumpkin or Custard | 1/8 | 168 | 8 | 70 | 1 | 0 | 16 | 226 | 22 | 2 | 3 | 1 1/2 carb, 2 fat |
| **CAKE/PIE/CHEESECAKE** | | | | | | | | | | | | |
| ***Betty Crocker*** | | | | | | | | | | | | |
| Angel Food Mix | 1/12 recipe | 140 | 0 | 0 | 0 | 0 | 0 | 310 | 32 | 0 | 2 | 2 carb |
| Brownie Mix, Chocolate Fudge | 1/20 recipe | 170 | 9 | 80 | 1.5 | 0 | 20 | 95 | 23 | 1 | 2 | 1 1/2 carb, 2 fat |
| Brownie Mix, Low-Fat Fudge | 1/16 recipe | 140 | 2.5 | 25 | 1 | 0.5 | 10 | 130 | 28 | 1 | 2 | 2 carb, 1 fat |
| Cake Mix, Super Moist Chocolate Fudge | 1/12 recipe | 260 | 12 | 110 | 2.5 | 0 | 55 | 380 | 35 | 1 | 3 | 2 carb, 2 fat |

DESSERTS, CAKE, PIE, CHEESECAKE, COOKIES, BROWNIES

| | Serving | Calories | Fat (g) | Cal. from Fat | Sat. Fat (g) | Trans Fat (g) | Chol. (mg) | Sod. (mg) | Carb. (g) | Fiber (g) | Prot. (g) | Servings/Exchanges |
|---|---|---|---|---|---|---|---|---|---|---|---|---|
| Cake Mix, Super Moist French Vanilla | 1/12 recipe | 230 | 9 | 80 | 2 | 0 | 55 | 300 | 35 | 0 | 1 | 2 carb, 2 fat |
| Dessert Bar Mix | 1/16 recipe | 140 | 4 | 40 | 1 | 1 | 40 | 90 | 24 | 0 | 2 | 1 1/2 carb, 1 fat |
| Frosting, Rich & Creamy Butter Cream | 2 Tbsp | 140 | 5 | 45 | 1 | 2 | 0 | 70 | 23 | 0 | 0 | 1 1/2 carb, 1 fat |
| Frosting, Rich & Creamy Chocolate | 2 Tbsp | 130 | 5 | 45 | 1.5 | 2 | 0 | 95 | 21 | <1 | 0 | 1 1/2 carb, 1 fat |
| Pound Cake Mix | 1/8 recipe | 260 | 8 | 70 | 3 | 1.5 | 55 | 210 | 45 | 0 | 4 | 3 carb, 2 fat |
| ***Claim Jumper*** | | | | | | | | | | | | |
| Chocolate Motherlode 6-layer Cake | 1 slice | 500 | 24 | 210 | 8 | 2.5 | 45 | 430 | 71 | 2 | 6 | 4 1/2 carb, 5 fat |
| Original Carrot Cake | 1/6 cake | 460 | 25 | 230 | 8 | 2 | 60 | 510 | 54 | 2 | 5 | 3 1/2 carb, 5 fat |

| | | | | | | | | | | | | |
|---|---|---|---|---|---|---|---|---|---|---|---|---|
| ***Comstock*** | | | | | | | | | | | | |
| Pie Filling, Cherry, No Sugar Added | 1/3 cup | 35 | 0 | 0 | 0 | 0 | 0 | 10 | 8 | 0 | 0 | 1/2 carb |
| Pie Filling, Country Cherry | 1/3 cup | 90 | 0 | 0 | 0 | 0 | 0 | 25 | 23 | 1 | 0 | 1 1/2 carb |
| Pie Filling, More Fruit, Apple | 1/3 cup | 80 | 0 | 0 | 0 | 0 | 0 | 40 | 20 | 1 | 0 | 1 carb |
| Pie Filling, More Fruit, Blueberry | 1/3 cup | 100 | 0 | 0 | 0 | 0 | 0 | 10 | 24 | 1 | 0 | 1 1/2 carb |
| Pie Filling, More Fruit, Cherry | 1/3 cup | 100 | 0 | 0 | 0 | 0 | 0 | 15 | 23 | 1 | 0 | 1 1/2 carb |
| Pie Filling, More Fruit, Peach | 1/3 cup | 100 | 0 | 0 | 0 | 0 | 0 | 15 | 26 | 1 | 1 | 2 carb |
| Pie Filling, Premium Strawberry | 1/3 cup | 100 | 0 | 0 | 0 | 0 | 0 | 25 | 23 | 1 | 0 | 1 1/2 carb |
| ***Duncan Hines*** | | | | | | | | | | | | |

DESSERTS, CAKE, PIE, CHEESECAKE, COOKIES, BROWNIES

| | Serving | Calories | Fat (g) | Cal. from Fat | Sat. Fat (g) | Trans Fat (g) | Chol. (mg) | Sod. (mg) | Carb. (g) | Fiber (g) | Prot. (g) | Servings/Exchanges |
|---|---|---|---|---|---|---|---|---|---|---|---|---|
| Whipped Chocolate Frosting | 3 Tbsp | 140 | 7 | 60 | 2 | 1.5 | 0 | 70 | 20 | <1 | <1 | 1 carb, 1 fat |
| Whipped Vanilla Frosting | 3 Tbsp | 150 | 7 | 60 | 2 | 1.5 | 0 | 60 | 22 | 0 | 0 | 1 1/2 carb, 1 fat |
| ***Edwards*** | | | | | | | | | | | | |
| Boston Cream Pie | 1/10 pie | 210 | 10 | 90 | 5 | 0 | 25 | 170 | 31 | <1 | 3 | 2 carb, 2 fat |
| Cookies & Crème | 1/6 pie | 470 | 27 | 240 | 18 | 0 | 10 | 310 | 53 | 2 | 4 | 3 1/2 carb, 5 fat |
| Georgia Pecan Pie | 1/8 pie | 470 | 25 | 220 | 7 | 0 | 80 | 260 | 60 | 2 | 4 | 4 carb, 5 fat |
| Hershey's Crème Pie | 1/6 pie | 450 | 27 | 240 | 17 | 0 | 10 | 330 | 48 | 1 | 5 | 3 carb, 5 fat |
| Key Lime Pie | 1/8 pie | 450 | 22 | 200 | 16 | 0 | 50 | 310 | 57 | <1 | 6 | 4 carb, 4 fat |
| Singles, Apple Pie | 1 | 380 | 20 | 180 | 10 | 0 | 10 | 370 | 47 | 1 | 3 | 3 carb, 4 fat |
| Singles, Hot Fudge Brownie | 1 | 340 | 17 | 150 | 8 | 0 | 20 | 200 | 46 | 2 | 4 | 3 carb, 3 fat |
| Turtle Pie | 1/8 pie | 390 | 22 | 200 | 13 | 1 | 10 | 270 | 46 | 1 | 4 | 3 carb, 4 fat |

| ***Entenmann's*** | | | | | | | | | | | | |
|---|---|---|---|---|---|---|---|---|---|---|---|---|
| All Butter Loaf Cake | 1/6 cake | 220 | 9 | 80 | 5 | 0 | 70 | 270 | 30 | 0 | 3 | 2 carb, 2 fat |
| Banana Crunch Cake | 1/8 cake | 230 | 10 | 90 | 3 | 0 | 30 | 270 | 33 | <1 | 2 | 2 carb, 2 fat |
| Deluxe French Cheesecake | 1/6 cake | 390 | 24 | 220 | 12 | 0 | 40 | 400 | 39 | <1 | 6 | 2 1/2 carb, 5 fat |
| Fudge Chocolate Cake | 1 slice | 270 | 11 | 100 | 4 | 0 | 25 | 230 | 40 | 2 | 3 | 2 1/2 carb, 2 fat |
| Homestyle Apple Pie | 1/6 pie | 380 | 16 | 140 | 8 | 0 | 0 | 400 | 57 | 2 | 3 | 4 carb, 3 fat |
| Lemon Crunch Cake | 1/9 cake | 330 | 14 | 130 | 4 | 0 | 45 | 300 | 49 | <1 | 3 | 3 carb, 3 fat |
| Louisana Crunch Cake | 1 slice | 330 | 14 | 130 | 4 | 0 | 45 | 300 | 49 | <1 | 3 | 3 carb, 3 fat |
| Marble Loaf Cake | 1/8 cake | 180 | 8 | 70 | 2 | 0 | 35 | 240 | 26 | <1 | 2 | 2 carb, 2 fat |
| ***Hostess*** | | | | | | | | | | | | |
| Ding Dongs | 2 | 360 | 19 | 170 | 13 | 0 | 10 | 230 | 47 | 1 | 2 | 3 carb, 4 fat |
| Ho Ho's | 3 | 370 | 17 | 150 | 13 | 0 | 30 | 220 | 54 | 1 | 2 | 3 1/2 carb, 3 fat |
| Twinkies | 1 | 150 | 4.5 | 40 | 2.5 | 0 | 20 | 220 | 27 | 0 | 1 | 2 carb, 1 fat |
| ***Little Debbie*** | | | | | | | | | | | | |
| Chocolate Cupcakes | 1 | 210 | 8 | 70 | 2 | 0 | 30 | 170 | 33 | <1 | 2 | 2 carb, 2 fat |

DESSERTS, CAKE, PIE, CHEESECAKE, COOKIES, BROWNIES

| | Serving | Calories | Fat (g) | Cal. from Fat | Sat. Fat (g) | Trans Fat (g) | Chol. (mg) | Sod. (mg) | Carb. (g) | Fiber (g) | Prot. (g) | Servings/Exchanges |
|---|---|---|---|---|---|---|---|---|---|---|---|---|
| Chocolate Marshmallow Pie | 1 | 180 | 7 | 60 | 4 | 0 | 0 | 105 | 28 | 0 | 2 | 2 carb, 1 fat |
| Devil Squares | 2 | 260 | 11 | 100 | 6 | 0 | 0 | 160 | 38 | 1 | 2 | 2 1/2 carb, 2 fat |
| ***Marie Callender's*** | | | | | | | | | | | | |
| Apple Crumb Cobbler | 1/8 pie | 330 | 17 | 150 | 4 | 4.5 | 0 | 160 | 44 | 1 | 2 | 3 carb, 3 fat |
| Banana Cream Pie | 1/10 pie | 290 | 17 | 150 | 8 | 2 | 40 | 210 | 30 | <1 | 3 | 2 carb, 3 fat |
| Cherry Crunch Pie | 1/10 pie | 350 | 15 | 140 | 3.5 | 4.5 | 0 | 250 | 51 | 1 | 2 | 3 1/2 carb, 3 fat |
| Chocolate Satin Pie | 1/8 pie | 410 | 29 | 260 | 14 | 4.5 | 50 | 200 | 36 | 2 | 4 | 2 1/2 carb, 6 fat |
| Coconut Cream Pie | 1/10 pie | 310 | 18 | 170 | 10 | 2 | 35 | 220 | 32 | <1 | 3 | 2 carb, 4 fat |
| Dutch Apple Pie | 1/10 pie | 320 | 15 | 130 | 3.5 | 4 | 0 | 170 | 47 | 2 | 2 | 3 carb, 3 fat |
| I Love Chocolate Cream Pie | 1/8 pie | 350 | 19 | 170 | 9 | 2 | 40 | 190 | 42 | 2 | 4 | 3 carb, 4 fat |
| Lattice Apple Pie | 1/10 pie | 330 | 18 | 160 | 4 | 5 | 0 | 160 | 42 | 2 | 2 | 3 carb, 4 fat |
| Lattice Peach Pie | 1/10 pie | 330 | 18 | 160 | 4 | 5 | 0 | 140 | 38 | 0 | 3 | 2 1/2 carb, 4 fat |

| | | | | | | | | | | | | |
|---|---|---|---|---|---|---|---|---|---|---|---|---|
| Lemon Meringue Pie | 1/10 pie | 260 | 9 | 80 | 2.5 | 2 | 40 | 190 | 44 | <1 | 2 | 3 carb, 2 fat |
| Peach Cobbler | 1/8 pie | 330 | 19 | 170 | 4 | 5 | 0 | 160 | 38 | 1 | 3 | 2 1/2 carb, 4 fat |
| Razzleberry Pie | 1/9 pie | 360 | 18 | 160 | 4 | 4.5 | 0 | 300 | 47 | 2 | 3 | 3 carb, 4 fat |
| Turtle Pie | 1/8 pie | 400 | 27 | 240 | 11 | 4.5 | 40 | 210 | 39 | 2 | 4 | 2 1/2 carb, 5 fat |
| ***Pepperidge Farm*** | | | | | | | | | | | | |
| Apple Turnover | 1 | 270 | 15 | 135 | 8 | 0 | 0 | 230 | 31 | 1 | 4 | 2 carb, 3 fat |
| Cherry Turnover | 1 | 270 | 15 | 135 | 8 | 0 | 0 | 230 | 31 | 1 | 4 | 2 carb, 3 fat |
| Chocolate Fudge 3-Layer Cake | 1/8 cake | 230 | 10 | 90 | 2 | 1.5 | 20 | 130 | 33 | 1 | 2 | 2 carb, 2 fat |
| Coconut 3-Layer Cake | 1/8 cake | 240 | 10 | 90 | 3 | 1.5 | 20 | 120 | 35 | <1 | 2 | 2 carb, 2 fat |
| Devil's Food Cake | 1/8 cake | 220 | 9 | 80 | 2 | 1.5 | 20 | 170 | 34 | <1 | 2 | 2 carb, 2 fat |
| German Chocolate Cake | 1/8 cake | 240 | 10 | 90 | 3 | 2 | 15 | 200 | 34 | <1 | 2 | 2 carb, 2 fat |
| ***Pillsbury*** | | | | | | | | | | | | |
| Frosting, Chocolate Fudge | 2 Tbsp | 140 | 6 | 50 | 1.5 | 2 | 0 | 90 | 21 | <1 | 0 | 1 1/2 carb, 1 fat |
| Frosting, Vanilla | 2 Tbsp | 150 | 6 | 50 | 1.5 | 2 | 0 | 70 | 24 | 0 | 0 | 1 1/2 carb, 1 fat |

DESSERTS, CAKE, PIE, CHEESECAKE, COOKIES, BROWNIES

| | Serving | Calories | Fat (g) | Cal. from Fat | Sat. Fat (g) | Trans Fat (g) | Chol. (mg) | Sod. (mg) | Carb. (g) | Fiber (g) | Prot. (g) | Servings/Exchanges |
|---|---|---|---|---|---|---|---|---|---|---|---|---|
| Sweet Moments Caramel Pecan Crumble | 1 | 390 | 21 | 190 | 9 | 0.5 | 40 | 190 | 46 | 1 | 4 | 3 carb, 4 fat |
| ***Sara Lee*** | | | | | | | | | | | | |
| All Butter Pound Cake | 1/4 cake | 300 | 16 | 140 | 9 | 0 | 110 | 220 | 35 | <1 | 4 | 2 carb, 3 fat |
| Apple Pie | 1/8 pie | 340 | 16 | 140 | 7 | 0 | 0 | 330 | 47 | 2 | 3 | 3 carb, 3 fat |
| Blueberry Pie | 1/6 pie | 350 | 16 | 150 | 7 | 0 | 0 | 350 | 50 | 2 | 3 | 3 carb, 3 fat |
| Cherry Pie | 1/8 pie | 340 | 16 | 150 | 7 | 0 | 0 | 350 | 45 | 2 | 3 | 3 carb, 3 fat |
| Chocolate Dream Pie | 1/8 pie | 420 | 24 | 220 | 12 | 3.5 | 0 | 270 | 47 | 2 | 4 | 3 carb, 5 fat |
| Cinnamon French Apple Pie | 1/10 pie | 330 | 13 | 120 | 6 | 0 | 0 | 250 | 51 | 2 | 2 | 3 1/2 carb, 3 fat |
| Crumb Coffee Cake | 1/6 cake | 190 | 9 | 80 | 5 | 0.5 | 40 | 200 | 24 | <1 | 3 | 1 1/2 carb, 2 fat |
| Dutch Apple Pie | 1/8 pie | 340 | 14 | 130 | 6 | 0 | 0 | 290 | 52 | 2 | 3 | 3 1/2 carb, 3 fat |
| French Cheesecake | 1/5 cake | 410 | 26 | 230 | 13 | 2.5 | 20 | 250 | 39 | 0 | 5 | 2 1/2 carb, 5 fat |

| | | | | | | | | | | | | |
|---|---|---|---|---|---|---|---|---|---|---|---|---|
| Fruits of the Forest Deep Dish Pie | 1/9 pie | 350 | 19 | 180 | 8 | 0 | 0 | 310 | 42 | 2 | 3 | 3 carb, 4 fat |
| Original Cheesecake Bites | 25 | 440 | 27 | 240 | 13 | 0.5 | 60 | 390 | 44 | 1 | 7 | 3 carb, 5 fat |
| Original Cheesecake | 1/4 cake | 320 | 17 | 150 | 8 | 2 | 70 | 250 | 36 | <1 | 7 | 2 1/2 carb, 3 fat |
| Pumpkin Pie | 1/8 pie | 260 | 10 | 90 | 4 | 0 | 40 | 320 | 39 | 2 | 4 | 2 1/2 carb, 2 fat |
| Southern Pecan Pie | 1 piece | 470 | 23 | 210 | 8 | 2 | 75 | 440 | 62 | 2 | 5 | 4 carb, 5 fat |
| ***Weight Watchers Smart Ones*** | | | | | | | | | | | | |
| Brownie à La Mode | 1 | 200 | 2.5 | 35 | 2.5 | 0 | 25 | 160 | 36 | 3 | 5 | 2 1/2 carb, 1 fat |
| Chocolate Chip Cookie Dough Sundae | 1 | 170 | 3 | 30 | 1.5 | 0 | 5 | 100 | 32 | 1 | 3 | 2 carb, 1 fat |
| Chocolate Éclair | 1 | 140 | 4 | 35 | 1 | 0 | 30 | 180 | 24 | 1 | 3 | 1 1/2 carb, 1 fat |
| Chocolate Mousse | 1 | 180 | 4 | 40 | 3.5 | 0 | <5 | 100 | 28 | 3 | 7 | 2 carb, 1 fat |
| Key Lime Pie | 1 | 190 | 4.5 | 40 | 2 | 0 | 10 | 85 | 33 | <1 | 4 | 2 carb, 1 fat |
| **COOKIES/BROWNIES** | | | | | | | | | | | | |
| ***Archway*** | | | | | | | | | | | | |

DESSERTS, CAKE, PIE, CHEESECAKE, COOKIES, BROWNIES

| | Serving | Calories | Fat (g) | Cal. from Fat | Sat. Fat (g) | Trans Fat (g) | Chol. (mg) | Sod. (mg) | Carb. (g) | Fiber (g) | Prot. (g) | Servings/Exchanges |
|---|---|---|---|---|---|---|---|---|---|---|---|---|
| Coconut Macaroon | 2 | 160 | 8 | 70 | 7 | 0 | 0 | 85 | 22 | 2 | 1 | 1 1/2 carb, 2 fat |
| Date Oatmeal | 1 | 90 | 3 | 25 | 0.5 | 1 | 0 | 75 | 16 | 0 | 1 | 1 carb, 1 fat |
| Frosted Lemon | 1 | 110 | 4.5 | 40 | 1.5 | 1 | 0 | 105 | 18 | 0 | 1 | 1 carb, 1 fat |
| Ginger Snap | 4 | 140 | 5 | 45 | 1 | 0 | 0 | 105 | 22 | 0 | 1 | 1 1/2 carb, 1 fat |
| Ginger Snap, Reduced Fat | 4 | 130 | 3.5 | 30 | 1 | 0 | 0 | 125 | 23 | 0 | 1 | 1 1/2 carb, 1 fat |
| Iced Oatmeal | 1 | 110 | 4.5 | 40 | 1 | 1 | <5 | 100 | 17 | <1 | 1 | 1 carb, 1 fat |
| Oatmeal | 1 | 110 | 4 | 35 | 1 | 1 | <5 | 105 | 18 | <1 | 1 | 1 carb, 1 fat |
| Windmill | 2 | 160 | 6 | 50 | 1.5 | 1.5 | 0 | 160 | 25 | <1 | 2 | 1 1/2 carb, 1 fat |
| ***Duncan Hines*** | | | | | | | | | | | | |
| Oven Ready! Homestyle Brownies | 1/12 pan | 170 | 8 | 70 | 2 | 1 | 20 | 85 | 23 | <1 | 2 | 1 1/2 carb, 2 fat |
| ***Estee*** | | | | | | | | | | | | |
| Chocolate Chip | 4 | 150 | 7 | 63 | 2 | 0 | 0 | 30 | 21 | 0 | 2 | 1 1/2 carb, 1 fat |

| | | | | | | | | | | | | |
|---|---|---|---|---|---|---|---|---|---|---|---|---|
| Coconut | 4 | 140 | 6 | 54 | 2 | 0 | 0 | 25 | 19 | 0 | 2 | 1 carb, 1 fat |
| Fudge | 4 | 150 | 7 | 63 | 1 | 0 | 0 | 45 | 19 | 0 | 2 | 1 carb, 1 fat |
| Lemon | 4 | 140 | 6 | 54 | 0 | 0 | 0 | 25 | 19 | 0 | 2 | 1 carb, 1 fat |
| Oatmeal Raisin | 4 | 130 | 5 | 45 | 1 | 0 | 0 | 25 | 19 | 1 | 2 | 1 carb, 1 fat |
| Shortbread | 4 | 130 | 4 | 36 | 1 | 0 | 0 | 150 | 22 | 0 | 2 | 1 1/2 carb, 1 fat |
| Vanilla Sandwich | 3 | 160 | 5 | 45 | 1 | 0 | 0 | 35 | 35 | 0 | 2 | 2 carb, 1 fat |
| Sugar Free Vanilla Crème Wafers | 5 | 155 | 8 | 72 | 2 | 0 | 0 | 10 | 21 | 0 | 1 | 1 1/2 carb, 2 fat |
| ***Famous Amos*** | | | | | | | | | | | | |
| Chocolate Chip | 4 | 150 | 7 | 60 | 3 | 0 | <5 | 105 | 20 | <1 | 1 | 1 1/2 carb, 1 fat |
| Chocolate Chip & Pecans | 4 | 150 | 8 | 70 | 3 | 0 | 0 | 95 | 18 | 1 | 2 | 1 carb, 2 fat |
| Fifty50 | | | | | | | | | | | | |
| Butter | 4 | 190 | 9 | 80 | 6 | 0 | 30 | 50 | 24 | <1 | 2 | 1 1/2 carb, 2 fat |
| Chocolate Chip | 4 | 170 | 9 | 80 | 2.5 | 0 | 0 | 35 | 22 | 1 | 2 | 1 1/2 carb, 2 fat |
| Hearty Oatmeal | 4 | 160 | 7 | 60 | 1.5 | 0 | 0 | 60 | 24 | 1 | 2 | 1 1/2 carb, 1 fat |

DESSERTS, CAKE, PIE, CHEESECAKE, COOKIES, BROWNIES

| | Serving | Calories | Fat (g) | Cal. from Fat | Sat. Fat (g) | Trans Fat (g) | Chol. (mg) | Sod. (mg) | Carb. (g) | Fiber (g) | Prot. (g) | Servings/Exchanges |
|---|---|---|---|---|---|---|---|---|---|---|---|---|
| Sugar Free Vanilla Crème Wafers | 6 | 160 | 9 | 80 | 4 | 0 | 0 | 30 | 22 | 0 | 1 | 1 1/2 carb, 2 fat |
| ***Girl Scout*** | | | | | | | | | | | | |
| Do-Si-Dos | 2 | 120 | 5 | 45 | 1.5 | 0 | 0 | 75 | 16 | <1 | 2 | 1 carb, 1 fat |
| Lemon Chalet Cremes | 3 | 170 | 7 | 60 | 2.5 | 0 | 0 | 95 | 26 | <1 | 1 | 2 carb, 1 fat |
| Peanut Butter Patties or Tagalongs | 2 | 140 | 9 | 80 | 5 | 0 | 0 | 95 | 13 | <1 | 2 | 1 carb, 2 fat |
| Samoas | 2 | 150 | 8 | 70 | 6 | 0 | 0 | 50 | 18 | <1 | 1 | 1 carb, 2 fat |
| Sugar Free Chocolate Chip | 3 | 160 | 9 | 80 | 3 | 0 | 0 | 140 | 22 | 2 | 1 | 1 1/2 carb, 2 fat |
| Thin Mints | 4 | 160 | 8 | 70 | 5 | 0 | 0 | 115 | 22 | <1 | 1 | 1 1/2 carb, 2 fat |
| Trefoils | 5 | 170 | 8 | 70 | 2.5 | 0 | 0 | 115 | 23 | <1 | 2 | 1 1/2 carb, 2 fat |
| ***Health Valley Organic*** | | | | | | | | | | | | |
| Mini Chocolate Chip | 4 | 120 | 6 | 60 | 2 | 0 | 5 | 125 | 16 | 1 | 1 | 1 carb, 1 fat |

| | | | | | | | | | | | | |
|---|---|---|---|---|---|---|---|---|---|---|---|---|
| Oatmeal Raisin | 1 | 90 | 3.5 | 30 | 0 | 0 | 0 | 50 | 14 | 1 | 2 | 1 carb, 1 fat |
| Vanilla Sandwich Cremes | 2 | 130 | 5 | 45 | 3 | 0 | 0 | 110 | 20 | 0 | 1 | 1 carb, 1 fat |
| ***Kashi*** | | | | | | | | | | | | |
| Happy Trail Cookies | 1 | 130 | 5 | 45 | 1 | 0 | 0 | 80 | 21 | 4 | 2 | 1 1/2 carb, 1 fat |
| Oatmeal Dark Chocolate | 1 | 130 | 5 | 45 | 1.5 | 0 | 0 | 70 | 21 | 3 | 2 | 1 1/2 carb, 1 fat |
| Oatmeal Raisin Flax | 1 | 130 | 5 | 45 | 0.5 | 0 | 0 | 75 | 20 | 4 | 2 | 1 carb, 1 fat |
| ***Keebler*** | | | | | | | | | | | | |
| Chips Deluxe Chocolate Lovers | 1 | 80 | 4.5 | 65 | 2 | 0 | 0 | 65 | 10 | <1 | <1 | 1/2 carb, 1 fat |
| Chips Deluxe Chocolate Peanut Butter | 1 | 80 | 4.5 | 40 | 2 | 0 | 0 | 65 | 10 | <1 | 1 | 1/2 carb, 1 fat |
| Chips Deluxe Coconut | 2 | 160 | 9 | 80 | 4.5 | 0 | 0 | 85 | 18 | 1 | 2 | 1 carb, 2 fat |
| Chips Deluxe Original | 2 | 170 | 9 | 80 | 3.5 | 0 | <5 | 105 | 19 | <1 | 2 | 1 carb, 2 fat |
| Chips Deluxe Soft 'N Chewy | 1 | 80 | 4.5 | 30 | 1.5 | 0 | 0 | 55 | 11 | <1 | <1 | 1 carb, 1 fat |

DESSERTS, CAKE, PIE, CHEESECAKE, COOKIES, BROWNIES

| | Serving | Calories | Fat (g) | Cal. from Fat | Sat. Fat (g) | Trans Fat (g) | Chol. (mg) | Sod. (mg) | Carb. (g) | Fiber (g) | Prot. (g) | Servings/Exchanges |
|---|---|---|---|---|---|---|---|---|---|---|---|---|
| E.L. Fudge Double Stuffed | 2 | 180 | 9 | 80 | 3.5 | 0 | <5 | 95 | 24 | 1 | 2 | 1 1/2 carb, 2 fat |
| E.L. Fudge Fudge Original | 1 | 90 | 3.5 | 30 | 1.5 | 0 | 5 | 50 | 13 | <1 | 1 | 1 carb, 1 fat |
| Fudge Shoppe Deluxe Grahams | 3 | 140 | 7 | 60 | 4.5 | 1.5 | 0 | 70 | 17 | <1 | 1 | 1 carb, 1 fat |
| Fudge Shoppe Fudge Sticks | 3 | 150 | 8 | 70 | 5 | 0 | 0 | 30 | 20 | 0 | <1 | 1 carb, 2 fat |
| Fudge Shoppe Fudge Stripes | 3 | 150 | 7 | 60 | 4.5 | 0 | 0 | 110 | 21 | <1 | 1 | 1 1/2 carb, 2 fat |
| Fudge Shoppe Grasshopper | 4 | 140 | 7 | 60 | 4.5 | 1.5 | 0 | 75 | 19 | <1 | 1 | 1 carb, 1 fat |
| Sandies Fudge Drops | 4 | 140 | 7 | 60 | 3.5 | 0 | 0 | 60 | 18 | <1 | 1 | 1 carb, 1 fat |
| Sandies Pecan Shortbread | 2 | 160 | 10 | 90 | 3 | 0 | <5 | 105 | 18 | <1 | 1 | 1 carb, 2 fat |

| | | | | | | | | | | | | |
|---|---|---|---|---|---|---|---|---|---|---|---|---|
| Sandies Simply Shortbread | 2 | 160 | 9 | 80 | 4 | 0 | 15 | 90 | 19 | 0 | 2 | 1 carb, 2 fat |
| Soft Batch Chocolate Chip | 1 | 80 | 3.5 | 30 | 1.5 | 0 | 0 | 55 | 11 | <1 | <1 | 1 carb, 1 fat |
| Soft Batch Peanut Butter | 1 | 80 | 3.5 | 30 | 1.5 | 0 | 0 | 50 | 10 | 0 | <1 | 1/2 carb, 1 fat |
| Vienna Fingers | 2 | 150 | 6 | 50 | 2 | 0 | 0 | 95 | 23 | <1 | 1 | 1 1/2 carb, 1 fat |
| Vienna Fingers Reduced Fat | 2 | 140 | 4.5 | 40 | 1.5 | 0 | 0 | 115 | 24 | <1 | 1 | 1 1/2 carb, 1 fat |
| ***Little Debbie*** | | | | | | | | | | | | |
| Oatmeal Creme Pie | 1 | 170 | 7 | 60 | 2 | 0 | 0 | 170 | 26 | <1 | 1 | 2 carb, 1 fat |
| ***Mother's*** | | | | | | | | | | | | |
| Chocolate Chip | 2 | 160 | 7 | 60 | 2 | 1 | <5 | 150 | 22 | <1 | 2 | 1 1/2 carb, 1 fat |
| Circus Animal | 6 | 150 | 7 | 70 | 7 | 0 | 0 | 60 | 20 | <1 | 1 | 1 carb, 1 fat |
| Coconut Cocadas | 5 | 160 | 8 | 70 | 3.5 | 1.5 | <5 | 140 | 21 | 1 | 2 | 1 1/2 carb, 2 fat |
| Double Fudge | 2 | 170 | 7 | 60 | 2.5 | 2 | 0 | 95 | 27 | 1 | 2 | 2 carb, 1 fat |

DESSERTS, CAKE, PIE, CHEESECAKE, COOKIES, BROWNIES

| | Serving | Calories | Fat (g) | Cal. from Fat | Sat. Fat (g) | Trans Fat (g) | Chol. (mg) | Sod. (mg) | Carb. (g) | Fiber (g) | Prot. (g) | Servings/Exchanges |
|---|---|---|---|---|---|---|---|---|---|---|---|---|
| English Tea | 2 | 180 | 7 | 60 | 2.5 | 2 | 0 | 100 | 27 | <1 | 2 | 2 carb, 1 fat |
| Iced Lemonade | 4 | 140 | 7 | 60 | 1.5 | 0 | 0 | 75 | 19 | <1 | 1 | 1 carb, 1 fat |
| Iced Oatmeal | 4 | 130 | 5 | 45 | 1 | 0 | 0 | 135 | 20 | <1 | 1 | 1 1/2 carb, 1 fat |
| Macaroons | 2 | 170 | 11 | 100 | 5 | 2 | 0 | 90 | 17 | 1 | 2 | 1 carb, 2 fat |
| Oatmeal | 2 | 130 | 5 | 45 | 1 | 1.5 | 0 | 170 | 19 | <1 | 2 | 1 carb, 1 fat |
| Taffy Sandwich | 2 | 180 | 8 | 70 | 4 | 1.5 | 0 | 125 | 27 | <1 | 1 | 2 carb, 2 fat |
| Vanilla Crèmes | 2 | 180 | 7 | 70 | 3 | 2 | 0 | 105 | 26 | <1 | 2 | 2 carb, 1 fat |
| Murray Sugar Free | | | | | | | | | | | | |
| Chocolate Chip | 3 | 160 | 9 | 80 | 3.5 | 0 | <5 | 130 | 20 | 1 | 2 | 1 carb, 2 fat |
| Chocolate Sandwich Creme | 3 | 130 | 7 | 60 | 2.5 | 0 | 0 | 55 | 19 | 1 | 1 | 1 carb, 1 fat |
| Fudge Dipped Grahams | 4 | 150 | 8 | 70 | 6 | 0 | 0 | 80 | 19 | 1 | 2 | 1 carb, 2 fat |
| Oatmeal | 3 | 140 | 7 | 60 | 2.5 | 0 | 0 | 130 | 21 | 3 | 2 | 1 1/2 carb, 1 fat |
| Peanut Butter | 3 | 150 | 9 | 80 | 2.5 | 0 | <5 | 130 | 16 | 1 | 3 | 1 carb, 2 fat |

| | | | | | | | | | | | | |
|---|---|---|---|---|---|---|---|---|---|---|---|---|
| Shortbread | 8 | 130 | 5 | 45 | 1.5 | 0 | 0 | 140 | 21 | 2 | 2 | 1 1/2 carb, 1 fat |
| Vanilla Sandwich Creme | 3 | 130 | 6 | 60 | 2 | 0 | 0 | 55 | 20 | <1 | 1 | 1 carb, 1 fat |
| Vanilla Sugar Wafer | 9 | 130 | 5 | 50 | 1.5 | 0 | 0 | 90 | 24 | 2 | 2 | 1 1/2 carb, 1 fat |
| ***Nabisco*** | | | | | | | | | | | | |
| Barnum's Animals | 8 | 120 | 3.5 | 30 | 1 | 0 | 0 | 140 | 22 | 1 | 2 | 1 1/2 carb, 1 fat |
| Biscos Sugar Wafers | 8 | 140 | 6 | 50 | 2.5 | 0 | 0 | 25 | 21 | 0 | <1 | 1 1/2 carb, 1 fat |
| Cameo Creme Sandwich | 1 oz | 130 | 5 | 40 | 1 | 0 | 0 | 105 | 21 | 0 | 1 | 1 1/2 carb, 1 fat |
| Chips Ahoy! Chewy | 2 | 120 | 6 | 50 | 3 | 0 | 0 | 80 | 18 | 1 | 1 | 1 carb, 1 fat |
| Chips Ahoy! Chocolate Chip | 3 | 160 | 8 | 70 | 2.5 | 0 | 0 | 105 | 21 | 1 | 2 | 1 1/2 carb, 2 fat |
| Chips Ahoy! Chunky Chocolate | 1 | 80 | 4.5 | 40 | 1.5 | 0 | 0 | 55 | 11 | 1 | 1 | 1 carb, 1 fat |
| Chips Ahoy! Chunky White Fudge | 1 | 90 | 4.5 | 40 | 1.5 | 0 | 0 | 60 | 11 | 0 | 2 | 1 carb, 1 fat |
| Chips Ahoy! Peanut Butter Chunky | 1 | 90 | 5 | 45 | 2.5 | 0 | 0 | 75 | 10 | 0 | 1 | 1/2 carb, 1 fat |

DESSERTS, CAKE, PIE, CHEESECAKE, COOKIES, BROWNIES

| | Serving | Calories | Fat (g) | Cal. from Fat | Sat. Fat (g) | Trans Fat (g) | Chol. (mg) | Sod. (mg) | Carb. (g) | Fiber (g) | Prot. (g) | Servings/Exchanges |
|---|---|---|---|---|---|---|---|---|---|---|---|---|
| Chips Ahoy! White Fudge Chewy | 1 | 120 | 5 | 50 | 3 | 0 | 0 | 120 | 18 | 1 | 1 | 1 carb, 1 fat |
| Ginger Snaps | 4 | 120 | 2.5 | 20 | 0 | 0 | 0 | 190 | 23 | 0 | 11 | 1/2 carb, 1 fat |
| Lorna Doone Shortbread | 4 | 140 | 7 | 60 | 2 | 0 | 0 | 150 | 20 | 0 | 1 | 1 carb, 1 fat |
| Mallomars | 2 | 120 | 5 | 45 | 3 | 0 | 0 | 40 | 18 | 1 | 1 | 1 carb, 1 fat |
| Newtons, Fig | 2 | 110 | 2 | 20 | 0 | 0 | 0 | 125 | 22 | 1 | 1 | 1 1/2 carb |
| Newtons, Fig, 100% Whole Grain | 1 oz | 110 | 2 | 20 | 0 | 0 | 0 | 115 | 21 | 2 | 1 | 1 1/2 carb |
| Newtons, Fig, Fat Free | 2 | 90 | 0 | 0 | 0 | 0 | 0 | 125 | 22 | 1 | 1 | 1 1/2 carb |
| Newtons, Fruit Crisps, Apple Cinnamon | 2 pieces | 100 | 2 | 15 | 0 | 0 | 0 | 90 | 20 | 0 | <1 | 1 carb |
| Newtons, Minis | 1 pkg | 130 | 3 | 30 | 0.5 | 0 | 0 | 140 | 26 | 2 | 2 | 2 carb, 1 fat |
| Newtons, Raspberry | 2 | 100 | 1.5 | 15 | 0 | 0 | 0 | 110 | 21 | 0 | 1 | 1 1/2 carb |

| | | | | | | | | | | | | |
|---|---|---|---|---|---|---|---|---|---|---|---|---|
| Newtons, Strawberry | 2 | 100 | 1.5 | 15 | 0 | 0 | 0 | 110 | 21 | 0 | 1 | 1 1/2 carb |
| Nilla Wafers, Mini | 1 oz | 140 | 6 | 50 | 1.5 | 0 | 5 | 115 | 21 | 0 | 1 | 1 1/2 carb, 1 fat |
| Nilla Wafers, Original | 8 | 140 | 6 | 50 | 1.5 | 0 | 5 | 115 | 21 | 0 | 1 | 1 1/2 carb, 1 fat |
| Nilla Wafers, Reduced Fat | 8 | 110 | 2 | 2 | 0 | 0 | 0 | 110 | 24 | 0 | 1 | 1 1/2 carb |
| Nutter Butter | 2 | 130 | 5 | 45 | 1 | 0.5 | 0 | 110 | 20 | 1 | 2 | 1 carb, 1 fat |
| Nutter Butter Bites | 10 | 120 | 5 | 45 | 2 | 0 | 0 | 90 | 17 | 1 | 2 | 1 carb, 1 fat |
| Oreo Cakesters, Golden | 1 pkg | 220 | 10 | 90 | 2 | 0 | 5 | 135 | 32 | 0 | 2 | 2 carb, 2 fat |
| Oreo Cakesters, Original | 1 pkg | 250 | 12 | 100 | 2.5 | 0 | 5 | 250 | 36 | 1 | 2 | 2 1/2 carb, 2 fat |
| Oreo Fun Stix | 1 pkg | 90 | 3.5 | 35 | 3.5 | 0 | 0 | 50 | 13 | 0 | <1 | 1 carb, 1 fat |
| Oreo Sandwich Cookies, Chocolate | 3 | 160 | 7 | 60 | 2 | 0 | 0 | 160 | 25 | 1 | 1 | 1 1/2 carb, 1 fat |
| Oreo Sandwich Cookies, Chocolate Crème | 2 | 150 | 7 | 60 | 2.5 | 0 | 0 | 110 | 21 | 1 | 1 | 1 1/2 carb, 1 fat |
| Oreo Sandwich Cookies, Chocolate Fudge Mint Covered | 1 | 90 | 4 | 36 | 1 | 0 | 0 | 70 | 12 | <1 | 1 | 1 carb, 1 fat |

DESSERTS, CAKE, PIE, CHEESECAKE, COOKIES, BROWNIES

| | Serving | Calories | Fat (g) | Cal. from Fat | Sat. Fat (g) | Trans Fat (g) | Chol. (mg) | Sod. (mg) | Carb. (g) | Fiber (g) | Prot. (g) | Servings/Exchanges |
|---|---|---|---|---|---|---|---|---|---|---|---|---|
| Oreo Sandwich Cookies, Golden Original | 3 | 170 | 4 | 60 | 2 | 0 | 0 | 120 | 25 | 0 | 1 | 1 1/2 carb, 1 fat |
| Oreo Sandwich Cookies, Reduced Fat, Chocolate | 3 | 150 | 4.5 | 40 | 1 | 0 | 0 | 160 | 27 | 1 | 1 | 2 carb, 1 fat |
| Teddy Grahams, Chocolate | 24 | 130 | 4.5 | 40 | 1 | 0 | 0 | 160 | 22 | 2 | 2 | 1 1/2 carb, 1 fat |
| Teddy Grahams, Honey | 24 | 130 | 4 | 35 | 1 | 0 | 0 | 150 | 23 | 1 | 2 | 1 1/2 carb, 1 fat |
| ***Nabisco SnackWell's*** | | | | | | | | | | | | |
| Cookie Cake, Black Forest | 1/2 oz | 50 | 0.5 | 5 | 0 | 0 | 0 | 40 | 12 | 0 | 1 | 1 carb, 1 fat |
| Cookie Cakes, Chocolate Mint | 1/2 oz | 50 | 0.5 | 5 | 0 | 0 | 0 | 40 | 12 | 0 | 1 | 1 carb |
| Cookie Cakes, Devil's Food, Fat Free | 50 | 0 | 0 | 0 | 0 | 0 | 25 | 12 | 0 | 1 | 1 | 1 carb |

| | | | | | | | | | | | |
|---|---|---|---|---|---|---|---|---|---|---|---|
| Creme Sandwich | 2 | 110 | 3 | 25 | 0.5 | 0 | 0 | 130 | 20 | 0 | 1 | 1 carb, 1 fat |
| Lemon Creme Sandwich Cookies, Sugar Free | 3 | 130 | 6 | 50 | 2 | 0 | 0 | 135 | 23 | 2 | 1 | 1 1/2 carb, 1 fat |
| Shortbread Cookies, Sugar Free | 3 | 130 | 6 | 50 | 1.5 | 0 | 5 | 140 | 21 | 2 | 2 | 1 1/2 carb, 1 fat |
| ***Pepperidge Farm*** | | | | | | | | | | | | |
| Bordeaux | 3 | 130 | 5 | 45 | 3.5 | 0 | 10 | 95 | 19 | <1 | 2 | 1 carb, 1 fat |
| Brussels | 3 | 150 | 7 | 65 | 4 | 0 | 5 | 65 | 20 | 1 | 2 | 1 carb, 1 fat |
| Chessmen | 3 | 120 | 5 | 45 | 3 | 0 | 20 | 80 | 18 | <1 | 2 | 1 carb, 1 fat |
| Chewy Granola, Fruit & Nut | 1 | 140 | 6 | 55 | 1.5 | 0 | 5 | 80 | 20 | 2 | 3 | 1 carb, 1 fat |
| Chocolate Chunk, Nantucket | 1 | 140 | 7 | 65 | 4 | 10 | 0 | 80 | 16 | 0 | 2 | 1 carb, 1 fat |
| Chocolate Chunk, Sausalito | 1 | 140 | 8 | 70 | 3.5 | 0 | 10 | 80 | 16 | 0 | 2 | 1 carb, 2 fat |

DESSERTS, CAKE, PIE, CHEESECAKE, COOKIES, BROWNIES

| | Serving | Calories | Fat (g) | Cal. from Fat | Sat. Fat (g) | Trans Fat (g) | Chol. (mg) | Sod. (mg) | Carb. (g) | Fiber (g) | Prot. (g) | Servings/Exchanges |
|---|---|---|---|---|---|---|---|---|---|---|---|---|
| Chocolate Chunk, Tahoe | 1 | 130 | 6 | 55 | 4 | 0 | <5 | 85 | 17 | <1 | 1 | 1 carb, 1 fat |
| Geneva | 3 | 160 | 9 | 80 | 4 | 0 | 0 | 95 | 19 | 1 | 2 | 1 carb, 2 fat |
| Milano, Black & White | 1 | 180 | 10 | 90 | 5 | 0 | <5 | 85 | 21 | 1 | 2 | 1 1/2 carb, 2 fat |
| Milano, Original | 3 | 180 | 10 | 90 | 5 | 0 | 10 | 80 | 21 | <1 | 2 | 1 1/2 carb, 2 fat |
| Milano, Raspberry | 1 | 130 | 7 | 65 | 4.5 | 0 | <5 | 40 | 16 | <1 | 1 | 1 carb, 1 fat |
| Petite Cinnamon Twists | 3 | 130 | 4.5 | 45 | 2 | 0 | 0 | 100 | 21 | 1 | 2 | 1 1/2 carb, 1 fat |
| Pirouette, Chocolate Hazelnut | 2 | 120 | 5 | 45 | 2 | 0 | 5 | 40 | 19 | 1 | 1 | 1 carb, 1 fat |
| Shortbread | 2 | 140 | 7 | 65 | 4 | 0 | 10 | 105 | 16 | <1 | 2 | 1 carb, 1 fat |
| Soft Baked, Dark Chocolate Chunk | 1 | 140 | 7 | 65 | 3 | 0 | 10 | 80 | 18 | 1 | 2 | 1 carb, 1 fat |
| Soft Baked, Milk Chocolate Caramel | 1 | 140 | 6 | 55 | 3 | 0 | 5 | 75 | 21 | <1 | 1 | 1 1/2 carb, 1 fat |
| Soft Baked, Oatmeal Raisin | 1 | 130 | 4.5 | 45 | 1.5 | 0 | <5 | 90 | 23 | 2 | 2 | 1 1/2 carb, 1 fat |

| | | | | | | | | | | | | |
|---|---|---|---|---|---|---|---|---|---|---|---|---|
| Soft Baked, Sugar | 1 | 140 | 5 | 45 | 2.5 | 0 | 10 | 90 | 22 | 0 | 2 | 1 1/2 carb, 1 fat |
| Sugar | 3 | 140 | 6 | 55 | 2.5 | 0 | 15 | 90 | 20 | <1 | 2 | 1 carb, 1 fat |
| Tahiti | 2 | 170 | 10 | 90 | 6 | 0 | 5 | 40 | 17 | 2 | 2 | 1 carb, 2 fat |
| Verona, Apricot Raspberry | 3 | 140 | 5 | 45 | 2.5 | 0 | 10 | 100 | 22 | <1 | 2 | 1 1/2 carb, 1 fat |
| Verona, Strawberry | 3 | 140 | 5 | 45 | 2.5 | 0 | 10 | 100 | 22 | <1 | 2 | 1 1/2 carb, 1 fat |
| Pillsbury | | | | | | | | | | | | |
| Brownie Mix, Traditional Chocolate Fudge | 1/12 recipe | 150 | 6 | 50 | 1 | 1.5 | 0 | 120 | 24 | <1 | 2 | 1 1/2 carb, 1 fat |
| Milk Chocolate Chip Cookies | 3 | 150 | 7 | 60 | 3 | 0 | 5 | 90 | 20 | 0 | 1 | 1 carb, 1 fat |
| Soft Baked Chocolate Chunk | 1 | 190 | 9 | 80 | 4.5 | 0 | 15 | 140 | 25 | 0 | 2 | 1 1/2 carb, 2 fat |

# DIPS, SPREADS, SALSA

| | Serving | Calories | Fat (g) | Cal. from Fat | Sat. Fat (g) | Trans Fat (g) | Chol (mg) | Sod. (mg) | Carb. (g) | Fiber (g) | Prot. (g) | Servings/Exchanges |
|---|---|---|---|---|---|---|---|---|---|---|---|---|
| ***Alouette*** | | | | | | | | | | | | |
| Soft Spreadable Cheese, All Varietites | 2 Tbsp | 60–80 | 6–8 | 55–70 | 3–5 | 0 | 15–30 | 60–160 | 1 | 0 | 1–2 | 1 fat |
| Light Soft Spreadable Cheese | 2 Tbsp | 50 | 4 | 35 | 2.5 | 0 | 15 | 60 | 2 | 0 | 2 | 1 fat |
| ***Athenos*** | | | | | | | | | | | | |
| Hummus, All Varieties | 2 Tbsp | 50–60 | 3 | 25 | 0 | 0 | 0 | 150–210 | 4–5 | <1 | 2 | 1 fat |
| NeoClassic Hummus, All Varieties | 2 Tbsp | 80 | 5–6 | 45–55 | 1 | 0 | 0 | 130–200 | 5 | 1 | 2 | 1 fat |
| ***Dean's*** | | | | | | | | | | | | |
| French Onion or Ranch Dip | 2 Tbsp | 60 | 5 | 45 | 2.5 | 0 | 0 | 170 | 2 | 0 | 1 | 1 fat |

| | | | | | | | | | | | | |
|---|---|---|---|---|---|---|---|---|---|---|---|---|
| Guacamole Flavored Dip | 2 Tbsp | 90 | 9 | 80 | 2.5 | 0 | <5 | 170 | 2 | 0 | 1 | 2 fat |
| Skinny Dip Light French Onion | 2 Tbsp | 35 | 1.5 | 15 | 1 | 0 | 5 | 210 | 4 | 0 | 2 | 1 fat |
| No Fat French Onion | 2 Tbsp | 30 | 0 | 0 | 0 | 0 | 0 | 240 | 5 | 0 | 2 | 1/2 carb |
| Veggie Dip | 2 Tbsp | 60 | 5 | 45 | 2.5 | 0 | 0 | 170 | 3 | 0 | 1 | 1 fat |
| Bacon & Horseradish | 2 Tbsp | 60 | 5 | 45 | 2.5 | 0 | 0 | 240 | 2 | 0 | 1 | 1 fat |
| Cheddar Cheese Pretzel Dip | 2 Tbsp | 90 | 9 | 80 | 2 | 0 | 15 | 200 | 3 | 0 | 1 | 2 fat |
| Honey Mustard Pretzel Dip | 2 Tbsp | 50 | 1.5 | 15 | 0 | 0 | 0 | 190 | 9 | 0 | 0 | 1/2 carb |
| Creamy Taco Dip | 2 Tbsp | 60 | 5 | 45 | 2 | 0 | 0 | 190 | 4 | 1 | 1 | 1 fat |
| ***Fritos*** | | | | | | | | | | | | |
| Chili Cheese Dip | 2 Tbsp | 45 | 3 | 30 | 1 | 0 | <5 | 310 | 3 | 0 | 1 | 1 fat |
| Hot Bean Dip | 2 Tbsp | 40 | 1 | 10 | 0 | 0 | 0 | 210 | 5 | 1 | 2 | 1/2 carb |
| Jalapeño Cheddar Flavor Cheese | 2 Tbsp | 45 | 4 | 35 | 1 | 0 | <5 | 300 | 4 | 0 | 1 | 1 fat |

| | Serving | Calories | Fat (g) | Cal. from Fat | Sat. Fat (g) | Trans Fat (g) | Chol. (mg) | Sod. (mg) | Carb. (g) | Fiber (g) | Prot. (g) | Servings/Exchanges |
|---|---|---|---|---|---|---|---|---|---|---|---|---|
| Original Flavor Bean Dip | 2 Tbsp | 40 | 1 | 10 | 0 | 0 | 0 | 170 | 5 | 1 | 2 | 1/2 carb |
| ***Guiltless Gourmet*** | | | | | | | | | | | | |
| Mild or Spicy Black Bean Dip | 2 Tbsp | 40 | 0 | 0 | 0 | 0 | 0 | 100 | 7 | 1 | 2 | 1/2 carb |
| ***Herdez*** | | | | | | | | | | | | |
| Salsa Casera | 2 tsp | 10 | 0 | 0 | 0 | 0 | 0 | 270 | 1 | 0 | 0 | free |
| Salsa Verde | 2 tsp | 10 | 0 | 0 | 0 | 0 | 0 | 310 | 1 | 0 | 0 | free |
| Kaukauna/WisPride | | | | | | | | | | | | |
| Garden Vegetable Cheese Spread | 2 Tbsp | 90 | 8 | 70 | 5 | 0 | 25 | 190 | 2 | 0 | 2 | 2 fat |
| Lite Smokey Cheddar Cheese Spread | 2 Tbsp | 70 | 3.5 | 30 | 2 | 0 | 15 | 190 | 5 | 0 | 5 | 1 lean meat |
| Port Wine Cheese Spread | 2 Tbsp | 90 | 7 | 60 | 3.5 | 0 | 20 | 190 | 4 | 0 | 5 | 1 med–fat meat |

| | | | | | | | | | | | | |
|---|---|---|---|---|---|---|---|---|---|---|---|---|
| Extremely Creamy Horseradish Spread | 2 Tbsp | 100 | 8 | 70 | 4 | 0 | 20 | 170 | 3 | 0 | 3 | 2 fat |
| Extremely Creamy Mozarella Spread | 2 Tbsp | 90 | 9 | 80 | 3.5 | 0 | 20 | 220 | 1 | 0 | 2 | 2 fat |
| ***Kraft*** | | | | | | | | | | | | |
| Pimento Cheese Spread | 2 Tbsp | 70 | 6 | 60 | 4 | 0 | 20 | 220 | 3 | 0 | 2 | 1 fat |
| Bacon Cheese Spread | 2 Tbsp | 90 | 8 | 70 | 5 | 0 | 25 | 570 | 1 | 0 | 5 | 1 high fat meat |
| Sharp Old English Spread | 2 Tbsp | 90 | 5 | 70 | 5 | 0 | 25 | 520 | 1 | 0 | 5 | 1 med–fat meat |
| Roka Blue Cheese Spread | 2 Tbsp | 80 | 7 | 60 | 5 | 0 | 20 | 340 | 2 | 0 | 3 | 1 med–fat meat |
| Cheez Whiz Light | 2 Tbsp | 80 | 3.5 | 30 | 2 | 0 | 20 | 500 | 6 | 0 | 6 | 1/2 carb, 1 fat |
| Cheez Whiz Salsa Con Queso | 2 Tbsp | 90 | 7 | 60 | 4.5 | 0 | 30 | 500 | 4 | 0 | 3 | 2 fat |
| Cheeze Whiz Original | 2 Tbsp | 90 | 7 | 60 | 4.5 | 0 | 30 | 490 | 4 | 0 | 3 | 2 fat |
| Creamy Ranch Dip | 2 Tbsp | 60 | 4.5 | 40 | 3 | 0 | 0 | 190 | 3 | 0 | 1 | 1 fat |

DIPS, SPREADS, SALSA

| | Serving | Calories | Fat (g) | Cal. from Fat | Sat. Fat (g) | Trans Fat (g) | Chol. (mg) | Sod. (mg) | Carb. (g) | Fiber (g) | Prot. (g) | Servings/Exchanges |
|---|---|---|---|---|---|---|---|---|---|---|---|---|
| French Onion Dip Onion Dip | 2 Tbsp | 60 | 4.5 | 40 | 3 | 0 | 0 | 220 | 3–4 | 0 | 1 | 1 fat |
| Easy Cheese Cheddar | 2 Tbsp | 90 | 6 | 60 | 3 | 0 | 20 | 410 | 2 | 0 | 5 | 1 med–fat meat |
| Easy Cheese Cheddar 'N Bacon | 2 Tbsp | 90 | 7 | 60 | 4.5 | 0 | 25 | 400 | 2 | 0 | 5 | 1 med–fat meat |
| Pineapple Cheese Spread | 2 Tbsp | 70 | 5 | 50 | 3.5 | 0 | 15 | 120 | 4 | 0 | 2 | 1 fat |
| Blue Cheese Spread | 2 Tbsp | 80 | 7 | 65 | 4 | 0 | 30 | 290 | 2 | 0 | 3 | 2 fat |
| ***La Victoria*** | | | | | | | | | | | | |
| Salsa (All Varieties) | 2 Tbsp | 10 | 0 | 0 | 0 | 0 | 0 | 105–190 | 2 | 0 | 0 | free |
| ***Litehouse*** | | | | | | | | | | | | |
| Avacado Dip | 2 Tbsp | 140 | 15 | 140 | 2 | 0 | 15 | 210 | 2 | 0 | 1 | 3 fat |
| Low Fat Caramel Dip | 2 Tbsp | 110 | 0 | 0 | 0 | 0 | 0 | 140 | 27 | 0 | 1 | 2 carb |

| | | | | | | | | | | | | |
|---|---|---|---|---|---|---|---|---|---|---|---|---|
| Lite Ranch Veggie Dip | 2 Tbsp | 60 | 6 | 50 | 0.5 | 0 | 10 | 230 | 3 | 0 | 1 | 1 fat |
| Caramel Dip | 2 Tbsp | 110 | 1.5 | 15 | 1.5 | 0 | 25 | 125 | 25 | 0 | 1 | 1 1/2 carb |
| Ranch Veggie Dip | 2 Tbsp | 130 | 13 | 120 | 1 | 0 | 10 | 230 | 3 | 0 | 1 | 3 fat |
| Spinach Parmesan Veggie Dip | 2 Tbsp | 120 | 13 | 110 | 1.5 | 0 | 15 | 240 | 2 | 0 | 1 | 3 fat |
| Chocolate Dip | 1.4 oz | 100 | 1.5 | 15 | 0 | 0 | 0 | 45 | 25 | 4 | 0 | 1 1/2 carb |
| Vanilla Yogurt Fruit Dip | 2 Tbsp | 60 | 1.5 | 15 | 0 | 0 | 0 | 50 | 10 | 0 | 1 | 1/2 carb |
| Chocolate Yogurt Fruit Dip | 2 Tbsp | 110 | 6 | 50 | 0 | 0 | 0 | 95 | 14 | 0 | 1 | 1 carb, 1 fat |
| Strawberry Glaze | 3 Tbsp | 70 | 0 | 0 | 0 | 0 | 0 | 50 | 17 | 0 | 0 | 1 carb |
| Chocolate Caramel Dip | 2 Tbsp | 120 | 3 | 30 | 2.5 | 0 | 0 | 120 | 23 | 0 | 1 | 1 1/2 carb, 1 fat |
| ***Maria's Dip*** | | | | | | | | | | | | |
| Creamy Dill | 2 Tbsp | 100 | 10 | 90 | 3 | 0 | 15 | 140 | 2 | 0 | 1 | 2 fat |
| Roasted French Onion | 2 Tbsp | 100 | 10 | 90 | 3 | 0 | 15 | 220 | 2 | 0 | 1 | 2 fat |
| Guacamole Dip | 2 Tbsp | 40 | 3 | 30 | 1.5 | 0 | 5 | 140 | 3 | 1 | 1 | 1 fat |
| Lite Buttermilk Ranch | 2 Tbsp | 60 | 5 | 45 | 1.5 | 0 | 10 | 310 | 3 | 0 | 2 | 1 fat |

| | Serving | Calories | Fat (g) | Cal. from Fat | Sat. Fat (g) | Trans Fat (g) | Chol. (mg) | Sod. (mg) | Carb. (g) | Fiber (g) | Prot. (g) | Servings/Exchanges |
|---|---|---|---|---|---|---|---|---|---|---|---|---|
| Spinach Parmesan | 2 Tbsp | 90 | 9 | 80 | 3 | 0 | 15 | 200 | 2 | 0 | 2 | 2 fat |
| Honey Vanilla Cream | 2 Tbsp | 60 | 4.5 | 40 | 2.5 | 0 | 15 | 20 | 5 | 0 | 1 | 1 fat |
| ***Newman's Own*** | | | | | | | | | | | | |
| Bandito Salsa | 2 Tbsp | 10 | 0 | 0 | 0 | 0 | 0 | 105 | 2 | 1 | 0 | free |
| Mango Salsa | 2 Tbsp | 20 | 0 | 0 | 0 | 0 | 0 | 140 | 5 | 2 | 1 | free |
| Pineapple Salsa | 2 Tbsp | 15 | 0 | 0 | 0 | 0 | 0 | 90 | 3 | 1 | 0 | free |
| Black Bean & Corn Salsa | 2 Tbsp | 20 | 0 | 0 | 0 | 0 | 0 | 140 | 5 | 2 | 1 | free |
| ***Old El Paso*** | | | | | | | | | | | | |
| Thick 'n Chunky Salsa | 2 Tbsp | 10 | 0 | 0 | 0 | 0 | 0 | 230 | 3 | 0 | 0 | free |
| Cheese 'n Salsa | 2 Tbsp | 35 | 3 | 25 | 0.5 | 1 | 0 | 280 | 3 | 0 | 0 | 1 fat |
| ***Ortega*** | | | | | | | | | | | | |
| Thick & Chunky Salsa | 2 Tbsp | 10 | 0 | 0 | 0 | 0 | 0 | 170 | 2 | 0 | 0 | free |
| Salsa Con Queso | 2 Tbsp | 45 | 3 | 25 | 1 | 0 | 0 | 280 | 4 | 0 | 1 | 1 fat |

| | | | | | | | | | | | | |
|---|---|---|---|---|---|---|---|---|---|---|---|---|
| ***Pace*** | | | | | | | | | | | | |
| Chunky Salsa | 2 Tbsp | 10 | 0 | 0 | 0 | 0 | 0 | 230 | 2 | 0 | 0 | free |
| Black Bean & Roasted Corn Salsa | 2 Tbsp | 25 | 0 | 0 | 0 | 0 | 0 | 150 | 5 | 1 | 1 | free |
| Pineapple Mango Chipotle Salsa | 2 Tbsp | 20 | 0 | 0 | 0 | 0 | 0 | 130 | 4 | 0 | 0 | free |
| Mexican Four Cheese Con Queso | 2 Tbsp | 90 | 7 | 65 | 1.5 | 0 | 5 | 430 | 5 | 0 | 2 | 1 fat |
| ***Rojos Salsa*** | | | | | | | | | | | | |
| Chunky Salsa | 2 Tbsp | 10 | 0 | 0 | 0 | 0 | 0 | 230 | 2 | 0 | 0 | free |
| ***Rondele*** | | | | | | | | | | | | |
| Garlic & Herb Spreadable Cheese | 2 Tbsp | 70 | 7 | 60 | 5 | 0 | 20 | 150 | 1 | 0 | 2 | 1 fat |
| Lite Garlic & Herbs Spreadable Cheese | 2 Tbsp | 60 | 4.5 | 40 | 3 | 0 | 15 | 190 | 2 | 0 | 3 | 1 fat |
| Cheddar Horseradish Spreadable Cheese | 2 Tbsp | 70 | 7 | 60 | 4.5 | 0 | 25 | 150 | 1 | 0 | 2 | 1 fat |

| | Serving | Calories | Fat (g) | Cal. from Fat | Sat. Fat (g) | Trans Fat (g) | Chol. (mg) | Sod. (mg) | Carb. (g) | Fiber (g) | Prot. (g) | Servings/Exchanges |
|---|---|---|---|---|---|---|---|---|---|---|---|---|
| ***Ruffles*** | | | | | | | | | | | | |
| Sour Cream & Chives Dip | 2 Tbsp | 60 | 5 | 50 | 0.5 | 0 | <5 | 240 | 2 | <1 | 1 | 1 fat |
| Smokey Bacon & Cheddar Dip | 2 Tbsp | 70 | 8 | 50 | 1 | 0 | <5 | 100 | 2 | <1 | 2 | 2 fat |
| ***T. Marzetti's*** | | | | | | | | | | | | |
| Blue Cheese Veggie Dip | 2 Tbsp | 140 | 15 | 130 | 3 | 0 | 15 | 250 | 1 | 0 | 1 | 3 fat |
| Dill Veggie Dip | 2 Tbsp | 120 | 13 | 110 | 3.5 | 0 | 20 | 200 | 2 | 0 | 1 | 3 fat |
| Fat Free Ranch Veggie Dip | 2 Tbsp | 30 | 0 | 0 | 0 | 0 | 0 | 330 | 6 | 0 | 1 | 1/2 carb |
| French Onion Veggie Dip | 2 Tbsp | 120 | 12 | 110 | 3 | 0 | 20 | 220 | 2 | 0 | 1 | 3 fat |
| Light Ranch Veggie Dip | 2 Tbsp | 60 | 6 | 50 | 1 | 0 | 5 | 240 | 6 | 0 | 0 | 1/2 carb, 1 fat |
| Light Caramel Apple Dip | 2 Tbsp | 100 | 1.5 | 10 | 1 | 0 | 5 | 75 | 26 | 0 | 1 | 2 carb |

| | | | | | | | | | | | | |
|---|---|---|---|---|---|---|---|---|---|---|---|---|
| Chocolate Fruit Dip | 2 Tbsp | 110 | 2 | 15 | 0.5 | 0 | 0 | 85 | 23 | 1 | 1 | 1 1/2 carb |
| Cream Cheese Fruit Dip | 2 Tbsp | 70 | 3 | 30 | 2 | 0 | 15 | 85 | 10 | 0 | 0 | 1/2 carb, 1 fat |
| Garden Hummus Veggie Dip & Spread | 2 Tbsp | 70 | 4.5 | 40 | 0.5 | 0 | 0 | 170 | 5 | 1 | 2 | 1 fat |
| Old Fashioned Caramel Apple Dip | 2 Tbsp | 140 | 6 | 50 | 3 | 0 | 5 | 75 | 22 | 0 | 0 | 1 1/2 carb, 1 fat |
| Peanut Butter Caramel Apple Dip | 2 Tbsp | 120 | 5 | 25 | 1 | 0 | 0 | 120 | 17 | 1 | 2 | 1 carb, 1 fat |
| Ranch Veggie Dip | 2 Tbsp | 120 | 12 | 110 | 3.5 | 0 | 20 | 210 | 2 | 0 | 1 | 2 fat |
| Spinach Veggie Dip | 2 Tbsp | 130 | 13 | 120 | 3 | 0 | 20 | 250 | 2 | 0 | 1 | 3 fat |
| ***Tostitos*** | | | | | | | | | | | | |
| Chunky Salsa | 2 Tbsp | 10 | 0 | 0 | 0 | 0 | 0 | 250 | 2 | <1 | 0 | free |
| Salsa Con Queso | 2 Tbsp | 40 | 2.5 | 25 | 1 | 0 | <5 | 280 | 5 | <1 | <1 | 1 fat |
| Creamy Spinach Dip | 2 Tbsp | 50 | 4 | 35 | 0 | 0 | <5 | 200 | 2 | <1 | 1 | 1 fat |

## EGGS, EGG DISHES, EGG PRODUCTS

| | Serving | Calories | Fat (g) | Cal. from Fat | Sat. Fat (g) | Trans Fat (g) | Chol. (mg) | Sod. (mg) | Carb. (g) | Fiber (g) | Prot. (g) | Servings/Exchanges |
|---|---|---|---|---|---|---|---|---|---|---|---|---|
| 1-Egg Omelet with Cheese & Ham | 1 | 142 | 11 | 100 | 4 | 0 | 231 | 368 | <1 | 0 | 10 | 1 med-fat meat, 1 fat |
| 1-Egg Omelet with Chicken | 1 | 149 | 10 | 90 | 3 | 0 | 287 | 222 | <1 | 0 | 13 | 2 med-fat meat |
| 1-Egg Omelet with Fish | 1 | 132 | 9 | 80 | 3 | 0 | 267 | 277 | <1 | 0 | 10 | 2 med-fat meat |
| 1-Egg Omelet with Mushroom | 1 | 91 | 7 | 65 | 2 | 0 | 204 | 158 | 1 | <1 | 6 | 1 med-fat meat |
| 1-Egg Omelet with Onion, Pepper, Tomato & Mushroom | 1 | 125 | 9 | 80 | 2 | 0 | 126 | 251 | 7 | 2 | 5 | 1 vegetable, 1 med-fat meat, 1 fat |
| 1-Egg Omelet with Sausage & Mushroom | 1 | 172 | 13 | 115 | 4 | 0 | 254 | 454 | 1 | <1 | 11 | 2 med-fat meat, 1 fat |
| 1-Egg Omelet with Spinach | 1 | 95 | 7 | 65 | 2 | 0 | 201 | 201 | 2 | <1 | 7 | 1 med-fat meat |

| | | | | | | | | | | | | |
|---|---|---|---|---|---|---|---|---|---|---|---|---|
| 1-Egg Omelet, Plain | 1 | 96 | 7 | 65 | 2 | 0 | 217 | 98 | <1 | 0 | 6 | 1 med-fat meat |
| Deviled Egg | 1/2 egg & filling | 63 | 5 | 45 | 1 | 0 | 121 | 94 | <1 | 0 | 4 | 1 med-fat meat |
| Egg, Boiled/Cooked | 1 extra large | 90 | 6 | 55 | 2 | 0 | 246 | 72 | <1 | 0 | 7 | 1 med-fat meat |
| Egg, Boiled/Cooked | 1 jumbo | 99 | 7 | 65 | 2 | 0 | 271 | 79 | <1 | 0 | 8 | 1 med-fat meat |
| Egg, Boiled/Cooked | 1 large | 78 | 5 | 45 | 2 | 0 | 212 | 62 | <1 | 0 | 6 | 1 med-fat meat |
| Egg, Boiled/Cooked | 1 medium | 68 | 5 | 45 | 1 | 0 | 187 | 55 | <1 | 0 | 6 | 1 med-fat meat |
| Egg, Boiled/Cooked | 1 small | 57 | 4 | 35 | 1 | 0 | 157 | 46 | <1 | 0 | 5 | 1 med-fat meat |
| Egg, Fried in Margarine | 1 large | 90 | 7 | 65 | 2 | 0 | 210 | 94 | <1 | 0 | 6 | 1 high-fat meat |
| Egg, Scrambled, Plain | 1 | 102 | 7 | 65 | 2 | 0 | 215 | 171 | 1 | 0 | 7 | 2 med-fat meat |
| Egg Substitute | 1/4 cup | 30 | 0 | 0 | 0 | 0 | 0 | 115 | 1 | 0 | 6 | 1 lean meat |
| Egg Whites | 2 | 32 | 0 | 0 | 0 | 0 | 0 | 110 | <1 | 0 | 7 | 1 lean meat |
| Souffle, Cheese | 1 cup | 197 | 14 | 125 | 6 | 0 | 194 | 299 | 6 | <1 | 12 | 1/2 reduced-fat milk, 1 med-fat meat, 1 fat |
| Souffle, Spinach | 1 cup | 234 | 18 | 165 | 8 | 0 | 160 | 770 | 8 | 1 | 11 | 1/2 reduced-fat milk, 1 med-fat meat, 2 fat |

EGGS, EGG DISHES, EGG PRODUCTS

| | Serving | Calories | Fat (g) | Cal. from Fat | Sat. Fat (g) | Trans Fat (g) | Chol. (mg) | Sod. (mg) | Carb. (g) | Fiber (g) | Prot. (g) | Servings/Exchanges |
|---|---|---|---|---|---|---|---|---|---|---|---|---|
| **Brands** | | | | | | | | | | | | |
| ***ConAgra*** | | | | | | | | | | | | |
| Egg Beaters, Cheese & Chive | 1/4 cup | 35 | 1 | 10 | 0.5 | 0 | <5 | 210 | 1 | 0 | 5 | 1 lean meat |
| Egg Beaters, Garden Vegetable | 1/4 cup | 30 | 0 | 0 | 0 | 0 | 0 | 160 | 1 | 0 | 5 | 1 lean meat |
| Egg Beaters, Original | 1/4 cup | 30 | 0 | 0 | 0 | 0 | 0 | 115 | 1 | 0 | 6 | 1 lean meat |
| Egg Beaters, Whites | 3 Tbsp | 25 | 0 | 0 | 0 | 0 | 0 | 75 | 1 | 0 | 5 | 1 lean meat |
| Egg Beaters. Southwestern | 1/4 cup | 30 | 0 | 0 | 0 | 0 | 0 | 180 | 1 | 0 | 5 | 1 lean meat |
| ***Crystal Farms*** | | | | | | | | | | | | |
| All Whites | 1/4 cup | 30 | 0 | 0 | 0 | 0 | 0 | 95 | 1 | 0 | 6 | 1 lean meat |
| Better'n Eggs | 1/4 cup | 30 | 0 | 0 | 0 | 0 | 0 | 120 | 1 | 0 | 6 | 1 lean meat |
| Better'n Eggs Plus | 1/4 cup | 35 | 0 | 0 | 0 | 0 | 0 | 105 | 0 | 0 | 6 | 1 lean meat |

# ETHNIC FOODS

| | Serving | Calories | Fat (g) | Cal. from Fat | Sat. Fat (g) | Trans Fat (g) | Chol. (mg) | Sod. (mg) | Carb. (g) | Fiber (g) | Prot. (g) | Servings/Exchanges |
|---|---|---|---|---|---|---|---|---|---|---|---|---|
| **ALASKA NATIVE** | | | | | | | | | | | | |
| Beach Asparagus | 1 cup | 15 | <1 | 0 | NA | 0 | 0 | 23 | 2 | NA | 1 | free |
| Caribou, Cooked | 1 oz | 47 | 1 | 10 | <1 | 0 | 31 | 17 | 0 | 0 | 8 | 1 lean meat |
| Dried Fish/King Salmon | 1/2 oz | 60 | 5 | 45 | NA | 0 | NA | NA | 0 | 0 | 7 | 1 med-fat meat |
| Fiddlehead Fern, Raw | 1 cup | 34 | <1 | 0 | NA | 0 | 0 | 84 | 5 | NA | 3 | 1 vegetable |
| Gumboots/Leathery Chiton | 2 oz | 46 | <1 | 0 | NA | 0 | NA | NA | 0 | 0 | 10 | 1 lean meat |
| Halibut, Cooked | 1 oz | 39 | <1 | 0 | <1 | 0 | 12 | 20 | 0 | 0 | 8 | 1 lean meat |
| Herring Eggs, Plain | 1/2 cup | 48 | <1 | 0 | NA | 0 | NA | 52 | 4 | 0 | 8 | 1 lean meat |
| Highbush Cranberries | 1 1/4 cup | 58 | <1 | 0 | NA | 0 | 0 | 1 | 15 | NA | <1 | 1 fruit |
| Hooligan, Smoked | 1 oz | 86 | 7 | 65 | NA | 0 | NA | NA | 0 | 0 | 6 | 1 high-fat meat |
| Huckleberries | 1 cup | 56 | <1 | 0 | NA | 0 | 0 | 15 | 13 | NA | <1 | 1 fruit |
| Moose, Cooked | 1 oz | 38 | <1 | 0 | <1 | 0 | 22 | 19 | 0 | 0 | 8 | 1 lean meat |

## ETHNIC FOODS

| | Serving | Calories | Fat (g) | Cal. from Fat | Sat. Fat (g) | Trans Fat (g) | Chol. (mg) | Sod. (mg) | Carb. (g) | Fiber (g) | Prot. (g) | Servings/Exchanges |
|---|---|---|---|---|---|---|---|---|---|---|---|---|
| Muktuk with Skin and Fat | 1x1x2 inches | 138 | 12 | 110 | NA | 0 | NA | NA | 0 | 0 | 8 | 1 high-fat meat, 1 fat |
| Muskrat, Cooked | 1 oz | 67 | 3 | 25 | 0 | 0 | 34 | 27 | 0 | 0 | 9 | 1 lean meat |
| Pike, Cooked | 1 oz | 33 | <1 | 0 | 0 | 0 | 14 | 13 | 0 | 0 | 7 | 1 lean meat |
| Pilot Bread | 1,4-inch round | 104 | 2 | 20 | NA | 0 | NA | 142 | 18 | NA | 2 | 1 starch |
| Salmon, Sockeye | 1 oz | 60 | 3 | 25 | <1 | 0 | 24 | 18 | 0 | 0 | 8 | 1 lean meat |
| Salmonberries | 1 1/2 cup | 55 | <1 | 0 | NA | 0 | 0 | 52 | 13 | NA | 1 | 1 fruit |
| Seal Meat, Raw | 1 oz | 41 | <1 | 0 | <1 | 0 | NA | NA | 0 | 0 | 9 | 1 lean meat |
| Seal Oil | 1 tsp | 45 | 5 | 45 | <1 | 0 | 8 | NA | 0 | 0 | 0 | 1 fat |
| Seaweed, Dried Black | 1 cup | 39 | <1 | 0 | NA | 0 | NA | 0 | 39 | 40 | NA | 4 Vegetable |
| Sour Dock, Cooked | 1/2 cup | 19 | <1 | 0 | NA | 0 | 0 | NA | 4 | NA | 1 | 1 vegetable |
| Venison, Cooked | 1 oz | 44 | <1 | 0 | <1 | 0 | 31 | 15 | 0 | 0 | 9 | 1 lean meat |
| Walrus, Raw | 1 oz | 56 | 4 | 35 | <1 | 0 | 22 | NA | 0 | 0 | 5 | 1 lean meat |

| | | | | | | | | | | | | |
|---|---|---|---|---|---|---|---|---|---|---|---|---|
| Whale, Bonehead, Raw | 1 oz | 37 | <1 | 0 | <1 | 0 | NA | 17 | 0 | 0 | 7 | 1 lean meat |
| Willow Greens, Cooked | 1 /2 cup | 28 | <1 | 0 | NA | 0 | 0 | NA | 6 | NA | 2 | 1 vegetable |
| **CAJUN & CREOLE** | | | | | | | | | | | | |
| Alligator, Cooked | 1 oz | 42 | 0.5 | 5 | <1 | 0 | 19 | 22 | 0 | 0 | 9 | 1 lean meat |
| Beef Tasso | 1 oz | 47 | 1 | 10 | 0.5 | 0 | 12 | NA | 0 | 0 | 8 | 1 lean meat |
| Cafe au Lait | 8 oz | 76 | 4 | 35 | 3 | 0 | 17 | 59 | 6 | 0 | 4 | 1/2 whole milk |
| Couche-Couche, No Fat Added | 1/2 cup | 82 | <1 | 0 | NA | 0 | 0 | 4 | 17 | 1 | 3 | 1 starch |
| Cracklins | 1/4 cup | 131 | 11 | 100 | 4 | 0 | 19 | 362 | 0 | 0 | 7 | 1 high-fat meat, 1 fat |
| Crawfish, Cooked | 2 oz | 46 | 0.5 | 5 | <1 | 0 | 81 | 107 | 0 | 0 | 10 | 1 lean meat |
| Cushaw Squash | 1/2 cup | 41 | 0.5 | 5 | <1 | 0 | 0 | 2 | 9 | 3 | 1 | 1 vegetable |
| Dewberries/ Blackberries | 3/4 cup | 60 | <1 | 0 | 0 | 0 | 0 | 0 | 15 | 6 | <1 | 1 fruit |
| Dove, Cooked | 1 oz | 62 | 4 | 35 | 1 | 0 | 33 | 82 | 0 | 0 | 7 | 1 med-fat meat |
| Frog Legs, Steamed | 2 legs | 45 | <1 | 0 | NA | 0 | 31 | 36 | 0 | 0 | 10 | 1 lean meat |
| Goat, Baked or Roasted | 1 oz | 45 | 2 | 18 | <1 | 0 | 38 | 96 | 0 | 0 | 7 | 1 lean meat |

ETHNIC FOODS

| | Serving | Calories | Fat (g) | Cal. from Fat | Sat. Fat (g) | Trans Fat (g) | Chol. (mg) | Sod. (mg) | Carb. (g) | Fiber (g) | Prot. (g) | Servings/Exchanges |
|---|---|---|---|---|---|---|---|---|---|---|---|---|
| Guinea, Flesh Only | 1 oz | 42 | 1 | 9 | <1 | 0 | 24 | 26 | 0 | 0 | 8 | 1 lean meat |
| Hogshead Cheese | 1/4 cup | 77 | 6 | 55 | 2 | 0 | 29 | 455 | 0 | 0 | 6 | 1 med-fat meat |
| Kumquats | 5 | 60 | 0 | 0 | 0 | 0 | 0 | 6 | 16 | 4 | 1 | 1 fruit |
| Lamb, Cooked | 1 oz | 83 | 6 | 55 | 3 | 0 | 28 | 20 | 0 | 0 | 7 | 1 med-fat meat |
| Mirliton/Chayote, Cooked | 1/2 cup | 24 | 0.5 | 5 | 0 | 0 | 0 | 1 | 5 | 3 | <1 | 1 vegetable |
| Muscadines | 17 | 60 | 0.5 | 5 | 0 | 0 | 0 | 2 | 15 | <1 | <1 | 1 fruit |
| Passionfruit (Maypops) | 3 | 52 | 0 | 0 | 0 | 0 | 0 | 17 | 13 | 1 | 1 | 1 fruit |
| Peas, Crowder, Purple Hull | 1/2 cup | 92 | <1 | 0 | <1 | 0 | 0 | 8 | 15 | 4 | 7 | 1 starch |
| Persimmons (Japanese) | 1/2 of 2 1/2 inches | 59 | 0 | 0 | 0 | 0 | 0 | 1 | 16 | 1 | 0.5 | 1 fruit |
| Pickled Pigs Feet | 1/2 foot | 88 | 7 | 65 | 2 | 0 | 40 | 402 | 0 | 0 | 6 | 1 high-fat meat |

| | | | | | | | | | | | | |
|---|---|---|---|---|---|---|---|---|---|---|---|---|
| Pork Sausage, Cooked | 1 oz | 105 | 9 | 80 | 3 | 0 | 24 | 367 | 0 | 0 | 6 | 1 high-fat meat |
| Pumpkin, Cooked | 1/2 cup | 20 | 0 | 0 | 0 | 0 | 0 | 1 | 5 | 2 | <1 | 1 vegetable |
| Remoulade Sauce | 1 Tbsp | 52 | 6 | 50 | 2 | 0 | 7 | 54 | <1 | 0 | <1 | 1 fat |
| Salt Pork or Fatback | 1/2-inch | 45 | 5 | 45 | 2 | 0 | 5 | 80 | 0 | 0 | <1 | 1 fat |
| Satsuma/Mandarin | 2 small | 62 | 0 | 0 | 0 | 0 | 0 | 1 | 16 | 1 | <1 | 1 fruit |
| Shrimp, Dried | 36 | 55 | 1 | 9 | <1 | 0 | 79 | 77 | 0.5 | 0 | 11 | 2 lean meat |
| Smoked Beef Sausage | 1 oz | 89 | 8 | 70 | 3 | 0 | 19 | 321 | <1 | 0 | 4 | 1 high-fat meat |
| Smoked Pork Sausage | 1 oz | 110 | 9 | 80 | 3 | 0 | 19 | 426 | 0 | 0 | 6 | 1 high-fat meat |
| Squab, Flesh Only, Cooked | 1 oz | 60 | 3 | 25 | <1 | 0 | 38 | 22 | 0 | 0 | 7 | 1 lean meat |
| Tongue, Beef, Cooked | 1 oz | 80 | 6 | 55 | 3 | 0 | 30 | 17 | 0 | 0 | 6 | 1 med-fat meat |
| Tripe, Cooked | 2 oz | 57 | 1 | 10 | <1 | 0 | 54 | 41 | 0 | 0 | 11 | 2 lean meat |
| Turtle, Cooked | 1.5 oz | 57 | 2 | 18 | <1 | 0 | 26 | 170 | 0 | 0 | 10 | 1 lean meat |
| **CHINESE AMERICAN** | | | | | | | | | | | | |
| Amaranth/Chinese Spinach, Cooked | 1/2 cup | 14 | <1 | 0 | 0 | 0 | 0 | 14 | 3 | NA | 1 | 1 vegetable |

| | Serving | Calories | Fat (g) | Cal. from Fat | Sat. Fat (g) | Trans Fat (g) | Chol. (mg) | Sod. (mg) | Carb. (g) | Fiber (g) | Prot. (g) | Servings/Exchanges |
|---|---|---|---|---|---|---|---|---|---|---|---|---|
| Amaranth/Chinese Spinach, Raw | 1 cup | 7 | <1 | 0 | 0 | 0 | 0 | 6 | 1 | NA | <1 | 1 vegetable |
| Arrowheads/Fresh Corn, Large | 1 | 25 | <1 | 0 | NA | 0 | NA | 6 | 5 | NA | 1 | 1 vegetable |
| Baby Corn, Canned | 1/2 cup | 13 | <1 | 0 | NA | 0 | 0 | 730 | 2 | NA | 2 | 1 vegetable |
| Bamboo Shoots, Canned | 1/2 cup | 13 | <1 | 0 | 0 | 0 | 0 | 5 | 2 | <1 | 1 | 1 vegetable |
| Beef Jerky | 1/2 oz | 57 | 4 | 35 | 2 | NA | 7 | 310 | 2 | <1 | 5 | 1 lean meat |
| Beef Tongue | 1 oz | 81 | 6 | 55 | 3 | 0 | 30 | 17 | <1 | 0 | 6 | 1 med-fat meat |
| Bitter Melon/Bitter Gourd/Balsam-Pear Pods | 1 cup | 16 | <1 | 0 | 0 | 0 | 0 | 5 | 3 | 3 | <1 | 1 vegetable |
| Bok Choy/Chinese Cabbage/Pakchoi | 1/2 cup | 9 | <1 | 0 | 0 | 0 | 0 | 46 | 2 | <1 | 1 | 1 vegetable |
| Carambola/Star Fruit | 2 | 60 | <1 | 0 | 0 | 0 | 0 | 4 | 14 | 5 | 1 | 1 fruit |

| | | | | | | | | | | | | |
|---|---|---|---|---|---|---|---|---|---|---|---|---|
| Cellophane/Mung Bean Noodles, Cooked | 1/2 cup | 67 | NA | NA | 0 | 0 | 0 | 2 | 16 | <1 | NA | 1 starch |
| Cha Shu Bun, Frozen, Steamed | 2 | 360 | 13 | 115 | 5 | 0 | 20 | 410 | 50 | 1 | 8 | 2 starch, 3 fat |
| Chayote, Raw | 1 cup | 32 | <1 | 0 | 0 | 0 | 0 | 5 | 7 | 4 | 1 | 1 vegetable |
| Chinese Banana, Dwarf | 1 | 72 | <1 | 0 | NA | 0 | 0 | 18 | 18 | NA | 2 | 1 fruit |
| Chinese Celery, Raw | 1 cup | 26 | <1 | 0 | 0 | 0 | 0 | 116 | 5 | 0 | 2 | 1 vegetable |
| Chinese Eggplant, Purple, Cooked | 1/2 cup | 17 | <1 | 0 | NA | 0 | 0 | NA | 4 | 2 | <1 | 1 vegetable |
| Chinese Eggplant, White, Cooked | 1/2 cup | 20 | <1 | 0 | NA | 0 | 0 | NA | 5 | 2 | <1 | 1 vegetable |
| Chinese Sausage | 1 oz | 100 | 8 | 70 | 3 | NA | NA | 246 | 2 | NA | 6 | 1 high-fat meat |
| Chinese/Black Mushrooms, Dried | 2 | 21 | <1 | 0 | 0 | 0 | 0 | 1 | 5 | <1 | <1 | 1 vegetable |
| Chinese/Peking/Pe-tsai/ Napa Cabbage, Raw | 1 cup | 12 | <1 | 0 | 0 | 0 | 0 | 1 | 3 | <1 | <1 | 1 vegetable |

ETHNIC FOODS

| | Serving | Calories | Fat (g) | Cal. from Fat | Sat. Fat (g) | Trans Fat (g) | Chol. (mg) | Sod. (mg) | Carb. (g) | Fiber (g) | Prot. (g) | Servings/Exchanges |
|---|---|---|---|---|---|---|---|---|---|---|---|---|
| Choy Sum/Chinese Flowering Cabbage | 1 cup | 9 | NA | NA | NA | 0 | 0 | NA | 2 | NA | 1 | 1 vegetable |
| Coconut Milk | 1 Tbsp | 35 | 4 | 35 | 3 | 0 | 0 | 2 | <1 | <1 | 2 | 1 fat |
| Coriander, Raw | 1 cup | 3 | <1 | 0 | 0 | 0 | 0 | 4 | <1 | <1 | <1 | free |
| Dried Mung Beans/ Grean Beans, Cooked | 1/2 cup | 106 | <1 | 0 | <1 | 0 | o | 2 | 19 | 8 | 7 | 1 starch, 1 lean meat |
| Dried Red Beans, Cooked | 1/3 cup | 99 | <1 | 0 | 0 | 0 | 0 | 6 | 19 | 1 | 6 | 1 starch, 1 lean meat |
| Garland Chrysanthemum, Raw | 1 cup | 4 | 0 | 0 | NA | 0 | NA | 13 | 1 | NA | <1 | free |
| Ginger Root, Raw | 1/4 cup | 17 | <1 | 0 | NA | 0 | NA | 3 | 4 | NA | <1 | free |
| Gingko Seeds, Canned | 1/2 cup | 86 | 1 | 10 | <1 | 0 | 0 | 238 | 17 | 7 | 2 | 1 starch |
| Guava, Medium | 1 1/2 | 69 | <1 | 0 | <1 | 0 | 0 | 4 | 16 | 7 | 1 | 1 fruit |
| Hairy Melon/Hairy Cucumber, Raw | 1 cup | 22 | NA | NA | NA | 0 | NA | NA | 5 | 2 | 1 | 1 vegetable |

| | | | | | | | | | | | | |
|---|---|---|---|---|---|---|---|---|---|---|---|---|
| Kumquat, Medium | 5 | 30 | <1 | 0 | 0 | 0 | 0 | 6 | 16 | 6 | <1 | 1 fruit |
| Leeks, Cooked | 1/2 cup | 16 | <1 | 0 | 0 | 0 | 0 | 5 | 4 | <1 | <1 | 1 vegetable |
| Litchi/Lychee, Canned | 1/2 cup | 57 | <1 | 0 | NA | 0 | 0 | 27 | 15 | <1 | <1 | 1 fruit |
| Litchi/Lychee, Raw | 10 | 63 | <1 | 0 | <1 | 0 | 0 | 1 | 16 | 1 | <1 | 1 fruit |
| Longan, Canned | 3/4 cup | 68 | <1 | 0 | NA | 0 | 0 | 54 | 18 | NA | <1 | 1 fruit |
| Longan, Raw | 30 | 58 | <1 | 0 | 0 | 0 | 0 | 0 | 15 | 1 | 1 | 1 fruit |
| Lotus Root | 10 slices | 45 | <1 | 0 | <1 | 0 | 0 | 33 | 14 | 4 | 2 | 1 starch |
| Luffa, Angled, Raw | 1 cup | 30 | <1 | 0 | NA | 0 | 0 | 2 | 7 | NA | 1 | 1 vegetable |
| Luffa, Smooth/Sponge, Raw | 1 cup | 34 | <1 | 0 | NA | 0 | 0 | 6 | 8 | NA | 2 | 1 vegetable |
| Mango, Small | 1/2 cup | 68 | <1 | 0 | <1 | 0 | 0 | 2 | 18 | 2 | <1 | 1 fruit |
| Moon Cake, Plain Lotus Seed Paste | 1/4 | 169 | 8 | 70 | NA | 0 | 2 | NA | 24 | <1 | 2 | 1 1/2 carb, 2 fat |
| Mung Bean Sprouts, Seed Attached, Raw | 1 cup | 31 | <1 | 0 | 0 | 0 | 0 | 6 | 6 | 2 | 3 | 1 vegetable |
| Mustard Greens, Cooked | 1/2 cup | 11 | <1 | 0 | 0 | 0 | 0 | 11 | 2 | 1 | 2 | 1 vegetable |

ETHNIC FOODS

| | Serving | Calories | Fat (g) | Cal. from Fat | Sat. Fat (g) | Trans Fat (g) | Chol. (mg) | Sod. (mg) | Carb. (g) | Fiber (g) | Prot. (g) | Servings/Exchanges |
|---|---|---|---|---|---|---|---|---|---|---|---|---|
| Mustard Greens, Salted | 2 Tbsp | 14 | <1 | 0 | NA | 0 | 0 | NA | 4 | NA | <1 | free |
| Oriental Radish/Daikon, Raw | 1 cup | 16 | <1 | 0 | 0 | 0 | 0 | 18 | 4 | 1 | <1 | 1 vegetable |
| Papaya, Medium | 1/2 | 59 | <1 | 0 | <1 | 0 | 0 | 5 | 15 | 3 | <1 | 1 fruit |
| Peapods/Sugar Peas, Cooked | 1/2 cup | 34 | <1 | 0 | 0 | 0 | 0 | 3 | 6 | 2 | 3 | 1 vegetable |
| Pepper, Chili, Raw | 1 cup | 60 | <1 | 0 | 0 | 0 | 0 | 11 | 14 | 2 | 3 | 3 vegetables |
| Persimmon | 1/2 | 59 | <1 | 0 | 0 | 0 | 0 | 1 | 16 | 3 | <1 | 1 fruit |
| Pummelo | 3/4 cup | 58 | <1 | 0 | NA | 0 | 0 | 1 | 14 | <1 | 1 | 1 fruit |
| Rice Noodles, Fresh | 1/2 cup | 99 | <1 | 0 | 0 | 0 | 0 | NA | 23 | NA | 1 | 1 1/2 starch |
| Rice Vermicelli, Cooked | 1/2 cup | 56 | 0 | 0 | 0 | 0 | 0 | NA | 13 | NA | 1 | 1 starch |
| Salted Duck Egg | 1 | 137 | 7 | 65 | NA | 0 | NA | NA | <1 | 0 | 10 | 1 high-fat meat |
| Scallop, Dried, Large | 1 | 44 | <1 | 0 | NA | 0 | NA | NA | 1 | NA | 9 | 1 lean meat |
| Sesame Paste | 2 tsp | 60 | 5 | 45 | 1 | 0 | 0 | 12 | 2 | <1 | 2 | 1 fat |

| | | | | | | | | | | | | |
|---|---|---|---|---|---|---|---|---|---|---|---|---|
| Sesame Seeds, Whole, Dried | 1 Tbsp | 52 | 5 | 45 | <1 | 0 | 0 | 1 | 2 | 1 | 2 | 1 fat |
| Shrimp, Dried, Medium | 10 | 40 | <1 | 0 | NA | 0 | NA | NA | 2 | NA | 7 | 1 lean meat |
| Soybean Milk, Unsweetened | 1 cup | 81 | 5 | 45 | <1 | 0 | 0 | 29 | 4 | 3 | 7 | 1 med-fat meat |
| Soybean Sprouts, Seed Attached, Raw | 1 cup | 86 | 5 | 45 | <1 | 0 | 0 | 10 | 7 | <1 | 9 | 1 vegetable, 1 med-fat meat |
| Soybeans, Cooked | 3 Tbsp | 56 | 3 | 25 | <1 | 0 | 0 | 0 | 3 | 2 | 5 | 1 lean meat |
| Squid, Raw | 2 oz | 52 | <1 | 0 | <1 | 0 | 132 | 26 | 2 | 0 | 9 | 1 lean meat |
| Straw Mushrooms, Canned | 1/2 cup | 20 | <1 | 0 | NA | 0 | 0 | 172 | 4 | NA | 2 | 1 vegetable |
| Sweet Rice Dough Ball | 3 | 220 | 10 | 90 | 6 | NA | 0 | 0 | 29 | 1 | 3 | 2 carb, 2 fat |
| Taro, Cooked | 1/2 cup | 94 | <1 | 0 | <1 | 0 | 0 | 10 | 23 | 3 | <1 | 1 1/2 starch |
| Tofu/Soybean Curd | 4 oz | 91 | 6 | 55 | <1 | NA | 0 | 8 | 2 | 1 | 10 | 1 med-fat meat |
| Tripe, Beef, Raw | 2 oz | 56 | 2 | 20 | 1 | 0 | 54 | 26 | 0 | 0 | 8 | 1 lean meat |
| Turnip, Raw | 1 cup | 35 | <1 | 0 | 0 | 0 | 0 | 87 | 8 | 2 | 1 | 1 vegetable |

| | Serving | Calories | Fat (g) | Cal. from Fat | Sat. Fat (g) | Trans Fat (g) | Chol. (mg) | Sod. (mg) | Carb. (g) | Fiber (g) | Prot. (g) | Servings/Exchanges |
|---|---|---|---|---|---|---|---|---|---|---|---|---|
| Water Chestnuts, Chinese | 1/2 cup | 66 | <1 | 0 | 0 | 0 | 0 | 9 | 15 | 2 | <1 | 1 starch |
| Watercress, Raw | 1 cup | 4 | 0 | 0 | 0 | 0 | 0 | 14 | <1 | <1 | <1 | free |
| Winter Melon/Wax Gourd/Chinese Preserving Melon | 1 cup | 17 | <1 | 0 | 0 | 0 | 0 | 147 | 4 | 4 | <1 | 1 vegetable |
| Won Ton, Cantonese Style | 5 | 83 | <1 | 0 | 0 | 0 | 0 | 850 | 13 | 2 | 6 | 1 starch |
| Yard-Long Beans, Cooked | 1/2 cup | 24 | <1 | 0 | 0 | 0 | 0 | 2 | 5 | NA | 1 | 1 vegetable |
| Yard-Long Beans, Raw | 1 cup | 43 | <1 | 0 | <1 | 0 | 0 | 4 | 8 | NA | 3 | 1 vegetable |
| **FILIPINO AMERICAN** | | | | | | | | | | | | |
| Bamboo Shoots, Canned | 1/2 cup | 13 | <1 | 0 | <1 | 0 | 0 | 5 | 2 | 1 | 1 | 1 vegetable |

| | | | | | | | | | | | | |
|---|---|---|---|---|---|---|---|---|---|---|---|---|
| Banana Sauce | 1 tsp | 11 | NA | NA | NA | 0 | 0 | NA | 3 | 0 | 0 | free |
| Banana Squash, Cooked | 1/2 cup | 24 | <1 | 0 | <1 | 0 | 0 | 2 | 6 | 1 | <1 | 1 vegetable |
| Banana, Native, Small | 1 | 46 | <1 | 0 | <1 | 0 | 0 | 0 | 12 | <1 | <1 | 1 fruit |
| Beef Shank, Lean, Cooked | 1 oz | 57 | 2 | 20 | <1 | 0 | 22 | 18 | 0 | 0 | 10 | 1 lean meat |
| Beef Tongue | 1 oz | 80 | 6 | 55 | 3 | 0 | 30 | 17 | <1 | 0 | 6 | 1 med-fat meat |
| Bitter Melon, Cooked | 1/2 cup | 12 | <1 | 0 | NA | 0 | 0 | 4 | 3 | NA | <1 | 1 vegetable |
| Bottle Gourd, Cooked | 1/2 cup | 9 | <1 | 0 | NA | 0 | 0 | NA | 2 | <1 | <1 | free |
| Cassava Tuber, Cooked | 1/2 cup | 60 | <1 | 0 | <1 | 0 | 0 | 4 | 15 | <1 | <1 | 1 starch |
| Ceylon Moss Bar, Dried | 1/4 | 8 | 0 | 0 | 0 | 0 | 0 | 3 | 2 | <1 | <1 | free |
| Chayote, Cooked | 1/2 cup | 19 | <1 | 0 | 0 | 0 | 0 | 1 | 4 | <1 | <1 | 1 vegetable |
| Chicken Gizzard, Cooked | 1 oz | 43 | 1 | 10 | <1 | 0 | 55 | 19 | <1 | 0 | 8 | 1 lean meat |
| Chinese Celery, Raw | 1 cup | 32 | 2 | 20 | NA | 0 | NA | 48 | 5 | <1 | 3 | 1 vegetable |
| Chinese Sausage | 1 oz | 100 | 8 | 70 | 3 | NA | 30 | 249 | 2 | NA | 6 | 1 high-fat meat |
| Chinese Spinach, Raw | 1 cup | 7 | <1 | 0 | <1 | 0 | 0 | 5 | 1 | NA | <1 | free |

ETHNIC FOODS

| | Serving | Calories | Fat (g) | Cal. from Fat | Sat. Fat (g) | Trans Fat (g) | Chol. (mg) | Sod. (mg) | Carb. (g) | Fiber (g) | Prot. (g) | Servings/Exchanges |
|---|---|---|---|---|---|---|---|---|---|---|---|---|
| Clam, Cooked | 1oz | 42 | <1 | 0 | <1 | 0 | 19 | 32 | 2 | 0 | 7 | 1 lean meat |
| Coconut Milk, Canned | 1 Tbsp | 35 | 4 | 35 | 3 | 0 | 0 | 2 | <1 | 0 | <1 | 1 fat |
| Corned Beef, Canned | 1 oz | 71 | 4 | 35 | 2 | 0 | 24 | 285 | 0 | 0 | 8 | 1 med-fat meat |
| Cracklings, Crushed | 2 Tbsp | 42 | 3 | 25 | <1 | 0 | 9 | 3 | 0 | 0 | 4 | 1 fat |
| Fish Sauce | 1 Tbsp | 4 | <1 | 0 | NA | 0 | NA | 1088 | 0 | 0 | <1 | free |
| Guava, Raw | 1 1/2 | 61 | <1 | 0 | <1 | 0 | 0 | 3 | 14 | 7 | 1 | 1 fruit |
| Horseradish Leaves, Cooked | 1/2 cup | 13 | <1 | 0 | NA | 0 | 0 | 2 | 2 | NA | 1 | 1 vegetable |
| Indian Sardines, Dried | 1 oz | 57 | 1 | 10 | NA | 0 | NA | NA | 0 | 0 | 11 | 1 lean meat |
| Jicama, Cooked | 1/2 cup | 19 | 0 | 0 | 0 | 0 | 0 | 2 | 4 | <1 | <1 | 1 vegetable |
| Long-Jawed Anchovy, Dried | 2 Tbsp | 64 | 1 | 10 | NA | 0 | NA | 26 | 0 | 0 | 12 | 1 lean meat |
| Mango, Small | 1/2 | 61 | <1 | 0 | <1 | 0 | 0 | 2 | 18 | 3 | <1 | 1 fruit |
| Mung Beans, Cooked | 1/3 cup | 71 | <1 | 0 | <1 | 0 | 0 | 1 | 13 | NA | 5 | 1 starch |

| | | | | | | | | | | | | |
|---|---|---|---|---|---|---|---|---|---|---|---|---|
| Mung Bean Noodles, Cooked | 3/4 cup | 73 | 0 | 0 | 0 | 0 | 0 | 9 | 18 | NA | 0 | 1 starch |
| Native Sausage, Raw | 1 oz | 167 | 17 | 155 | NA | NA | NA | NA | <1 | 0 | 3 | 1 high-fat meat, 1 fat |
| Oriental Radish/Daikon, Raw | 1 cup | 16 | 0 | 0 | 0 | 0 | 0 | 9 | 2 | NA | <1 | free |
| Oyster, Cooked, Medium | 1 | 41 | 1 | 9 | <1 | 0 | 38 | 53 | 3 | 0 | 5 | 1 lean meat |
| Papaya, Unripe, Cooked | 1/2 cup | 20 | <1 | 0 | NA | 0 | 0 | 3 | 5 | <1 | 1 | 1 vegetable |
| Papaya, Yellow, Raw, Cubed | 1 cup | 54 | <1 | 0 | <1 | 0 | 0 | 4 | 14 | 2 | <1 | 1 fruit |
| Peapods, Cooked | 1/2 cup | 34 | <1 | 0 | <1 | 0 | 0 | 3 | 6 | 1 | 3 | 1 vegetable |
| Plantain, Cooked, Sliced | 1/2 cup | 89 | <1 | 0 | NA | 0 | 0 | 4 | 24 | 2 | <1 | 1 1/2 starch |
| Pummelo | 3/4 cup | 62 | <1 | 0 | NA | 0 | 0 | 0 | 15 | 2 | 1 | 1 fruit |
| Rice Sticks/Noodles, Cooked | 3/4 cup | 91 | 1 | 10 | NA | 0 | 0 | 1 | 19 | <1 | 1 | 1 starch |
| Sausage, Simulated | 1 oz | 72 | 5 | 45 | <1 | NA | 0 | 251 | 3 | 0 | 5 | 1 med-fat meat |
| Sesame Seeds, Dried | 1 Tbsp | 52 | 5 | 45 | <1 | 0 | 0 | 1 | 2 | <1 | 2 | 1 fat |

ETHNIC FOODS

| | Serving | Calories | Fat (g) | Cal. from Fat | Sat. Fat (g) | Trans Fat (g) | Chol. (mg) | Sod. (mg) | Carb. (g) | Fiber (g) | Prot. (g) | Servings/Exchanges |
|---|---|---|---|---|---|---|---|---|---|---|---|---|
| Shrimp, Fermented, Small | 1 Tbsp | 12 | <1 | 0 | <1 | 0 | 0 | 734 | 0 | <1 | 3 | free |
| Soy Bean Curd/Tofu | 1/2 cup | 94 | 6 | 55 | <1 | 0 | 0 | 9 | 2 | 2 | 10 | 1 med-fat meat |
| Spanish Sausage | 1 oz | 125 | 11 | 100 | 4 | NA | 30 | 367 | NA | 0 | 7 | 1 high-fat meat, 1 fat |
| Swamp Cabbage, Cooked | 1/2 cup | 9 | <1 | 0 | NA | 0 | 0 | 63 | <1 | <1 | 1 | free |
| Taro, Cooked | 1/3 cup | 62 | <1 | 0 | <1 | 0 | 0 | 6 | 15 | NA | <1 | 1 starch |
| Watermelon Seeds, Dried | 1 Tbsp | 38 | 3 | 25 | <1 | 0 | 0 | 6 | 1 | <1 | 2 | 1 fat |
| Yard-Long Beans, Cooked | 1/2 cup | 24 | <1 | 0 | <1 | 0 | 0 | 2 | 5 | NA | 1 | 1 vegetable |
| **HMONG** | | | | | | | | | | | | |
| Asian Pear | 1 | 51 | <1 | 0 | 0 | 0 | 0 | 0 | 13 | 4 | <1 | 1 fruit |
| Bamboo Shoots, Canned | 1/2 cup | 13 | <1 | 0 | <1 | 0 | 0 | 4 | 2 | <1 | 1 | 1 vegetable |

| | | | | | | | | | | | | |
|---|---|---|---|---|---|---|---|---|---|---|---|---|
| Beef Tallow | 1 tsp | 39 | 4 | 35 | 2 | NA | 5 | 0 | 0 | 0 | 0 | 1 fat |
| Bitter Melon, Raw | 1 cup | 16 | <1 | 0 | 0 | 0 | 0 | 5 | 3 | 3 | <1 | 1 vegetable |
| Cellophane/Mung Bean Noodles, Cooked | 1/2 cup | 67 | NA | NA | 0 | 0 | 0 | 2 | 16 | <1 | NA | 1 starch |
| Chicken Fat | 1 tsp | 39 | 4 | 35 | 1 | 0 | 4 | 0 | 0 | 0 | 0 | 1 fat |
| Chitterlings, Boiled | 2 Tbsp | 42 | 4 | 35 | 1 | 0 | 20 | 6 | 0 | 0 | 1 | 1 fat |
| Coconut Cream, Canned | 1 Tbsp | 36 | 3 | 35 | 3 | 0 | 0 | 10 | 2 | <1 | <1 | 1 fat |
| Coconut Milk, Canned | 1 Tbsp | 30 | 3 | 25 | 3 | 0 | 0 | 2 | <1 | 0 | <1 | 1 fat |
| Coconut Milk, Raw | 1 Tbsp | 35 | 4 | 35 | 3 | 0 | 0 | 2 | <1 | <1 | <1 | 1 fat |
| Coconut, Raw | 2 Tbsp | 35 | 3 | 25 | 3 | 0 | 0 | 2 | 2 | <1 | <1 | 1 fat |
| Condensed Milk, Sweetened | 2 Tbsp | 123 | 3 | 25 | 2 | 0 | 13 | 46 | 21 | 0 | 3 | 1 1/2 carb, 1 fat |
| Coriander/Chinese Parsely, Raw | 1 cup | 3 | <1 | 0 | 0 | 0 | 0 | 4 | <1 | <1 | <1 | free |
| Cucuzzi Squash, Cooked | 1/2 cup | 23 | <1 | 0 | 0 | 0 | 0 | 14 | 5 | 1 | <1 | 1 vegetable |

ETHNIC FOODS

| | Serving | Calories | Fat (g) | Cal. from Fat | Sat. Fat (g) | Trans Fat (g) | Chol. (mg) | Sod. (mg) | Carb. (g) | Fiber (g) | Prot. (g) | Servings/Exchanges |
|---|---|---|---|---|---|---|---|---|---|---|---|---|
| Fish Sauce | 1 Tbsp | 6 | 0 | 0 | 0 | 0 | 0 | 1390 | <1 | 0 | <1 | free |
| Guava, Medium | 1 | 69 | <1 | 0 | <1 | 0 | 0 | 4 | 16 | 7 | 1 | 1 fruit |
| Jackfruit | 1/2 cup | 78 | <1 | 0 | 0 | 0 | 0 | 2 | 20 | 1 | 1 | 1 fruit |
| Leeks, Cooked | 1/2 cup | 16 | <1 | 0 | 0 | 0 | 0 | 6 | 4 | NA | <1 | 1 vegetable |
| Luffa Gourd/Squash, Raw | 1 cup | 30 | <1 | 0 | NA | 0 | 0 | 6 | 7 | NA | 2 | 1 vegetable |
| Mango, Small | 1/2 | 68 | <1 | 0 | <1 | 0 | 0 | 2 | 18 | 2 | <1 | 1 fruit |
| Mung Bean Sprouts with Seeds, Cooked | 1/2 cup | 13 | <1 | 0 | 0 | 0 | 0 | 6 | 3 | <1 | 1 | 1 vegetable |
| Mustard Greens | 1/2 cup | 10 | <1 | 0 | 0 | 0 | 0 | 11 | 2 | 1 | 2 | 1 vegetable |
| Papaya, Medium | 1/2 | 59 | <1 | 0 | <1 | 0 | 9 | 4 | 15 | 3 | <1 | 1 fruit |
| Peas, Podded, Cooked | 1/2 cup | 24 | <1 | 0 | 0 | 0 | 0 | 3 | 6 | 2 | 3 | 1 vegetable |
| Peas, Podded, Raw | 1/2 cup | 26 | <1 | 0 | 0 | 0 | 0 | 3 | 5 | 2 | 2 | 1 vegetable |
| Pheasant, No Skin, Raw | 1 oz | 38 | 1 | 0 | <1 | 0 | 19 | 10 | 0 | 0 | 7 | 1 lean meat |

| | | | | | | | | | | | | |
|---|---|---|---|---|---|---|---|---|---|---|---|---|
| Pig's Feet | 1/2 foot | 68 | 4 | 35 | 1.5 | 0 | 35 | 11 | 0 | 0 | 7 | 1 med-fat meat |
| Pork Lard | 1 tsp | 39 | 4 | 35 | 2 | NA | 4 | 0 | 0 | 0 | 0 | 1 fat |
| Pork, Ground | 1 oz | 84 | 6 | 55 | 2 | 0 | 27 | 21 | 0 | 0 | 7 | 1 high-fat meat |
| Pumpkin Blossom, Cooked | 1 cup | 20 | <1 | 0 | 0 | 0 | 0 | 8 | 4 | 1 | 2 | free |
| Pumpkin, Cooked | 1/2 cup | 24 | <1 | 0 | 0 | 0 | 0 | 2 | 6 | 1 | <1 | 1 vegetable |
| Rice Noodles, Fresh | 1/2 cup | 99 | <1 | 0 | 0 | 0 | 0 | NA | 23 | <1 | 1 | 1 starch |
| Squirrel, Roasted | 1 oz | 49 | 1 | 10 | <1 | 0 | 34 | 34 | 0 | 0 | 9 | 1 lean meat |
| Tofu/Soybean Curd | 4 oz, 1/2 cup | 94 | 6 | 55 | <1 | 0 | 0 | 9 | 2 | 2 | 10 | 1 med-fat meat |
| Venison | 1 oz | 45 | <1 | 0 | <1 | 0 | 32 | 15 | 0 | 0 | 9 | 1 lean meat |
| Vinespinach, Raw | 1 cup | 11 | <1 | 0 | 0 | 0 | 0 | 13 | 2 | 0 | 1 | free |
| Yard-Long Beans, Cooked | 1/2 cup | 102 | <1 | 0 | <1 | 0 | 0 | 4 | 18 | NA | 7 | 1 starch, 1 lean meat |
| **INDIAN & PAKISTANI** | | | | | | | | | | | | |
| Aviyal | 1/2 cup | 81 | 2 | 20 | 1 | 0 | NA | 412 | 14 | NA | 2 | 1 starch |

| | Serving | Calories | Fat (g) | Cal. from Fat | Sat. Fat (g) | Trans Fat (g) | Chol. (mg) | Sod. (mg) | Carb. (g) | Fiber (g) | Prot. (g) | Servings/Exchanges |
|---|---|---|---|---|---|---|---|---|---|---|---|---|
| Brinjal, Cooked | 1/2 cup | 13 | 0 | 0 | 0 | 0 | 0 | 1 | 3 | 1 | 0 | 1 vegetable |
| Chai Masala | 1/2 cup | 14 | 0 | 0 | 0 | 0 | 0 | 0 | 3 | NA | 1 | free |
| Chicken Tikka | 3 1-inch pieces | 54 | 2 | 20 | <1 | 0 | 23 | 156 | 0 | 0 | 9 | 1 lean meat |
| Chickpeas, Cooked | 1/2 cup | 134 | 2 | 20 | <1 | 0 | 0 | 6 | 23 | 4 | 7 | 1 1/2 starch, 1 lean meat |
| Coconut, Fresh, Shredded | 3 Tbsp | 53 | 5 | 45 | 4 | 0 | 0 | 3 | 2 | 1 | 1 | 1 fat |
| Coriander, Fresh | 1/2 cup | 2 | 0 | 0 | 0 | 0 | 0 | 2 | 0 | <1 | 0 | free |
| Cucumber Raita | 1/2 cup | 21 | 0 | 0 | 0 | 0 | 0 | 22 | 3 | NA | 1 | 1 vegetable |
| Dhakla, Khaman | 1-inch square | 104 | 5 | 45 | 0 | 0 | NA | 539 | 12 | NA | 5 | 1 starch, 1 fat |
| Dhansak | 1/2 cup | 104 | 4 | 35 | 0.5 | 0 | NA | 137 | 15 | NA | 4 | 1 starch, 1 fat |
| Fresh Shredded Coconut | 3 Tbsp | 53 | 5 | 45 | 4 | 0 | 0 | 3 | 2 | 1 | 1 | 1 fat |

| | | | | | | | | | | | | |
|---|---|---|---|---|---|---|---|---|---|---|---|---|
| Ghee | 1 tsp | 45 | 5 | 45 | 3 | 0 | 20 | 0 | 0 | 0 | 0 | 1 fat |
| Ginger, Fresh | 1/4 cup | 17 | <1 | 0 | 0 | 0 | 0 | 3 | 4 | 0.5 | 0 | free |
| Green Plantain, Cooked | 1/3 cup | 60 | <1 | 0 | 0 | 0 | 0 | 3 | 16 | 1 | 0 | 1 starch |
| Guava, Medium, Raw | 1 1/2 | 61 | <1 | 0 | <1 | 0 | 0 | 3 | 14 | 7 | 1 | 1 fruit |
| Idli | 3 inches | 70 | 0 | 0 | 0 | 0 | 0 | 12 | 12 | NA | 2 | 1 starch |
| Jheera Pani | 1/2 cup | 16 | 0.5 | 5 | 0.5 | 0 | NA | 104 | 3 | NA | 1 | free |
| Karela, Cooked | 1/2 cup | 12 | 0 | 0 | 0 | 0 | 0 | 4 | 3 | 1 | 1 | 1 vegetable |
| Lassi | 1 cup | 90 | 0 | 0 | 0 | 0 | 4 | 128 | 13 | 0 | 10 | 1 skim milk |
| Mango, Small, Raw | 1/2 | 68 | <1 | 0 | 0 | 0 | 0 | 2 | 18 | 2 | 1 | 1 fruit |
| Matki Usual | 1/2 cup | 104 | 6 | 55 | 4 | 0 | 0 | 192 | 10 | NA | 3 | 1 starch, 1 fat |
| Mung Bean Sprouts, Cooked | 1/2 cup | 13 | <1 | 0 | 0 | 0 | 0 | 6 | 3 | 0.5 | 1 | 1 vegetable |
| Mung Dhal, Cooked | 1/2 cup | 107 | <1 | 0 | <1 | 0 | 0 | 2 | 19 | 8 | 7 | 1 starch, 1 lean meat |
| Naan | 1/4 of 8 x 2 inches | 75 | 2 | 20 | <1 | 0 | 9 | 90 | 13 | <1 | 2 | 1 starch |
| Cooked | 1/2 cup | 34 | <1 | 0 | 0 | 0 | 0 | 3 | 8 | 3 | 2 | 1 vegetable |

| | Serving | Calories | Fat (g) | Cal. from Fat | Sat. Fat (g) | Trans Fat (g) | Chol. (mg) | Sod. (mg) | Carb. (g) | Fiber (g) | Prot. (g) | Servings/Exchanges |
|---|---|---|---|---|---|---|---|---|---|---|---|---|
| Paneer | 1 oz | 103 | 3 | 25 | 2 | 0 | NA | 246 | 12 | 0 | 8 | 1 2% milk |
| Pesarattu | 9 inches | 127 | 5 | 45 | 1 | 0 | NA | 372 | 14 | NA | 5 | 1 starch, 1 fat |
| Phulka/Chappathi | 6 inches | 68 | <1 | 0 | <1 | 0 | 0 | 179 | 15 | 2 | 3 | 1 starch |
| Poha | 1/2 cup | 140 | 6 | 55 | 1 | 0 | NA | 405 | 18 | NA | 2 | 1 starch, 1 fat |
| Puri | 5 inches | 128 | 7 | 65 | <1 | 0 | 0 | 1 | 16 | 2 | 3 | 1 starch, 1 fat |
| Rasam | 1 cup | 22 | 1 | 10 | <1 | 0 | NA | 255 | 2 | NA | 1 | free |
| Sambar | 1/2 cup | 88 | 1 | 10 | 0 | 0 | NA | 263 | 16 | NA | 5 | 1 starch |
| Tandoori Chicken | 1 oz | 75 | 4 | 35 | 1 | 0 | NA | 152 | 2 | NA | 8 | 1 med-fat meat |
| Tomato, Dhal | 1/2 cup | 132 | 3 | 25 | 2 | 0 | NA | 262 | 18 | NA | 7 | 1 starch, 1 lean meat |
| Toor Dhal, Cooked | 1/2 cup | 103 | <1 | 0 | <1 | 0 | 0 | 4 | 20 | 5 | 6 | 1 starch, 1 lean meat |
| **JEWISH** | | | | | | | | | | | | |
| Bagel | 1/2 | 78 | <1 | 0 | <1 | 0 | 0 | 151 | 15 | <1 | 3 | 1 starch |
| Beef Brisket | 1 oz | 52 | 2 | 20 | <1 | 0 | 16 | 28 | 1 | 0 | 6 | 1 lean meat |
| Beef Tongue | 1 oz | 80 | 6 | 55 | 3 | 0 | 30 | 17 | <1 | 0 | 6 | 1 med-fat meat |

| | | | | | | | | | | | | |
|---|---|---|---|---|---|---|---|---|---|---|---|---|
| Bialy | 1/2 | 69 | 0 | 0 | 0 | 0 | 0 | 167 | 16 | 1 | 7 | 1 starch |
| Blintzes | 2 1/4 oz | 80 | 2 | 20 | <1 | 0 | 118 | 135 | 13 | 0 | 6 | 1 carb |
| Borekas | 1/2 pie | 114 | 11 | 100 | 5 | 0 | 45 | 191 | 15 | <1 | 5 | 1 starch, 2 fat |
| Borscht | 1/2 cup | 26 | <1 | 0 | <1 | 0 | 0 | 473 | 5 | 1 | 2 | 1 vegetable |
| Bulgur, Cooked | 1/2 cup | 76 | <1 | 0 | 0 | 0 | 0 | 5 | 17 | 4 | 3 | 1 starch |
| Bulke Roll | 1/2 roll | 78 | <1 | 0 | NA | 0 | 0 | 137 | 15 | <1 | 4 | 1 starch |
| Challah | 1 oz | 81 | 2 | 20 | <1 | 0 | 15 | 139 | 14 | <1 | 3 | 1 starch |
| Chicken Liver | 1 oz | 45 | 2 | 20 | <1 | 0 | 179 | 15 | <1 | 0 | 7 | 1 lean meat |
| Chickpeas | 1/2 cup | 135 | 2 | 20 | <1 | 0 | 0 | 6 | 23 | 6 | 7 | 1 1/2 starch, 1 lean meat |
| Corned Beef | 1 oz | 71 | 5 | 45 | 2 | NA | 28 | 321 | <1 | 0 | 5 | 1 med-fat meat |
| Couscous | 1/2 cup | 88 | <1 | 0 | 0 | 0 | 0 | 4 | 18 | 1 | 3 | 1 starch |
| Cream Cheese | 1 Tbsp | 51 | 5 | 45 | 3 | 0 | 16 | 43 | <1 | 0 | 1 | 1 fat |
| Farfel | 1/2 cup | 73 | <1 | 0 | 0 | 0 | 0 | 0 | 15 | <1 | 2 | 1 starch |
| Flanken, Raw | 1 oz | 51 | 3 | 25 | 1 | 0 | 15 | 20 | 0 | 0 | 6 | 1 lean meat |
| Gefilte Fish | 2 pieces | 71 | 2 | 20 | <1 | 0 | 25 | 440 | 6 | 0 | 8 | 1/2 carb, 1 lean meat |

| | Serving | Calories | Fat (g) | Cal. from Fat | Sat. Fat (g) | Trans Fat (g) | Chol. (mg) | Sod. (mg) | Carb. (g) | Fiber (g) | Prot. (g) | Servings/Exchanges |
|---|---|---|---|---|---|---|---|---|---|---|---|---|
| Herring in Wine Sauce | 1/4 cup | 90 | 4 | 35 | 1 | 0 | 25 | 420 | 7 | 0 | 5 | 1/2 carb, 1 med-fat meat |
| Herring, Pickled | 1 oz | 74 | 5 | 45 | <1 | 0 | 4 | 247 | 3 | 0 | 4 | 1 med-fat meat |
| Horseradish, Root | 1 Tbsp | 7 | <1 | 0 | 0 | 0 | 0 | 47 | 2 | <1 | <1 | free |
| Kasha, Cooked | 1/2 cup | 77 | <1 | 0 | <1 | 0 | 0 | 3 | 17 | 2 | 3 | 1 starch |
| Kasha, Dry | 2 Tbsp | 71 | <1 | 0 | <1 | 0 | 0 | 2 | 15 | 2 | 2 | 1 starch |
| Kichlach | 2-3 | 106 | 4 | 35 | <1 | 0 | 42 | 13 | 15 | <1 | 3 | 1 carb, 1 fat |
| Knishes | 1 1/2 oz | 114 | 5 | 45 | <1 | 0 | 35 | 162 | 15 | 1 | 3 | 1 starch, 1 fat |
| Kreplach | 2 oz | 128 | 4 | 35 | 1 | 0 | 62 | 70 | 13 | <1 | 10 | 1 carb, 1 lean meat |
| Kugel | 1/2 cup | 113 | 2 | 20 | <1 | 0 | 31 | 277 | 17 | <1 | 7 | 1 carb |
| Leckach | 1 oz | 84 | 2 | 20 | <1 | 0 | 13 | 43 | 16 | <1 | 1 | 1 starch |
| Lentils, Cooked | 1/2 cup | 115 | <1 | 0 | 0 | 0 | 0 | 2 | 20 | 8 | 9 | 1 starch, 1 lean meat |
| Lox | 1 oz | 33 | 1 | 10 | <1 | 0 | 7 | 567 | 0 | 0 | 5 | 1 lean meat |
| Matzoh | 3/4 oz | 84 | <1 | 0 | 0 | 0 | 0 | 0 | 18 | <1 | 2 | 1 starch |

| | | | | | | | | | | | | |
|---|---|---|---|---|---|---|---|---|---|---|---|---|
| Matzoh Ball | 3 balls | 212 | 13 | 115 | 4 | NA | 127 | 678 | 16 | <1 | 6 | 1 carb, 2 1/2 fat |
| Matzoh Meal | 2 Tbsp | 65 | <1 | 0 | 0 | 0 | 0 | 0 | 0 | <1 | 2 | 1 starch |
| Pastrami | 1 oz | 99 | 8 | 70 | 3 | NA | 26 | 348 | <1 | 0 | 5 | 1 high-fat meat |
| Pickles, Dill, Large | 1 1/2 | 36 | <1 | 0 | <1 | 0 | 0 | 2596 | 8 | 2 | 1 | 1 vegetable |
| Potato Flour | 2 Tbsp | 71 | <1 | 0 | <1 | 0 | 0 | 11 | 14 | 1 | 1 | 1 starch |
| Potato Pancakes, Medium | 1 | 124 | 7 | 65 | 1 | 0 | 13 | 232 | 13 | <1 | 3 | 1 starch, 1 fat |
| Pumpernickel Bread | 1 oz | 71 | <1 | 0 | <1 | 0 | 0 | 190 | 14 | 2 | 3 | 1 starch |
| Rye Bread | 1 oz | 73 | <1 | 0 | <1 | 0 | 0 | 187 | 14 | 2 | 2 | 1 starch |
| Sablefish | 1 oz | 73 | 6 | 55 | 1 | 0 | 18 | 209 | 0 | 0 | 5 | 1 med-fat meat |
| Salmon, Canned | 1 oz | 39 | 2 | 20 | <1 | 0 | 16 | 157 | 0 | 0 | 6 | 1 lean meat |
| Sardines, Medium, in Oil, Drained | 2 | 60 | 3 | 25 | <1 | 0 | 41 | 145 | 0 | 0 | 7 | 1 lean meat |
| Schmaltz | 1 tsp | 38 | 4 | 35 | 1 | 0 | 4 | 0 | 0 | 0 | 0 | 1 fat |
| Smelt | 1 oz | 35 | <1 | 0 | <1 | 0 | 26 | 22 | 0 | 0 | 6 | 1 lean meat |
| Sour Cream | 2 Tbsp | 52 | 5 | 45 | 3 | 0 | 11 | 13 | <1 | 0 | <1 | 1 fat |

ETHNIC FOODS

| | Serving | Calories | Fat (g) | Cal. from Fat | Sat. Fat (g) | Trans Fat (g) | Chol. (mg) | Sod. (mg) | Carb. (g) | Fiber (g) | Prot. (g) | Servings/Exchanges |
|---|---|---|---|---|---|---|---|---|---|---|---|---|
| Split Peas, Cooked | 1/2 cup | 116 | <1 | 0 | 0 | 0 | 0 | 2 | 21 | 8 | 8 | 1 1/2 starch, 1 lean meat |
| Sweet Wine | 4 oz | 173 | 13 | 115 | 0 | 0 | 0 | 0 | 173 | 10 | 0 | 2 |
| Tzimmes | 1/4 cup | 88 | <1 | 0 | 0 | 0 | 0 | 118 | 21 | 2 | 1 | 1 1/2 starch |
| Whitefish, Smoked | 1 oz | 31 | <1 | 0 | <1 | 0 | 9 | 289 | 0 | 0 | 7 | 1 lean meat |
| **MEXICAN AMERICAN** | | | | | | | | | | | | |
| Avocado, Medium | 1/8 | 40 | 4 | 35 | <1 | 0 | 0 | 3 | 2 | <1 | <1 | 1 fat |
| Bolillo, Large | 1/4 | 82 | <1 | 0 | <1 | 0 | 0 | 183 | 16 | <1 | 3 | 1 starch |
| Chayote, Boiled, Drained | 1/2 cup | 19 | <1 | 0 | 0 | 0 | 0 | 1 | 4 | 2 | <1 | 1 vegetable |
| Chorizo | 1 oz | 129 | 11 | 100 | 4 | NA | 25 | 351 | <1 | 0 | 7 | 1 high-fat meat, 1 fat |
| Corn Tortilla, 6-inch | 1 | 58 | <1 | 0 | <1 | 0 | 0 | 42 | 12 | 1 | 2 | 1 starch |
| Corn Tortilla, Fat Added, 6-inch | 1 | 102 | 6 | 55 | <1 | NA | 0 | 42 | 12 | 1 | 2 | 1 starch, 1 fat |

| | | | | | | | | | | | | |
|---|---|---|---|---|---|---|---|---|---|---|---|---|
| Flour Tortilla, 6-inch | 1 | 104 | 2 | 20 | <1 | 0 | 0 | 153 | 18 | 1 | 3 | 1 starch |
| Flour Tortilla, Fat Added, 6-inch | 1 | 148 | 7 | 65 | 1 | NA | 0 | 153 | 18 | 1 | 3 | 1 starch, 1 fat |
| Frijoles Cocidos | 1/2 cup | 117 | <1 | 0 | <1 | 0 | 0 | 2 | 22 | 7 | 7 | 1 starch, 1 lean meat |
| Frijoles Refritos, Fat Added | 1/2 cup | 161 | 5 | 45 | <1 | 0 | 0 | 378 | 22 | 7 | 7 | 1 starch, 1 lean meat, 1 fat |
| Jicama, Raw | 1 cup | 49 | <1 | 0 | 0 | 0 | 0 | 5 | 12 | 6 | <1 | 2 vegetable |
| Mango, Small, Raw | 1/2 | 68 | <1 | 0 | <1 | 0 | 0 | 2 | 18 | 2 | <1 | 1 fruit |
| Menudo | 1 cup | 170 | 9 | 65 | 4 | 0 | NA | 950 | 1 | NA | 20 | 3 lean meat |
| Nopales, Cooked | 1/2 cup | 11 | 0 | 0 | 0 | 0 | 0 | 15 | 3 | 2 | 1 | 1 vegetable |
| Nopales, Raw | 1 cup | 14 | <1 | 0 | <1 | 0 | 0 | 19 | 3 | 2 | 1 | 1 vegetable |
| Pan Dulce, 5-inch | 1 | 458 | 21 | 190 | NA | NA | NA | 389 | 59 | NA | 8 | 4 carb, 4 fat |
| Papaya, Raw, Cubed | 1 cup | 55 | <1 | 0 | <1 | 0 | 0 | 4 | 14 | 3 | <1 | 1 fruit |
| Peppers, Hot Green Chili, Chopped, Raw | 1 cup | 60 | <1 | 0 | 0 | 0 | 0 | 11 | 14 | 2 | 3 | 2 vegetable |
| Queso Anejo | 1 oz | 106 | 9 | 80 | 5 | 0 | 30 | 321 | 1 | 0 | 6 | 1 high-fat meat |

| | Serving | Calories | Fat (g) | Cal. from Fat | Sat. Fat (g) | Trans Fat (g) | Chol. (mg) | Sod. (mg) | Carb. (g) | Fiber (g) | Prot. (g) | Servings/Exchanges |
|---|---|---|---|---|---|---|---|---|---|---|---|---|
| Queso Asadero | 1 oz | 101 | 8 | 70 | 5 | 0 | 30 | 186 | <1 | 0 | 6 | 1 high-fat meat |
| Queso Chihuahua | 1 oz | 106 | 8 | 70 | 5 | 0 | 30 | 175 | 2 | 0 | 6 | 1 high-fat meat |
| Queso Fresco | 1 oz | 83 | 7 | 65 | 4 | 0 | NA | 200 | NA | 0 | 6 | 1 med-fat meat |
| Salsa De Chile | 1/4 cup | 14 | <1 | 0 | 0 | 0 | 0 | 166 | 3 | 1 | <1 | free |
| Taco Shell, 6-inch | 2 | 122 | 6 | 55 | <1 | 0 | 0 | 95 | 16 | 2 | 2 | 1 starch, 1 fat |
| Verdolagas, Cooked | 1/2 cup | 10 | <1 | 0 | 0 | 0 | 0 | 26 | 2 | 1 | <1 | 1 vegetable |
| **NAVAJO** | | | | | | | | | | | | |
| Blue Corn Mush | 3/4 cup | 94 | <1 | 0 | NA | 0 | 0 | 32 | 21 | NA | 3 | 1 starch |
| Corn Hominy, Steamed | 1/2 cup | 70 | 1 | 10 | <1 | 0 | 0 | 18 | 13 | 3 | 2 | 1 starch |
| Four Tortilla, 8-inch | 1/4 | 87 | <1 | 0 | NA | 0 | 0 | 211 | 19 | 1 | 3 | 1 starch |
| Mutton, Lean and Fat, Cooked | 1 oz | 96 | 9 | 80 | NA | 0 | NA | NA | 0 | 0 | 4 | 1 high-fat meat |
| Mutton, Lean, Cooked | 1 oz | 55 | 3 | 25 | 1 | 0 | 21 | 10 | 0 | 0 | 8 | 1 lean meat |
| Piñon Nuts, in Shell | 1 Tbsp | 60 | 6 | 55 | <1 | 0 | 0 | 7 | <1 | 1 | 1 | 1 fat |

**PLAINS INDIAN**

| | | | | | | | | | | | | |
|---|---|---|---|---|---|---|---|---|---|---|---|---|
| Beans, Dried, Cooked | 1/2 cup | 117 | <1 | 0 | <1 | 0 | 0 | 1 | 22 | 7 | 7 | 1 1/2 starch, 1 lean meat |
| Beef Fat, Raw | 1 tsp | 38 | 4 | 35 | 2 | 0 | 5 | 0 | 0 | 0 | 0 | 1 fat |
| Biscuit Mix, Dry | 1/4 cup | 129 | 5 | 45 | 1 | 0 | 19 | 383 | 19 | <1 | 2 | 1 starch, 1 fat |
| Buffalo/Bison | 1 oz | 40 | <1 | 0 | <1 | 0 | 23 | 16 | 0 | 0 | 8 | 1 lean meat |
| Chicken with Skin, Fried | 1 oz | 76 | 4 | 35 | 1 | 0 | 26 | 24 | <1 | 0 | 8 | 1 med-fat meat |
| Commodity Meat, Luncheon | 1 oz | 97 | 9 | 80 | NA | NA | NA | 420 | 1 | NA | 3 | 1 high-fat meat |
| Cracklings | 1/3 oz | 57 | 5 | 45 | 2 | 0 | 9 | 18 | 0 | 0 | 2 | 1 fat |
| Dry Meat | 1 oz | 47 | 1 | 10 | <1 | 0 | 12 | 984 | <1 | 0 | 8 | 1 lean meat |
| Eggs, Dried Powdered | 3 Tbsp | 81 | 7 | 65 | 2 | 0 | 351 | 12 | 0 | 0 | 4 | 1 med-fat meat |
| Elk, Roasted | 1 oz | 41 | <1 | 0 | <1 | 0 | 0 | 17 | 0 | 0 | 9 | 1 lean meat |
| Huckleberries | 1 cup | 56 | <1 | 0 | NA | 0 | NA | 15 | 13 | NA | <1 | 1 fruit |
| Indian Corn, Dried | 1/4 cup | 132 | 2 | 20 | NA | 0 | NA | 37 | 26 | <1 | 4 | 2 starch |
| Kidney, Raw | 1 oz | 30 | <1 | 0 | <1 | 0 | 81 | 51 | <1 | 0 | 5 | 1 lean meat |

ETHNIC FOODS

| | Serving | Calories | Fat (g) | Cal. from Fat | Sat. Fat (g) | Trans Fat (g) | Chol. (mg) | Sod. (mg) | Carb. (g) | Fiber (g) | Prot. (g) | Servings/Exchanges |
|---|---|---|---|---|---|---|---|---|---|---|---|---|
| Lemon, Raw, Peeled | 1 | 17 | <1 | 0 | NA | 0 | 0 | 1 | 5 | 0 | <1 | free |
| Liver, Beef | 1 oz | 46 | 1 | 10 | <1 | 0 | 110 | 20 | 1 | 0 | 7 | 1 lean meat |
| Pheasant, Skinless | 1 oz | 38 | 1 | 10 | <1 | 0 | 0 | 10 | 0 | 0 | 7 | 1 lean meat |
| Pilot Bread | 4-inch piece | 104 | 2 | 20 | NA | 0 | NA | 142 | 18 | NA | 2 | 1 starch |
| Potatoes, Fried | 1/2 cup | 163 | 11 | 100 | 4 | 0 | NA | 19 | 17 | 2 | 2 | 1 starch, 2 fat |
| Short Ribs | 1 oz | 83 | 5 | 45 | 2 | 0 | 0 | 16 | 0 | 0 | 9 | 1 med-fat meat |
| Sweetbreads, Fried | 1 oz | 108 | 8 | 70 | 3 | NA | NA | 126 | 1 | 0 | 7 | 1 high-fat meat |
| Venison | 1 oz | 45 | <1 | 0 | <1 | 0 | 32 | 15 | 0 | 0 | 9 | 1 lean meat |
| White Fish, Dry Heat Cooked | 1 oz | 49 | 2 | 20 | <1 | 0 | 22 | 19 | 0 | 0 | 7 | 1 lean meat |
| Wild Rice, | 1/2 cup | 82 | <1 | 0 | 0 | 0 | 0 | 3 | 17 | <1 | 3 | 1 starch |
| **SOUTHERN & SOUL** | | | | | | | | | | | | |
| Fatback, Raw | 1/4 oz | 58 | 6 | 55 | 2 | 0 | 4 | 1 | 0 | 0 | 0 | 1 fat |

| Ham Hock | 1 oz | 90 | 7 | 65 | 2 | 0 | 18 | 383 | 2 | 0 | 6 | 1 high-fat meat |
|---|---|---|---|---|---|---|---|---|---|---|---|---|
| Hog Jowl | 1 oz | 54 | 5 | 55 | 2 | 0 | 9 | 7 | 0 | 0 | 2 | 1 fat |
| Hog Maw | 1 oz | 45 | 3 | 25 | NA | 0 | 55 | 15 | 0 | 0 | 5 | 1 lean meat |
| Hominy | 3/4 cup | 86 | 1 | 10 | <1 | 0 | 0 | 252 | 17 | 3 | 2 | 1 starch |
| Kale, Cooked | 1/2 cup | 21 | 0 | 0 | 0 | 0 | 0 | 15 | 4 | 1 | 1 | 1 vegetable |
| Lard | 1 tsp | 38 | 4 | 40 | 2 | 0 | 4 | 0 | 0 | 0 | 0 | 1 fat |
| Muscadines | 17 | 60 | 0.5 | 5 | 0 | 0 | 0 | 2 | 15 | 1 | <1 | 1 fruit |
| Opossum | 1 oz | 63 | 3 | 25 | NA | 0 | 23 | 27 | 0 | 0 | 9 | 1 lean meat |
| Oxtail | 1 oz | 72 | 4 | 35 | 1 | 0 | 30 | 20 | 0 | 0 | 9 | 1 med-fat meat |
| Pig Ear | 1/4 ear | 47 | 3 | 25 | NA | 0 | 26 | 48 | 0 | 0 | 5 | 1 lean meat |
| Pigs Feet | 1/2 foot | 68 | 4 | 35 | 2 | 0 | 35 | 58 | 0 | 0 | 7 | 1 med-fat meat |
| Pig Tail | 1 oz or 1/3 tail | 113 | 10 | 90 | 4 | 0 | 37 | 48 | 0 | 0 | 5 | 1 high-fat meat |
| Poke Salad, Cooked | 1/2 cup | 16 | 0 | 0 | 0 | 0 | 0 | NA | 3 | 1 | 2 | 1 vegetable |
| Pork Brains | 1 oz | 39 | 3 | 25 | 0.5 | 0 | 727 | 26 | 0 | 0 | 4 | 1 lean meat |
| Pork Cracklings | 1 Tbsp | 57 | 5 | 45 | 2 | 0 | 9 | 18 | 0 | 0 | 2 | 1 fat |

ETHNIC FOODS

| | Serving | Calories | Fat (g) | Cal. from Fat | Sat. Fat (g) | Trans Fat (g) | Chol. (mg) | Sod. (mg) | Carb. (g) | Fiber (g) | Prot. (g) | Servings/Exchanges |
|---|---|---|---|---|---|---|---|---|---|---|---|---|
| Pork Neck Bones | 1 oz | 66 | 4 | 35 | 2 | 0 | 24 | 20 | 0 | 0 | 7 | 1 med-fat meat |
| Pork Skin (Rind), Fried | 1 cup | 68 | 4 | 35 | 2 | 0 | 17 | 231 | 0 | 0 | 8 | 1 med-fat meat |
| Pork Tongue | 1 oz, 1/3 tongue | 77 | 5 | 45 | 2 | 0 | 42 | 31 | 0 | 0 | 7 | 1 med-fat meat |
| Sousemeat (Headcheese) | 1 oz | 60 | 5 | 45 | 1 | 0 | 23 | 357 | 0 | 0 | 5 | 1 med-fat meat |
| Succotash | 1/2 cup | 79 | 1 | 10 | 0 | 0 | 0 | 38 | 17 | 5 | 4 | 1 starch |
| Tripe | 2 oz | 56 | 2 | 20 | 1 | 0 | 54 | 26 | 0 | 0 | 8 | 1 lean meat |

# FAST FOODS

| | Serving | Calories | Fat (g) | Cal. from Fat | Sat. Fat (g) | Trans Fat (g) | Chol. (mg) | Sod. (mg) | Carb. (mg) | Fiber (g) | Prot. (g) | Servings/Exchanges |
|---|---|---|---|---|---|---|---|---|---|---|---|---|
| **ARBY'S** | | | | | | | | | | | | |
| ***Roast Beef Sandwiches*** | | | | | | | | | | | | |
| Regular Roast Beef | 1 | 320 | 14 | 125 | 5 | 0.5 | 44 | 953 | 34 | 2 | 21 | 2 carb, 2 med-fat meat, 1 fat |
| Super Roast Beef | 1 | 399 | 19 | 170 | 6 | 1 | 40 | 1061 | 44 | 2 | 21 | 3 carb, 2 med-fat meat, 2 fat |
| Bacon & Bleu Roastburger | 1 | 466 | 23 | 210 | 9 | 1 | 52 | 1372 | 44 | 2 | 21 | 3 carb, 2 med-fat meat, 2 fat |
| Beef 'n Cheddar, Regular | 1 | 440 | 21 | 190 | 6 | 1 | 55 | 1275 | 43 | 2 | 22 | 3 carb, 2 med-fat meat, 2 fat |
| Ham & Swiss Melt | 1 | 268 | 8 | 70 | 3 | 0 | 25 | 1042 | 35 | 1 | 17 | 2 carb, 2 med-fat meat |
| ***Chicken*** | | | | | | | | | | | | |
| Chicken Bacon & Swiss, Crispy | 1 | 544 | 25 | 225 | 7 | 0 | 65 | 1632 | 50 | 2 | 32 | 3 carb, 3 med-fat meat, 2 fat |

| | Serving | Calories | Fat (g) | Cal. from Fat | Sat. Fat (g) | Trans Fat (g) | Chol. (mg) | Sod. (mg) | Carb. (g) | Fiber (g) | Prot. (g) | Servings/Exchanges |
|---|---|---|---|---|---|---|---|---|---|---|---|---|
| Chicken Breast Fillet, Roast | 1 | 383 | 16 | 145 | 3 | 0 | 51 | 921 | 37 | 2 | 23 | 2 1/2 carb, 2 med-fat meat, 1 fat |
| Popcorn Chicken, Regular | 1 | 363 | 16 | 145 | 3 | 0 | 54 | 930 | 27 | 2 | 24 | 2 1/2 carb, 2 med-fat meat, 1 fat |
| Roast Chicken Club | 1 | 498 | 20 | 180 | 7 | 0 | 65 | 1540 | 65 | 2 | 30 | 3 carb, 3 med-fat meat, 1 fat |
| ***Market Fresh Sandwiches*** | | | | | | | | | | | | |
| Corned Beef Reuben | 1 | 590 | 32 | 290 | 9 | 0.5 | 77 | 1685 | 55 | 3 | 32 | 3 1/2 carb, 3 med-fat meat, 3 fat |
| Pecan Chicken Salad Sandwich, Grilled | 1 | 870 | 44 | 400 | 6 | 0 | 65 | 1510 | 88 | 7 | 34 | 6 carb, 4 med-fat meat, 5 fat |
| Roast Ham & Swiss | 1 | 691 | 31 | 280 | 8 | 0.5 | 59 | 1952 | 75 | 5 | 33 | 5 carb, 3 med-fat meat, 3 fat |
| Roast Turkey & Swiss | 1 | 708 | 30 | 270 | 8 | 0.5 | 83 | 1677 | 74 | 5 | 41 | 5 carb, 4 med-fat meat, 2 fat |

| | | | | | | | | | | | | |
|---|---|---|---|---|---|---|---|---|---|---|---|---|
| Roast Turkey, Ranch & Bacon | 1 | 818 | 38 | 340 | 11 | 0.5 | 102 | 2146 | 75 | 5 | 46 | 5 carb, 5 med-fat meat, 3 fat |
| Ultimate BLT | 1 | 779 | 45 | 405 | 11 | 0.5 | 51 | 1571 | 75 | 6 | 23 | 5 carb, 1 med-fat meat, 8 fat |
| Toasted Subs | | | | | | | | | | | | |
| French Dip & Swiss | 1 | 533 | 19 | 170 | 8 | 1 | 54 | 2169 | 67 | 3 | 29 | 4 1/2 carb, 2 med-fat meat, 2 fat |
| Philly Beef | 1 | 610 | 30 | 270 | 9 | 1 | 63 | 1549 | 62 | 3 | 29 | 4 carb, 2 med-fat meat, 4 fat |
| Turkey Bacon Club | 1 | 605 | 34 | 305 | 6 | 0 | 67 | 1701 | 65 | 3 | 35 | 4 carb, 3 med-fat meat, 4 fat |
| ***Market Fresh Chopped Salads*** | | | | | | | | | | | | |
| Chopped Italian Salad | 1 | 386 | 28 | 250 | 12 | 1 | 78 | 1420 | 11 | 3 | 21 | 1 carb, 3 med-fat meat, 3 fat |
| Chopped Turkey Club Salad | 1 | 230 | 11 | 100 | 6 | 0.5 | 54 | 801 | 9 | 3 | 22 | 1/2 carb, 3 lean meat |

| | Serving | Calories | Fat (g) | Cal. from Fat | Sat. Fat (g) | Trans Fat (g) | Chol. (mg) | Sod. (mg) | Carb. (g) | Fiber (g) | Prot. (g) | Servings/Exchanges |
|---|---|---|---|---|---|---|---|---|---|---|---|---|
| Farmhouse Chicken Salad, Crispy | 1 | 395 | 19 | 170 | 7 | 0.5 | 65 | 857 | 25 | 4 | 25 | 1 1/2 carb, 3 med-fat meat, 1 fat |
| Farmhouse Chicken Salad, Grilled | 1 | 229 | 11 | 100 | 6 | 0.5 | 58 | 579 | 9 | 3 | 20 | 1/2 carb, 2 med-fat meat |
| ***Salad Dressing*** | | | | | | | | | | | | |
| Balsamic Vinaigrette | 1 pkg | 130 | 5 | 45 | 2 | 0 | 0 | 460 | 5 | 0 | 0 | 1 fat |
| Buttermilk Ranch | 1 pkg | 230 | 24 | 215 | 4 | 0 | 10 | 390 | 2 | 0 | 1 | 5 fat |
| Dijon Honey Mustard | 1 pkg | 180 | 17 | 155 | 3 | 0 | 15 | 240 | 8 | 0 | 1 | 2 fat |
| ***Sides & Sidekickers*** | | | | | | | | | | | | |
| Cheddar Cheese Sauce | 1 pkg | 25 | 2 | 20 | 2 | 0 | 5 | 182 | 2 | 0 | 0 | 1 fat |
| Curly Fries, Large | 1 order | 604 | 36 | 325 | 7 | 0.5 | 0 | 1413 | 70 | 7 | 8 | 5 carb, 7 fat |
| Curly Fries, Medium | 1 order | 496 | 29 | 260 | 5 | 0.5 | 0 | 1160 | 58 | 6 | 7 | 4 carb, 5 fat |
| Curly Fries, Small | 1 order | 338 | 20 | 180 | 4 | 0 | 0 | 790 | 39 | 4 | 4 | 2 1/2 carb, 4 fat |
| Jalapeño Bites, Large | 8 | 486 | 34 | 305 | 14 | 1.5 | 45 | 841 | 47 | 3 | 9 | 3 carb, 6 fat |

| | | | | | | | | | | | | |
|---|---|---|---|---|---|---|---|---|---|---|---|---|
| Jalapeño Bites, Regular | 5 | 305 | 21 | 190 | 9 | 1 | 28 | 526 | 29 | 2 | 5 | 2 carb, 4 fat |
| Mozarella Sticks, Large | 6 | 637 | 42 | 380 | 19 | 1.5 | 68 | 2047 | 56 | 3 | 27 | 4 carb, 2 med-fat meat, 6 fat |
| Mozzarella Sticks, Regular | 4 | 426 | 28 | 250 | 13 | 1 | 45 | 1370 | 38 | 2 | 16 | 2 1/2 carb, 2 med-fat meat, 3 fat |
| Onion Petals, Large | 1 order | 480 | 33 | 300 | 5 | 1 | 0 | 482 | 51 | 3 | 6 | 3 1/2 carb, 6 fat |
| Onion Petals, Regular | 1 order | 248 | 17 | 155 | 3 | 1 | 0 | 249 | 26 | 2 | 3 | 3 carb, 3 fat |
| Potato Cakes | 2 | 246 | 18 | 160 | 4 | 0 | 0 | 391 | 26 | 2 | 2 | 2 carb, 3 fat |
| ***Desserts*** | | | | | | | | | | | | |
| Apple Turnover | 1 | 380 | 14 | 125 | 7 | 0.5 | 287 | 58 | 3 | 3 | 4 | 4 carb, 2 fat |
| Cherry Turnover | 1 | 364 | 13 | 115 | 7 | 0.5 | 0 | 269 | 58 | 1 | 4 | 4 carb, 2 fat |
| **BOSTON MARKET** | | | | | | | | | | | | |
| ***Individual Meals*** | | | | | | | | | | | | |
| 1 Thigh & 1 Drumstick | 5 oz | 290 | 17 | 150 | 5 | 0 | 210 | 950 | 0 | 0 | 37 | 5 lean meat |
| 1/2 BBQ Chicken | 14.5 oz | 730 | 30 | 270 | 9 | 0 | 405 | 2360 | 28 | 1 | 90 | 2 carb, 12 lean meat |
| 1/4 White BBQ Chicken | 9 oz | 430 | 13 | 115 | 4 | 0 | 200 | 1400 | 28 | 1 | 52 | 2 carb, 6 med-fat meat |

FAST FOOD

| | Serving | Calories | Fat (g) | Cal. from Fat | Sat. Fat (g) | Trans Fat (g) | Chol. (mg) | Sod. (mg) | Carb. (g) | Fiber (g) | Prot. (g) | Servings/Exchanges |
|---|---|---|---|---|---|---|---|---|---|---|---|---|
| 1/4 White Rotisserie Chicken | 6.5 oz | 320 | 12 | 110 | 4 | 0 | 200 | 900 | 0 | 0 | 52 | 7 lean meat |
| 1/4 White Rotisserie Chicken, No Skin | 6.8 oz | 240 | 4 | 35 | 1 | 0 | 180 | 890 | 1 | 0 | 50 | 7 lean meat |
| 3 Piece BBQ Dark Chicken | 9 oz | 430 | 13 | 120 | 4 | 0 | 200 | 1400 | 28 | 1 | 52 | 2 carb, 7 lean meat |
| 3 Piece Dark Individual Meal | 7.3 oz | 390 | 22 | 190 | 6 | 0 | 290 | 1270 | 1 | 0 | 51 | 7 lean meat |
| 3 Piece Dark Skinless (2 Thighs & Drumstick) | 7 oz | 350 | 15 | 130 | 4.5 | 0 | 280 | 1210 | 0 | 0 | 52 | 7 lean meat |
| BBQ Brisket | 6.5 oz | 400 | 20 | 180 | 1.5 | 0 | 40 | 760 | 28 | 1 | 26 | 2 carb, 3 med-fat meat, 1 fat |
| Beef Brisket | 4 oz | 280 | 20 | 180 | 1.5 | 0 | 40 | 260 | 1 | 0 | 26 | 4 med-fat meat |
| Beef Shepherd's Pie | 14 oz | 480 | 25 | 230 | 9 | 0 | 55 | 1490 | 40 | 5 | 25 | 3 carb, 2 med-fat meat, 3 fat |

| | | | | | | | | | | | | |
|---|---|---|---|---|---|---|---|---|---|---|---|---|
| Crispy Country Chicken with Gravy | 8 oz | 480 | 23 | 200 | 4.5 | 0 | 80 | 1150 | 36 | 1 | 33 | 3 carb, 3 med-fat meat, 2 fat |
| Half Rotisserie Chicken | 12 oz | 610 | 29 | 260 | 9 | 0 | 405 | 1860 | 1 | 1 | 89 | 13 lean meat |
| Meatloaf | 7.6 oz | 520 | 36 | 320 | 16 | 1.5 | 145 | 1030 | 21 | 0 | 29 | 1 1/2 carb, 3 med-fat meat, 4 fat |
| Pastry Top Chicken Pot Pie | 15 oz | 800 | 48 | 430 | 18 | 7 | 140 | 1090 | 59 | 4 | 32 | 4 carb, 3 med-fat meat, 7 fat |
| Roasted Turkey | 4 oz | 150 | 2.5 | 25 | 1 | 0 | 55 | 500 | 0 | 0 | 31 | 4 lean meat |
| ***Soups & Sides*** | | | | | | | | | | | | |
| Baked Beans | 7.7 oz | 270 | 1.5 | 15 | 0 | 0 | 0 | 1000 | 53 | 11 | 11 | 3 1/2 carb |
| Beef Gravy | 3 oz | 35 | 1.5 | 15 | 0.5 | 0 | 0 | 500 | 4 | 0 | 1 | 1/2 carb |
| Caesar Salad Dressing | 2.5 oz | 360 | 38 | 340 | 6 | 0.5 | 30 | 910 | 4 | 1 | 2 | 8 fat |
| Caesar Side Salad | 3.2 oz | 180 | 17 | 150 | 3.5 | 0 | 15 | 410 | 4 | 1 | 4 | 1 vegetable, 3 fat |
| Caesar Side Salad, No Dressing | 2.2 oz | 40 | 2 | 20 | 1.5 | 0 | 5 | 75 | 3 | 1 | 3 | 1 med-fat meat |
| Chicken Noodle Soup | 14 oz | 250 | 8 | 70 | 2.5 | 0 | 95 | 1420 | 23 | 2 | 22 | 1 1/2 carb, 2 med-fat meat |

| | Serving | Calories | Fat (g) | Cal. from Fat | Sat. Fat (g) | Trans Fat (g) | Chol. (mg) | Sod. (mg) | Carb. (g) | Fiber (g) | Prot. (g) | Servings/Exchanges |
|---|---|---|---|---|---|---|---|---|---|---|---|---|
| Chicken Tortilla Soup with Toppings | 12.8 oz | 410 | 26 | 230 | 7 | 0 | 70 | 2100 | 30 | 2 | 17 | 2 carb, 2 med-fat meat, 3 fat |
| Cinnamon Apples | 5.1 oz | 210 | 3 | 25 | 0 | 0 | 0 | 15 | 47 | 3 | 0 | 3 carb, 1 fat |
| Coleslaw | 6.6 oz | 300 | 20 | 180 | 4.5 | 0 | 15 | 280 | 27 | 4 | 2 | 2 carb, 4 fat |
| Creamed Spinach | 6.7 oz | 280 | 23 | 210 | 15 | 0 | 70 | 580 | 12 | 4 | 9 | 1 carb, 1 med-fat meat, 4 fat |
| Fresh Steamed Vegetables, Lowfat | 4.8 oz | 60 | 2 | 20 | 0 | 0 | 0 | 40 | 8 | 3 | 2 | 2 vegetable |
| Fresh Vegetable Stuffing | 4.8 oz | 190 | 8 | 70 | 1 | 0 | 0 | 580 | 25 | 2 | 3 | 1 1/2 carb, 2 fat |
| Garlic Dill New Potatoes, Lowfat | 5.5 oz | 140 | 3 | 30 | 1 | 0 | 0 | 120 | 24 | 3 | 3 | 1 1/2 carb, 1 fat |
| Garlic Spinach | 6 oz | 130 | 9 | 80 | 6 | 0 | 20 | 200 | 9 | 5 | 5 | 2 vegetable, 2 fat |
| Green Beans | 3.2 oz | 60 | 3.5 | 35 | 1.5 | 0 | 0 | 180 | 7 | 3 | 2 | 1 vegetable, 1 fat |
| Macaroni & Cheese | 7.8 oz | 300 | 11 | 100 | 7 | 0 | 30 | 1110 | 35 | 2 | 11 | 2 carb, 1 med-fat meat, 1 fat |

| | | | | | | | | | | | | |
|---|---|---|---|---|---|---|---|---|---|---|---|---|
| Mashed Potatoes | 7.8 oz | 270 | 11 | 100 | 5 | 0 | 25 | 820 | 36 | 4 | 5 | 2 1/2 carb, 2 fat |
| Potato Salad | 7 oz | 390 | 29 | 260 | 7 | 0 | 20 | 640 | 26 | 3 | 3 | 2 carb, 6 fat |
| Poultry Gravy | 4 oz | 50 | 2 | 20 | 0.5 | 0 | 0 | 690 | 7 | 0 | 0 | 1/2 carb |
| Seasoned Fresh Fruit Salad, Lowfat | 5 oz | 60 | 0 | 5 | 0 | 0 | 0 | 20 | 15 | 1 | 1 | 1 fruit |
| Southern Style Squash Casserole | 8 oz | 300 | 19 | 170 | 7 | 0 | 30 | 1390 | 23 | 3 | 10 | 1 1/2 carb, 1 med-fat meat, 3 fat |
| Sweet Corn | 6.2 oz | 170 | 4 | 35 | 1 | 0 | 0 | 95 | 37 | 2 | 6 | 2 1/2 carb, 1 fat |
| Sweet Potato Casserole | 7 oz | 460 | 16 | 140 | 4.5 | 0 | 5 | 270 | 77 | 3 | 4 | 6 1/2 carb 3 fat |
| ***Sandwiches*** | | | | | | | | | | | | |
| BBQ Brisket Sandwich | 12 oz | 800 | 30 | 270 | 6 | 0 | 60 | 1840 | 90 | 3 | 43 | 6 carb, 4 med-fat meat, 2 fat |
| Boston Sirloin Dip Carver | 13 oz | 900 | 46 | 410 | 13 | 2 | 165 | 1610 | 62 | 3 | 57 | 4 carb, 6 med-fat meat, 3 fat |
| Boston Turkey Carver | 12 oz | 700 | 26 | 240 | 8 | 0.5 | 95 | 1710 | 65 | 3 | 50 | 4 carb, 5 med-fat meat |
| Classic Chicken Salad Sandwich | 12.8 oz | 800 | 41 | 370 | 7 | 5 | 145 | 1900 | 65 | 4 | 40 | 4 carb, 4 med-fat meat, 4 fat |

| | Serving | Calories | Fat (g) | Cal. from Fat | Sat. Fat (g) | Trans Fat (g) | Chol. (mg) | Sod. (mg) | Carb. (g) | Fiber (g) | Prot. (g) | Servings/Exchanges |
|---|---|---|---|---|---|---|---|---|---|---|---|---|
| Crispy Country Chicken Carver | 14 oz | 1020 | 42 | 380 | 7 | 0 | 90 | 2210 | 114 | 4 | 45 | 7 1/2 carb, 3 med-fat meat, 5 fat |
| Meatloaf Open-Faced Sandwich | 13 oz | 670 | 38 | 350 | 17 | 1.5 | 145 | 1760 | 48 | 1 | 34 | 3 carb, 4 med-fat meat, 4 fat |
| Roasted Sirloin Open-Faced Sandwich | 12 oz | 410 | 15 | 140 | 6 | 1 | 100 | 1640 | 32 | 1 | 35 | 2 carb, 4 lean meat |
| Rotisserie Chicken Open-Faced Sandwich | 10 oz | 320 | 8 | 70 | 2.5 | 0 | 95 | 1630 | 34 | 1 | 27 | 2 carb, 3 lean meat |
| ***Salads*** | | | | | | | | | | | | |
| Crispy Country Chicken | 3 oz | 220 | 11 | 90 | 2 | 0 | 40 | 480 | 16 | 1 | 16 | 1 carb, 2 med-fat meat |
| Market Chopped Salad | 14 oz | 480 | 40 | 360 | 8 | 1 | 10 | 1640 | 24 | 7 | 9 | 1 1/2 carb, 1 med-fat meat, 7 fat |
| Roasted Sirloin | 3 oz | 160 | 6 | 50 | 2 | 0 | 75 | 170 | 0 | 0 | 26 | 4 lean meat |
| Rotisserie Chicken | 5 oz | 180 | 3 | 25 | 0 | 125 | 620 | 0 | 0 | 0 | 39 | 6 lean meat |

| | | | | | | | | | | | | |
|---|---|---|---|---|---|---|---|---|---|---|---|---|
| ***Desserts*** | | | | | | | | | | | | |
| Apple Gallette | 4.73 oz | 420 | 22 | 190 | 12 | 0 | 25 | 280 | 54 | 3 | 3 | 4 1/2 carb, 4 fat |
| Chocolate Chip Fudge Brownie | 3 oz | 320 | 13 | 120 | 3 | 0 | 50 | 220 | 49 | 3 | 5 | 3 carb, 3 fat |
| Chocolate Chunk Cookie | 2.75 oz | 370 | 19 | 170 | 9 | 0 | 20 | 340 | 49 | 2 | 4 | 3 carb, 4 fat |
| Cornbread | 2 oz | 180 | 5 | 45 | 1.5 | 1.5 | 10 | 320 | 31 | 0 | 2 | 2 carb, 1 fat |
| Pecan Pie | 5.5 oz | 640 | 36 | 320 | 11 | 0 | 115 | 340 | 74 | 2 | 7 | 5 carb, 7 fat |
| **BURGER KING** | | | | | | | | | | | | |
| ***WHOPPER Sandwiches*** | | | | | | | | | | | | |
| WHOPPER | 1 | 670 | 40 | 360 | 11 | 1.5 | 75 | 1020 | 51 | 3 | 29 | 3 1/2 carb, 3 med-fat meat, 5 fat |
| WHOPPER with Cheese | 1 | 770 | 48 | 430 | 16 | 1.5 | 100 | 1450 | 52 | 3 | 33 | 3 1/2 carb, 4 med-fat meat, 6 fat |
| Double WHOPPER | 1 | 920 | 58 | 520 | 19 | 2.5 | 140 | 1090 | 51 | 3 | 48 | 3 1/2 carb, 6 med-fat meat, 6 fat |

| | Serving | Calories | Fat (g) | Cal. from Fat | Sat. Fat (g) | Trans Fat (g) | Chol. (mg) | Sod. (mg) | Carb. (g) | Fiber (g) | Prot. (g) | Servings/Exchanges |
|---|---|---|---|---|---|---|---|---|---|---|---|---|
| Double WHOPPER with Cheese | 1 | 1010 | 66 | 595 | 24 | 2.5 | 160 | 1530 | 53 | 3 | 53 | 3 1/2 carb, 6 med-fat meat, 7 fat |
| Triple WHOPPER | 1 | 1160 | 76 | 685 | 27 | 3 | 205 | 1170 | 51 | 3 | 68 | 3 1/2 carb, 8 med-fat meat, 7 fat |
| Triple WHOPPER with Cheese | 1 | 1250 | 84 | 755 | 32 | 3.5 | 225 | 1600 | 52 | 3 | 73 | 3 1/2 carb, 9 med-fat meat, 8 fat |
| WHOPPER JR. | 1 | 370 | 21 | 190 | 6 | 0.5 | 40 | 560 | 31 | 2 | 16 | 2 carb, 2 med-fat meat, 2 fat |
| WHOPPER JR. with Cheese | 1 | 420 | 25 | 225 | 8 | 1 | 50 | 780 | 31 | 2 | 18 | 2 carb, 2 med-fat meat, 3 fat |
| ***Flame Broiled Burgers*** | | | | | | | | | | | | |
| Hamburger | 1 | 290 | 12 | 110 | 4.5 | 0.5 | 35 | 550 | 30 | 1 | 15 | 2 carb, 2 med-fat meat, 1 fat |
| Cheeseburger | 1 | 340 | 16 | 145 | 7 | 0.5 | 45 | 770 | 31 | 1 | 18 | 2 carb, 2 med-fat meat, 1 fat |

| | | | | | | | | | | | | |
|---|---|---|---|---|---|---|---|---|---|---|---|---|
| Double Hamburger | 1 | 420 | 22 | 200 | 9 | 1 | 65 | 590 | 30 | 1 | 26 | 2 carb, 3 med-fat meat, 2 fat |
| Double Cheeseburger | 1 | 510 | 29 | 260 | 14 | 1.5 | 90 | 1020 | 31 | 1 | 30 | 2 carb, 3 med-fat meat, 3 fat |
| BK Double Stacker | 1 | 620 | 39 | 350 | 16 | 1.5 | 105 | 110 | 32 | 1 | 34 | 2 carb, 4 med-fat meat, 4 fat |
| BK Triple Stacker | 1 | 820 | 55 | 495 | 23 | 2 | 160 | 1450 | 33 | 1 | 49 | 2 carb, 6 med-fat meat, 5 fat |
| BK Quad Stacker | 1 | 1010 | 70 | 630 | 30 | 3 | 210 | 1800 | 34 | 1 | 64 | 2 carb, 8 med-fat meat, 6 fat |
| Steakhouse T | 1 | 970 | 61 | 550 | 23 | 1 | 135 | 1930 | 44 | 4 | 42 | 3 1/2 carb, 5 med-fat meat, 7 fat |
| Mushroom & Swiss Steakhouse T | 1 | 870 | 49 | 440 | 20 | 0.5 | 125 | 1890 | 54 | 4 | 43 | 3 1/2 carb, 5 med-fat meat, 5 fat |
| ***Chicken, Fish & Veggie*** | | | | | | | | | | | | |
| TENDERGRILL Chicken Sandwich | 1 | 490 | 21 | 190 | 4 | 0 | 55 | 1220 | 51 | 3 | 26 | 3 1/2 carb, 2 med-fat meat, 2 fat |

FAST FOOD

| | Serving | Calories | Fat (g) | Cal. from Fat | Sat. Fat (g) | Trans Fat (g) | Chol. (mg) | Sod. (mg) | Carb. (g) | Fiber (g) | Prot. (g) | Servings/Exchanges |
|---|---|---|---|---|---|---|---|---|---|---|---|---|
| TENDERCRISP Chicken Sandwich | 1 | 800 | 46 | 415 | 8 | 0.5 | 70 | 1640 | 68 | 3 | 32 | 4 1/2 carb, 3 med-fat meat, 6 fat |
| Original Chicken Sandwich | 1 | 630 | 39 | 350 | 7 | 0.5 | 65 | 1390 | 46 | 3 | 24 | 3 carb, 2 med-fat meat, 6 fat |
| Chicken Tenders | 4 pieces | 180 | 11 | 100 | 3 | 0 | 30 | 310 | 13 | 0 | 9 | 1 carb, 1 med-fat meat, 1 fat |
| Chicken Tenders | 6 pieces | 270 | 16 | 145 | 3.5 | 0 | 45 | 460 | 19 | 0 | 14 | 1 carb, 2 med-fat meat, 1 fat |
| Chicken Tenders | 8 pieces | 360 | 21 | 190 | 4 | 0 | 60 | 610 | 25 | 0 | 18 | 1 1/2 carb, 2 med-fat meat, 2 fat |
| Kraft Macaroni & Cheese | 1 order | 160 | 5 | 45 | 1.5 | 0 | 10 | 340 | 22 | 1 | 7 | 1 1/2 carb, 1 med-fat meat |
| BK Chicken Fries | 9 pieces | 380 | 22 | 200 | 4 | 0 | 40 | 1220 | 24 | 2 | 21 | 1 1/2 carb, 2 med-fat meat, 2 fat |

| | | | | | | | | | | | | |
|---|---|---|---|---|---|---|---|---|---|---|---|---|
| BK BIG FISH Sandwich | 1 | 640 | 32 | 290 | 5 | 0.5 | 45 | 1540 | 66 | 3 | 23 | 4 1/2 carb, 1 med-fat meat, 5 fat |
| BK VEGGIE Burger | 1 | 420 | 16 | 145 | 2.5 | 0 | 10 | 1090 | 46 | 7 | 23 | 3 carb, 2 med-fat meat, 1 fat |
| ***Side Orders*** | | | | | | | | | | | | |
| BK Fresh Apple Fries | 1 order | 25 | 0 | 0 | 0 | 0 | 0 | 0 | 6 | 1 | 0 | 1/2 fruit |
| Caramel Sauce | 1 order | 45 | 0.5 | 5 | 0 | 0 | 0 | 35 | 10 | 0 | 0 | 1 carb |
| Cheesy TOTS Potatoes | 9 pieces | 330 | 18 | 160 | 6 | 0 | 20 | 950 | 31 | 3 | 11 | 2 carb, 1 med-fat meat, 3 fat |
| French Fries, Small, Salted | 1 order | 340 | 17 | 155 | 3.5 | 0 | 0 | 590 | 44 | 4 | 4 | 3 carb, 3 fat |
| French Fries, Small, Salt Not Added | 1 order | 340 | 17 | 155 | 3.5 | 0 | 0 | 380 | 44 | 4 | 4 | 3 carb, 3 fat |
| French Fries, Medium, Salted | 1 order | 480 | 23 | 205 | 5 | 0 | 0 | 820 | 61 | 5 | 5 | 4 carb, 5 fat |
| French Fries, Medium, Salt Not Added | 1 order | 480 | 23 | 205 | 5 | 0 | 0 | 530 | 61 | 5 | 5 | 4 carb, 5 fat |

FAST FOOD

| | Serving | Calories | Fat (g) | Cal. from Fat | Sat. Fat (g) | Trans Fat (g) | Chol. (mg) | Sod. (mg) | Carb. (g) | Fiber (g) | Prot. (g) | Servings/Exchanges |
|---|---|---|---|---|---|---|---|---|---|---|---|---|
| French Fries, Large, Salted | 1 order | 580 | 28 | 250 | 6 | 0 | 0 | 990 | 74 | 6 | 6 | 5 carb, 6 fat |
| French Fries, Large, Salt Not Added | 1 order | 580 | 28 | 250 | 6 | 0 | 0 | 640 | 74 | 6 | 6 | 5 carb, 6 fat |
| French Fries, Value, Salted | 1 order | 220 | 11 | 100 | 2.5 | 0 | 0 | 380 | 28 | 2 | 2 | 2 carb, 2 fat |
| Onion Rings, Small | 1 order | 310 | 17 | 155 | 3 | 0 | 0 | 490 | 36 | 3 | 4 | 2 1/2 carb, 3 fat |
| Onion Rings, Medium | 1 order | 450 | 24 | 215 | 4 | 0 | 0 | 700 | 52 | 5 | 6 | 3 1/2 carb, 5 fat |
| Onion Rings, Large | 1 order | 510 | 27 | 245 | 4.5 | 0 | 0 | 810 | 60 | 5 | 7 | 4 carb, 5 fat |
| ***Dipping Sauces*** | | | | | | | | | | | | |
| BBQ Dipping Sauce | 1 oz | 40 | 0 | 0 | 0 | 0 | 0 | 310 | 11 | 0 | 0 | 1 carb |
| Honey Mustard Dipping Sauce | 1 oz | 90 | 6 | 55 | 1 | 0 | 10 | 180 | 8 | 0 | 0 | 1/2 carb, 1 fat |
| Sweet & Sour Dipping Sauce | 1 oz | 45 | 0 | 0 | 0 | 0 | 0 | 55 | 11 | 0 | 0 | 1 carb |

| | | | | | | | | | | | | |
|---|---|---|---|---|---|---|---|---|---|---|---|---|
| Ranch Dipping Sauce | 1 oz | 140 | 15 | 135 | 2.5 | 0 | 5 | 95 | 1 | 0 | 1 | 3 fat |
| Buffalo Dipping Sauce | 1 oz | 80 | 8 | 70 | 1.5 | 0 | 5 | 360 | 2 | 0 | 0 | 2 fat |
| Zesty Onion Ring Dipping Sauce | 1 oz | 150 | 15 | 135 | 2.5 | 0 | 15 | 210 | 3 | 1 | 0 | 3 fat |
| ***BK Salad Collection*** | | | | | | | | | | | | |
| Side Salad | 1 | 40 | 2 | 20 | 1 | 0 | 5 | 45 | 2 | 1 | 3 | 1 vegetable |
| TENDERGRILL Chicken Garden Salad | 1 | 210 | 7 | 65 | 3 | 0 | 75 | 780 | 8 | 3 | 29 | 1/2 carb, 4 lean meat |
| TENDERCRISP Chicken Garden Salad | 1 | 410 | 23 | 205 | 6 | 0 | 65 | 1060 | 27 | 4 | 27 | 2 carb, 3 med-fat meat, 2 fat |
| Garden Salad, No Chicken | 1 | 70 | 4 | 35 | 2.5 | 0 | 10 | 100 | 7 | 3 | 4 | 1 vegetable, 1 fat |
| ***Salad Dressings & Toppings*** | | | | | | | | | | | | |
| KEN's Creamy Caesar Dressing | 2 oz | 210 | 21 | 190 | 4 | 0 | 25 | 610 | 4 | 0 | 3 | 4 fat |
| KEN's Honey Mustard Dressing | 2 oz | 270 | 23 | 205 | 3 | 0 | 20 | 510 | 15 | 0 | 1 | 1 carb, 5 fat |

| | Serving | Calories | Fat (g) | Cal. from Fat | Sat. Fat (g) | Trans Fat (g) | Chol. (mg) | Sod. (mg) | Carb. (g) | Fiber (g) | Prot. (g) | Servings/Exchanges |
|---|---|---|---|---|---|---|---|---|---|---|---|---|
| KEN's Light Italian Dressing | 2 oz | 120 | 11 | 100 | 1.5 | 0 | 0 | 440 | 5 | 0 | 0 | 2 fat |
| KEN's Ranch Dressing | 2 oz | 190 | 20 | 180 | 3 | 0 | 20 | 550 | 2 | 0 | 1 | 4 fat |
| ***Desserts*** | | | | | | | | | | | | |
| Dutch Apple Pie | 1 | 320 | 13 | 115 | 5 | 0 | 0 | 290 | 47 | 1 | 2 | 3 carb, 3 fat |
| HERSHEY's Sundae Pie | 1 | 310 | 19 | 170 | 12 | 0 | 10 | 220 | 32 | 1 | 3 | 2 carb, 4 fat |
| ***Breakfast*** | | | | | | | | | | | | |
| BK Breakfast Shots, Sausage & Cheese | 2 pkg | 420 | 31 | 280 | 10 | 0.5 | 215 | 910 | 18 | 1 | 18 | 1 carb, 2 med-fat meat, 4 fat |
| BK Breakfast Shots, Ham & Cheese | 2 pkg | 270 | 16 | 145 | 5 | 0 | 190 | 840 | 18 | 1 | 13 | 1 carb, 1 med-fat meat, 2 fat |
| Croissan'wich with Bacon, Egg & Cheese | 1 | 350 | 19 | 170 | 8 | 0 | 155 | 870 | 27 | 0 | 15 | 2 carb, 1 med-fat meat, 1 fat |
| Croissan'wich with Ham, Egg & Cheese | 1 | 340 | 17 | 155 | 7 | 0 | 160 | 1200 | 28 | 0 | 18 | 2 carb, 2 med-fat meat, 1 fat |

| Croissan'wich with Sausage, Egg & Cheese | 1 | 470 | 31 | 280 | 11 | 0.5 | 175 | 1030 | 28 | 0 | 20 | 2 carb, 2 med-fat meat, 4 fat |
|---|---|---|---|---|---|---|---|---|---|---|---|---|
| Croissan'wich with Sausage & Cheese | 1 | 380 | 24 | 215 | 10 | 0 | 50 | 780 | 26 | 0 | 14 | 2 carb, 1 med-fat meat, 4 fat |
| Croissan'wich with Egg & Cheese | 1 | 310 | 16 | 145 | 7 | 0 | 145 | 730 | 27 | 0 | 12 | 2 carb, 1 med-fat meat, 2 fat |
| Double Croissan'wich with Sausage, Egg & Cheese | 1 | 690 | 50 | 450 | 19 | 1 | 220 | 1560 | 30 | 0 | 30 | 2 carb, 3 med-fat meat, 8 fat |
| Double Croissan'wich with Ham, Egg & Cheese | 1 | 420 | 21 | 190 | 10 | 0.5 | 190 | 1890 | 30 | 0 | 26 | 2 carb, 3 med-fat meat, 1 fat |
| French Toast Sticks | 5 pieces | 380 | 18 | 160 | 3 | 0 | 0 | 430 | 49 | 2 | 5 | 3 carb, 4 fat |
| Hash Browns, Small | 1 | 420 | 27 | 245 | 6 | 0 | 0 | 680 | 40 | 6 | 3 | 2 1/2 carb, 5 fat |
| Hash Browns, Medium | 1 | 610 | 39 | 350 | 8 | 0 | 0 | 980 | 58 | 8 | 5 | 4 carb, 8 fat |

| | Serving | Calories | Fat (g) | Cal. from Fat | Sat. Fat (g) | Trans Fat (g) | Chol. (mg) | Sod. (mg) | Carb. (g) | Fiber (g) | Prot. (g) | Servings/Exchanges |
|---|---|---|---|---|---|---|---|---|---|---|---|---|
| ***Drinks*** | | | | | | | | | | | | |
| Mocha BK Joe Iced Coffee | 1 | 360 | 10 | 90 | 6 | 0 | 40 | 290 | 66 | 1 | 6 | 4 1/2 carb, 1 fat |
| Chocolate Shake | 12 oz | 310 | 11 | 100 | 7 | 0 | 45 | 220 | 53 | 1 | 6 | 3 1/2 carb, 2 fat |
| Chocolate Shake | 22 oz | 670 | 21 | 190 | 13 | 0.5 | 80 | 510 | 119 | 2 | 11 | 8 carb, 4 fat |
| Chocolate Shake | 32 oz | 990 | 31 | 280 | 20 | 1 | 120 | 750 | 178 | 3 | 17 | 12 carb, 6 fat |
| Vanilla Shake | 12 oz | 270 | 11 | 100 | 7 | 0 | 45 | 180 | 42 | 0 | 6 | 3 carb, 2 fat |
| Vanilla Shake | 22 oz | 480 | 20 | 180 | 13 | 0.5 | 80 | 320 | 76 | 0 | 11 | 5 carb, 4 fat |
| Vanilla Shake | 32 oz | 720 | 29 | 260 | 19 | 1 | 120 | 480 | 113 | 1 | 16 | 7 1/2 carb, 6 fat |
| Oreo BK Sundae Shake, Medium | 22 oz | 1010 | 35 | 315 | 21 | 1 | 95 | 800 | 171 | 3 | 15 | 11 carb, 7 fat |
| **CARL'S JR.** | | | | | | | | | | | | |
| Big Hamburger | 1 | 460 | 17 | 160 | 8 | 0.5 | 50 | 1090 | 54 | 3 | 24 | 3 1/2 carb, 2 med-fat meat, 1 fat |

| | | | | | | | | | | | | |
|---|---|---|---|---|---|---|---|---|---|---|---|---|
| Famous Star with Cheese | 1 | 660 | 39 | 340 | 13 | 1 | 80 | 1300 | 53 | 3 | 27 | 3 1/2 carb, 2 med-fat meat, 6 fat |
| Super Star with Cheese | 1 | 920 | 58 | 510 | 23 | 1.5 | 145 | 1640 | 54 | 3 | 47 | 3 1/2 carb, 5 med-fat meat, 7 fat |
| Chili Cheeseburger | 1 | 780 | 41 | 370 | 19 | 1.5 | 105 | 1650 | 58 | 4 | 41 | 4 carb, 4 med-fat meat, 5 fat |
| Double Western Bacon Cheeseburger | 1 | 960 | 52 | 470 | 23 | 2 | 140 | 1750 | 70 | 3 | 52 | 4 1/2 carb, 5 med-fat meat, 5 fat |
| Jalapeno Burger | 1 | 720 | 46 | 410 | 15 | 0.5 | 85 | 1340 | 50 | 3 | 27 | 3 carb, 3 med-fat meat, 6 fat |
| Western Bacon Cheeseburger | 1 | 710 | 33 | 300 | 13 | 1 | 75 | 1410 | 69 | 3 | 32 | 4 1/2 carb, 3 med-fat meat, 3 fat |
| Charbroiled BBQ Chicken Sandwich | 1 | 380 | 7 | 60 | 1.5 | 0 | 60 | 1010 | 49 | 2 | 34 | 3 carb, 4 lean meat |
| Charbroiled Chicken Club Sandwich | 1 | 560 | 27 | 240 | 7 | 0 | 90 | 1280 | 44 | 2 | 39 | 3 carb, 4 med-fat meat, 1 fat |

FAST FOOD

| | Serving | Calories | Fat (g) | Cal. from Fat | Sat. Fat (g) | Trans Fat (g) | Chol. (mg) | Sod. (mg) | Carb. (g) | Fiber (g) | Prot. (g) | Servings/Exchanges |
|---|---|---|---|---|---|---|---|---|---|---|---|---|
| Charbroiled Sante Fe Chicken Sandwich | 1 | 630 | 35 | 310 | 8 | 0 | 95 | 1410 | 44 | 2 | 36 | 3 carb, 4 med-fat meat, 3 fat |
| Bacon Swiss Crispy Chicken Sandwich | 1 | 750 | 40 | 360 | 9 | 1.5 | 70 | 1990 | 62 | 4 | 36 | 6 carb, 3 med-fat meat, 5 fat |
| Spicy Chicken Sandwich | 1 | 420 | 27 | 230 | 5 | 0 | 25 | 930 | 33 | 2 | 12 | 2 carb, 1 med-fat meat, 5 fat |
| Chicken Strips | 3 pieces | 370 | 26 | 230 | 6 | 0 | 30 | 620 | 19 | 2 | 14 | 1 carb, 2 med-fat meat, 3 fat |
| Carl's Catch Fish Sandwich | 1 | 710 | 37 | 330 | 6 | 0 | 40 | 1280 | 74 | 4 | 20 | 5 carb, 1 med-fat meat, 6 fat |
| Low Carb Six Dollar Burger | 1 | 570 | 43 | 380 | 18 | 2 | 120 | 1480 | 7 | 1 | 38 | 1/2 carb, 5 med-fat meat, 4 fat |
| Original Six Dollar Burger | 1 | 890 | 54 | 480 | 20 | 2 | 130 | 2040 | 58 | 3 | 45 | 4 carb, 5 med-fat meat, 6 fat |

| | | | | | | | | | | | | |
|---|---|---|---|---|---|---|---|---|---|---|---|---|
| Western Bacon Six Dollar Burger | 1 | 1020 | 53 | 480 | 22 | 2.5 | 130 | 2520 | 81 | 3 | 53 | 5 carb, 5 med-fat meat, 6 fat |
| Kid's Hamburger | 1 | 230 | 10 | 90 | 3.5 | 0.5 | 25 | 550 | 24 | 1 | 9 | 1 1/2 carb, 1 med-fat meat, 1 fat |
| Kid's Cheeseburger | 1 | 290 | 15 | 140 | 7 | 0.5 | 40 | 830 | 24 | 1 | 12 | 1 1/2 carb, 1 med-fat meat, 2 fat |
| ***Sides*** | | | | | | | | | | | | |
| Natural-Cut French Fries, Kids | 1 order | 220 | 11 | 100 | 2 | 0 | 0 | 580 | 29 | 2 | 3 | 2 carb, 2 fat |
| Natural-Cut Fries, Small | 1 order | 320 | 15 | 140 | 3 | 0 | 0 | 830 | 42 | 4 | 4 | 3 carb, 3 fat |
| Natural-Cut Fries, Medium | 1 order | 460 | 22 | 200 | 4.5 | 0 | 0 | 1180 | 60 | 5 | 5 | 4 carb, 4 fat |
| Natural-Cut Fries, Large | 1 order | 500 | 24 | 210 | 5 | 0 | 0 | 1290 | 65 | 5 | 6 | 4 carb, 5 fat |
| Chicken Stars | 6 pieces | 320 | 24 | 220 | 6 | 0 | 35 | 460 | 14 | 2 | 12 | 1 carb, 1 med-fat meat, 4 fat |
| Chili Cheese Fries | 1 order | 990 | 56 | 510 | 19 | 1 | 70 | 2380 | 89 | 8 | 28 | 6 carb, 2 med-fat meat, 9 fat |

| | Serving | Calories | Fat (g) | Cal. from Fat | Sat. Fat (g) | Trans Fat (g) | Chol. (mg) | Sod. (mg) | Carb. (g) | Fiber (g) | Prot. (g) | Servings/Exchanges |
|---|---|---|---|---|---|---|---|---|---|---|---|---|
| CrissCut Fries | 1 order | 450 | 29 | 260 | 5 | 0 | 0 | 900 | 42 | 4 | 5 | 3 carb, 6 fat |
| Fish & Chips | 1 order | 730 | 39 | 350 | 7 | 0 | 25 | 1630 | 72 | 6 | 22 | 5 carb, 1 med-fat meat, 7 fat |
| Fried Zucchini | 1 order | 330 | 18 | 160 | 3 | 0 | 0 | 610 | 36 | 2 | 6 | 2 1/2 carb, 4 fat |
| Onion Rings | 1 order | 530 | 28 | 250 | 4.5 | 0 | 0 | 590 | 61 | 3 | 8 | 4 carb, 6 fat |
| ***Salads (without Dressing)*** | | | | | | | | | | | | |
| Grilled Chicken Salad | 1 | 200 | 6 | 60 | 3 | 0 | 70 | 610 | 13 | 3 | 24 | 1 carb, 3 lean meat |
| Garden Side Salad | 1 | 50 | 2.5 | 20 | 1.5 | 0 | 5 | 75 | 5 | 2 | 3 | 1 vegetable, 1 fat |
| Green Burrito Taco Salad | 1 | 970 | 58 | 530 | 19 | 1.5 | 85 | 1850 | 76 | 17 | 42 | 5 carb, 4 med-fat meat, 8 fat |
| ***Salad Dressings*** | | | | | | | | | | | | |
| Blue Cheese Dressing | 2-oz pkt | 320 | 34 | 310 | 7 | 0 | 20 | 410 | 1 | 0 | 2 | 7 fat |
| House Dressing | 2-oz pkt | 220 | 22 | 200 | 3.5 | 0 | 20 | 440 | 3 | 0 | 1 | 4 fat |
| Low Fat Balsamic Dressing | 2-oz pkt | 35 | 1.5 | 15 | 0 | 0 | 0 | 480 | 4 | 0 | 0 | 1 fat |

| | | | | | | | | | | | | |
|---|---|---|---|---|---|---|---|---|---|---|---|---|
| Thousand Island Dressing | 2-oz pkt | 240 | 23 | 210 | 3.5 | 0 | 20 | 460 | 7 | 0 | 0 | 1/2 carb, 5 fat |
| ***Breakfast*** | | | | | | | | | | | | |
| Bacon & Egg Burrito | 1 | 550 | 32 | 290 | 10 | 0 | 500 | 990 | 37 | 1 | 29 | 2 1/2 carb, 3 med-fat meat, 3 fat |
| Breakfast Burger | 1 | 780 | 41 | 370 | 15 | 1 | 305 | 1460 | 64 | 3 | 38 | 4 carb, 4 med-fat meat, 4 fat |
| Croissant Sunrise Sandwich | 1 | 590 | 44 | 390 | 17 | 0 | 285 | 810 | 27 | 1 | 20 | 2 carb, 2 med-fat meat, 7 fat |
| French Toast Dips, No Syrup | 5 pieces | 460 | 21 | 190 | 4 | 0 | 0 | 570 | 60 | 3 | 9 | 4 carb, 4 fat |
| Hash Brown Nuggets | 1 order | 350 | 23 | 210 | 4 | 0 | 0 | 440 | 32 | 3 | 3 | 2 carb, 5 fat |
| Loaded Breakfast Burrito | 1 | 780 | 49 | 440 | 16 | 0 | 510 | 1480 | 51 | 3 | 36 | 3 carb, 3 med-fat meat, 7 fat |
| Sourdough Breakfast Sandwich | 1 | 450 | 21 | 190 | 8 | 0 | 270 | 1470 | 38 | 1 | 29 | 2 1/2 carb, 3 med-fat meat, 1 fat |

| | Serving | Calories | Fat (g) | Cal. from Fat | Sat. Fat (g) | Trans Fat (g) | Chol. (mg) | Sod. (mg) | Carb. (g) | Fiber (g) | Prot. (g) | Servings/Exchanges |
|---|---|---|---|---|---|---|---|---|---|---|---|---|
| Steak & Egg Burrito | 1 | 650 | 36 | 330 | 14 | 0 | 535 | 1750 | 43 | 1 | 41 | 3 carb, 4 med-fat meat, 3 fat |
| **CHIPOTLE** | | | | | | | | | | | | |
| Flour Tortilla, Burrito | 1 | 290 | 9 | 80 | 3 | 0 | 0 | 970 | 44 | 2 | 7 | 3 carb, 2 fat |
| Flour Tortilla, Taco | 1 | 90 | 2.5 | 25 | 1 | 0 | 0 | 200 | 13 | <1 | 2 | 1 carb, 1 fat |
| Crispy Taco Shell | 1 | 60 | 2 | 20 | 0.5 | 0 | 0 | 10 | 9 | 1 | <1 | 1/2 carb |
| Cilantro-Lime Rice | 3 oz | 130 | 3 | 30 | 0.5 | 0 | 0 | 150 | 23 | 0 | 2 | 1 1/2 carb |
| Black Beans | 4 oz | 120 | 1 | 10 | 0 | 0 | 0 | 250 | 23 | 11 | 7 | 1 1/2 carb |
| Pinto Beans | 4 oz | 120 | 1 | 10 | 0 | 0 | 5 | 330 | 22 | 10 | 7 | 1 1/2 carb |
| Fajita Vegetables | 2.5 oz | 20 | 0.5 | 5 | 0 | 0 | 0 | 170 | 4 | 1 | 1 | 1 vegetable |
| Barbacoa | 4 oz | 170 | 7 | 60 | 2.5 | 0 | 60 | 510 | 2 | 0 | 24 | 3 lean meat |
| Chicken | 4 oz | 190 | 6.5 | 60 | 2 | 0 | 115 | 370 | 1 | 0 | 32 | 5 lean meat |
| Carnitas | 4 oz | 190 | 8 | 70 | 2.5 | 0 | 70 | 540 | 1 | 0 | 27 | 4 lean meat |
| Steak | 4 oz | 190 | 6.5 | 60 | 2 | 0 | 65 | 320 | 2 | 0 | 30 | 4 lean meat |

| | | | | | | | | | | | | |
|---|---|---|---|---|---|---|---|---|---|---|---|---|
| Tomato Salsa | 3.5 oz | 20 | 0 | 0 | 0 | 0 | 0 | 470 | 4 | <1 | 1 | free |
| Corn Salsa | 3.5 oz | 80 | 1.5 | 15 | 0 | 0 | 0 | 410 | 15 | 3 | 3 | 1 carb |
| Red Tomatillo Salsa | 2 oz | 40 | 1 | 10 | 0 | 0 | 0 | 510 | 8 | 4 | 2 | 2 vegetable |
| Green Tomatillo Salsa | 2 oz | 15 | 0 | 5 | 0 | 0 | 0 | 230 | 3 | 1 | 1 | free |
| Cheese | 1 oz | 100 | 8.5 | 80 | 5 | 0 | 30 | 180 | 0 | 0 | 8 | 1 med-fat meat |
| Sour Cream | 2 oz | 120 | 10 | 90 | 7 | 0 | 40 | 30 | 2 | 0 | 2 | 2 fat |
| Guacamole | 3.5 oz | 150 | 13 | 120 | 2 | 0 | 0 | 190 | 8 | 6 | 2 | 1/2 carb, 3 fat |
| Romaine Lettuce, in Salad | 2.5 oz | 10 | 0 | 0 | 0 | 0 | 0 | 5 | 2 | 1 | 1 | free |
| Romaine Lettuce, in Taco | 1 oz | 5 | 0 | 0 | 0 | 0 | 0 | 0 | 1 | 1 | 0 | free |
| Chips | 4 oz | 570 | 27 | 240 | 3.5 | 0 | 0 | 420 | 73 | 8 | 8 | 4 1/2 carb, 5 fat |
| Vinaigrette | 2 oz | 260 | 24.5 | 220 | 4 | 0 | 0 | 700 | 12 | 1 | 0 | 1 carb, 5 fat |
| **CINNABON** | | | | | | | | | | | | |
| Caramel Pecanbon | 1 | 1100 | 56 | 505 | 10 | 5 | 63 | 600 | 141 | 8 | 16 | 9 carb, 11 fat |
| Cinnabon Classic | 1 | 813 | 32 | 290 | 8 | 5 | 67 | 801 | 117 | 4 | 15 | 7 1/2 carb, 6 fat |

| | Serving | Calories | Fat (g) | Cal. from Fat | Sat. Fat (g) | Trans Fat (g) | Chol. (mg) | Sod. (mg) | Carb. (g) | Fiber (g) | Prot. (g) | Servings/Exchanges |
|---|---|---|---|---|---|---|---|---|---|---|---|---|
| Cinnabon Stix | 5 sticks | 379 | 21 | 190 | 6 | 4 | 16 | 413 | 41 | 1 | 6 | 3 1/2 carb, 4 fat |
| Minibon | 1 | 339 | 13 | 115 | 3 | 2 | 27 | 337 | 49 | 2 | 6 | 3 carb, 3 fat |
| **DUNKIN DONUTS** | | | | | | | | | | | | |
| ***Donuts*** | | | | | | | | | | | | |
| Apple Crumb | 1 | 460 | 14 | 130 | 8 | 0 | 0 | 330 | 80 | 2 | 4 | 5 carb, 3 fat |
| Bavarian Crème | 1 | 250 | 12 | 110 | 5 | 0 | 0 | 330 | 31 | 1 | 3 | 2 carb, 2 fat |
| Blueberry Cake | 1 | 330 | 18 | 160 | 8 | 0 | 25 | 460 | 38 | 1 | 3 | 2 1/2 carb, 4 fat |
| Boston Kreme | 1 | 280 | 12 | 110 | 5 | 0 | 0 | 350 | 38 | 1 | 3 | 2 1/2 carb, 2 fat |
| Chocolate Frosted Cake | 1 | 340 | 19 | 170 | 8 | 0 | 25 | 330 | 38 | 1 | 3 | 2 1/2 carb, 4 fat |
| Chocolate Glazed Cake | 1 | 280 | 15 | 140 | 7 | 0 | 0 | 400 | 33 | 1 | 3 | 2 carb, 3 fat |
| Chocolate Kreme Filled | 1 | 310 | 16 | 140 | 7 | 0 | 0 | 340 | 37 | 1 | 4 | 2 1/2carb, 3 fat |
| Glazed | 1 | 220 | 9 | 80 | 4 | 0 | 0 | 320 | 31 | 1 | 3 | 2 carb, 2 fat |
| Glazed Cake | 1 | 320 | 18 | 160 | 8 | 0 | 25 | 310 | 37 | 1 | 3 | 2 1/2 carb, 4 fat |
| Jelly Filled | 1 | 260 | 11 | 100 | 5 | 0 | 0 | 330 | 36 | 1 | 3 | 2 1/2carb, 2 fat |

| | | | | | | | | | | | | |
|---|---|---|---|---|---|---|---|---|---|---|---|---|
| Maple Frosted | 1 | 230 | 10 | 90 | 4 | 0 | 0 | 330 | 33 | 1 | 3 | 2 carb, 2 fat |
| Old Fashioned Cake | 1 | 280 | 18 | 160 | 8 | 0 | 25 | 310 | 27 | 1 | 3 | 2 carb, 1 fat |
| Powdered Cake | 1 | 300 | 18 | 160 | 8 | 0 | 25 | 310 | 30 | 1 | 3 | 2 carb, 4 fat |
| Sugar Raised | 1 | 190 | 9 | 80 | 4 | 0 | 0 | 320 | 22 | 1 | 3 | 1 1/2 carb, 2 fat |
| Toffee for Your Coffee | 1 | 400 | 24 | 220 | 11 | 0 | 10 | 330 | 42 | 1 | 4 | 3 carb, 5 fat |
| Vanilla Kreme Filled | 1 | 320 | 17 | 160 | 8 | 0 | 0 | 340 | 37 | 1 | 3 | 2 1/2 carb, 3 fat |
| ***Fancies*** | | | | | | | | | | | | |
| Apple Fritter | 1 | 400 | 15 | 130 | 6 | 0 | 0 | 530 | 63 | 2 | 5 | 4 carb, 3 fat |
| Coffee Roll | 1 | 370 | 18 | 160 | 7 | 0 | 0 | 510 | 49 | 2 | 5 | 3 carb, 4 fa |
| Éclair | 1 | 350 | 14 | 120 | 5 | 0 | 0 | 460 | 53 | 1 | 4 | 3 1/2 carb, 3 fat |
| Glazed Fritter | 1 | 400 | 15 | 130 | 6 | 0 | 0 | 530 | 63 | 2 | 5 | 4 carb, 3 fat |
| Maple Frosted Coffee Roll | 1 | 380 | 18 | 160 | 8 | 0 | 0 | 520 | 50 | 2 | 5 | 3 carb, 4 fat |
| ***Munchkins*** | | | | | | | | | | | | |
| Glazed | 1 | 50 | 2.5 | 20 | 1 | 0 | 0 | 65 | 7 | 0 | 1 | 1/2 carb, 1 fat |
| Glazed Cake | 1 | 60 | 3 | 30 | 1.5 | 0 | 5 | 65 | 8 | 0 | 1 | 1/2 carb, 1 fat |
| Jelly Filled | 1 | 60 | 2.5 | 20 | 1 | 0 | 0 | 65 | 8 | 0 | 1 | 1/2 carb, 1 fat |

| | Serving | Calories | Fat (g) | Cal. from Fat | Sat. Fat (g) | Trans Fat (g) | Chol. (mg) | Sod. (mg) | Carb. (g) | Fiber (g) | Prot. (g) | Servings/Exchanges |
|---|---|---|---|---|---|---|---|---|---|---|---|---|
| Plain Cake | 1 | 50 | 3 | 30 | 1.5 | 0 | 5 | 60 | 5 | 0 | 1 | 1 fat |
| Powdered Cake | 1 | 60 | 3.5 | 30 | 1.5 | 0 | 5 | 60 | 6 | 0 | 1 | 1/2 carb, 1 fat |
| ***Sticks*** | | | | | | | | | | | | |
| Cinnamon Cake | 1 | 310 | 20 | 180 | 9 | 0 | 25 | 300 | 30 | 1 | 3 | 2 carb, 4 fat |
| Glazed Cake | 1 | 340 | 20 | 180 | 9 | 0 | 25 | 300 | 38 | 1 | 3 | 2 1/2 carb, 4 fat |
| Plain Cake | 1 | 300 | 20 | 180 | 9 | 0 | 25 | 300 | 26 | 1 | 3 | 2 1/2 carb, 4 fat |
| ***Muffins*** | | | | | | | | | | | | |
| Banana Walnut | 1 | 540 | 23 | 205 | 6 | 0 | 75 | 550 | 73 | 3 | 10 | 5 carb, 5 fat |
| Blueberry | 1 | 510 | 16 | 140 | 1.5 | 0 | 15 | 490 | 87 | 3 | 6 | 6 carb, 3 fat |
| Chocolate Chip | 1 | 630 | 23 | 210 | 6 | 0 | 20 | 520 | 98 | 5 | 8 | 6 1/2 carb, 5 fat |
| Coffee Cake | 1 | 620 | 25 | 230 | 7 | 0 | 20 | 530 | 93 | 2 | 7 | 6 carb, 5 fat |
| Corn | 1 | 510 | 17 | 150 | 2 | 0 | 20 | 860 | 84 | 2 | 6 | 5 1/2 carb, 3 fat |
| Honey Bran Raisin | 1 | 500 | 14 | 130 | 1.5 | 0 | 15 | 450 | 86 | 9 | 7 | 5 1/2 carb, 3 fat |
| Reduced Fat Blueberry | 1 | 450 | 10 | 90 | 1.5 | 0 | 15 | 670 | 86 | 3 | 6 | 5 1/2 carb, 2 fat |

| | | | | | | | | | | | | |
|---|---|---|---|---|---|---|---|---|---|---|---|---|
| ***Danish*** | | | | | | | | | | | | |
| Apple Cheese | 1 | 330 | 16 | 150 | 7 | 0 | 0 | 270 | 41 | 1 | 4 | 3 carb, 3 fat |
| Cheese | 1 | 330 | 17 | 150 | 8 | 0 | 5 | 270 | 39 | 1 | 5 | 2 1/2 carb, 3 fat |
| Strawberry Cheese | 1 | 320 | 16 | 150 | 7 | 0 | 0 | 260 | 40 | 1 | 4 | 2 1/2 carb, 3 fat |
| ***Bagels*** | | | | | | | | | | | | |
| Cinnamon Raisin | 1 | 370 | 4 | 35 | 0.5 | 0 | 0 | 530 | 72 | 3 | 13 | 5 starch, 1 fat |
| Everything | 1 | 430 | 7 | 65 | 0.5 | 0 | 0 | 780 | 75 | 3 | 17 | 5 starch, 1 fat |
| Garlic | 1 | 350 | 3.5 | 30 | 0.5 | 0 | 0 | 780 | 76 | 4 | 15 | 5 starch, 1 fat |
| Plain | 1 | 330 | 3 | 30 | 0.5 | 0 | 0 | 780 | 71 | 3 | 14 | 4 1/2 starch, 1 fat |
| Wheat | 1 | 350 | 4 | 35 | 0.5 | 0 | 5 | 650 | 66 | 5 | 13 | 4 1/2 starch, 1 fat |
| ***Cream Cheese*** | | | | | | | | | | | | |
| Plain Cream Cheese | 1.8 oz | 150 | 15 | 130 | 9 | 0.5 | 40 | 250 | 3 | 0 | 3 | 3 fat |
| Reduced Fat Cream Cheese | 1.8 oz | 100 | 8 | 70 | 5 | 0 | 25 | 250 | 5 | 0 | 4 | 2 fat |
| Reduced Fat Smoked Salmon Cream Cheese | 1.8 oz | 140 | 11 | 100 | 7 | 0 | 35 | 260 | 6 | 0 | 4 | 1/2 carb, 2 fat |

| | Serving | Calories | Fat (g) | Cal. from Fat | Sat. Fat (g) | Trans Fat (g) | Chol. (mg) | Sod. (mg) | Carb. (g) | Fiber (g) | Prot. (g) | Servings/Exchanges |
|---|---|---|---|---|---|---|---|---|---|---|---|---|
| ***Oven Toasted Breakfast Sandwiches*** | | | | | | | | | | | | |
| Bacon, Egg & Cheese Bagel | 1 | 530 | 18 | 160 | 6 | 0 | 195 | 1370 | 76 | 3 | 26 | 5 starch, 2 med-fat meat, 2 fat |
| Bacon, Egg & Cheese on English Muffin | 1 | 360 | 16 | 150 | 6 | 0 | 195 | 920 | 35 | 2 | 18 | 2 starch, 2 med-fat meat, 1fat |
| Egg & Cheese on Biscuit | 1 | 430 | 26 | 240 | 13 | 0 | 195 | 1010 | 36 | 1 | 13 | 2 1/2 starch, 1 med-fat meat, 4 fat |
| Egg & Cheese on English Muffin | 1 | 320 | 13 | 120 | 5 | 0 | 190 | 730 | 34 | 2 | 14 | 2 starch, 1 med-fat meat, 2 fat |
| Ham, Egg & Cheese on Bagel | 1 | 520 | 17 | 150 | 6 | 0 | 210 | 1480 | 75 | 3 | 28 | 5 starch, 2 med-fat meat, 1 fat |
| Ham, Egg & Cheese on Croissant | 1 | 510 | 30 | 270 | 12 | 0 | 210 | 1050 | 39 | 1 | 21 | 2 1/2 starch, 2 med-fat meat, 4 fat |
| Sausage Biscuit | 1 | 450 | 28 | 250 | 14 | 0 | 45 | 1020 | 33 | 1 | 12 | 2 starch, 1 med-fat meat, 5 fat |

| | | | | | | | | | | | | |
|---|---|---|---|---|---|---|---|---|---|---|---|---|
| Sausage, Egg & Cheese on English Muffin | 1 | 490 | 28 | 250 | 10 | 0 | 235 | 1130 | 35 | 2 | 22 | 2 starch, 2 med-fat meat, 4 fat |
| ***Favorites Sandwiches*** | | | | | | | | | | | | |
| Steak & Cheese | 1 | 470 | 16 | 140 | 6 | 0 | 75 | 2040 | 50 | 2 | 31 | 3 starch, 3 med-fat meat |
| Toasted Italian | 1 | 560 | 25 | 220 | 9 | 0 | 75 | 2630 | 52 | 3 | 33 | 3 1/2 starch, 3 med-fat meat, 2 fat |
| Tuna Melt | 1 | 770 | 30 | 270 | 7 | 0 | 70 | 1560 | 57 | 3 | 36 | 4 starch, 3 med-fat meat, 3 fat |
| Turkey & Bacon Club | 1 | 440 | 13 | 110 | 3 | 0 | 45 | 1800 | 51 | 3 | 35 | 3 1/2 starch, 3 med-fat meat |
| ***Beverages*** | | | | | | | | | | | | |
| Cappucino | 10 oz | 80 | 4 | 35 | 2.5 | 0 | 15 | 70 | 7 | 0 | 4 | 1/2 carb, 1 fat |
| Caramel Swirl Latte | 10 oz | 230 | 6 | 50 | 3.5 | 0 | 25 | 150 | 35 | 0 | 8 | 2 carb, 1 fat |
| Coffee Coolatta with Cream | 16 oz | 330 | 23 | 210 | 14 | 0.5 | 80 | 60 | 28 | 0 | 3 | 2 carb, 5 fat |

| | Serving | Calories | Fat (g) | Cal. from Fat | Sat. Fat (g) | Trans Fat (g) | Chol. (mg) | Sod. (mg) | Carb. (g) | Fiber (g) | Prot. (g) | Servings/Exchanges |
|---|---|---|---|---|---|---|---|---|---|---|---|---|
| Coffee Coolatta with Milk | 16 oz | 170 | 4 | 35 | 2.5 | 0 | 15 | 75 | 29 | 0 | 4 | 2 carb, 1 fat |
| Coffee Coolatta with Skim Milk | 16 oz | 140 | 0 | 0 | 0 | 0 | 0 | 75 | 30 | 0 | 4 | 2 carb |
| Espresso | 1.75 oz | 0 | 0 | 0 | 0 | 0 | 0 | 5 | 1 | 0 | 0 | free |
| Iced Latte | 16 oz | 120 | 6 | 50 | 3.5 | 0 | 25 | 105 | 10 | 0 | 6 | 1/2 carb, 1 fat |
| Iced Mocha Spice Latte | 16 oz | 220 | 6 | 60 | 4 | 0 | 25 | 95 | 34 | 1 | 7 | 2 carb, 1 fat |
| Latte | 10 oz | 120 | 6 | 50 | 3.5 | 0 | 25 | 105 | 10 | 0 | 6 | 1/2 carb, 1 fat |
| Tropicana Orange Coolatta | 16 oz | 220 | 0 | 0 | 0 | 0 | 0 | 35 | 52 | 0 | 1 | 3 1/2 carb |
| Vanilla Bean Coolatta | 16 oz | 430 | 6 | 50 | 3.5 | 0 | 20 | 170 | 90 | 0 | 3 | 6 carb, 1 fat |
| **DAIRY QUEEN** | | | | | | | | | | | | |
| ***Burgers*** | | | | | | | | | | | | |
| Original Hamburger | 1 | 350 | 14 | 130 | 7 | 0.5 | 50 | 680 | 33 | 1 | 17 | 2 carb, 2 med-fat meat, 1 fat |

| | | | | | | | | | | | | |
|---|---|---|---|---|---|---|---|---|---|---|---|---|
| Original Cheeseburger | 1 | 400 | 18 | 160 | 7 | 0.5 | 65 | 920 | 34 | 1 | 19 | 2 carb, 2 med-fat meat, 2 fat |
| Original Double Cheeseburger | 1 | 640 | 34 | 310 | 18 | 1 | 125 | 1230 | 34 | 1 | 34 | 2 carb, 4 med-fat meat, 3 fat |
| Original Bacon Double Cheeseburger | 1 | 730 | 41 | 370 | 21 | 1 | 150 | 1550 | 35 | 1 | 41 | 2 carb, 5 med-fat meat, 3 fat |
| Classic GrillBurger | 1 | 470 | 21 | 190 | 8 | 0.5 | 50 | 950 | 42 | 2 | 24 | 3 carb, 2 med-fat meat, 2 fat |
| 1/4 lb Bacon Cheddar GrillBurger | 1 | 650 | 35 | 320 | 15 | 1 | 95 | 1410 | 41 | 2 | 36 | 3 carb, 4 med-fat meat, 3 fat |
| 1/2 lb GrillBurger | 1 | 720 | 40 | 360 | 15 | 1.5 | 105 | 1240 | 42 | 2 | 42 | 3 carb, 5 med-fat meat, 3 fat |
| 1/2 lb GrillBurger with Cheese | 1 | 870 | 51 | 460 | 23 | 1.5 | 140 | 1440 | 42 | 2 | 51 | 3 carb, 6 med-fat meat, 4 fat |
| 1/2 lb Flame Thrower Grillburger | 1 | 1060 | 75 | 680 | 26 | 2 | 165 | 1980 | 41 | 2 | 54 | 3 carb, 6 med-fat meat, 9 fat |

| | Serving | Calories | Fat (g) | Cal. from Fat | Sat. Fat (g) | Trans Fat (g) | Chol. (mg) | Sod. (mg) | Carb. (g) | Fiber (g) | Prot. (g) | Servings/Exchanges |
|---|---|---|---|---|---|---|---|---|---|---|---|---|
| ***Hot Dogs*** | | | | | | | | | | | | |
| All-Beef Hot Dog | 1 | 250 | 14 | 130 | 5 | 0 | 25 | 770 | 21 | 1 | 9 | 1 1/2 carb, 1 med-fat meat, 2 fat |
| All-Beef Chili Cheese Dog | 1 | 430 | 22 | 220 | 10 | 0 | 50 | 1010 | 39 | 2 | 18 | 2 1/2 carb, 2 med-fat meat, 2 fat |
| ***Sandwiches/Baskets*** | | | | | | | | | | | | |
| Grilled Chicken Sandwich | 1 | 370 | 16 | 150 | 2.5 | 0 | 55 | 780 | 32 | 1 | 24 | 2 carb, 3 med-fat meat |
| Crispy Chicken Sandwich | 1 | 560 | 28 | 250 | 3.5 | 0 | 35 | 980 | 48 | 3 | 20 | 3 carb, 2 med-fat meat, 4 fat |
| Chicken Strip Basket with Gravy | 4 pieces | 1360 | 63 | 570 | 11 | 1 | 100 | 2910 | 103 | 8 | 39 | 7 carb, 3 med-fat meat, 10 fat |
| ***Side Items*** | | | | | | | | | | | | |
| French Fries, Kid's | 1 | 190 | 8 | 70 | 1 | 0 | 0 | 400 | 27 | 2 | 2 | 2 carb, 2 fat |
| French Fries Regular | 1 | 310 | 13 | 120 | 2 | 0 | 0 | 640 | 43 | 3 | 4 | 3 carb, 3 fat |

| | | | | | | | | | | | | |
|---|---|---|---|---|---|---|---|---|---|---|---|---|
| French Fries, Large | 1 | 500 | 21 | 190 | 3.5 | 0 | 0 | 1040 | 70 | 5 | 6 | 4 1/2 carb, 4 fat |
| Onion Rings | 1 order | 360 | 16 | 140 | 2 | 0 | 0 | 840 | 47 | 2 | 6 | 3 carb, 3 fat |
| Side Salad | 1 | 45 | 0 | 0 | 0 | 0 | 0 | 50 | 11 | 3 | 2 | 2 vegetable |
| ***Cones*** | | | | | | | | | | | | |
| Vanilla Cone, Kids | 1 | 140 | 14 | 35 | 2.5 | 0 | 15 | 60 | 22 | 0 | 4 | 1 1/2 carb, 3 fat |
| Vanilla Cone, Small | 1 | 230 | 7 | 60 | 4.5 | 0 | 25 | 100 | 31 | 0 | 6 | 2 carb, 1 fat |
| Vanilla Cone, Medium | 1 | 330 | 10 | 90 | 6 | 0.5 | 30 | 140 | 53 | 0 | 9 | 3 1/2 carb, 2 fat |
| Vanilla Cone, Large | 1 | 470 | 14 | 130 | 9 | 0.5 | 45 | 200 | 74 | 0 | 12 | 5 carb, 3 fat |
| Dipped Cone, Chocolate, Small | 1 | 330 | 15 | 140 | 6 | 0 | 25 | 105 | 36 | 0 | 6 | 3 carb, 3 fat |
| Dipped Cone, Chocolate, Medium | 1 | 470 | 22 | 200 | 9 | 0.5 | 30 | 150 | 60 | 1 | 9 | 4 carb, 4 fat |
| Dipped Cone, Chocolate, Large | 1 | 660 | 30 | 270 | 13 | 0.5 | 45 | 220 | 84 | 1 | 13 | 5 1/2 carb, 6 fat |
| ***Malts, Shakes, and Arctic Rush*** | | | | | | | | | | | | |
| Chocolate Malt, Small | 1 | 650 | 16 | 150 | 10 | 1 | 55 | 310 | 110 | 0 | 15 | 7 1/2 carb, 3 fat |

| | Serving | Calories | Fat (g) | Cal. from Fat | Sat. Fat (g) | Trans Fat (g) | Chol. (mg) | Sod. (mg) | Carb. (g) | Fiber (g) | Prot. (g) | Servings/Exchanges |
|---|---|---|---|---|---|---|---|---|---|---|---|---|
| Chocolate Malt, Medium | 1 | 900 | 22 | 200 | 14 | 1 | 70 | 430 | 154 | 0 | 20 | 10 carb, 4 fat |
| Chocolate Malt, Large | 1 | 1310 | 33 | 290 | 21 | 1.5 | 105 | 630 | 220 | 0 | 30 | 14 1/2 carb, 7 fat |
| Chocolate Shake, Small | 1 | 570 | 15 | 140 | 10 | 0.5 | 50 | 250 | 92 | 0 | 13 | 6 carb, 3 fat |
| Chocolate Shake, Medium | 1 | 790 | 21 | 190 | 13 | 1 | 70 | 350 | 130 | 0 | 18 | 8 1/2 carb, 4 fat |
| Chocolate Shake, Large | 1 | 1130 | 31 | 280 | 20 | 1.5 | 100 | 510 | 184 | 0 | 26 | 12 carb, 6 fat |
| Arctic Rush, All Flavors, Small | 1 | 240 | 0 | 0 | 0 | 0 | 0 | 0 | 48 | 0 | 0 | 3 carb |
| Arctic Rush, All Flavors, Medium | 1 | 310 | 0 | 0 | 0 | 0 | 0 | 0 | 63 | 0 | 0 | 4 carb |
| ***MooLatte Frozen Blended Coffee*** | | | | | | | | | | | | |
| Cappuccino MooLatte | 16 oz | 500 | 18 | 160 | 15 | 0.5 | 35 | 170 | 71 | 0 | 8 | 4 1/2 carb, 4 fat |
| Caramel MooLatte | 16 oz | 630 | 19 | 170 | 15 | 0.5 | 40 | 240 | 101 | 0 | 9 | 6 1/2 carb, 4 fat |
| French Vanilla MooLatte | 16 oz | 560 | 18 | 160 | 14 | 0.5 | 35 | 160 | 88 | 0 | 8 | 6 carb, 4 fat |

| | | | | | | | | | | | | |
|---|---|---|---|---|---|---|---|---|---|---|---|---|
| Mocha MooLatte | 16 oz | 590 | 23 | 200 | 15 | 0.5 | 35 | 190 | 82 | 0 | 9 | 5 1/2 carb, 5 fat |
| ***Sundaes*** | | | | | | | | | | | | |
| Chocolate Sundae, Small | 1 | 280 | 7 | 60 | 4.5 | 0 | 25 | 115 | 48 | 0 | 5 | 3 carb, 1 fat |
| Chocolate Sundae, Medium | 1 | 400 | 10 | 90 | 6 | 0.5 | 30 | 170 | 70 | 0 | 8 | 4 1/2 carb, 2 fat |
| Chocolate Sundae, Large | 1 | 570 | 14 | 120 | 9 | 0.5 | 45 | 240 | 98 | 0 | 11 | 6 1/2 carb, 3 fat |
| ***Treats*** | | | | | | | | | | | | |
| Banana Split | 1 | 520 | 13 | 120 | 10 | 0.5 | 30 | 160 | 94 | 3 | 9 | 6 1/2 carb, 3 fat |
| Oreo Brownie Earthquake | 1 | 760 | 27 | 240 | 16 | 0 | 60 | 400 | 117 | 2 | 11 | 8 carb, 5 fat |
| Peanut Buster Parfait | 1 | 700 | 30 | 270 | 16 | 0.5 | 35 | 360 | 94 | 2 | 16 | 6 carb, 6 fat |
| Plain Waffle Cone with Soft Serve | 1 | 420 | 13 | 110 | 7 | 0.5 | 40 | 140 | 67 | 0 | 10 | 4 1/2 carb, 3 fat |
| Turtle Waffle Bowl Sundae | 1 | 810 | 34 | 310 | 18 | 0.5 | 40 | 320 | 116 | 2 | 12 | 7 1/2 carb, 7 fat |
| ***Novelties*** | | | | | | | | | | | | |
| Buster Bar Treat | 1 | 480 | 31 | 280 | 15 | 0 | 20 | 220 | 45 | 2 | 11 | 3 carb, 6 fat |

| | Serving | Calories | Fat (g) | Cal. from Fat | Sat. Fat (g) | Trans Fat (g) | Chol. (mg) | Sod. (mg) | Carb. (g) | Fiber (g) | Prot. (g) | Servings/Exchanges |
|---|---|---|---|---|---|---|---|---|---|---|---|---|
| Cherry StarKiss Bar | 1 | 80 | 0 | 0 | 0 | 0 | 0 | 10 | 21 | 0 | 0 | 1 1/2 carb |
| Chocolate Dilly Bar | 1 | 240 | 15 | 140 | 9 | 0 | 15 | 70 | 24 | 1 | 4 | 1 1/2 carb, 3 fat |
| Dilly Bar, No Sugar Added | 1 | 190 | 13 | 120 | 10 | 0 | 15 | 60 | 24 | 5 | 3 | 1 1/2 carb, 3 fat |
| DQ Fudge Bar, No Sugar Added | 1 | 50 | 0 | 0 | 0 | 0 | 0 | 70 | 13 | 6 | 4 | 1 carb |
| DQ Sandwich | 1 | 190 | 5 | 45 | 3 | 0 | 10 | 135 | 31 | 1 | 4 | 2 carb, 1 fat |
| DQ Vanilla Orange Bar, No Sugar Added | 1 | 60 | 0 | 0 | 0 | 0 | 0 | 45 | 18 | 6 | 2 | 1 carb |
| ***Blizzard Treats*** | | | | | | | | | | | | |
| Oreo Cookies Blizzard, Small | 1 | 550 | 20 | 180 | 10 | 0.5 | 40 | 410 | 81 | 1 | 12 | 5 1/2 carb, 4 fat |
| Oreo Cookies Blizzard, Medium | 1 | 820 | 35 | 320 | 19 | 1 | 105 | 610 | 108 | 1 | 16 | 7 carb, 7 fat |

| | | | | | | | | | | | | |
|---|---|---|---|---|---|---|---|---|---|---|---|---|
| Oreo Cookies Blizzard, Large | 1 | 1140 | 49 | 440 | 26 | 1 | 140 | 840 | 151 | 1 | 23 | 10 carb, 10 fat |
| Chocolate Chip Cookie Dough Blizzard, Small | 1 | 710 | 27 | 250 | 14 | 3 | 55 | 350 | 103 | 1 | 13 | 7 carb, 6 fat |
| Chocolate Chip Cookie Dough Blizzard, Medium | 1 | 1010 | 40 | 360 | 20 | 4.5 | 75 | 500 | 148 | 1 | 18 | 10 carb, 8 fat |
| Chocolate Chip Cookie Dough Blizzard, Large | 1 | 1300 | 51 | 460 | 26 | 6 | 95 | 640 | 189 | 2 | 22 | 12 1/2 carb, 10 fat |
| DQ Cake (8" round cake) | 1/8 cake | 410 | 15 | 140 | 10 | 1 | 30 | 210 | 59 | 1 | 9 | 4 carb, 3 fat |
| **DOMINO'S** | | | | | | | | | | | | |
| ***Hand-Tossed, Large*** | | | | | | | | | | | | |
| Cheese | 1/8 pizza | 240 | 8 | 70 | 3 | 0 | 10 | 490 | 34 | 2 | 10 | 2 carb, 1 med-fat meat, 1 fat |
| Pepperoni | 1/8 pizza | 290 | 13 | 110 | 5 | 0 | 20 | 680 | 34 | 2 | 12 | 2 1/2 carb, 1 med-fat meat, 1 fat |

| | Serving | Calories | Fat (g) | Cal. from Fat | Sat. Fat (g) | Trans Fat (g) | Chol. (mg) | Sod. (mg) | Carb. (g) | Fiber (g) | Prot. (g) | Servings/Exchanges |
|---|---|---|---|---|---|---|---|---|---|---|---|---|
| Sausage | 1/8 pizza | 300 | 13 | 120 | 5 | 0 | 20 | 670 | 36 | 3 | 12 | 2 1/2 carb, 1 med-fat meat, 2 fat |
| Ham | 1/8 pizza | 255 | 9 | 75 | 3 | 0 | 15 | 625 | 34 | 2 | 12 | 2 carb, 1 med-fat meat, 1 fat |
| Beef | 1/8 pizza | 290 | 13 | 110 | 5 | 0 | 20 | 590 | 34 | 2 | 13 | 2 carb, 1 med-fat meat, 2 fat |
| ***Deep Dish, Large*** | | | | | | | | | | | | |
| Cheese | 1/8 pizza | 330 | 14 | 130 | 5 | 0 | 15 | 760 | 40 | 5 | 12 | 2 1/2 carb,1 med-fat meat, 2 fat |
| Pepperoni | 1/8 pizza | 380 | 15 | 170 | 7 | 0 | 25 | 950 | 40 | 5 | 12 | 2 1/2 carb, 1 med-fat meat, 2 fat |
| Sausage | 1/8 pizza | 390 | 19 | 180 | 7 | 0 | 25 | 940 | 42 | 6 | 14 | 3 carb, 1 med-fat meat, 4 fat |
| Ham | 1/8 pizza | 345 | 16 | 135 | 5 | 0 | 20 | 895 | 40 | 5 | 14 | 2 1/2 carb, 1 med-fat meat, 2 fat |

| | | | | | | | | | | | | |
|---|---|---|---|---|---|---|---|---|---|---|---|---|
| Beef | 1/8 pizza | 380 | 19 | 170 | 7 | 0 | 25 | 860 | 40 | 5 | 12 | 2 1/2 carb, 1 med-fat meat, 3 fat |
| ***Thin Crust, Large*** | | | | | | | | | | | | |
| Cheese | 1/8 pizza | 180 | 10 | 90 | 4 | 0 | 15 | 340 | 19 | 1 | 7 | 1 carb, 1 med-fat meat, 1 fat |
| Pepperoni | 1/8 pizza | 230 | 15 | 130 | 5 | 0 | 25 | 530 | 19 | 1 | 9 | 1 carb, 1 med-fat meat, 2 fat |
| Sausage | 1/8 pizza | 240 | 15 | 140 | 6 | 0 | 25 | 520 | 19 | 2 | 9 | 1 carb, 1 med-fat meat, 2 fat |
| Ham | 1/8 pizza | 195 | 11 | 95 | 4 | 0 | 20 | 475 | 19 | 1 | 9 | 1 carb, 1 med-fat meat, 1 fat |
| ***Breadbowl Pasta*** | | | | | | | | | | | | |
| Chicken Alfredo | 1/2 | 700 | 25 | 230 | 11 | 0.5 | 50 | 1070 | 93 | 3 | 26 | 6 carb, 1 med-fat meat, 4 fat |
| Italian Sausage Marinara | 1/2 | 730 | 26 | 240 | 11 | 0 | 35 | 1410 | 97 | 4 | 26 | 6 1/2 carb, 1 med-fat meat, 4 fat |
| Three Cheese Mac-N-Cheese | 1/2 | 730 | 28 | 250 | 14 | 1 | 55 | 1420 | 95 | 3 | 27 | 6 1/2 carb, 1 med-fat meat, 5 fat |

| | Serving | Calories | Fat (g) | Cal. from Fat | Sat. Fat (g) | Trans Fat (g) | Chol. (mg) | Sod. (mg) | Carb. (g) | Fiber (g) | Prot. (g) | Servings/Exchanges |
|---|---|---|---|---|---|---|---|---|---|---|---|---|
| ***Oven Baked Sandwiches*** | | | | | | | | | | | | |
| Chicken Bacon Ranch | 1 | 890 | 45 | 400 | 16 | 1 | 115 | 2210 | 72 | 2 | 49 | 5 carb, 5 med-fat meat, 4 fat |
| Italian | 1 | 880 | 45 | 410 | 22 | 1 | 120 | 2560 | 71 | 3 | 47 | 4 1/2 carb, 5 med-fat meat, 4 fat |
| Philly Cheese Steak | 1 | 690 | 27 | 250 | 14 | 1 | 90 | 2080 | 72 | 3 | 41 | 5 carb, 4 med-fat meat, 1 fat |
| ***Salads (no dressing)*** | | | | | | | | | | | | |
| Garden Fresh | 1/2 salad | 70 | 4 | 35 | 3 | 0 | 10 | 80 | 5 | 2 | 4 | 1 vegetable, 1 fat |
| Grilled Chicken Caesar | 1/2 salad | 100 | 5 | 40 | 2 | 0 | 20 | 310 | 6 | 2 | 10 | 1 vegetable, 1 med-fat meat |
| ***Side Items*** | | | | | | | | | | | | |
| Barbeque Buffalo Wings | 2 pieces | 230 | 14 | 130 | 3.5 | 0 | 50 | 410 | 6 | 0 | 17 | 1/2 carb, 2 med-fat meat, 1 fat |

| | | | | | | | | | | | | |
|---|---|---|---|---|---|---|---|---|---|---|---|---|
| Blue Cheese Dipping Sauce | 1 container | 210 | 22 | 200 | 4 | 0 | 20 | 390 | 2 | 0 | 1 | 4 fat |
| Breadsticks | 1 | 110 | 6 | 60 | 2 | 0 | 0 | 100 | 11 | 0 | 2 | 1 carb, 1 fat |
| Buffalo Chicken Kickers | 2 pieces | 100 | 5 | 40 | 0.5 | 0 | 20 | 280 | 7 | 1 | 9 | 1/2 carb, 1 med-fat meat |
| Cheesy Bread | 1 | 120 | 6 | 60 | 2 | 0 | 5 | 150 | 11 | 0 | 4 | 1 carb, 1 fat |
| Cinna Stix | 1 | 120 | 6 | 60 | 1 | 0 | 0 | 85 | 14 | 1 | 2 | 1 carb, 1 fat |
| Garlic Dipping Sauce | 1 container | 250 | 28 | 250 | 5 | 0 | 0 | 160 | 0 | 0 | 0 | 6 fat |
| Hot Buffalo Wings | 2 pieces | 200 | 14 | 120 | 3.5 | 0 | 50 | 690 | 2 | 0 | 16 | 2 med-fat meat, 1 fat |
| Hot Dipping Sauce | 1 container | 50 | 5 | 40 | 5 | 0 | 0 | 1480 | 3 | 0 | 0 | 1 fat |
| Marinara Dipping Sauce | 1 container | 25 | 0 | 0 | 0 | 0 | 0 | 270 | 5 | 1 | 1 | free |
| Ranch Dipping Sauce | 1 container | 190 | 21 | 190 | 3 | 0 | 10 | 390 | 2 | 0 | 1 | 4 fat |
| Sweet Icing | 1 container | 250 | 3 | 25 | 1 | 0 | 0 | 0 | 57 | 0 | 0 | 4 carb, 1 fat |

| | Serving | Calories | Fat (g) | Cal. from Fat | Sat. Fat (g) | Trans Fat (g) | Chol. (mg) | Sod. (mg) | Carb. (g) | Fiber (g) | Prot. (g) | Servings/Exchanges |
|---|---|---|---|---|---|---|---|---|---|---|---|---|
| **EINSTEIN BROS. BAGELS** | | | | | | | | | | | | |
| ***Bagels*** | | | | | | | | | | | | |
| Asiago Cheese | 1 | 330 | 5 | 50 | 3 | 0 | 15 | 660 | 59 | 2 | 15 | 4 starch, 1 fat |
| Blueberry | 1 | 290 | 1.5 | 10 | 0 | 0 | 0 | 480 | 64 | 3 | 9 | 4 starch |
| Chocolate Chip | 1 | 290 | 3 | 25 | 1 | 0 | 0 | 460 | 60 | 3 | 10 | 4 starch , 1 fat |
| Cinnamon Raisin Swirl | 1 | 290 | 1 | 10 | 0 | 0 | 0 | 450 | 64 | 3 | 10 | 4 starch |
| Cinnamon Sugar Bagel, Chicago Style | 1 | 310 | 2.5 | 20 | 0.5 | 0 | 0 | 510 | 66 | 3 | 10 | 4 1/2 starch, 1 fat |
| Cranberry | 1 | 290 | 1 | 10 | 0 | 0 | 0 | 450 | 64 | 3 | 9 | 4 starch |
| Egg | 1 | 300 | 6 | 50 | 1.5 | 0 | 150 | 480 | 52 | 2 | 12 | 3 1/2 starch, 1 fat |
| Everything | 1 | 270 | 2 | 15 | 0 | 0 | 0 | 610 | 56 | 2 | 10 | 3 1/2 starch |
| Garlic Dip'd | 1 | 290 | 2.5 | 20 | 0 | 0 | 0 | 490 | 60 | 2 | 10 | 4 starch, 1 fat |
| Good Grains | 1 | 290 | 2.5 | 20 | 0 | 0 | 0 | 480 | 62 | 4 | 10 | 4 starch, 1 fat |
| Honey Whole Wheat | 1 | 270 | 1 | 10 | 0 | 0 | 0 | 480 | 61 | 3 | 9 | 4 starch |

| | | | | | | | | | | | | |
|---|---|---|---|---|---|---|---|---|---|---|---|---|
| Onion Dip'd | 1 | 270 | 1 | 10 | 0 | 0 | 0 | 460 | 59 | 2 | 9 | 4 starch |
| Plain | 1 | 260 | 1 | 10 | 0 | 0 | 0 | 460 | 56 | 2 | 9 | 3 1/2 starch |
| Poppy Dip'd | 1 | 280 | 3 | 25 | 0 | 0 | 0 | 460 | 56 | 2 | 10 | 3 1/2 starch, 1 fat |
| Potato | 1 | 260 | 1 | 10 | 0 | 0 | 0 | 540 | 58 | 2 | 9 | 4 starch |
| Power Bagel, Fruit & Nut | 1 | 380 | 6 | 50 | 1 | 0 | 0 | 330 | 72 | 5 | 13 | 5 starch, 1 fat |
| Pumpernickel | 1 | 250 | 1.5 | 10 | 0 | 0 | 0 | 710 | 55 | 3 | 9 | 3 1/2 starch |
| Sesame Dip'd | 1 | 280 | 3 | 25 | 0 | 0 | 0 | 460 | 56 | 2 | 10 | 3 1/2 starch, 1 fat |
| Sun-Dried Tomato | 1 | 270 | 1.5 | 15 | 0 | 0 | 0 | 570 | 58 | 3 | 10 | 4 starch |
| ***Gourmet Bagels*** | | | | | | | | | | | | |
| Dutch Apple | 1 | 340 | 7 | 60 | 1.5 | 0 | 0 | 540 | 66 | 2 | 8 | 4 1/2 starch, 1 fat |
| Green Chile | 1 | 370 | 8 | 70 | 4.5 | 0 | 25 | 710 | 62 | 2 | 16 | 4 starch, 2 fat |
| Six Cheese | 1 | 350 | 6 | 60 | 3.5 | 0 | 15 | 680 | 60 | 2 | 16 | 4 starch, 1 fat |
| Spinach Florentine | 1 | 360 | 8 | 70 | 4 | 0 | 20 | 620 | 61 | 2 | 16 | 4 starch, 2 fat |
| ***Bagel Pretzels*** | | | | | | | | | | | | |
| Asiago Cheese | 1 | 300 | 7 | 70 | 2.5 | 0 | 5 | 710 | 52 | 2 | 11 | 3 1/2 starch, 1 fat |

| | Serving | Calories | Fat (g) | Cal. from Fat | Sat. Fat (g) | Trans Fat (g) | Chol. (mg) | Sod. (mg) | Carb. (g) | Fiber (g) | Prot. (g) | Servings/Exchanges |
|---|---|---|---|---|---|---|---|---|---|---|---|---|
| Cinnamon Sugar | 1 | 320 | 5 | 50 | 1 | 0 | 0 | 630 | 66 | 3 | 8 | 4 1/2 starch, 1 fat |
| Plain | 1 | 270 | 5 | 50 | 1 | 0 | 0 | 630 | 52 | 2 | 8 | 3 1/2 starch, 1 fat |
| ***Cream Cheese*** | | | | | | | | | | | | |
| Whipped Plain | 2 Tbsp | 70 | 7 | 60 | 4.5 | 0 | 20 | 65 | 1 | 0 | 1 | 1 fat |
| Whipped Plain, Reduced Fat | 2 Tbsp | 60 | 5 | 45 | 3.5 | 0 | 15 | 100 | 2 | 0 | 1 | 1 fat |
| Whipped Blueberry, Reduced Fat | 2 Tbsp | 70 | 5 | 45 | 3.5 | 0 | 15 | 50 | 6 | 0 | 1 | 1/2 carb, 1 fat |
| Whipped Garlic Herb, Reduced Fat | 2 Tbsp | 60 | 5 | 45 | 3.5 | 0 | 15 | 100 | 3 | 0 | 1 | 1 fat |
| Whipped Garden Vegetable, Reduced Fat | 2 Tbsp | 60 | 5 | 45 | 3.5 | 0 | 15 | 100 | 3 | 0 | 1 | 1 fat |
| Whipped Honey Almond, Reduced Fat | 2 Tbsp | 70 | 5 | 45 | 3 | 0 | 15 | 45 | 6 | 0 | 1 | 1/2 carb, 1 fat |

| | | | | | | | | | | | | |
|---|---|---|---|---|---|---|---|---|---|---|---|---|
| Whipped Jalapeño Salsa Reduced Fat | 2 Tbsp | 60 | 5 | 45 | 3.5 | 0 | 15 | 105 | 3 | 0 | 1 | 1 fat |
| Whipped Smoked Salmon | 2 Tbsp | 60 | 6 | 50 | 3.5 | 0 | 20 | 120 | 2 | 0 | 1 | 1 fat |
| Whipped Strawberry, Reduced Fat | 2 Tbsp | 70 | 5 | 45 | 3.5 | 0 | 15 | 50 | 5 | 0 | 1 | 1 fat |
| Whipped Sundried Tomato, Reduced Fat | 2 Tbsp | 60 | 5 | 45 | 3.5 | 0 | 15 | 100 | 2 | 0 | 1 | 1 fat |
| ***Wraps*** | | | | | | | | | | | | |
| California Chicken Wrap | 13.1 oz | 630 | 28 | 250 | 8 | 0 | 110 | 1170 | 63 | 8 | 33 | 4 carb, 3 med-fat meat, 3 fat |
| Chipotle Turkey Wrap | 13 oz | 730 | 37 | 330 | 12 | 0 | 75 | 1990 | 70 | 9 | 34 | 4 1/2 carb, 3 med-fat meat, 4 fat |
| ***Salads (and Half Salads)*** | | | | | | | | | | | | |
| Bros. Bistro House Salad | 10.5 oz | 820 | 68 | 610 | 11 | 0 | 25 | 320 | 38 | 7 | 14 | 2 1/2 carb, 1 med-fat meat, 13 fat |

FAST FOOD

| | Serving | Calories | Fat (g) | Cal. from Fat | Sat. Fat (g) | Trans Fat (g) | Chol. (mg) | Sod. (mg) | Carb. (g) | Fiber (g) | Prot. (g) | Servings/Exchanges |
|---|---|---|---|---|---|---|---|---|---|---|---|---|
| Bros. Bistro House Salad with Chicken | 14 oz | 940 | 71 | 630 | 12 | 0 | 105 | 810 | 39 | 7 | 36 | 2 1/2 carb, 4 med-fat meat, 10 fat |
| Caesar Salad | 10 oz | 690 | 63 | 570 | 15 | 0 | 55 | 1730 | 18 | 4 | 18 | 1 carb, 2 med-fat meat, 11 fat |
| Caesar Salad with Chicken | 14 oz | 820 | 66 | 600 | 16 | 0 | 145 | 2290 | 20 | 4 | 42 | 1 carb, 6 med-fat meat, 7 fat |
| Chicken Chipotle Salad | 15.2 oz | 710 | 41 | 370 | 9 | 0 | 95 | 1960 | 54 | 10 | 34 | 3 1/2 carb, 2 med-fat meat, 6 fat |
| Chipotle Salad | 11.7 oz | 590 | 38 | 340 | 8 | 0 | 20 | 1470 | 53 | 10 | 13 | 3 1/2 carb, 1 med-fat meat, 7 fat |
| Half Caesar Salad | 4.5 oz | 280 | 27 | 240 | 6 | 0 | 2 | 680 | 7 | 2 | 6 | 1/2 carb carb, 1 med-fat meat, 4 fat |
| Half Caesar Salad with Chicken | 6.5 oz | 350 | 28 | 260 | 6 | 0 | 65 | 960 | 8 | 2 | 18 | 1/2 carb, 2 med-fat meat, 4 fat |

| | | | | | | | | | | | | |
|---|---|---|---|---|---|---|---|---|---|---|---|---|
| Half Chicken Chipotle Salad | 7.8 oz | 360 | 21 | 190 | 4.5 | 0 | 40 | 970 | 27 | 5 | 18 | 2 carb, 2 med-fat meat, 2 fat |
| Half Chipotle Salad | 5.8 oz | 290 | 18 | 170 | 4 | 0 | 10 | 730 | 26 | 5 | 6 | 2 carb, 4 fat |
| ***Sandwiches*** | | | | | | | | | | | | |
| Deli Chicken Salad | 9.7 oz | 460 | 18 | 160 | 4 | 0.5 | 75 | 890 | 47 | 4 | 28 | 3 1/2 carb, 3 med-fat meat, 1 fat |
| Deli Ham | 9.2 oz | 520 | 26 | 230 | 5 | 0.5 | 45 | 1550 | 48 | 4 | 26 | 3 carb, 2 med-fat meat, 3 fat |
| Deli Pastrami | 10.9 oz | 630 | 33 | 300 | 9 | 1 | 80 | 1860 | 53 | 5 | 34 | 3 1/2 carb, 3 med-fat meat, 4 fat |
| Deli Tuna Salad | 9.5 oz | 440 | 15 | 130 | 2.5 | 0 | 35 | 920 | 50 | 4 | 29 | 3 carb, 3 med-fat meat |
| Deli Turkey | 9.6 oz | 510 | 15 | 130 | 8 | 0 | 75 | 1430 | 62 | 3 | 38 | 4 carb, 4 lean meat |
| Egg Way Original | 8.7 oz | 530 | 20 | 180 | 9 | 0 | 395 | 840 | 62 | 2 | 30 | 4 carb, 3 med-fat meat, 1 fat |
| Egg Way with Black Forest Ham | 10.1 oz | 570 | 21 | 190 | 9 | 0 | 410 | 1270 | 62 | 2 | 37 | 4 carb, 3 med-fat meat, 1 fat |

FAST FOOD

| | Serving | Calories | Fat (g) | Cal. from Fat | Sat. Fat (g) | Trans Fat (g) | Chol. (mg) | Sod. (mg) | Carb. (g) | Fiber (g) | Prot. (g) | Servings/Exchanges |
|---|---|---|---|---|---|---|---|---|---|---|---|---|
| Egg Way with Sausage | 10.1 oz | 600 | 24 | 210 | 10 | 0 | 425 | 1020 | 63 | 2 | 38 | 4 carb, 4 med-fat meat, 1 fat |
| Original Asiago Bagel Dog | 6.8 oz | 490 | 21 | 190 | 8 | 1 | 60 | 1230 | 56 | 2 | 22 | 3 1/2 carb, 2 med-fat meat, 2 fat |
| Original Bagel Dog | 6.7 oz | 470 | 20 | 180 | 7 | 1 | 55 | 1190 | 56 | 2 | 20 | 3 1/2 carb, 2 med-fat meat, 2 fat |
| Pepperoni Pizza Bagel | 6.6 oz | 470 | 16 | 140 | 8 | 0 | 45 | 1120 | 63 | 3 | 24 | 4 carb, 2 med-fat meat, 1 fat |
| Rachel, Regular Size | 10.1 oz | 910 | 64 | 580 | 16 | 1.5 | 130 | 2210 | 51 | 2 | 36 | 3 1/2 carb, 4 med-fat meat, 9 fat |
| Reuben, Regular Size | 9.9 oz | 650 | 38 | 340 | 12 | 1 | 105 | 2360 | 47 | 3 | 34 | 3 carb, 3 med-fat meat, 5 fat |
| Roasted Turkey & Swiss | 10.9 oz | 690 | 41 | 370 | 9 | 1 | 80 | 1460 | 49 | 4 | 35 | 5 carb, 2 lean meat |
| Sausage Ranchero Panini | 12.2 oz | 680 | 29 | 260 | 12 | 0 | 435 | 1360 | 64 | 4 | 32 | 4 1/2 carb, 3 med-fat meat, 3 fat |

| | | | | | | | | | | | | |
|---|---|---|---|---|---|---|---|---|---|---|---|---|
| Veg Out, on Sesame Seed Bagel | 9.5 oz | 440 | 14 | 120 | 7 | 0 | 30 | 760 | 66 | 4 | 17 | 4 1/2 carb, 1 med-fat meat, 2 fat |
| ***Paninis*** | | | | | | | | | | | | |
| Italian Chicken | 12.6 oz | 800 | 40 | 360 | 12 | 0 | 120 | 2450 | 66 | 5 | 35 | 4 1/2 carb, 3 med-fat meat, 5 fat |
| Turkey Club | 13.3 oz | 790 | 41 | 370 | 11 | 1 | 100 | 2200 | 66 | 6 | 34 | 4 1/2 carb, 3 med-fat meat, 5 fat |
| ***Soups (Cup)*** | | | | | | | | | | | | |
| Chicken Noodle | 8.75 oz | 120 | 3.5 | 35 | 1 | 0 | 30 | 770 | 14 | 1 | 5 | 1 carb, 1 fat |
| Corn Crab Chowder | 8.75 oz | 280 | 18 | 160 | 15 | 0 | 30 | 940 | 18 | 1 | 8 | 1 carb, 1 med-fat meat, 3 fat |
| Italian Wedding | 8.75 oz | 160 | 6 | 50 | 1.5 | 0 | 20 | 1060 | 15 | 2 | 11 | 1 carb, 1 med-fat meat |
| Seafood Minestrone | 8.75 oz | 130 | 4.5 | 40 | 1 | 0 | 40 | 1010 | 16 | 2 | 8 | 1 carb, 1 med-fat meat |
| Turkey Chili | 8.75 oz | 220 | 7 | 60 | 1.5 | 0 | 35 | 930 | 24 | 5 | 20 | 1 1/2 carb, 2 lean meat |
| Vegetarian Broccoli Cheese | 8.75 oz | 290 | 20 | 180 | 10 | 0 | 45 | 990 | 16 | 2 | 14 | 1 carb, 2 med-fat meat, 2 fat |

| | Serving | Calories | Fat (g) | Cal. from Fat | Sat. Fat (g) | Trans Fat (g) | Chol. (mg) | Sod. (mg) | Carb. (g) | Fiber (g) | Prot. (g) | Servings/Exchanges |
|---|---|---|---|---|---|---|---|---|---|---|---|---|
| **HARDEE'S** | | | | | | | | | | | | |
| ***Breakfast*** | | | | | | | | | | | | |
| Made from Scratch Biscuit | 1 | 370 | 23 | 210 | 5 | NA | 0 | 890 | 35 | 0 | 5 | 2 carb, 5 fat |
| Bacon, Egg & Cheese Biscuit | 1 | 530 | 36 | 320 | 11 | NA | 195 | 1390 | 36 | 0 | 15 | 2 1/2 carb, 1 med-fat meat, 6 fat |
| Biscuit 'N' Gravy | 1 | 530 | 33 | 300 | 8 | NA | 10 | 1510 | 48 | 1 | 9 | 3 carb, 7 fat |
| Chicken Fillet Biscuit | 1 | 600 | 34 | 310 | 7 | NA | 55 | 1680 | 50 | 1 | 24 | 3 carb, 2 med-fat meat, 5 fat |
| Country Ham Biscuit | 1 | 440 | 26 | 240 | 6 | NA | 35 | 1710 | 36 | 0 | 14 | 2 1/2 carb, 1 med-fat meat, 4 fat |
| Country Steak Biscuit | 1 | 630 | 43 | 390 | 11 | NA | 35 | 1330 | 45 | 0 | 16 | 3 carb, 1 med-fat meat, 8 fat |
| Frisco Breakfast Sandwich | 1 | 400 | 18 | 160 | 7 | NA | 215 | 1350 | 27 | 2 | 23 | 2 carb, 2 med-fat meat, 2 fat |

| | | | | | | | | | | | | |
|---|---|---|---|---|---|---|---|---|---|---|---|---|
| Loaded Biscuit 'N' Gravy Breakfast Bowl | 1 | 740 | 52 | 460 | 14 | NA | 220 | 1920 | 49 | 1 | 20 | 3 carb, 2 med-fat meat, 8 fat |
| Loaded Breakfast Burrito | 1 | 760 | 49 | 440 | 21 | NA | 445 | 1700 | 39 | 1 | 39 | 2 1/2 carb, 5 med-fat meat, 5 fat |
| Low Carb Breakfast Bowl | 1 | 620 | 50 | 450 | 21 | NA | 325 | 1380 | 6 | 2 | 36 | 1/2 carb, 5 med-fat meat, 5 fat |
| Monster Biscuit | 1 | 770 | 55 | 500 | 18 | NA | 250 | 2310 | 37 | 0 | 29 | 2 1/2 carb, 3 med-fat meat, 8 fat |
| Pancakes | 3 | 300 | 5 | 45 | 1 | NA | 25 | 830 | 55 | 2 | 8 | 3 1/2 carb, 1 fat |
| Sausage & Egg Biscuit | 1 | 590 | 42 | 380 | 11 | NA | 210 | 1300 | 36 | 0 | 16 | 2 1/2 carb, 2 med-fat meat, 6 fat |
| Sausage Biscuit | 1 | 530 | 38 | 340 | 10 | NA | 30 | 1240 | 36 | 0 | 11 | 2 1/2 carb, 1 med-fat meat, 7 fat |
| Smoked Sausage Biscuit | 1 | 620 | 46 | 420 | 15 | NA | 40 | 1680 | 37 | 0 | 14 | 2 1/2 carb, 1 med-fat meat, 8 fat |
| Sunrise Croissant with Ham | 1 | 400 | 23 | 210 | 10 | NA | 225 | 1070 | 27 | 1 | 21 | 2 carb, 2 med-fat meat, 3 fat |

FAST FOOD

| | Serving | Calories | Fat (g) | Cal. from Fat | Sat. Fat (g) | Trans Fat (g) | Chol. (mg) | Sod. (mg) | Carb. (g) | Fiber (g) | Prot. (g) | Servings/Exchanges |
|---|---|---|---|---|---|---|---|---|---|---|---|---|
| ***Sandwiches*** | | | | | | | | | | | | |
| Small Hamburger | 1 | 310 | 15 | 140 | 4 | NA | 35 | 500 | 32 | 1 | 14 | 2 carb, 1 med-fat meat, 2 fat |
| Small Cheeseburger | 1 | 350 | 19 | 170 | 4 | NA | 45 | 730 | 32 | 1 | 16 | 2 carb, 1 med-fat meat, 3 fat |
| Little Thickburger | 1 | 570 | 39 | 350 | 12 | NA | 80 | 1140 | 35 | 3 | 24 | 2 carb, 3 med-fat meat, 5 fat |
| 1/3 lb Original Thickburger | 1 | 770 | 48 | 430 | 16 | NA | 95 | 1560 | 53 | 4 | 35 | 3 1/2 carb, 3 med-fat meat, 8 fat |
| 1/3 lb Low Carb Thickburger | 1 | 420 | 32 | 280 | 12 | NA | 115 | 1010 | 5 | 2 | 30 | 4 med-fat meat, 2 fat |
| 1/3 lb Cheeseburger | 1 | 620 | 33 | 290 | 13 | NA | 80 | 1580 | 51 | 3 | 35 | 3 1/2 carb, 3 med-fat meat, 4 fat |
| 1/3 lb Mushroom 'N Swiss Thickburger | 1 | 650 | 36 | 320 | 14 | NA | 90 | 1620 | 47 | 3 | 39 | 3 carb, 4 med-fat meat, 3 fat |

| | | | | | | | | | | | | |
|---|---|---|---|---|---|---|---|---|---|---|---|---|
| 1/3 lb Bacon Cheese Thickburger | 1 | 850 | 57 | 520 | 19 | NA | 105 | 1650 | 49 | 3 | 38 | 3 carb, 4 med-fat meat, 7 fat |
| 2/3 lb Monster Thickburger | 1 | 1320 | 95 | 860 | 36 | NA | 210 | 3020 | 46 | 2 | 70 | 3 carb, 9 med-fat meat, 10 fat |
| 2/3 lb Bacon Cheese Thickburger | 1 | 1200 | 84 | 750 | 30 | NA | 185 | 2450 | 50 | 3 | 65 | 3 carb, 8 med-fat meat, 9 fat |
| 2/3 lb Double Thickburger | 1 | 1150 | 78 | 700 | 28 | NA | 180 | 2410 | 53 | 4 | 62 | 3 1/2 carb, 7 med-fat meat, 9 fat |
| BBQ Chicken Sandwich | 1 | 400 | 6 | 50 | 1 | NA | 45 | 1370 | 62 | 5 | 27 | 4 carb, 2 lean meat |
| Six Dollar Thickburger | 1 | 930 | 59 | 530 | 21 | NA | 130 | 1960 | 57 | 4 | 46 | 4 carb, 5 med-fat meat, 7 fat |
| Charbroiled Chicken Club Sandwich | 1 | 630 | 32 | 280 | 8 | NA | 80 | 1730 | 54 | 4 | 32 | 3 1/2 carb, 3 med-fat meat, 3 fat |
| Low Carb Charbroiled Chicken Club Sandwich | 1 | 360 | 23 | 200 | 7 | NA | 75 | 1290 | 14 | 1 | 24 | 1 carb, 3 med-fat meat, 4 fat |
| Big Chicken Fillet Sandwich | 1 | 710 | 38 | 350 | 7 | NA | 55 | 1610 | 62 | 5 | 33 | 4 carb, 3 med-fat meat, 5 fat |

| | Serving | Calories | Fat (g) | Cal. from Fat | Sat. Fat (g) | Trans Fat (g) | Chol. (mg) | Sod. (mg) | Carb. (g) | Fiber (g) | Prot. (g) | Servings/Exchanges |
|---|---|---|---|---|---|---|---|---|---|---|---|---|
| Spicy Chicken Sandwich | 1 | 440 | 21 | 180 | 5 | NA | 50 | 1140 | 41 | 3 | 11 | 3 carb, 1 med-fat meat, 3 fat |
| Regular Roast Beef | 1 | 310 | 15 | 130 | 5 | NA | 40 | 860 | 28 | 1 | 17 | 2 carb, 2 med-fat meat, 1 fat |
| Big Roast Beef | 1 | 400 | 21 | 190 | 7 | NA | 60 | 1180 | 28 | 1 | 25 | 2 carb, 3 med-fat meat, 1 fat |
| Hot Ham 'N Cheese | 1 | 280 | 12 | 100 | 4 | NA | 35 | 1090 | 29 | 1 | 18 | 2 carb, 2 med-fat meat |
| Big Hot Ham 'N Cheese | 1 | 460 | 20 | 180 | 8 | NA | 75 | 2040 | 40 | 2 | 36 | 4 carb, 4 med-fat meat, 1 fat |
| Jumbo Hot Dog | 1 | 400 | 26 | 240 | 9 | NA | 55 | 1170 | 25 | 1 | 16 | 2 carb, 2 med-fat meat, 3 fat |
| 3 Piece Chicken Strips | 1 order | 370 | 26 | 230 | 6 | NA | 30 | 620 | 19 | 2 | 14 | 1 carb, 2 med-fat meat, 3 fat |
| 5 Piece Chicken Strips | 1 order | 610 | 43 | 390 | 9 | NA | 50 | 1030 | 32 | 3 | 23 | 2 carb, 2 med-fat meat, 7 fat |

| | | | | | | | | | | | | |
|---|---|---|---|---|---|---|---|---|---|---|---|---|
| ***Fried Chicken & Sides*** | | | | | | | | | | | | |
| Fried Chicken Breast | 1 | 370 | 15 | 130 | 4 | NA | 75 | 1190 | 29 | 0 | 29 | 2 carb, 3 med-fat meat |
| Fried Chicken Leg | 1 | 170 | 7 | 60 | 2 | NA | 45 | 570 | 15 | 0 | 13 | 1 carb, 1 med-fat meat |
| Fried Chicken Thigh | 1 | 330 | 15 | 130 | 4 | NA | 60 | 1000 | 30 | 0 | 19 | 2 carb, 2 med-fat meat, 1 fat |
| Fried Chicken Wing | 1 | 200 | 8 | 70 | 2 | NA | 30 | 740 | 23 | 0 | 10 | 1 1/2 carb, 1 med-fat meat, 1 fat |
| Natural-Cut French Fries, Small | 1 order | 320 | 14 | 130 | 3 | NA | 0 | 710 | 45 | 3 | 4 | 3 carb, 3 fat |
| Natural-Cut French Fries, Medium | 1 order | 430 | 19 | 170 | 4 | NA | 5 | 960 | 60 | 4 | 5 | 4 carb, 4 fat |
| Natural-Cut French Fries, Large | 1 order | 470 | 21 | 190 | 4 | NA | 5 | 1640 | 65 | 5 | 5 | 4 1/2 carb, 4 fat |
| Crispy Curls, Small | 1 order | 340 | 17 | 150 | 4 | NA | 0 | 840 | 43 | 4 | 4 | 3 carb, 3 fat |
| Crispy Curls, Medium | 1 order | 410 | 20 | 180 | 5 | NA | 0 | 1020 | 52 | 4 | 5 | 3 1/2 carb, 4 fat |
| Crispy Curls, Large | 1 order | 480 | 23 | 210 | 6 | NA | 0 | 1190 | 60 | 5 | 6 | 4 carb, 5 fat |
| Coleslaw, Small | 1 order | 170 | 10 | 90 | 2 | NA | 10 | 140 | 20 | 2 | 1 | 1 carb, 2 fat |

| | Serving | Calories | Fat (g) | Cal. from Fat | Sat. Fat (g) | Trans Fat (g) | Chol. (mg) | Sod. (mg) | Carb. (g) | Fiber (g) | Prot. (g) | Servings/Exchanges |
|---|---|---|---|---|---|---|---|---|---|---|---|---|
| Mashed Potatoes, Small | 1 order | 90 | 2 | 15 | 0 | NA | 0 | 410 | 17 | 0 | 1 | 1 carb |
| Side Salad, No Dressing | 1 | 120 | 7 | 70 | 5 | NA | 20 | 160 | 7 | 2 | 7 | 1 carb, 1 med-fat meat |
| **IN-N-OUT BURGER** | | | | | | | | | | | | |
| Hamburger with Onion | 1 | 390 | 19 | 170 | 5 | 0 | 40 | 650 | 39 | 3 | 16 | 2 1/2 carb, 2 med-fat meat, 2 fat |
| Hamburger, Protein Style | 1 | 240 | 17 | 150 | 4 | 0 | 40 | 370 | 11 | 3 | 13 | 2 vegetable, 2 med-fat meat, 1 fat |
| Cheeseburger with Onion | 1 | 480 | 27 | 240 | 10 | 0.5 | 60 | 1000 | 39 | 3 | 22 | 2 1/2 carb, 2 med-fat meat, 3 fat |
| Cheeseburger, Protein Style | 1 | 330 | 25 | 220 | 9 | 0 | 60 | 720 | 11 | 3 | 18 | 2 vegetable, 2 med-fat meat, 3 fat |
| Double-Double with Onion | 1 | 670 | 41 | 370 | 18 | 1 | 120 | 1440 | 39 | 3 | 37 | 2 1/2 carb, 4 med-fat meat, 4 fat |
| Double-Double, Protein Style | 1 | 520 | 39 | 350 | 17 | 1 | 120 | 1160 | 11 | 3 | 33 | 2 vegetable, 4 med-fat meat, 4 fat |

| | | | | | | | | | | | | |
|---|---|---|---|---|---|---|---|---|---|---|---|---|
| French Fries | 1 order | 400 | 18 | 160 | 5 | 0 | 0 | 245 | 54 | 2 | 7 | 3 1/2 carb, 4 fat |
| Chocolate Shake | 15 oz | 690 | 36 | 320 | 24 | 1 | 95 | 350 | 83 | 0 | 9 | 5 1/2 carb, 7 fat |
| Vanilla Shake | 15 oz | 680 | 37 | 330 | 25 | 1 | 90 | 390 | 78 | 0 | 9 | 5 carb, 7 fat |
| Strawberry Shake | 15 oz | 690 | 33 | 300 | 22 | 0.5 | 85 | 280 | 91 | 0 | 9 | 6 carb, 7 fat |
| **JACK IN THE BOX** | | | | | | | | | | | | |
| ***Healthy Dining*** | | | | | | | | | | | | |
| Chicken Fajita Pita | 1 | 320 | 11 | 100 | 5 | 0.5 | 65 | 1110 | 33 | 4 | 24 | 2 carb, 2 med-fat meat |
| Chicken Teriyaki Bowl | 1 | 580 | 5 | 50 | 1 | 0 | 35 | 1460 | 106 | 4 | 26 | 7 carb, 1 med-fat meat |
| Grilled Chicken Strip | 1 order | 180 | 2 | 20 | 0.5 | 0 | 125 | 700 | 3 | 0 | 37 | 5 lean meat |
| Hamburger Delue | 1 | 340 | 18 | 170 | 6 | 1 | 40 | 550 | 31 | 2 | 14 | 2 carb, 1 med-fat meat, 3 fat |
| Steak Teriyaki Bowl | 1 | 650 | 10 | 90 | 3 | 0 | 45 | 1740 | 106 | 4 | 30 | 7 carb, 1 med-fat meat, 1 fat |
| ***Burgers*** | | | | | | | | | | | | |
| Big Cheeseburger | 1 | 650 | 40 | 360 | 15 | 1.5 | 70 | 1170 | 50 | 2 | 24 | 3 carb, 2 med-fat meat, 6 fat |

FAST FOOD

| | Serving | Calories | Fat (g) | Cal. from Fat | Sat. Fat (g) | Trans Fat (g) | Chol. (mg) | Sod. (mg) | Carb. (g) | Fiber (g) | Prot. (g) | Servings/Exchanges |
|---|---|---|---|---|---|---|---|---|---|---|---|---|
| Bacon Ultimate Cheeseburger | 1 | 980 | 67 | 600 | 27 | 3 | 135 | 1880 | 52 | 2 | 43 | 3 1/2 carb, 5 med-fat meat, 8 fat |
| Hamburger | 1 | 280 | 12 | 100 | 4.5 | 0.5 | 30 | 540 | 29 | 5 | 14 | 2 carb, 1 med-fat meat, 1 fat |
| Hamburger with Cheese | 1 | 320 | 15 | 140 | 7 | 1 | 45 | 730 | 30 | 5 | 16 | 2 carb, 1 med-fat meat, 3 fat |
| Hamburger Deluxe | 1 | 362 | 18 | 171 | 5 | 1 | 38 | 579 | 33 | 1 | 14 | 2 carb, 1 med-fat meat, 3 fat |
| Hamburger Deluxe with Cheese | 1 | 430 | 25 | 230 | 10 | 1 | 65 | 920 | 33 | 7 | 19 | 2 carb, 2 med-fat meat, 3 fat |
| Jumbo Jack | 1 | 580 | 33 | 300 | 11 | 1 | 50 | 920 | 51 | 10 | 20 | 3 1/2 carb, 1 med-fat meat, 6 fat |
| Junior Bacon Cheeseburger | 1 | 400 | 23 | 210 | 8 | 1 | 55 | 800 | 30 | 1 | 18 | 2 carb, 2 med-fat meat, 3 fat |

| | | | | | | | | | | | | |
|---|---|---|---|---|---|---|---|---|---|---|---|---|
| Sourdough Jack | 1 | 680 | 46 | 410 | 17 | 1.5 | 75 | 1200 | 41 | 6 | 26 | 2 1/2 carb, 3 med-fat meat, 6 fat |
| Ultimate Cheeseburger | 1 | 920 | 63 | 560 | 26 | 2.5 | 120 | 1530 | 52 | 11 | 38 | 3 1/2 carb, 4 med-fat meat, 9 fat |
| Sirloin Cheeseburger | 1 | 950 | 60 | 540 | 19 | 2 | 145 | 1920 | 61 | 4 | 41 | 4 carb, 4 med-fat meat, 8 fat |
| ***Chicken & Fish*** | | | | | | | | | | | | |
| Chicken Breast Strips | 4 | 500 | 25 | 220 | 6 | 6 | 80 | 1260 | 36 | 3 | 35 | 2 1/2 carb, 4 med-fat meat, 1 fat |
| Chicken Fajita Pita | 1 | 326 | 10 | 95 | 6 | 0 | 64 | 987 | 35 | 3 | 23 | 2 carb, 2 med-fat meat |
| Chicken Sandwich | 1 | 400 | 21 | 190 | 4.5 | 2.5 | 35 | 740 | 38 | 2 | 15 | 2 1/2 carb, 1 med-fat meat, 3 fat |
| Jack's Spicy Chicken | 1 | 550 | 24 | 220 | 5 | 3 | 50 | 1050 | 59 | 8 | 24 | 4 carb, 2 med-fat meat, 3 fat |
| Sourdough Grilled Chicken Club | 1 | 530 | 28 | 250 | 7 | 2 | 90 | 1440 | 34 | 3 | 36 | 2 carb, 4 med-fat meat, 2 fat |

| | Serving | Calories | Fat (g) | Cal. from Fat | Sat. Fat (g) | Trans Fat (g) | Chol. (mg) | Sod. (mg) | Carb. (g) | Fiber (g) | Prot. (g) | Servings/Exchanges |
|---|---|---|---|---|---|---|---|---|---|---|---|---|
| Fish & Chips | Small order | 630 | 35 | 310 | 8 | 10 | 40 | 1290 | 61 | 5 | 19 | 4 carb, 1 med-fat meat, 6 fat |
| ***Snacks & Sides*** | | | | | | | | | | | | |
| Bacon Cheddar Potato Wedges | 1 order | 760 | 52 | 470 | 16 | 13 | 45 | 960 | 53 | 4 | 21 | 3 1/2 carb, 2 med-fat meat, 8 fat |
| Egg Roll | 1 | 130 | 6 | 60 | 2 | 1 | 5 | 310 | 15 | 1 | 5 | 1 carb, 1 fat |
| French Fries, Small | 1 | 290 | 15 | 140 | 3.5 | 4.5 | 0 | 540 | 35 | 1 | 4 | 2 carb, 3 fat |
| French Fries, Medium | 1 | 460 | 24 | 210 | 6 | 7 | 0 | 850 | 55 | 1 | 6 | 3 1/2 carb, 5 fat |
| French Fries, Large | 1 | 620 | 32 | 290 | 7 | 9 | 0 | 1150 | 75 | 8 | 9 | 5 carb, 6 fat |
| Mozzarella Cheese Sticks | 3 | 240 | 14 | 120 | 6 | 2 | 25 | 510 | 20 | 1 | 10 | 1 1/2 carb, 1 med-fat meat, 2 fat |
| Onion Rings | 8 | 500 | 30 | 270 | 6 | 10 | 0 | 420 | 51 | 3 | 6 | 3 1/2 carb, 6 fat |
| Seasoned Curly Fries, Small | 1 | 280 | 15 | 140 | 3 | 5 | 0 | 600 | 30 | 3 | 4 | 2 carb, 3 fat |

| | | | | | | | | | | | | |
|---|---|---|---|---|---|---|---|---|---|---|---|---|
| Seasoned Curly Fries, Medium | 1 | 420 | 24 | 210 | 5 | 7 | 0 | 920 | 46 | 5 | 6 | 3 carb, 5 fat |
| Seasoned Curly Fries, Large | 1 | 570 | 32 | 290 | 7 | 10 | 0 | 1260 | 63 | 7 | 8 | 4 carb, 6 fat |
| Stuffed Jalapeños | 3 | 230 | 13 | 110 | 6 | 2 | 20 | 690 | 22 | 2 | 7 | 1 1/2 carb, 3 fat |
| Jack's Ultimate Salads | | | | | | | | | | | | |
| Asian Chicken Salad with Grilled Chicken | 1 | 180 | 1.5 | 15 | 0 | 0 | 65 | 380 | 22 | 6 | 22 | 1 1/2 carb, 3 lean meat |
| Chicken Club Salad with Grilled Chicken | 1 | 320 | 16 | 140 | 7 | 0 | 100 | 780 | 12 | 4 | 34 | 1 carb, 4 lean meat |
| Side Salad | 1 | 50 | 3 | 25 | 1.5 | 0 | 10 | 60 | 5 | 2 | 3 | 1 vegetable, 1 fat |
| Southwest Chicken Salad | 1 | 310 | 12 | 110 | 5 | 0 | 90 | 820 | 28 | 7 | 31 | 2 carb, 4 lean meat |
| ***Breakfast*** | | | | | | | | | | | | |
| Bacon, Egg, & Cheese Biscuit | 1 | 440 | 26 | 230 | 11 | 1 | 220 | 1030 | 37 | 2 | 16 | 2 1/2 carb, 1 med-fat meat, 4 fat |
| Breakfast Jack | 1 | 290 | 12 | 110 | 4.5 | 0 | 220 | 760 | 29 | 1 | 17 | 2 carb, 2 med-fat meat |

| | Serving | Calories | Fat (g) | Cal. from Fat | Sat. Fat (g) | Trans Fat (g) | Chol. (mg) | Sod. (mg) | Carb. (g) | Fiber (g) | Prot. (g) | Servings/Exchanges |
|---|---|---|---|---|---|---|---|---|---|---|---|---|
| Extreme Sausage Sandwich | 1 | 670 | 48 | 430 | 17 | 1.5 | 290 | 1300 | 31 | 2 | 29 | 2 carb, 3 med-fat meat, 7 fat |
| Sausage Breakfast Jack | 1 | 450 | 28 | 250 | 10 | 1 | 245 | 840 | 29 | 1 | 20 | 2 carb, 2 med-fat meat, 4 fat |
| Sausage Croissant | 1 | 580 | 39 | 350 | 13 | 4 | 255 | 770 | 37 | 2 | 21 | 2 1/2 carb, 2 med-fat meat, 6 fat |
| Sausage, Egg & Cheese Biscuit | 1 | 590 | 40 | 360 | 16 | 1.5 | 245 | 1140 | 38 | 2 | 20 | 2 1/2 carb, 1 med-fat meat, 7 fat |
| Sourdough Breakfast Sandwich | 1 | 420 | 24 | 220 | 8 | 2 | 230 | 980 | 31 | 2 | 20 | 2 carb, 2 med-fat meat, 3 fat |
| Supreme Croissant | 1 | 450 | 25 | 230 | 9 | 3.5 | 235 | 860 | 36 | 1 | 20 | 2 1/2 carb, 2 med-fat meat, 3 fat |
| Ultimate Breakfast Sandwich | 1 | 570 | 27 | 240 | 10 | 1 | 445 | 1700 | 49 | 2 | 34 | 3 carb, 4 med-fat meat, 1 fat |

| KFC | | | | | | | | | | | | |
|---|---|---|---|---|---|---|---|---|---|---|---|---|
| ***Salads*** | | | | | | | | | | | | |
| Crispy BLT Salad, with Chicken | 1 | 340 | 19 | 170 | 5 | 0 | 70 | 840 | 14 | 3 | 30 | 1 carb, 4 med-fat meat |
| Crispy Caesar Salad, with Chicken | 1 | 320 | 19 | 170 | 6 | 0 | 65 | 660 | 12 | 3 | 28 | 1 carb, 4 med-fat meat |
| House Side Salad | 1 | 15 | 0 | 0 | 0 | 0 | 0 | 10 | 10 | 2 | 1 | free |
| Roasted Caesar Salad | 1 | 190 | 6 | 50 | 3 | 0 | 75 | 530 | 5 | 2 | 29 | 1 vegetable, 4 lean meat |
| Roasted Chicken BLT Salad | 1 | 200 | 7 | 60 | 2 | 0 | 80 | 720 | 7 | 3 | 30 | 1/2 carb, 4 lean meat |
| ***Sandwiches & Wraps*** | | | | | | | | | | | | |
| Crispy Twister with Crispy Strip | 1 | 580 | 30 | 270 | 7 | 0 | 60 | 1250 | 49 | 3 | 28 | 3 carb, 3 med-fat meat, 3 fat |
| Crispy Twister with Original Strip | 1 | 540 | 26 | 230 | 7 | 0 | 65 | 1430 | 48 | 4 | 29 | 3 carb, 3 med-fat meat, 2 fat |

| | Serving | Calories | Fat (g) | Cal. from Fat | Sat. Fat (g) | Trans Fat (g) | Chol. (mg) | Sod. (mg) | Carb. (g) | Fiber (g) | Prot. (g) | Servings/Exchanges |
|---|---|---|---|---|---|---|---|---|---|---|---|---|
| Double Crunch, Original Strip | 1 | 470 | 23 | 200 | 6 | 0 | 65 | 1020 | 35 | 2 | 27 | 2 carb, 3 med-fat meat, 2 fat |
| Honey BBQ Sandwich | 1 | 310 | 4 | 35 | 1 | 0 | 70 | 810 | 42 | 1 | 23 | 3 carb, 2 lean meat |
| KFC Snacker with Crispy Strip | 1 | 300 | 14 | 120 | 3 | 0 | 30 | 470 | 28 | 2 | 15 | 2 carb, 2 med-fat meat, 1 fat |
| KFC Snacker with Original Strip | 1 | 270 | 12 | 100 | 3 | 0 | 30 | 560 | 28 | 2 | 15 | 2 carb, 1 med-fat meat, 1 fat |
| KFC Snacker, Fish | 1 | 320 | 14 | 130 | 3 | 0 | 60 | 640 | 31 | 2 | 16 | 2 carb, 1 med-fat meat, 2 fat |
| KFC Snacker, Honey BBQ | 1 | 210 | 3 | 30 | 1 | 0 | 35 | 470 | 32 | 2 | 13 | 2 carb, 1 med-fat meat |
| Oven Roast Filet Sandwich | 1 | 480 | 23 | 210 | 4 | 0 | 85 | 1230 | 38 | 2 | 25 | 2 1/2 carb, 3 med-fat meat, 2 fat |
| Tender Roast | 1 | 440 | 18 | 160 | 4 | 0 | 70 | 1120 | 42 | 2 | 29 | 3 carb, 3 med-fat meat, 1 fat |

| | | | | | | | | | | | | |
|---|---|---|---|---|---|---|---|---|---|---|---|---|
| Tender Roast Sandwich | 1 | 400 | 15 | 130 | 3 | 0 | 90 | 810 | 29 | 1 | 34 | 2 carb, 4 lean meat |
| Toasted Wrap with Crispy Strip | 1 | 360 | 20 | 180 | 6 | 0 | 40 | 730 | 27 | 2 | 17 | 2 carb, 2 med-fat meat, 2 fat |
| Toasted Wrap with Tender Roast Filet | 1 | 310 | 14 | 130 | 5 | 0 | 60 | 740 | 24 | 1 | 22 | 1 1/2 carb, 2 med-fat meat, 1 fat |
| ***Chicken*** | | | | | | | | | | | | |
| Original Chicken, Breast | 1 | 370 | 21 | 190 | 5 | 0 | 120 | 1050 | 7 | 0 | 38 | 1/2 carb, 5 lean meat |
| Original Chicken, Breast without Skin or Breading | 1 | 140 | 2 | 20 | 0 | 0 | 65 | 510 | 1 | 0 | 29 | 4 lean meat |
| Original Chicken, Drumstick | 1 | 110 | 7 | 60 | 1.5 | 0 | 55 | 290 | 2 | 0 | 10 | 1 med-fat meat |
| Original Chicken, Thigh | 1 | 260 | 19 | 170 | 5 | 0 | 85 | 670 | 6 | 0 | 16 | 1/2 carb, 3 med-fat meat, 2 fat |
| Original Chicken, Whole Wing | 1 | 110 | 7 | 60 | 1.5 | 0 | 45 | 310 | 3 | 0 | 9 | 1 med-fat meat |

| | Serving | Calories | Fat (g) | Cal. from Fat | Sat. Fat (g) | Trans Fat (g) | Chol. (mg) | Sod. (mg) | Carb. (g) | Fiber (g) | Prot. (g) | Servings/Exchanges |
|---|---|---|---|---|---|---|---|---|---|---|---|---|
| Extra Crispy Chicken, Breast | 1 | 490 | 31 | 280 | 7 | 0 | 120 | 1080 | 17 | 0 | 38 | 1 carb, 5 med-fat meat, 1 fat |
| Extra Crispy Chicken, Drumstick | 1 | 150 | 9 | 80 | 2 | 0 | 50 | 360 | 6 | 0 | 11 | 1/2 carb, 1 med-fat meat, 1 fat |
| Extra Crispy Chicken, Thigh | 1 | 370 | 27 | 250 | 6 | 0 | 85 | 840 | 12 | 0 | 18 | 1 carb, 2 med-fat meat, 3 fat |
| Extra Crispy Chicken, Whole Wing | 1 | 150 | 10 | 90 | 2 | 0 | 50 | 320 | 6 | 1 | 11 | 1/2 carb, 1 med-fat meat, 1 fat |
| Grilled Chicken, Breast | 1 | 180 | 4 | 35 | 1 | 0 | 110 | 440 | 0 | 0 | 35 | 5 lean meat |
| Grilled Chicken, Drumstick | 1 | 70 | 4 | 35 | 1 | 0 | 50 | 200 | 0 | 0 | 10 | 1 med-fat meat |
| Grilled Chicken, Thigh | 1 | 140 | 9 | 80 | 2.5 | 0 | 80 | 320 | 0 | 0 | 15 | 2 med-fat meat |
| Grilled Chicken, Wing | 1 | 80 | 4 | 40 | 1 | 0 | 50 | 160 | 0 | 0 | 10 | 1 med-fat meat |
| Strips, Crispy strips | 3 | 380 | 22 | 200 | 6 | 0 | 80 | 720 | 12 | 1 | 33 | 1 carb, 4 med-fat meat |
| Original Strips | 3 | 310 | 15 | 140 | 5 | 0 | 80 | 990 | 11 | 2 | 32 | 1 carb, 4 lean meat |

| | | | | | | | | | | | | |
|---|---|---|---|---|---|---|---|---|---|---|---|---|
| ***Popcorn Chicken*** | | | | | | | | | | | | |
| Individual | 1 order | 400 | 26 | 230 | 4.5 | 0 | 60 | 1160 | 22 | 3 | 21 | 1 1/2 carb, 3 med-fat meat, 2 fat |
| Large | 1 order | 550 | 35 | 320 | 6 | 0 | 80 | 1600 | 30 | 3 | 29 | 2 carb, 3 med-fat meat, 4 fat |
| ***Pot Pie & Bowls*** | | | | | | | | | | | | |
| Chicken Pot Pie | 1 | 690 | 40 | 360 | 31 | 0 | 95 | 1760 | 57 | 3 | 27 | 4 carb, 2 med-fat meat, 6 fat |
| KFC Famous Bowls, Rice | 1 | 790 | 28 | 250 | 7 | 1 | 55 | 2690 | 106 | 5 | 29 | 7 carb, 1 med-fat meat, 5 fat |
| KFC Famous Bowls, Mashed Potato | 1 | 700 | 32 | 290 | 8 | 1 | 55 | 2260 | 77 | 6 | 26 | 5 carb, 2 med-fat meat, 4 fat |
| ***Wings*** | | | | | | | | | | | | |
| Honey BBQ Wings | 1 | 80 | 5 | 45 | 1 | 0 | 20 | 170 | 5 | 1 | 4 | 1 med-fat meat |
| Honey BBQ Wings, Boneless | 1 | 80 | 3.5 | 35 | 0.5 | 0 | 10 | 340 | 7 | 1 | 5 | 1/2 carb, 1 med-fat meat |
| Hot Wings | 1 | 70 | 5 | 45 | 1 | 0 | 20 | 150 | 3 | 0 | 4 | 1 med-fat meat |

| | Serving | Calories | Fat (g) | Cal. from Fat | Sat. Fat (g) | Trans Fat (g) | Chol. (mg) | Sod. (mg) | Carb. (g) | Fiber (g) | Prot. (g) | Servings/Exchanges |
|---|---|---|---|---|---|---|---|---|---|---|---|---|
| ***Sides (Individual)*** | | | | | | | | | | | | |
| Baked Beans | 1 | 200 | 1.5 | 10 | 0 | 0 | 0 | 680 | 39 | 9 | 8 | 2 1/2 carb |
| Biscuit | 1 | 180 | 8 | 70 | 6 | 0 | 0 | 530 | 23 | 1 | 4 | 1 1/2 carb, 2 fat |
| Coleslaw | 1 | 180 | 10 | 90 | 1.5 | 0 | 5 | 270 | 22 | 3 | 1 | 1 1/2 carb, 2 fat |
| Corn on the Cob | 3 inches | 70 | 1.5 | 5 | 0.5 | 0 | 0 | 0 | 16 | 2 | 2 | 1 carb |
| Green Beans | 1 | 25 | 0 | 0 | 0 | 0 | 0 | 380 | 5 | 2 | 1 | 1 vegetable |
| KFC Red Beans with Sausage & Rice | 1 | 160 | 2.5 | 25 | 0.5 | 0 | 5 | 340 | 26 | 4 | 24 | 2 carb, 3 lean meat |
| Macaroni & Cheese | 1 | 180 | 9 | 80 | 3 | 0 | 5 | 880 | 20 | 2 | 6 | 1 carb, 1 med-fat meat, 2 fat |
| Macaroni Salad | 1 | 180 | 9 | 80 | 2 | 0 | 5 | 400 | 20 | 1 | 3 | 1 carb, 2 fat |
| Mashed Potatoes with Gravy | 1 | 130 | 4.5 | 40 | 1 | 0 | 0 | 550 | 20 | 1 | 2 | 1 carb, 1 fat |
| Mashed Potatoes without Gravy | 1 | 100 | 3 | 25 | 0.5 | 0 | 0 | 350 | 16 | 1 | 2 | 1 carb, 1 fat |

| | | | | | | | | | | | | |
|---|---|---|---|---|---|---|---|---|---|---|---|---|
| Potato Salad | 1 | 200 | 10 | 90 | 2 | 0 | 5 | 540 | 24 | 3 | 2 | 1 1/2 carb, 2 fat |
| Potato Wedges | 1 | 260 | 13 | 110 | 2.5 | 0 | 0 | 740 | 33 | 3 | 4 | 2 carb, 3 fat |
| Seasoned Rice | 1 | 140 | 0.5 | 5 | 0 | 0 | 0 | 560 | 31 | 1 | 3 | 2 carb |
| **KRISPY KREME DONUTS** | | | | | | | | | | | | |
| Apple Fritter | 1 | 380 | 20 | 180 | 10 | 0 | 5 | 220 | 47 | 2 | 4 | 3 carb, 4 fat |
| Caramel Kreme Crunch | 1 | 381 | 19 | 170 | 9 | 0 | 10 | 170 | 49 | <1 | 4 | 3 carb, 4 fat |
| Chocolate Iced Custard Filled | 1 | 300 | 17 | 150 | 8 | 0 | 5 | 150 | 35 | <1 | 3 | 2 carb, 3 fat |
| Chocolate Iced Glazed | 1 | 250 | 12 | 110 | 6 | 0 | 5 | 100 | 33 | <1 | 3 | 2 carb, 2 fat |
| Chocolate Iced Kreme Filled | 1 | 350 | 20 | 180 | 11 | 0 | 5 | 140 | 38 | <1 | 3 | 2 1/2 carb, 4 fat |
| Cinnamon Bun | 1 | 260 | 16 | 140 | 8 | 0 | 5 | 125 | 28 | <1 | 3 | 2 carb, 3 fat |
| Cinnamon Twist | 1 | 240 | 15 | 140 | 7 | 0 | 5 | 130 | 25 | <1 | 3 | 1 1/2 carb, 3 fat |
| Glazed Chocolate Cake | 1 | 300 | 15 | 130 | 7 | 0 | 20 | 250 | 42 | 2 | 3 | 3 carb, 3 fat |
| Glazed Cinnamon | 1 | 210 | 12 | 110 | 6 | 0 | 5 | 100 | 24 | <1 | 2 | 1 1/2 carb, 2 fat |
| Glazed Kreme Filled | 1 | 340 | 20 | 180 | 10 | 0 | 5 | 140 | 39 | <1 | 3 | 2 1/2 carb, 4 fat |

| | Serving | Calories | Fat (g) | Cal. from Fat | Sat. Fat (g) | Trans Fat (g) | Chol. (mg) | Sod. (mg) | Carb. (g) | Fiber (g) | Prot. (g) | Servings/Exchanges |
|---|---|---|---|---|---|---|---|---|---|---|---|---|
| Glazed Lemon Filled | 1 | 290 | 16 | 140 | 8 | 0 | 5 | 135 | 35 | <1 | 3 | 2 carb, 3 fat |
| Original Glazed | 1 | 200 | 12 | 100 | 6 | 0 | 5 | 95 | 22 | <1 | 2 | 1 1/2 carb, 2 fat |
| Powdered Cake | 1 | 290 | 14 | 130 | 6 | 0 | 20 | 320 | 37 | <1 | 3 | 2 1/2 carb, 3 fat |
| **LONG JOHN SILVER'S** | | | | | | | | | | | | |
| ***Fish & Seafood*** | | | | | | | | | | | | |
| Battered Fish | 1 piece | 260 | 16 | 140 | 4 | 4.5 | 35 | 790 | 17 | 0 | 12 | 1 carb, 1 med-fat meat, 2 fat |
| Baked Cod | 1 piece | 120 | 4.5 | 120 | 1 | 0 | 90 | 240 | 1 | 0 | 22 | 3 lean meat |
| Battered Shrimp | 3 pieces | 130 | 9 | 80 | 2.5 | 2.5 | 45 | 480 | 8 | 0 | 5 | 1/2 carb, 2 fat |
| Alaskan Flounder | 1 piece | 250 | 11 | 100 | 2.5 | 3 | 35 | 910 | 26 | 2 | 12 | 2 carb, 1 med-fat meat, 1 fat |
| Buttered Lobster Bites | 1 snack box | 230 | 9 | 80 | 3 | 3 | 60 | 520 | 24 | 2 | 13 | 1 1/2 carb, 2 med-fat meat |
| Grilled Pacific Salmon | 2 filets | 150 | 5 | 45 | 1 | 0 | 50 | 440 | 2 | 0 | 24 | 3 lean meat |

| | | | | | | | | | | | | |
|---|---|---|---|---|---|---|---|---|---|---|---|---|
| Grilled Tilapia | 1 filet | 110 | 2.5 | 20 | 1 | 0 | 55 | 250 | 1 | 0 | 22 | 3 lean meat |
| Shrimp Scampi | 8 pieces | 110 | 5 | 45 | 1 | 0.5 | 150 | 610 | 1 | 0 | 16 | 2 lean meat |
| Lobster Stuffed Crab Cake | 1 cake | 170 | 9 | 80 | 2 | 0 | 30 | 390 | 16 | 1 | 6 | 1 carb, 1 med-fat meat, 1 fat |
| Breaded Clam Strips | 1 snack box | 320 | 19 | 170 | 4.5 | 7 | 35 | 1190 | 29 | 2 | 9 | 2 carb, 1 med-fat meat, 3 fat |
| ***Chicken*** | | | | | | | | | | | | |
| Chicken Plank | 1 piece | 140 | 8 | 70 | 2 | 2.5 | 20 | 480 | 9 | 0 | 8 | 1/2 carb, 1 med-fat meat, 1 fat |
| Sandwiches | | | | | | | | | | | | |
| Fish Sandwich | 1 | 470 | 23 | 210 | 5 | 4.5 | 45 | 1210 | 48 | 3 | 18 | 3 carb, 1 med-fat meat, 4 fat |
| Ultimate Fish Sandwich | 1 | 530 | 28 | 250 | 8 | 5 | 60 | 1400 | 49 | 3 | 21 | 3 carb, 2 med-fat meat, 4 fat |
| Chicken Sandwich | 1 | 360 | 15 | 140 | 3.5 | 2.5 | 25 | 900 | 40 | 3 | 14 | 2 1/2 carb, 1 med-fat meat, 2 fat |

| | Serving | Calories | Fat (g) | Cal. from Fat | Sat. Fat (g) | Trans Fat (g) | Chol. (mg) | Sod. (mg) | Carb. (g) | Fiber (g) | Prot. (g) | Servings/Exchanges |
|---|---|---|---|---|---|---|---|---|---|---|---|---|
| Baja Fish Taco | 1 taco | 350 | 22 | 200 | 5 | 3.5 | 20 | 840 | 29 | 1 | 9 | 2 carb, 1 med-fat meat, 3 fat |
| Freshside Grille Smart Choice, Salmon | 1 plate | 280 | 7 | 60 | 2 | 0 | 50 | 1010 | 27 | 3 | 27 | 2 carb, 3 lean meat |
| Freshside Grille Smart Choice, Scampi | 1 plate | 250 | 7 | 60 | 2 | 0.5 | 155 | 1180 | 27 | 3 | 19 | 2 carb, 1 lean meat |
| Freshside Grille Smart Choice, Tilapia | 1 plate | 250 | 4.5 | 40 | 2 | 0 | 60 | 820 | 27 | 3 | 25 | 2 carb, 3 lean meat |
| Salmon Bowl with Sauce | 1 bowl | 460 | 8 | 70 | 2.5 | 0 | 50 | 1660 | 65 | 4 | 30 | 4 1/2 carb, 2 med-fat meat |
| Shrimp Bowl with Sauce | 1 bowl | 380 | 4.5 | 40 | 1.5 | 0 | 145 | 1580 | 64 | 4 | 21 | 4 carb, 1 med-fat meat |
| ***Sauces*** | | | | | | | | | | | | |
| Cocktail Sauce | 1 oz | 25 | 0 | 0 | 0 | 0 | 0 | 250 | 6 | 0 | 0 | 1/2 carb |

| | | | | | | | | | | | | |
|---|---|---|---|---|---|---|---|---|---|---|---|---|
| Tartar Sauce | 1 oz | 100 | 9 | 80 | 1.5 | 0 | 15 | 250 | 4 | 0 | 0 | 2 fat |
| ***Sides*** | | | | | | | | | | | | |
| Breadsticks | 1 | 170 | 3.5 | 30 | 1 | 1 | 0 | 290 | 29 | 1 | 6 | 2 carb, 1 fat |
| Broccoli Cheese Soup | 1 bowl | 220 | 18 | 160 | 8 | 0 | 30 | 650 | 8 | 1 | 5 | 1/2 carb, 1 med-fat meat, 3 fat |
| Coleslaw | 4 oz | 200 | 15 | 130 | 2.5 | 0 | 20 | 340 | 15 | 3 | 1 | 1 carb, 3 fat |
| Corn Cobbette with Butter Oil | 1 | 150 | 10 | 90 | 2 | 0 | 0 | 30 | 14 | 3 | 3 | 1 carb, 2 fat |
| Crumblies | 1 oz | 170 | 12 | 110 | 2.5 | 4 | 0 | 410 | 14 | 1 | 1 | 1 carb, 2 fat |
| Fries, Basket Combo Portion | 4 oz | 310 | 14 | 120 | 3.5 | 3.5 | 0 | 460 | 45 | 4 | 3 | 3 carb, 3 fat |
| Fries, Platter Portion | 3 oz | 230 | 10 | 90 | 2.5 | 3 | 0 | 350 | 34 | 3 | 3 | 2 carb, 2 fat |
| Hushpuppy | 1 | 60 | 2.5 | 20 | 0.5 | 1 | 0 | 200 | 9 | 1 | 1 | 1/2 carb, 1 fat |
| Rice | 5 oz | 180 | 1 | 10 | 0.5 | 0 | 0 | 470 | 37 | 2 | 4 | 2 1/2 carb |
| ***Desserts*** | | | | | | | | | | | | |
| Chocolate Cream Pie | 1 slice | 310 | 22 | 200 | 14 | 2 | 15 | 170 | 24 | 1 | 5 | 1 1/2 carb, 4 fat |

| | Serving | Calories | Fat (g) | Cal. from Fat | Sat. Fat (g) | Trans Fat (g) | Chol. (mg) | Sod. (mg) | Carb. (g) | Fiber (g) | Prot. (g) | Servings/Exchanges |
|---|---|---|---|---|---|---|---|---|---|---|---|---|
| Pecan Pie | 1 slice | 370 | 15 | 140 | 3 | 2 | 40 | 190 | 55 | 2 | 4 | 3 1/2 carb, 3 fat |
| Pineapple Cream Pie | 1 slice | 290 | 13 | 110 | 7 | 2 | 15 | 210 | 39 | 1 | 4 | 2 1/2 carb, 3 fat |
| **McDONALD'S** | | | | | | | | | | | | |
| ***Sandwiches*** | | | | | | | | | | | | |
| Hamburger | 1 | 250 | 9 | 80 | 3.5 | 0.5 | 25 | 520 | 31 | 2 | 12 | 2 carb, 1 med-fat meat, 1 fat |
| Cheeseburger | 1 | 300 | 12 | 110 | 6 | 0.5 | 40 | 750 | 33 | 2 | 15 | 2 carb, 1 med-fat meat, 1 fat |
| McDouble | 1 | 390 | 19 | 170 | 8 | 1 | 65 | 920 | 33 | 2 | 22 | 2 carb, 2 med-fat meat, 2 fat |
| Double Cheeseburger | 1 | 440 | 23 | 210 | 11 | 1.5 | 80 | 1150 | 34 | 2 | 25 | 2 carb, 3 med-fat meat, 2 fat |
| Quarter Pounder | 1 | 410 | 19 | 170 | 7 | 1 | 65 | 730 | 37 | 2 | 24 | 2 1/2 carb, 2 med-fat meat, 2 fat |

| | | | | | | | | | | | | |
|---|---|---|---|---|---|---|---|---|---|---|---|---|
| Quarter Pounder with Cheese | 1 | 510 | 26 | 230 | 12 | 1.5 | 90 | 1190 | 40 | 3 | 29 | 2 1/2 carb, 3 med-fat meat, 2 fat |
| Double Quarter Pounder with Cheese | 1 | 740 | 42 | 380 | 19 | 2.5 | 155 | 1380 | 40 | 3 | 48 | 2 1/2 carb, 6 med-fat meat, 2 fat |
| Big Mac | 1 | 540 | 29 | 260 | 10 | 1.5 | 75 | 1040 | 45 | 3 | 25 | 3 carb, 2 med-fat meat, 4 fat |
| Big N' Tasty | 1 | 460 | 24 | 220 | 8 | 1.5 | 70 | 720 | 37 | 3 | 24 | 2 1/2 carb, 2 med-fat meat, 3 fat |
| Angus Bacon & Cheese | 1 | 790 | 39 | 350 | 17 | 2 | 145 | 2070 | 63 | 4 | 45 | 4 carb, 5 med-fat meat, 3 fat |
| Angus Deluxe | 1 | 750 | 39 | 350 | 16 | 2 | 135 | 1700 | 61 | 4 | 40 | 4 carb, 5 med-fat meat, 3 fat |
| Angus Mushroom & Swiss | 1 | 770 | 40 | 360 | 17 | 2 | 135 | 1170 | 59 | 4 | 44 | 4 carb, 5 med-fat meat, 3 fat |
| Filet-O-Fish | 1 | 380 | 18 | 170 | 3.5 | 0 | 40 | 640 | 38 | 2 | 15 | 2 1/2 carb, 1 med-fat meat, 3 fat |

| | Serving | Calories | Fat (g) | Cal. from Fat | Sat. Fat (g) | Trans Fat (g) | Chol. (mg) | Sod. (mg) | Carb. (g) | Fiber (g) | Prot. (g) | Servings/Exchanges |
|---|---|---|---|---|---|---|---|---|---|---|---|---|
| McRib | 1 | 500 | 26 | 240 | 10 | 0 | 70 | 980 | 44 | 3 | 22 | 3 carb, 2 med-fat meat, 3 fat |
| McChicken | 1 | 360 | 16 | 150 | 3 | 0 | 35 | 830 | 40 | 2 | 15 | 2 1/2 carb, 1 med-fat meat, 2 fat |
| Premium Grilled Chicken Classic | 1 | 420 | 10 | 90 | 2 | 0 | 70 | 1190 | 51 | 3 | 32 | 3 1/2 carb, 3 lean meat |
| Premium Crispy Chicken Classic | 1 | 530 | 20 | 180 | 3.5 | 0 | 50 | 1150 | 59 | 3 | 28 | 4 carb, 2 med-fat meat, 2 fat |
| Premium Grilled Chicken Club | 1 | 530 | 17 | 160 | 6 | 0 | 95 | 1410 | 52 | 4 | 39 | 3 1/2 carb, 4 lean meat |
| Premium Crispy Chicken Club | 1 | 630 | 28 | 250 | 7 | 0 | 75 | 1360 | 60 | 4 | 35 | 4 carb, 2 med-fat meat, 4 fat |
| Premium Grilled Chicken Ranch BLT | 1 | 470 | 12 | 110 | 3 | 0 | 80 | 1440 | 54 | 3 | 36 | 3 1/2 carb, 4 lean meat |

| | | | | | | | | | | | | |
|---|---|---|---|---|---|---|---|---|---|---|---|---|
| Premium Crispy Chicken Ranch BLT | 1 | 580 | 23 | 200 | 4.5 | 0 | 65 | 1400 | 62 | 3 | 31 | 4 carb, 3 med-fat meat, 2 fat |
| Southern Style Crispy Chicken | 1 | 400 | 17 | 150 | 3 | 0 | 45 | 1030 | 39 | 1 | 24 | 2 1/2 carb, 2 med-fat meat, 1 fat |
| Honey Mustard Snack Wrap, Grilled | 1 | 260 | 9 | 80 | 3.5 | 0 | 45 | 800 | 27 | 1 | 18 | 2 carb, 2 med-fat meat |
| Honey Mustard Snack Wrap, Crispy | 1 | 330 | 16 | 140 | 4.5 | 0 | 30 | 780 | 34 | 1 | 14 | 2 carb, 1 med-fat meat, 2 fat |
| Ranch Snack Wrap, Grilled | 1 | 270 | 10 | 90 | 4 | 0 | 45 | 830 | 26 | 1 | 18 | 2 carb, 2 med-fat meat |
| Ranch Snack Wrap, Crispy | 1 | 340 | 17 | 150 | 4.5 | 0 | 30 | 810 | 33 | 1 | 14 | 2 carb, 1 med-fat meat, 2 fat |
| ***French Fries*** | | | | | | | | | | | | |
| French Fries, Small | 1 | 230 | 11 | 100 | 1.5 | 0 | 0 | 160 | 29 | 3 | 3 | 2 carb, 2 fat |
| French Fries, Medium | 1 | 380 | 19 | 170 | 2.5 | 0 | 0 | 270 | 48 | 5 | 4 | 3 carb, 4 fat |
| French Fries, Large | 1 | 500 | 25 | 220 | 3.5 | 0 | 0 | 350 | 63 | 6 | 6 | 4 carb, 5 fat |

| | Serving | Calories | Fat (g) | Cal. from Fat | Sat. Fat (g) | Trans Fat (g) | Chol. (mg) | Sod. (mg) | Carb. (g) | Fiber (g) | Prot. (g) | Servings/Exchanges |
|---|---|---|---|---|---|---|---|---|---|---|---|---|
| ***Chicken McNuggets, Chicken Strips, Sauces*** | | | | | | | | | | | | |
| Chicken McNuggets | 4 pieces | 190 | 12 | 100 | 2 | 0 | 30 | 400 | 11 | 0 | 10 | 1 carb, 1 med-fat meat, 1 fat |
| Chicken McNuggets | 10 pieces | 460 | 29 | 260 | 5 | 0 | 70 | 1000 | 27 | 0 | 24 | 2 carb, 3 med-fat meat, 3 fat |
| Chicken Selects Premium Breast Strips | 3 pieces | 400 | 24 | 210 | 3.5 | 0 | 17 | 1010 | 23 | 0 | 23 | 1 1/2 carb, 3 med-fat meat, 2 fat |
| Chicken Selects Premiun Breast Strips | 5 pieces | 660 | 40 | 360 | 6 | 0 | 85 | 1680 | 39 | 0 | 38 | 2 1/2 carb, 4 med-fat meat, 4 fat |
| BBQ Sauce | 1 pkg | 50 | 0 | 0 | 0 | 0 | 0 | 260 | 12 | 0 | 0 | 1 carb |
| Honey | 1 pkg | 50 | 0 | 0 | 0 | 0 | 0 | 12 | 0 | 0 | 0 | 1 carb |
| Sweet 'N Sour Sauce | 1 pkg | 50 | 0 | 0 | 0 | 0 | 0 | 150 | 12 | 0 | 0 | 1 carb |
| Creamy Ranch Sauce | 1.5 oz | 200 | 22 | 200 | 3.5 | 0 | 10 | 320 | 2 | 0 | 0 | 4 fat |

| | | | | | | | | | | | | |
|---|---|---|---|---|---|---|---|---|---|---|---|---|
| Premium Bacon Ranch Salad with Grilled Chicken | 1 | 260 | 9 | 90 | 4 | 0 | 90 | 1010 | 12 | 3 | 33 | 1 carb, 4 lean meat |
| Premium Bacon Ranch Salad with Crispy Chicken | 1 | 370 | 20 | 180 | 6 | 0 | 75 | 970 | 20 | 3 | 29 | 1 carb, 4 med-fat meat |
| Premium Caesar Salad | 1 | 90 | 4 | 35 | 2.5 | 0 | 10 | 180 | 9 | 3 | 7 | 1/2 carb, 1 med-fat meat |
| Premium Caesar Salad with Grilled Chicken | 1 | 220 | 6 | 60 | 3 | 0 | 75 | 890 | 12 | 3 | 30 | 1 carb, 4 lean meat |
| Premium Caesar Salad with Crispy Chicken | 1 | 330 | 17 | 150 | 4.5 | 0 | 60 | 840 | 20 | 3 | 26 | 1 carb, 3 med-fat meat |
| Premium Southwest Salad with Grilled Chicken | 1 | 320 | 9 | 80 | 3 | 0 | 70 | 960 | 30 | 6 | 30 | 2 carb, 1 1/2 lean meat |
| Premium Southwest Salad with Crispy Chicken | 1 | 430 | 20 | 180 | 4 | 0 | 55 | 920 | 38 | 6 | 26 | 2 1/2 carb, 3 med-fat meat, 1 fat |

| | Serving | Calories | Fat (g) | Cal. from Fat | Sat. Fat (g) | Trans Fat (g) | Chol. (mg) | Sod. (mg) | Carb. (g) | Fiber (g) | Prot. (g) | Servings/Exchanges |
|---|---|---|---|---|---|---|---|---|---|---|---|---|
| Side Salad | 1 | 20 | 0 | 0 | 0 | 0 | 0 | 10 | 4 | 1 | 1 | 1 vegetable |
| Snack Size Fruit & Walnut Salad | 1 | 210 | 8 | 70 | 1.5 | 0 | 5 | 60 | 31 | 2 | 4 | 2 carb, 2 fat |
| ***Salad Dressings*** | | | | | | | | | | | | |
| Newman's Own Creamy Caesar | 2 oz | 190 | 18 | 170 | 3.5 | 0 | 20 | 500 | 4 | 0 | 2 | 4 fat |
| Newman's Own Creamy Southwest | 1.5 oz | 100 | 6 | 50 | 1 | 0 | 20 | 340 | 11 | 0 | 1 | 1 carb, 1 fat |
| Newman's Own Low Fat Balsamic | 1.5 oz | 40 | 3 | 25 | 0 | 0 | 0 | 730 | 4 | 0 | 0 | 1 fat |
| Newman's Own Low Fat Italian | 1.5 oz | 60 | 2.5 | 20 | 0 | 0 | 0 | 730 | 8 | 0 | 1 | 1/2 carb, 1 fat |
| Newman's Own Ranch | 2 oz | 170 | 15 | 130 | 2.5 | 0 | 20 | 530 | 9 | 0 | 1 | 1/2 carb, 3 fat |
| ***Breakfast*** | | | | | | | | | | | | |

| | | | | | | | | | | | | |
|---|---|---|---|---|---|---|---|---|---|---|---|---|
| Egg McMuffin | 1 | 300 | 12 | 110 | 5 | 0 | 260 | 820 | 30 | 2 | 18 | 2 carb, 2 med-fat meat |
| Sausage McMuffin | 1 | 370 | 22 | 200 | 8 | 0 | 45 | 850 | 29 | 2 | 14 | 2 carb, 1 med-fat meat, 3 fat |
| Sausage McMuffin with Egg | 1 | 450 | 27 | 250 | 10 | 0 | 285 | 920 | 30 | 2 | 21 | 2 carb, 2 med-fat meat. 3 fat |
| English Muffin | 1 | 160 | 3 | 30 | 0.5 | 0 | 0 | 280 | 27 | 2 | 5 | 2 carb |
| Biscuit | Regular size | 260 | 12 | 110 | 7 | 0 | 0 | 740 | 33 | 2 | 5 | 2 carb, 2 fat |
| Bacon, Egg & Cheese Biscuit | Regular size | 420 | 23 | 210 | 12 | 0 | 235 | 1160 | 37 | 2 | 15 | 2 1/2 carb, 1 med-fat meat, 4 fat |
| Sausage Biscuit with Egg | Regular size | 510 | 33 | 290 | 14 | 0 | 250 | 1170 | 36 | 2 | 18 | 2 1/2 carb, 2 med-fat meat, 5 fat |
| Sausage Biscuit | Regular size | 430 | 27 | 240 | 12 | 0 | 30 | 1080 | 34 | 2 | 11 | 2 carb, 1 med-fat meat, 4 fat |
| Southern Style Chicken Biscuit | Regular size | 410 | 20 | 180 | 8 | 0 | 30 | 1180 | 41 | 2 | 17 | 3 carb, 1 med-fat meat, 1 fat |

FAST FOOD

| | Serving | Calories | Fat (g) | Cal. from Fat | Sat. Fat (g) | Trans Fat (g) | Chol. (mg) | Sod. (mg) | Carb. (g) | Fiber (g) | Prot. (g) | Servings/Exchanges |
|---|---|---|---|---|---|---|---|---|---|---|---|---|
| Bacon, Egg & Cheese McGriddle | 1 | 420 | 18 | 160 | 8 | 0 | 240 | 1110 | 48 | 2 | 15 | 3 carb, 1 med-fat meat, 3 fat |
| Sausage McGriddle | 1 | 420 | 22 | 200 | 8 | 0 | 35 | 1030 | 44 | 2 | 11 | 3 carb, 4 fat |
| Sausage, Egg & Cheese McGriddle | 1 | 560 | 32 | 290 | 12 | 0 | 265 | 1360 | 48 | 2 | 20 | 3 carb, 2 med-fat meat, 4 fat |
| Big Breakfast | Regular size | 740 | 48 | 430 | 17 | 0 | 555 | 1560 | 51 | 3 | 28 | 3 1/2 carb, 3 med-fat meat, 7 fat |
| Deluxe Breakfast | Regular size | 1090 | 56 | 510 | 19 | 0 | 575 | 2150 | 111 | 6 | 36 | 7 1/2 carb, 2 med-fat meat, 9 fat |
| Hash Browns | 2 oz | 150 | 9 | 80 | 1.5 | 0 | 0 | 310 | 15 | 2 | 1 | 4 carb, 3 fat |
| Hotcakes & Sausage | 1 | 520 | 24 | 210 | 7 | 0 | 50 | 930 | 61 | 3 | 15 | 4 carb, 5 fat |
| McSkillet Burrito with Sausage | 1 | 610 | 36 | 320 | 14 | 0.5 | 410 | 1390 | 44 | 3 | 27 | 3 carb, 3 med-fat meat, 4 fat |
| Sausage Burrito | 1 | 300 | 16 | 140 | 7 | 0.5 | 130 | 830 | 26 | 1 | 12 | 2 carb, 1 med-fat meat, 2 fat |

| | | | | | | | | | | | | |
|---|---|---|---|---|---|---|---|---|---|---|---|---|
| Scrambled Eggs | 3.3 oz | 170 | 11 | 100 | 4 | 0 | 520 | 180 | 1 | 0 | 15 | 2 med-fat meat |
| ***Desserts/Shakes*** | | | | | | | | | | | | |
| Apple Dippers | 1 pkg | 35 | 0 | 0 | 0 | 0 | 0 | 0 | 8 | 0 | 0 | 1/2 fruit |
| Baked Hot Apple Pie | 1 | 250 | 13 | 110 | 7 | 0 | 0 | 170 | 32 | 4 | 2 | 2 carb, 3 fat |
| Cinnamon Melts | 4 oz | 460 | 19 | 170 | 9 | 0 | 15 | 370 | 66 | 3 | 6 | 4 1/2 carb, 4 fat |
| Fruit ‘n Yogurt Parfait | 5.3 oz | 160 | 2 | 20 | 1 | 0 | 5 | 85 | 31 | 1 | 4 | 2 carb |
| Hot Caramel Sundae | 6.4 oz | 340 | 8 | 70 | 5 | 0 | 30 | 160 | 60 | 1 | 7 | 4 carb, 2 fat |
| Hot Fudge Sundae | 6.3 oz | 330 | 10 | 90 | 7 | 0 | 25 | 180 | 54 | 2 | 8 | 3 1/2 carb, 2 fat |
| Kiddie Cone | 1 oz | 45 | 1 | 10 | 0.5 | 0 | 5 | 20 | 8 | 0 | 1 | 1/2 carb |
| Low Fat Caramel Dip | 0.8 oz | 70 | 0.5 | 5 | 0 | 0 | 5 | 35 | 15 | 0 | 0 | 1 carb |
| M&M'S McFlurry | 12.3 oz | 620 | 20 | 180 | 12 | 1 | 55 | 190 | 96 | 1 | 14 | 6 1/2 carb, 4 fat |
| OREO McFlurry | 11.9 oz | 550 | 17 | 150 | 9 | 1 | 50 | 250 | 88 | 0 | 13 | 6 carb, 3 fat |
| Vanilla Reduced Fat Ice Cream Cone | 3.2 oz | 150 | 3.5 | 35 | 2 | 0 | 15 | 60 | 24 | 0 | 4 | 1 1/2 carb, 1 fat |
| Chocolate Triple Thick Shake, Small | 12 oz | 440 | 10 | 90 | 6 | 0.5 | 40 | 190 | 76 | 1 | 10 | 5 carb, 2 fat |

| | Serving | Calories | Fat (g) | Cal. from Fat | Sat. Fat (g) | Trans Fat (g) | Chol. (mg) | Sod. (mg) | Carb. (g) | Fiber (g) | Prot. (g) | Servings/Exchanges |
|---|---|---|---|---|---|---|---|---|---|---|---|---|
| Chocolate Triple Thick Shake, Medium | 16 oz | 580 | 14 | 120 | 8 | 1 | 50 | 250 | 102 | 1 | 13 | 7 carb, 3 fat |
| Chocolate Triple Thick Shake, Large | 21 oz | 770 | 18 | 160 | 11 | 1 | 70 | 330 | 134 | 1 | 18 | 9 carb, 4 fat |
| Vanilla Triple Thick Shake, Small | 12 oz | 420 | 10 | 90 | 6 | 0.5 | 40 | 140 | 72 | 0 | 9 | 5 carb, 2 fat |
| Vanilla Triple Thick Shake, Medium | 16 oz | 550 | 13 | 120 | 8 | 1 | 50 | 190 | 96 | 0 | 13 | 6 1/2 carb, 3 fat |
| Vanilla Triple Thick Shake, Large | 21 oz | 740 | 18 | 160 | 11 | 1 | 70 | 250 | 128 | 0 | 17 | 8 1/2 carb, 4 fat |
| McDonaldland Cookies | 2 oz | 260 | 8 | 70 | 2.5 | 0 | 0 | 300 | 43 | 1 | 4 | 3 carb, 2 fat |
| Chocolate Chip Cookie | 1 | 160 | 8 | 70 | 3.5 | 0 | 10 | 90 | 21 | 1 | 2 | 1 1/2 carb, 2 fat |
| ***McCafe Coffee, Nonfat Milk*** | | | | | | | | | | | | |
| Nonfat Cappuccino, Small | 12 oz | 60 | 0 | 0 | 0 | 0 | 5 | 85 | 9 | 0 | 6 | 1 skim milk |

| | | | | | | | | | | | | |
|---|---|---|---|---|---|---|---|---|---|---|---|---|
| Nonfat Cappuccino, Medium | 16 oz | 80 | 0 | 0 | 0 | 0 | 5 | 110 | 12 | 0 | 8 | 1 skim milk |
| Nonfat Cappuccino, Large | 20 oz | 90 | 0 | 0 | 0 | 0 | 5 | 130 | 13 | 0 | 9 | 1 skim milk |
| Nonfat Latte, Small | 12 oz | 90 | 0 | 0 | 0 | 0 | 5 | 115 | 13 | 0 | 9 | 1 skim milk |
| Nonfat Latte, Medium | 16 oz | 110 | 0 | 0 | 0 | 0 | 5 | 140 | 15 | 0 | 10 | 1 1/2 skim milk |
| Nonfat Latte, Large | 20 oz | 120 | 0 | 0 | 0 | 0 | 5 | 160 | 18 | 0 | 12 | 1 1/2 skim milk |
| Nonfat Caramel Cappuccino, Medium | 16 oz | 190 | 0 | 0 | 0 | 0 | 5 | 150 | 41 | 0 | 6 | 1 skim milk, 2 carb |
| Nonfat Caramel Latte, Medium | 16 oz | 220 | 0 | 0 | 0 | 0 | 5 | 180 | 45 | 0 | 9 | 1 skim milk, 2 carb |
| Nonfat Vanilla Cappuccino, Medium | 16 oz | 190 | 0 | 0 | 0 | 0 | 5 | 90 | 42 | 0 | 6 | 1 skim milk, 2 carb |
| Nonfat Vanilla Latte, Medium | 16 oz | 220 | 0 | 0 | 0 | 0 | 5 | 115 | 46 | 0 | 9 | 1 skim milk, 2 carb |
| Nonfat Cappuccino with Sugar Free Vanilla Syrup | 16 oz | 70 | 0 | 0 | 0 | 0 | 5 | 130 | 19 | 0 | 7 | 1 skim milk, 1/2 carb |

| | Serving | Calories | Fat (g) | Cal. from Fat | Sat. Fat (g) | Trans Fat (g) | Chol. (mg) | Sod. (mg) | Carb. (g) | Fiber (g) | Prot. (g) | Servings/Exchanges |
|---|---|---|---|---|---|---|---|---|---|---|---|---|
| Nonfat Latte with Sugar Free Vanilla Syrup | 16 oz | 90 | 0 | 0 | 0 | 0 | 5 | 160 | 22 | 0 | 9 | 1 skim milk, 1/2 carb |
| Iced Nonfat Latte, Medium | 16 oz | 60 | 0 | 0 | 0 | 0 | 5 | 90 | 9 | 0 | 6 | 1 skim milk |
| Iced Nonfat Caramel Latte, Medium | 16 oz | 150 | 0 | 0 | 0 | 0 | 5 | 120 | 32 | 0 | 5 | 1 skim milk, 1 carb |
| Iced Nonfat Vanilla Latte, Medium | 16 oz | 150 | 0 | 0 | 0 | 0 | 5 | 70 | 33 | 0 | 5 | 1 skim milk, 1 1/2 carb |
| Iced Nonfat Latte with Sugar Free Vanilla Syrup | 16 oz | 50 | 0 | 0 | 0 | 0 | 5 | 100 | 14 | 0 | 5 | 1 skim milk |
| ***McCafe Coffee, Whole Milk*** | | | | | | | | | | | | |
| Cappuccino, Small | 12 oz | 120 | 7 | 60 | 4 | 0 | 20 | 85 | 9 | 0 | 6 | 1 whole milk |
| Cappuccino, Medium | 16 oz | 140 | 8 | 70 | 4.5 | 0 | 25 | 105 | 11 | 0 | 8 | 1 whole milk |
| Cappuccino, Large | 20 oz | 180 | 10 | 90 | 6 | 0 | 30 | 130 | 13 | 0 | 9 | 1 whole milk |

| | | | | | | | | | | | | |
|---|---|---|---|---|---|---|---|---|---|---|---|---|
| Latte, Small | 12 oz | 150 | 8 | 70 | 4.5 | 0 | 25 | 105 | 11 | 0 | 8 | 1 whole milk |
| Latte, Medium | 16 oz | 180 | 10 | 90 | 6 | 0 | 30 | 130 | 13 | 0 | 10 | 1 whole milk |
| Latte, Large | 20 oz | 210 | 11 | 100 | 7 | 0 | 35 | 150 | 16 | 0 | 11 | 1 1/2 whole milk |
| Caramel Cappuccino, Medium | 16 oz | 240 | 6 | 50 | 3.5 | 0 | 20 | 150 | 41 | 0 | 6 | 1/2 whole milk, 2 carb |
| Caramel Latte, Medium | 16 oz | 280 | 8 | 70 | 4.5 | 0 | 25 | 170 | 43 | 0 | 8 | 1 whole milk, 2 carb |
| Vanilla Cappuccino, Medium | 16 oz | 240 | 6 | 50 | 3.5 | 0 | 20 | 85 | 42 | 0 | 6 | 1 whole milk, 2 carb |
| Vanilla Latte, Medium | 16 oz | 280 | 8 | 70 | 4.5 | 0 | 25 | 110 | 44 | 0 | 8 | 1 whole milk, 2 carb |
| Cappuccino with Sugar Free Vanilla Syrup, Medium | 16 oz | 120 | 6 | 60 | 3.5 | 0 | 20 | 130 | 18 | 0 | 6 | 1 whole milk |
| Latte with Sugar Free Vanilla Syrup, Medium | 16 oz | 160 | 8 | 70 | 5 | 0 | 25 | 150 | 21 | 0 | 8 | 1 whole milk, 1/2 carb |
| Iced Latte, Medium | 16 oz | 100 | 6 | 50 | 3.5 | 0 | 15 | 80 | 8 | 0 | 6 | 1/2 whole milk |
| Iced Caramel Latte, Medium | 16 oz | 180 | 4.5 | 40 | 2.5 | 0 | 15 | 120 | 31 | 0 | 4 | 1/2 whole milk, 1 1/2 carb |

| | Serving | Calories | Fat (g) | Cal. from Fat | Sat. Fat (g) | Trans Fat (g) | Chol. (mg) | Sod. (mg) | Carb. (g) | Fiber (g) | Prot. (g) | Servings/Exchanges |
|---|---|---|---|---|---|---|---|---|---|---|---|---|
| Iced Vanilla Latte, Medium | 16 oz | 190 | 4.5 | 40 | 2.5 | 0 | 15 | 70 | 33 | 0 | 5 | 1/2 whole milk, 2 carb |
| Iced Latte with Sugar Free Vanilla Syrup | 16 oz | 90 | 5 | 40 | 3 | 0 | 15 | 105 | 14 | 0 | 5 | 1/2 whole milk, 1/2 carb |
| **PANDA EXPRESS** | | | | | | | | | | | | |
| ***Chicken*** | | | | | | | | | | | | |
| Black Pepper Chicken | 5.5 oz | 200 | 11 | 100 | 2.5 | 0 | 90 | 740 | 11 | 2 | 14 | 1 carb, 2 med-fat meat |
| Broccoli Chicken | 5.5 oz | 180 | 9 | 80 | 2 | 0 | 65 | 630 | 11 | 3 | 13 | 1 carb, 1 med-fat meat, 1 fat |
| Kung Pao Chicken | 6.1 oz | 300 | 20 | 180 | 4 | 0 | 110 | 900 | 13 | 2 | 20 | 1 carb, 2 med-fat meat, 2 fat |
| Mandarin Chicken | 5.8 oz | 310 | 16 | 150 | 4 | 0 | 115 | 740 | 8 | 0 | 34 | 1/2 carb, 4 lean meat |
| Orange Chicken | 5.4 oz | 400 | 20 | 170 | 3.5 | 0 | 90 | 640 | 42 | 0 | 15 | 3 carb, 1 med-fat meat, 3 fat |

| | | | | | | | | | | | | |
|---|---|---|---|---|---|---|---|---|---|---|---|---|
| Pineapple Chicken | 6.5 oz | 230 | 10 | 90 | 2 | 0 | 75 | 710 | 21 | 2 | 13 | 1 1/2 carb, 1 med-fat meat, 1 fat |
| Pineapple Chicken Breast | 6.1 oz | 230 | 12 | 110 | 2 | 0 | 30 | 560 | 19 | 1 | 11 | 1 carb, 1 med-fat meat, 1 fat |
| Potato Chicken | 6 oz | 190 | 9 | 80 | 2 | 0 | 70 | 660 | 13 | 3 | 12 | 1 carb, 1 med-fat meat, 1 fat |
| String Bean Chicken | 6 oz | 190 | 9 | 80 | 2 | 0 | 70 | 660 | 13 | 3 | 12 | 1 carb, 1 med-fat meat, 1 fat |
| String Bean Chicken Breast | 6 oz | 200 | 12 | 100 | 2 | 0 | 30 | 550 | 12 | 2 | 10 | 1 carb, 1 med-fat meat, 1 fat |
| Sweet & Sour Chicken | 5.5 oz | 400 | 17 | 150 | 3 | 0 | 40 | 370 | 46 | 1 | 15 | 3 carb, 1 med-fat meat, 2 fat |
| Thai Cashew Chicken Breast | 6.3 oz | 330 | 22 | 190 | 3.5 | 0 | 35 | 630 | 17 | 2 | 15 | 1 carb, 2 med-fat meat, 2 fat |
| ***Beef*** | | | | | | | | | | | | |
| Beijing Beef | 4.9 oz | 660 | 41 | 360 | 7 | 0 | 60 | 860 | 52 | 4 | 24 | 3 1/2 carb, 2 med-fat meat, 6 fat |

FAST FOOD

| | Serving | Calories | Fat (g) | Cal. from Fat | Sat. Fat (g) | Trans Fat (g) | Chol. (mg) | Sod. (mg) | Carb. (g) | Fiber (g) | Prot. (g) | Servings/Exchanges |
|---|---|---|---|---|---|---|---|---|---|---|---|---|
| Broccoli Beef | 5.4 oz | 150 | 6 | 50 | 1.5 | 0 | 25 | 720 | 12 | 3 | 11 | 1 carb, 1 med-fat meat |
| Mongolian Beef | 6.1 oz | 200 | 9 | 80 | 2 | 0 | 40 | 830 | 16 | 3 | 15 | 1 carb, 2 med-fat meat |
| ***Pork*** | | | | | | | | | | | | |
| BBQ Pork | 4.6 oz | 360 | 19 | 180 | 8 | 0 | 120 | 1310 | 12 | 1 | 34 | 1 carb, 4 med-fat meat |
| Sweet & Sour Pork | 5.6 oz | 400 | 23 | 210 | 4.5 | 0 | 30 | 360 | 36 | 2 | 13 | 2 1/2 carb, 1 med-fat meat, 4 fat |
| ***Shrimp*** | | | | | | | | | | | | |
| Crispy Shrimp | 3.5 oz | 260 | 13 | 120 | 2.5 | 0 | 60 | 810 | 26 | 1 | 9 | 2 carb, 3 fat |
| Kung Pao Shrimp | 6.4 oz | 230 | 14 | 130 | 2.5 | 0 | 110 | 850 | 13 | 2 | 13 | 1 carb, 1 med-fat meat, 2 fat |
| Tangy Shrimp | 5.3 oz | 140 | 4.5 | 40 | 1 | 0 | 85 | 660 | 16 | 1 | 8 | 1 carb, 1 med-fat meat |
| ***Veggies*** | | | | | | | | | | | | |
| Eggplant & Tofu | 6.1 oz | 310 | 24 | 220 | 3 | 0 | 0 | 680 | 19 | 3 | 7 | 1 carb, 1 med-fat meat, 4 fat |

| | | | | | | | | | | | | |
|---|---|---|---|---|---|---|---|---|---|---|---|---|
| Mixed Veggies, Side | 4.8 oz | 100 | 6 | 60 | 1 | 0 | 0 | 220 | 7 | 3 | 3 | 1 vegetable. 1 fat |
| Mixed Veggies, Entrée | 9.6 oz | 190 | 13 | 120 | 2 | 0 | 0 | 440 | 14 | 5 | 5 | 3 vegetable, 3 fat |
| ***Rice & Noodles*** | | | | | | | | | | | | |
| Chow Mein | 8.3 oz | 400 | 12 | 110 | 2 | 0 | 0 | 1060 | 61 | 8 | 12 | 4 carb, 2 fat |
| Fried Rice | 10 oz | 570 | 18 | 160 | 4 | 0 | 130 | 900 | 85 | 8 | 16 | 5 1/2 carb, 4 fat |
| Steamed Rice | 8.7 oz | 420 | 0 | 0 | 0 | 0 | 0 | 0 | 93 | 0 | 8 | 6 carb |
| ***Appetizers*** | | | | | | | | | | | | |
| Chicken Egg Roll | 3 oz, 1 roll | 200 | 12 | 100 | 4 | 0 | 20 | 390 | 16 | 2 | 8 | 1 carb, 1 med-fat meat, 1 fat |
| Chicken Potsticker | 3.3 oz, 3 pcs | 220 | 11 | 100 | 2.5 | 0 | 20 | 280 | 23 | 1 | 7 | 1 1/2 carb, 1 med-fat meat, 1 fat |
| Cream Cheese Rangoon | 2.4 oz, 3 pcs | 190 | 8 | 70 | 5 | 0 | 35 | 180 | 24 | 2 | 5 | 1 1/2 carb, 2 fat |
| Veggie Spring Roll | 3.4 oz, 2 rolls | 160 | 7 | 60 | 1 | 0 | 0 | 540 | 22 | 4 | 4 | 1 1/2 carb, 1 fat |
| ***Soup*** | | | | | | | | | | | | |
| Hot & Sour Soup | 10.6 oz | 90 | 3.5 | 30 | 0.5 | 0 | 65 | 970 | 12 | 1 | 4 | 1 carb, 1 fat |

| | Serving | Calories | Fat (g) | Cal. from Fat | Sat. Fat (g) | Trans Fat (g) | Chol. (mg) | Sod. (mg) | Carb. (g) | Fiber (g) | Prot. (g) | Servings/Exchanges |
|---|---|---|---|---|---|---|---|---|---|---|---|---|
| ***Sauces & Cookie*** | | | | | | | | | | | | |
| Fortune Cookie | 1 | 32 | 0 | 2 | 0 | 0 | 0 | 8 | 7 | 0 | 1 | 1/2 carb |
| Mandarin Sauce | 1.8 oz | 160 | 0 | 0 | 0 | 0 | 0 | 340 | 40 | 0 | 0 | 2 1/2 carb |
| Sweet & Sour Sauce | 1.8 oz | 80 | 0 | 0 | 0 | 0 | 0 | 180 | 21 | 0 | 0 | 1 1/2 carb |
| **PAPA JOHN'S** | | | | | | | | | | | | |
| ***Original Crust, Large (14 inches)*** | | | | | | | | | | | | |
| Cheese | 1 slice | 280 | 10 | 90 | 3 | 0 | 15 | 700 | 38 | 2 | 12 | 2 1/2 carb, 1 med-fat meat, 1 fat |
| Pepperoni | 1 slice | 310 | 13 | 120 | 4 | 0 | 20 | 810 | 38 | 2 | 13 | 2 1/2 carb, 1 med-fat meat, 2 fat |
| Sausage | 1 slice | 330 | 15 | 130 | 4.5 | 0 | 20 | 810 | 37 | 3 | 13 | 2 1/2 carb, 1 med-fat meat, 2 fat |
| The Meats | 1 slice | 350 | 16 | 140 | 5 | 0 | 30 | 930 | 38 | 2 | 15 | 2 1/2 carb, 2 med-fat meat, 1 fat |

| | | | | | | | | | | | | |
|---|---|---|---|---|---|---|---|---|---|---|---|---|
| Garden Fresh | 1 slice | 280 | 9 | 80 | 2.5 | 0 | 15 | 680 | 39 | 2 | 11 | 2 1/2 carb, 1 med-fat meat, 1 fat |
| The Works | 1 slice | 330 | 11 | 100 | 6 | 0 | 25 | 890 | 39 | 3 | 14 | 2 1/2 carb, 1 med-fat meat, 1 fat |
| Spinach Alfredo | 1 slice | 280 | 11 | 100 | 4.5 | 0 | 20 | 630 | 36 | 2 | 11 | 2 1/2 carb, 1 med-fat meat, 1 fat |
| Tuscan Six Cheese | 1 slice | 320 | 13 | 110 | 4.5 | 0 | 25 | 780 | 38 | 2 | 15 | 2 1/2 carb, 1 med-fat meat, 2 fat |
| Spicy Italian | 1 slice | 370 | 11 | 100 | 10 | 0 | 30 | 960 | 38 | 4 | 15 | 2 1/2 carb, 1 med-fat meat, 1 fat |
| BBQ Chicken & Bacon | 1 slice | 340 | 11 | 100 | 3.5 | 0 | 30 | 960 | 44 | 2 | 15 | 3 carb, 1 med-fat meat, 1 fat |
| Hawaiian BBQ Chicken | 1 slice | 340 | 11 | 100 | 3.5 | 0 | 30 | 960 | 46 | 2 | 16 | 3 carb, 1 med-fat meat, 1 fat |
| ***Thin Crust, Large (14 inches)*** | | | | | | | | | | | | |
| Cheese | 1 slice | 220 | 12 | 100 | 3 | 0 | 15 | 490 | 21 | 1 | 9 | 1 1/2 carb, 1 med-fat meat, 1 fat |

| | Serving | Calories | Fat (g) | Cal. from Fat | Sat. Fat (g) | Trans Fat (g) | Chol. (mg) | Sod. (mg) | Carb. (g) | Fiber (g) | Prot. (g) | Servings/Exchanges |
|---|---|---|---|---|---|---|---|---|---|---|---|---|
| Sausage | 1 slice | 270 | 16 | 150 | 5 | 0 | 20 | 600 | 21 | 2 | 9 | 1 1/2 carb, 1 med-fat meat, 2 fat |
| The Meats | 1 slice | 280 | 17 | 160 | 5 | 0 | 30 | 720 | 21 | 1 | 12 | 1 1/2 carb, 1 med-fat meat, 2 fat |
| Garden Fresh | 1 slice | 210 | 11 | 90 | 2.5 | 0 | 15 | 470 | 23 | 2 | 8 | 1 1/2 carb, 1 med-fat meat, 1 fat |
| The Works | 1 slice | 260 | 13 | 110 | 6 | 0 | 25 | 680 | 22 | 2 | 11 | 1 1/2 carb, 1 med-fat meat, 2 fat |
| Spinach Alfredo | 1 slice | 220 | 13 | 110 | 4.5 | 0 | 20 | 420 | 19 | 1 | 8 | 1 carb, 1 med-fat meat, 2 fat |
| Tuscan Six Cheese | 1 slice | 250 | 14 | 130 | 5 | 0 | 25 | 580 | 21 | 1 | 12 | 1 1/2 carb, 1 med-fat meat, 2 fat |
| Spicy Italian | 1 slice | 310 | 13 | 110 | 11 | 0 | 30 | 760 | 22 | 3 | 12 | 1 1/2 carb, 1 med-fat meat, 2 fat |
| BBQ Chicken & Bacon | 1 slice | 270 | 13 | 110 | 3.5 | 0 | 30 | 750 | 27 | <1 | 12 | 2 carb, 1 med-fat meat, 2 fat |

| | | | | | | | | | | | | |
|---|---|---|---|---|---|---|---|---|---|---|---|---|
| Hawaiian BBQ Chicken | 1 slice | 290 | 14 | 120 | 3.5 | 0 | 30 | 740 | 31 | 1 | 13 | 2 carb, 1 med-fat meat, 2 fat |
| ***Pan Crust, Large (14 inches)*** | | | | | | | | | | | | |
| Cheese | 1 slice | 410 | 23 | 200 | 7 | 0 | 20 | 750 | 38 | 1 | 13 | 2 1/2 carb, 1 med-fat meat, 4 fat |
| Pepperoni | 1 slice | 410 | 24 | 210 | 8 | 0 | 20 | 820 | 37 | 1 | 13 | 2 1/2 carb, 1 med-fat meat, 4 fat |
| Sausage | 1 slice | 420 | 25 | 230 | 8 | 0 | 20 | 790 | 37 | 2 | 12 | 2 1/2 carb, 1 med-fat meat, 4 fat |
| The Meats | 1 slice | 440 | 8 | 230 | 8 | 0 | 30 | 890 | 37 | 1 | 15 | 2 1/2 carb, 1 med-fat meat, 1 fat |
| Garden Fresh | 1 slice | 370 | 19 | 170 | 6 | 0 | 15 | 660 | 39 | 2 | 11 | 2 1/2 carb, 1 med-fat meat, 3 fat |
| The Works | 1 slice | 420 | 21 | 190 | 9 | 0 | 25 | 860 | 38 | 2 | 14 | 2 1/2 carb, 1 med-fat meat, 3 fat |
| Spinach Alfredo | 1 slice | 380 | 22 | 200 | 8 | 0 | 20 | 610 | 35 | 1 | 11 | 2 carb, 1 med-fat meat, 3 fat |

| | Serving | Calories | Fat (g) | Cal. from Fat | Sat. Fat (g) | Trans Fat (g) | Chol. (mg) | Sod. (mg) | Carb. (g) | Fiber (g) | Prot. (g) | Servings/Exchanges |
|---|---|---|---|---|---|---|---|---|---|---|---|---|
| Tuscan Six Cheese | 1 slice | 410 | 23 | 200 | 8 | 0 | 25 | 760 | 37 | 1 | 15 | 2 1/2 carb, 1 med-fat meat, 4 fat |
| Spicy Italian | 1 slice | 470 | 21 | 190 | 14 | 0 | 30 | 950 | 38 | 3 | 15 | 2 1/2 carb, 1 med-fat meat, 3 fat |
| BBQ Chicken & Bacon | 1 slice | 430 | 22 | 200 | 7 | 0 | 30 | 940 | 43 | 1 | 15 | 3 carb, 1 med-fat meat, 3 fat |
| Hawaiian BBQ Chicken | 1 slice | 440 | 22 | 200 | 7 | 0 | 30 | 940 | 45 | 1 | 15 | 3 carb, 1 med-fat meat, 3 fat |
| ***Side Items*** | | | | | | | | | | | | |
| BBQ Wings | 2 | 160 | 10 | 90 | 3 | 0 | 85 | 560 | 4 | 0 | 14 | 2 med-fat meat |
| Bread Sticks | 2 | 290 | 4.5 | 40 | 0.5 | 0 | 0 | 540 | 53 | 2 | 9 | 3 1/2 carb, 1 fat |
| Buffalo Wings | 2 | 160 | 11 | 100 | 3.5 | 0 | 90 | 680 | 1 | 1 | 14 | 2 med-fat meat |
| Cheese Sticks | 4 | 370 | 16 | 150 | 4.5 | 0 | 25 | 830 | 42 | 2 | 15 | 3 carb, 1 med-fat meat, 2 fat |

| | | | | | | | | | | | | |
|---|---|---|---|---|---|---|---|---|---|---|---|---|
| Chicken Strips | 2 | 160 | 8 | 70 | 2 | 0 | 25 | 350 | 10 | 0 | 10 | 1/2 carb, 1 med-fat meat, 1 fat |
| Cinnamon Sweetsticks | 4 sticks | 580 | 16 | 140 | 4.5 | 0 | 0 | 740 | 98 | 3 | 11 | 6 1/2 carb, 3 fat |
| Cinnaple | 4 sticks | 560 | 19 | 170 | 6 | 0 | 0 | 540 | 90 | 2 | 8 | 6 carb, 4 fat |
| Garlic Parmesan Bread Sticks | 2 | 330 | 10 | 90 | 1.5 | 0 | 0 | 720 | 54 | 2 | 10 | 3 1/2 carb, 2 fat |
| Honey Chipotle Wings | 2 | 190 | 12 | 110 | 3 | 0 | 50 | 730 | 8 | 0 | 12 | 1/2 carb, 1 med-fat meat, 1 fat |
| Cheese Sauce | 1 | 40 | 3.5 | 30 | 1 | 0 | 0 | 160 | 2 | 0 | 1 | 1 fat |
| Garlic Sauce | 1 | 150 | 17 | 150 | 3 | 0 | 0 | 310 | 0 | 0 | 0 | 3 fat |
| Pizza Sauce | 1 | 20 | 1 | 10 | 0 | 0 | 0 | 230 | 3 | 0 | 0 | free |
| Ranch | 1 | 100 | 10 | 90 | 1.5 | 0 | 10 | 260 | 1 | 0 | 1 | 2 fat |
| Honey Mustard | 1 | 150 | 15 | 140 | 2.5 | 0 | 10 | 120 | 5 | 0 | 0 | 3 fat |
| **PIZZA HUT** | | | | | | | | | | | | |
| ***P'Zone*** | | | | | | | | | | | | |
| All Natural Pepperoni | 1/2 order | 630 | 24 | 220 | 11 | 0.5 | 70 | 1580 | 76 | 2 | 28 | 5 carb, 2 med-fat meat, 3 fat |

| | Serving | Calories | Fat (g) | Cal. from Fat | Sat. Fat (g) | Trans Fat (g) | Chol. (mg) | Sod. (mg) | Carb. (g) | Fiber (g) | Prot. (g) | Servings/Exchanges |
|---|---|---|---|---|---|---|---|---|---|---|---|---|
| Classic | 1/2 order | 630 | 23 | 210 | 11 | 0.5 | 65 | 1480 | 77 | 3 | 28 | 5 carb, 2 med-fat meat, 3 fat |
| Meaty | 1/2 order | 740 | 33 | 300 | 15 | 1 | 95 | 1840 | 76 | 3 | 34 | 5 carb, 3 med-fat meat, 4 fat |
| ***Appetizers*** | | | | | | | | | | | | |
| Baked Hot Wings | 2 | 120 | 7 | 70 | 2 | 0 | 65 | 500 | 1 | 0 | 11 | 2 lean meat |
| Bread Sticks | 1 | 140 | 6 | 60 | 1.5 | 0 | 0 | 240 | 18 | 1 | 4 | 1 carb, 1 fat |
| Cheese Breadsticks | 1 | 180 | 7 | 70 | 3.5 | 0 | 15 | 370 | 20 | 1 | 7 | 1 carb, 1 fat |
| Wing Ranch Dipping Sauce | 1.5 oz | 220 | 23 | 210 | 4 | 0 | 25 | 400 | 3 | 0 | 1 | 5 fat |
| Marinara Dipping Sauce | 3 oz | 60 | 0 | 0 | 0 | 0 | 0 | 440 | 12 | 2 | 2 | 1 carb |
| ***Desserts*** | | | | | | | | | | | | |
| Cinnamon Sticks | 2 pieces | 170 | 6 | 50 | 1.5 | 0 | 0 | 200 | 26 | 1 | 4 | 2 carb, 1 fat |
| White Icing Dipping Cup | 2 oz | 190 | 0 | 0 | 0 | 0 | 0 | 0 | 47 | 0 | 0 | 3 carb |

| 14-Inch Large Pan Pizzas | | | | | | | | | | | | |
|---|---|---|---|---|---|---|---|---|---|---|---|---|
| Cheese | 1 slice | 350 | 14 | 140 | 6 | 0 | 35 | 740 | 37 | 2 | 15 | 2 1/2 carb, 1 med-fat meat, 2 fat |
| All Natural Pepperoni | 1 slice | 370 | 18 | 160 | 7 | 0 | 35 | 850 | 37 | 2 | 15 | 2 1/2 carb, 1 med-fat meat, 3 fat |
| Ham & Pineapple | 1 slice | 320 | 13 | 110 | 5 | 0 | 25 | 740 | 38 | 2 | 14 | 2 1/2 carb, 1 med-fat meat, 2 fat |
| Supreme | 1 slice | 400 | 20 | 180 | 8 | 0 | 40 | 890 | 38 | 2 | 17 | 2 1/2 carb, 1 med-fat meat, 4 fat |
| Dan's Original | 1 slice | 400 | 20 | 180 | 8 | 0 | 40 | 890 | 37 | 2 | 17 | 2 1/2 carb, 1 med-fat meat, 3 fat |
| Meat Lover's | 1 slice | 470 | 27 | 240 | 10 | 0 | 60 | 1170 | 37 | 2 | 21 | 2 1/2 carb, 2 med-fat meat, 3 fat |
| Veggie Lover's | 1 slice | 320 | 13 | 120 | 4.5 | 0 | 20 | 690 | 38 | 2 | 13 | 2 1/2 carb, 1 med-fat meat, 2 fat |
| All Natural Pepperoni & Mushroom | 1 slice | 340 | 15 | 140 | 6 | 0 | 30 | 740 | 37 | 2 | 14 | 2 1/2 carb, 1 med-fat meat, 2 fat |

| | Serving | Calories | Fat (g) | Cal. from Fat | Sat. Fat (g) | Trans Fat (g) | Chol. (mg) | Sod. (mg) | Carb. (g) | Fiber (g) | Prot. (g) | Servings/Exchanges |
|---|---|---|---|---|---|---|---|---|---|---|---|---|
| Triple Meat Italiano | 1 slice | 410 | 21 | 190 | 8 | 0 | 45 | 1010 | 37 | 2 | 18 | 2 1/2 carb, 2 med-fat meat, 2 fat |
| ***14-Inch Large Thin 'N Crispy Pizzas*** | | | | | | | | | | | | |
| Cheese | 1 slice | 260 | 11 | 100 | 6 | 0 | 35 | 740 | 29 | 1 | 12 | 2 carb, 1 med-fat meat, 1 fat |
| All Natural Pepperoni | 1 slice | 290 | 14 | 120 | 6 | 0 | 35 | 860 | 28 | 1 | 12 | 2 carb, 1 med-fat meat, 2 fat |
| Ham & Pineapple | 1 slice | 240 | 9 | 80 | 4 | 0 | 25 | 750 | 31 | 1 | 11 | 2 carb, 1 med-fat meat, 1 fat |
| Supreme | 1 slice | 320 | 16 | 150 | 7 | 0 | 40 | 900 | 30 | 2 | 14 | 2 carb, 1 med-fat meat, 2 fat |
| Dan's Original | 1 slice | 320 | 16 | 150 | 7 | 0 | 40 | 900 | 29 | 2 | 15 | 2 carb, 1 med-fat meat, 2 fat |
| Meat Lover's | 1 slice | 400 | 23 | 210 | 9 | 0 | 60 | 1190 | 29 | 1 | 19 | 2 carb, 2 med-fat meat, 3 fat |

| | | | | | | | | | | | | |
|---|---|---|---|---|---|---|---|---|---|---|---|---|
| Veggie Lover's | 1 slice | 240 | 9 | 80 | 4 | 0 | 20 | 710 | 30 | 2 | 10 | 2 carb, 1 med-fat meat, 1 fat |
| All Natural Pepperoni & Mushroom | 1 slice | 260 | 11 | 100 | 5 | 0 | 30 | 740 | 29 | 1 | 12 | 2 carb, 1 med-fat meat, 1 fat |
| Triple Meat Italiano | 1 slice | 320 | 17 | 150 | 7 | 0 | 45 | 1010 | 28 | 1 | 15 | 2 carb, 1 med-fat meat, 2 fat |
| ***14-Inch Large Hand-Tossed Style Pizzas*** | | | | | | | | | | | | |
| Cheese | 1 slice | 320 | 12 | 110 | 6 | 0 | 35 | 820 | 38 | 2 | 15 | 2 1/2 carb, 1 med-fat meat, 1 fat |
| All Natural Pepperoni | 1 slice | 340 | 15 | 130 | 7 | 0 | 35 | 930 | 37 | 2 | 14 | 2 1/2 carb, 1 med-fat meat, 2 fat |
| Ham & Pineapple | 1 slice | 300 | 10 | 90 | 5 | 0 | 25 | 820 | 39 | 2 | 13 | 2 1/2 carb, 1 med-fat meat, 1 fat |
| Supreme | 1 slice | 380 | 17 | 160 | 8 | 0 | 40 | 970 | 39 | 3 | 16 | 2 1/2 carb, 1 med-fat meat, 2 fat |
| Dan's Original | 1 slice | 370 | 17 | 160 | 8 | 0 | 40 | 970 | 38 | 2 | 17 | 2 1/2 carb, 1 med-fat meat, 2 fat |

| | Serving | Calories | Fat (g) | Cal. from Fat | Sat. Fat (g) | Trans Fat (g) | Chol. (mg) | Sod. (mg) | Carb. (g) | Fiber (g) | Prot. (g) | Servings/Exchanges |
|---|---|---|---|---|---|---|---|---|---|---|---|---|
| Meat Lover's | 1 slice | 450 | 24 | 210 | 10 | 0 | 60 | 1250 | 38 | 2 | 20 | 2 1/2 carb, 2 med-fat meat, 3 fat |
| Veggie Lover's | 1 slice | 290 | 10 | 90 | 4.5 | 0 | 20 | 770 | 39 | 3 | 12 | 2 1/2 carb, 1 med-fat meat, 1 fat |
| Triple Meat Italiano | 1 slice | 380 | 18 | 160 | 8 | 0 | 45 | 1090 | 38 | 2 | 17 | 2 1/2 carb, 2 med-fat meat, 3 fat |
| All Natural Pepperoni & Mushroom | 1 slice | 310 | 12 | 110 | 6 | 0 | 30 | 820 | 38 | 2 | 14 | 2 1/2 carb, 1 med-fat meat, 1 fat |
| ***14-Inch Large Stuffed Crust Pizzas*** | | | | | | | | | | | | |
| Cheese | 1 slice | 340 | 14 | 130 | 8 | 0 | 40 | 910 | 39 | 2 | 15 | 2 1/2 carb, 1 med-fat meat, 2 fat |
| All Natural Pepperoni | 1 slice | 380 | 18 | 160 | 8 | 0 | 45 | 1060 | 39 | 2 | 16 | 2 1/2 carb, 1 med-fat meat, 3 fat |
| Ham & Pineapple | 1 slice | 330 | 13 | 110 | 7 | 0 | 35 | 940 | 41 | 2 | 15 | 2 1/2 carb, 1 med-fat meat, 2 fat |

| | | | | | | | | | | | | |
|---|---|---|---|---|---|---|---|---|---|---|---|---|
| Supreme | 1 slice | 410 | 20 | 180 | 9 | 0 | 50 | 1090 | 40 | 3 | 18 | 2 1/2 carb, 2 med-fat meat, 2 fat |
| Meat Lover's | 1 slice | 480 | 26 | 240 | 12 | 0.5 | 70 | 1370 | 39 | 2 | 22 | 2 1/2 carb, 2 med-fat meat, 3 fat |
| Veggie Lover's | 1 slice | 330 | 13 | 110 | 6 | 0 | 30 | 890 | 40 | 3 | 14 | 2 1/2 carb, 1 med-fat meat, 2 fat |
| Triple Meat Italiano | 1 slice | 440 | 23 | 200 | 11 | 0 | 65 | 1290 | 40 | 2 | 21 | 2 1/2 carb, 2 med-fat meat, 3 fat |
| All Natural Pepperoni & Mushroom | 1 slice | 350 | 15 | 130 | 7 | 0 | 40 | 940 | 39 | 2 | 15 | 2 1/2 carb, 1 med-fat meat, 2 fat |
| ***12 Large Fit 'N Delicious Pizzas*** | | | | | | | | | | | | |
| All Natural Chicken, Mushroom & Jalapeño | 1 slice | 180 | 4.5 | 40 | 1.5 | 0 | 25 | 710 | 22 | 1 | 12 | 1 1/2 carb, 1 med-fat meat |
| All Natural Chicken, Red Onion & Green Pepper | 1 slice | 180 | 4.5 | 40 | 1.5 | 0 | 25 | 500 | 24 | 1 | 11 | 1 1/2 carb, 1 med-fat meat |
| Green Pepper, Red Onion & Diced Tomato | 1 slice | 150 | 4 | 35 | 1.5 | 0 | 10 | 400 | 24 | 2 | 6 | 1 1/2 carb, 1 fat |

| | Serving | Calories | Fat (g) | Cal. from Fat | Sat. Fat (g) | Trans Fat (g) | Chol. (mg) | Sod. (mg) | Carb. (g) | Fiber (g) | Prot. (g) | Servings/Exchanges |
|---|---|---|---|---|---|---|---|---|---|---|---|---|
| Ham, Pineapple & Diced Red Tomato | 1 slice | 160 | 4.5 | 40 | 1.5 | 0 | 15 | 560 | 24 | 1 | 7 | 1 1/2 carb, 1 fat |
| Ham, Red Onion & Mushroom | 1 slice | 160 | 4.5 | 40 | 1.5 | 0 | 15 | 550 | 23 | 1 | 8 | 1 1/2 carb, 1 med-fat meat |
| Tomato, Mushroom & Jalapeño | 1 slice | 150 | 4 | 35 | 1.5 | 0 | 10 | 640 | 23 | 2 | 6 | 1 1/2 carb, 1 fat |
| ***Tuscani Pastas (1/4 Full Pan or 1/2 Half Pan)*** | | | | | | | | | | | | |
| All Natural Chicken Alfredo | 1 piece | 640 | 33 | 300 | 11 | 0.5 | 70 | 1190 | 56 | 4 | 28 | 3 1/2 carb, 3 med-fat meat, 4 fat |
| Bacon Mac 'N Cheese | 1 piece | 520 | 22 | 200 | 12 | 0.5 | 60 | 1170 | 54 | 4 | 24 | 3 1/2 carb, 2 med-fat meat, 2 fat |
| Lasagna | 1 piece | 570 | 30 | 270 | 13 | 1 | 105 | 1670 | 45 | 5 | 29 | 3 carb, 3 med-fat meat, 3 fat |
| Meaty Marinara | 1 piece | 510 | 24 | 220 | 10 | 1 | 80 | 1310 | 48 | 5 | 25 | 3 carb, 2 med-fat meat, 3 fat |

**RUBIOS**

| | | | | | | | | | | | | |
|---|---|---|---|---|---|---|---|---|---|---|---|---|
| ***Burritos*** | | | | | | | | | | | | |
| Baja Grill, Chicken | 1 | 620 | 26 | 230 | 9 | NA | 125 | 1890 | 53 | 4 | 46 | 3 1/2 carb, 5 med-fat meat |
| Baja Grill, Steak | 1 | 670 | 34 | 310 | 14 | NA | 100 | 2320 | 53 | 4 | 38 | 3 1/2 carb, 4 med-fat meat, 3 fat |
| Bean & Cheese | 1 | 700 | 33 | 290 | 17 | NA | 85 | 1750 | 75 | 12 | 29 | 5 carb, 2 med-fat meat, 5 fat |
| Big Burrito Especial Chicken | 1 | 830 | 32 | 290 | 7 | NA | 80 | 2030 | 99 | 7 | 38 | 6 1/2 carb, 3 med-fat meat, 3 fat |
| Big Burrito Especial Steak | 1 | 870 | 38 | 350 | 11 | NA | 65 | 2360 | 99 | 7 | 32 | 6 1/2 carb, 2 med-fat meat, 6 fat |
| Carnitas Rajas | 1 | 740 | 39 | 360 | 13 | NA | 85 | 1970 | 75 | 4 | 34 | 5 carb, 3 med-fat meat, 5 fat |
| Fish | 1 | 710 | 40 | 360 | 8 | NA | 80 | 1520 | 71 | 6 | 25 | 4 1/2 carb, 2 med-fat meat, 6 fat |
| Grilled Shrimp | 1 | 710 | 34 | 300 | 11 | NA | 220 | 2100 | 72 | 5 | 30 | 5 carb, 2 med-fat meat, 5 fat |

| | Serving | Calories | Fat (g) | Cal. from Fat | Sat. Fat (g) | Trans Fat (g) | Chol. (mg) | Sod. (mg) | Carb. (g) | Fiber (g) | Prot. (g) | Servings/Exchanges |
|---|---|---|---|---|---|---|---|---|---|---|---|---|
| Grilled Veggie | 1 | 630 | 29 | 260 | 9 | NA | 35 | 1290 | 73 | 4 | 19 | 5 carb, 6 fat |
| HealthMe, Chicken | 1 | 500 | 10 | 90 | 2.5 | NA | 70 | 1700 | 70 | 6 | 34 | 4 1/2 carb, 3 lean meat |
| HealthMe, Mahi Mahi | 1 | 510 | 15 | 130 | 3 | NA | 25 | 1190 | 68 | 6 | 29 | 4 1/2 carb, 2 med-fat meat, 1 fat |
| Mahi Mahi | 1 | 700 | 42 | 380 | 12 | NA | 65 | 1150 | 49 | 4 | 34 | 3 carb, 3 med-fat meat, 5 fat |
| ***Tacos*** | | | | | | | | | | | | |
| Carnitas Rajas | 1 | 210 | 11 | 100 | 2 | NA | 20 | 420 | 23 | 3 | 9 | 1 1/2 carb, 1 med-fat meat, 1 fat |
| Especial Fish | 1 | 330 | 20 | 180 | 4.5 | NA | 50 | 510 | 30 | 4 | 13 | 2 carb, 1 med-fat meat, 3 fat |
| Garlic Herb Shrimp | 1 | 360 | 22 | 200 | 7 | NA | 80 | 580 | 23 | 3 | 19 | 1 1/2 carb, 2 med-fat meat, 2 fat |
| Grilled Chicken | 1 | 280 | 15 | 130 | 4 | NA | 40 | 450 | 22 | 3 | 15 | 1 1/2 carb, 2 med-fat meat, 1 fat |

| | | | | | | | | | | | | |
|---|---|---|---|---|---|---|---|---|---|---|---|---|
| Grilled Chicken, Gourmet | 1 | 360 | 21 | 190 | 7 | NA | 65 | 670 | 23 | 3 | 22 | 1 1/2 carb, 3 med-fat meat, 1 fat |
| Grilled Mahi Mahi | 1 | 300 | 17 | 160 | 4 | NA | 25 | 250 | 22 | 4 | 15 | 1 1/2 carb, 2 med-fat meat, 1 fat |
| Grilled Portobello & Poblano | 1 | 310 | 19 | 170 | 6 | NA | 25 | 340 | 25 | 4 | 12 | 1 1/2 carb, 1 med-fat meat, 3 fat |
| Grilled Shrimp | 1 | 230 | 12 | 110 | 2 | NA | 90 | 540 | 22 | 3 | 9 | 1 1/2 carb, 1 med-fat meat, 1 fat |
| Grilled Steak | 1 | 220 | 10 | 90 | 4 | NA | 30 | 520 | 22 | 3 | 13 | 1 1/2 carb, 1 med-fat meat, 1 fat |
| Grilled Steak, Gourmet | 1 | 370 | 23 | 210 | 8 | NA | 55 | 800 | 23 | 3 | 20 | 1 1/2 carb, 3 med-fat meat, 2 |
| HealthMe, Chicken | 1 | 150 | 1.5 | 15 | 0 | NA | 30 | 400 | 21 | 3 | 12 | 1 1/2 carb, 1 lean meat |
| HealthMe, Mahi Mahi | 1 | 160 | 4 | 35 | 0.5 | NA | 10 | 200 | 21 | 3 | 12 | 1 1/2 carb, 1 med-fat meat |
| Street Taco, Carnitas | 1 | 100 | 5 | 45 | 1.5 | NA | 20 | 250 | 9 | 2 | 7 | 1/2 carb, 1 med-fat meat |
| Street Taco, Chicken | 1 | 100 | 4 | 30 | 0.5 | NA | 25 | 240 | 9 | 2 | 10 | 1/2 carb, 1 med-fat meat |

| | Serving | Calories | Fat (g) | Cal. from Fat | Sat. Fat (g) | Trans Fat (g) | Chol. (mg) | Sod. (mg) | Carb. (g) | Fiber (g) | Prot. (g) | Servings/Exchanges |
|---|---|---|---|---|---|---|---|---|---|---|---|---|
| Street Taco, Steak | 1 | 120 | 6 | 50 | 2 | NA | 20 | 380 | 9 | 2 | 8 | 1/2 carb, 1 med-fat meat |
| World Famous | 1 | 270 | 14 | 130 | 2 | NA | 35 | 420 | 29 | 3 | 10 | 2 carb, 1 med-fat meat, 2 fat |
| ***Kid's Meals*** | | | | | | | | | | | | |
| Bean & Cheese Burrito | 1 | 530 | 23 | 200 | 11 | NA | 50 | 1200 | 63 | 8 | 20 | 4 carb, 1 med-fat meat, 4 fat |
| Cheese Quesadilla | 1 | 500 | 27 | 240 | 14 | NA | 70 | 1030 | 44 | 1 | 23 | 3 carb, 2 med-fat meat, 3 fat |
| Taquitos | 2 | 230 | 10 | 90 | 4.5 | NA | 50 | 270 | 21 | 2 | 15 | 1 1/2 carb, 1 med-fat meat, 1 fat |
| ***Rubio's Favorites*** | | | | | | | | | | | | |
| Cheese Quesadilla | 1 | 1070 | 67 | 600 | 28 | NA | 125 | 1820 | 85 | 8 | 38 | 5 1/2 carb, 3 med-fat meat, 10 fat |
| Chicken Quesadilla | 1 | 1190 | 69 | 620 | 29 | NA | 195 | 2370 | 87 | 8 | 61 | 6 carb, 7 med-fat meat, 7 fat |

| | | | | | | | | | | | | |
|---|---|---|---|---|---|---|---|---|---|---|---|---|
| Chicken Taquitos | 3 | 270 | 8 | 70 | 2 | NA | 45 | 360 | 33 | 4 | 16 | 2 carb, 1 med-fat meat, 1 fat |
| Nachos Grande | 1 | 1270 | 78 | 710 | 27 | NA | 120 | 1850 | 112 | 20 | 37 | 7 carb, 2 med-fat meat, 14 fat |
| Nachos Grande Chicken | 1 | 1390 | 80 | 720 | 28 | NA | 190 | 2400 | 114 | 20 | 60 | 7 1/2 carb, 5 med-fat meat, 11 fat |
| Nachos Grande Steak | 1 | 1430 | 87 | 780 | 31 | NA | 175 | 2730 | 114 | 20 | 54 | 7 1/2 carb, 4 med-fat meat, 13 fat |
| Steak Quesadilla | 1 | 1230 | 75 | 680 | 32 | NA | 175 | 2710 | 87 | 8 | 55 | 6 carb, 5 med-fat meat, 10 fat |
| ***Sides*** | | | | | | | | | | | | |
| Black Beans, Regular | 1 | 100 | 1 | 5 | 1 | NA | 0 | 340 | 17 | 2 | 6 | 1 carb |
| Black Beans, Large | 1 | 280 | 0.5 | 5 | 0 | NA | 0 | 950 | 50 | 7 | 17 | 3 carb, 1 lean meat |
| Chips, Regular | 1 | 260 | 13 | 120 | 1 | NA | 0 | 290 | 33 | 4 | 3 | 2 carb, 3 fat |
| Chips, Large | 1 | 570 | 29 | 260 | 2.5 | NA | 0 | 650 | 74 | 9 | 7 | 5 carb, 6 fat |
| Churro | 1 | 170 | 8 | 70 | 2 | NA | 20 | 140 | 22 | 0 | 2 | 1 1/2 carb, 2 fat |
| Guacamole & Chips | 1 | 790 | 49 | 440 | 6 | NA | 0 | 920 | 85 | 16 | 10 | 5 1/2 carb, 5 fat |

| | Serving | Calories | Fat (g) | Cal. from Fat | Sat. Fat (g) | Trans Fat (g) | Chol. (mg) | Sod. (mg) | Carb. (g) | Fiber (g) | Prot. (g) | Servings/Exchanges |
|---|---|---|---|---|---|---|---|---|---|---|---|---|
| Pinto Beans, Regular | 1 | 110 | 2 | 10 | 0.5 | NA | 0 | 340 | 22 | 8 | 2 | 1 1/2 carb |
| Pinto Beans, Large | 1 | 300 | 2.5 | 25 | 1 | NA | 0 | 940 | 65 | 24 | 5 | 4 1/2 carb, 1 fat |
| Rice, Regular | 1 | 120 | 1 | 10 | 0 | NA | 0 | 220 | 25 | 1 | 2 | 1 1/2 carb |
| Rice, Large | 1 | 310 | 3 | 25 | 0 | NA | 0 | 580 | 67 | 2 | 5 | 4 1/2 carb, 1 fat |
| ***Salads, Wrapsalada, Bowls (dressing/sauce included)*** | | | | | | | | | | | | |
| Chicken Chipotle Ranch Salad | 1 | 520 | 35 | 310 | 6 | NA | 80 | 1460 | 24 | 6 | 30 | 1 1/2 carb, 4 med-fat meat, 3 fat |
| Chicken Chipotle Ranch Wrapsalada | 1 | 770 | 42 | 380 | 8 | NA | 80 | 2070 | 65 | 9 | 36 | 4 carb, 3 med-fat meat, 5 fat |
| Chicken Chopped Salad | 1 | 570 | 33 | 300 | 9 | NA | 100 | 1480 | 34 | 7 | 36 | 2 carb, 4 med-fat meat, 3 fat |
| Chicken Chopped Wrapsalada | 1 | 800 | 40 | 360 | 10 | NA | 100 | 2070 | 72 | 9 | 41 | 5 carb, 4 med-fat meat, 4 fat |
| Chicken Fiesta Salad | 1 | 590 | 46 | 410 | 11 | NA | 105 | 1130 | 13 | 4 | 32 | 1 carb, 4 med-fat meat, 5 fat |

| | | | | | | | | | | | | |
|---|---|---|---|---|---|---|---|---|---|---|---|---|
| Chicken Fiesta Wrapsalada | 1 | 830 | 53 | 480 | 12 | NA | 105 | 1740 | 53 | 8 | 38 | 3 1/2 carb, 4 med-fat meat, 7 fat |
| Chicken Tropical Salad | 1 | 410 | 23 | 200 | 3.5 | NA | 75 | 720 | 25 | 5 | 27 | 1 1/2 carb, 3 med-fat meat, 2 fat |
| Chicken Tropical Wrapsalada | 1 | 650 | 30 | 270 | 5 | NA | 75 | 1320 | 64 | 8 | 32 | 4 carb, 3 med-fat meat, 3 fat |
| **STARBUCKS** | | | | | | | | | | | | |
| ***Brewed Coffees*** | | | | | | | | | | | | |
| Caffè Misto/Caffè AuLait, 2% Milk | 12 oz | 80 | 3 | 30 | 2 | 0 | 15 | 70 | 7 | 0 | 5 | 1/2 low-fat milk |
| Iced Brewed Coffee | 12 oz | 60 | 0 | 0 | 0 | 0 | 0 | 0 | 15 | 0 | 0 | 1 carb |
| Iced Coffee, 2% Milk | 12 oz | 90 | 1 | 10 | 0.5 | 0 | 5 | 25 | 18 | 0 | 2 | 1 carb |
| ***Espresso, Hot*** | | | | | | | | | | | | |
| Caffè Americano | 12 oz | 10 | 0 | 0 | 0 | 0 | 0 | 0 | 5 | 2 | 1 | free |
| Caffè Latte, 2% Milk | 12 oz | 150 | 6 | 50 | 3.5 | 0 | 25 | 115 | 14 | 0 | 10 | 1 low-fat milk |
| Caffè Mocha, 2% Milk with Whipped Cream | 12 oz | 270 | 12 | 110 | 7 | 0 | 40 | 105 | 33 | 1 | 10 | 1 low-fat milk, 1 1/2 carb, 1 fat |

| | Serving | Calories | Fat (g) | Cal. from Fat | Sat. Fat (g) | Trans Fat (g) | Chol. (mg) | Sod. (mg) | Carb. (g) | Fiber (g) | Prot. (g) | Servings/Exchanges |
|---|---|---|---|---|---|---|---|---|---|---|---|---|
| Cappuccino, 2% Milk | 12 oz | 90 | 3.5 | 30 | 2 | 0 | 15 | 70 | 9 | 0 | 6 | 1 low-fat milk |
| Caramel Macchiato, 2% Milk | 12 oz | 180 | 5 | 45 | 3.5 | 0 | 20 | 100 | 25 | 0 | 8 | 1 low-fat milk, 1 carb |
| Espresso Solo | 1 oz | 5 | 0 | 0 | 0 | 0 | 0 | 0 | 1 | 0 | 0 | free |
| Espresso Truffle with Whipped Cream | 12 oz | 360 | 15 | 130 | 9 | 0 | 35 | 115 | 45 | 5 | 15 | 1 low-fat milk, 2 carb, 2 fat |
| Peppermint Mocha with Whipped Cream | 12 oz | 320 | 13 | 120 | 7 | 0 | 40 | 100 | 46 | 2 | 10 | 1 low-fat meat, 2 carb, 2 fat |
| Skinny Caramel Latte, Nonfat Milk | 12 oz | 130 | 0 | 0 | 0 | 0 | 5 | 170 | 19 | 0 | 12 | 1 skim milk, 1/2 carb |
| Skinny Latte, Nonfat Milk | 12 oz | 100 | 0 | 0 | 0 | 0 | 5 | 120 | 15 | 0 | 10 | 1 skim milk |
| Skinny Vanilla Latte, Nonfat Milk | 12 oz | 90 | 0 | 0 | 0 | 0 | 5 | 125 | 14 | 0 | 9 | 1 skim milk |
| Vanilla Latte, 2% Milk | 12 oz | 190 | 5 | 45 | 3.5 | 0 | 20 | 110 | 27 | 0 | 9 | 1 low-fat milk, 1 carb |

| | | | | | | | | | | | | |
|---|---|---|---|---|---|---|---|---|---|---|---|---|
| White Chocolate Mocha, 2% Milk with Whipped Cream | 12 oz | 370 | 15 | 130 | 10 | 0 | 45 | 190 | 48 | 0 | 12 | 1 low-fat milk, 2 1/2 carb, 2 fat |
| ***Espresso, Iced*** | | | | | | | | | | | | |
| Iced Caffè Americano | 12 oz | 10 | 0 | 0 | 0 | 0 | 0 | 5 | 2 | 0 | 1 | free |
| Iced Caffè Latte, 2% Milk | 12 oz | 100 | 3.5 | 30 | 2.5 | 0 | 15 | 80 | 10 | 0 | 6 | 1 low-fat milk |
| Iced Caffè Mocha, 2% Milk with Whipped Cream | 12 oz | 230 | 12 | 110 | 7 | 0 | 40 | 70 | 29 | 1 | 7 | 1 low-fat milk, 1 carb, 1 fat |
| Iced Caramel Macchiato, 2% Milk | 12 oz | 170 | 5 | 45 | 3 | 0 | 20 | 95 | 24 | 0 | 7 | 1 low-fat milk, 1 carb |
| Iced Espresso Truffle with Whipped Cream | 12 oz | 270 | 13 | 120 | 8 | 0 | 40 | 75 | 29 | 3 | 8 | 1 low-fat milk, 1 carb, 2 fat |
| Iced Sugar Free Syrup Latte, 2% Milk | 12 oz | 90 | 3 | 30 | 2 | 0 | 15 | 85 | 9 | 0 | 6 | 1 low-fat milk |

| | Serving | Calories | Fat (g) | Cal. from Fat | Sat. Fat (g) | Trans Fat (g) | Chol. (mg) | Sod. (mg) | Carb. (g) | Fiber (g) | Prot. (g) | Servings/Exchanges |
|---|---|---|---|---|---|---|---|---|---|---|---|---|
| Iced Vanilla Latte, 2% Milk | 12 oz | 140 | 3 | 30 | 2 | 0 | 15 | 70 | 23 | 0 | 6 | 1 low-fat milk, 1 carb |
| ***Frappuccino Blended Coffee*** | | | | | | | | | | | | |
| Caffè Vanilla with Whipped Cream | 12 oz | 320 | 10 | 90 | 6 | 0 | 40 | 190 | 52 | 0 | 4 | 3 carb, 2 fat |
| Caramel with Whipped Cream | 12 oz | 300 | 11 | 100 | 7 | 0 | 40 | 190 | 46 | 0 | 4 | 3 carb, 2 fat |
| Coffee | 12 oz | 180 | 2.5 | 20 | 1.5 | 0 | 10 | 170 | 37 | 0 | 4 | 2 1/2 carb, 1 fat |
| Mocha with Whipped Cream | 12 oz | 280 | 11 | 100 | 6 | 0 | 40 | 180 | 43 | 0 | 5 | 3 carb, 2 fat |
| Pumpkin Spice with Whipped Cream | 12 oz | 310 | 11 | 100 | 7 | 0 | 40 | 210 | 49 | 0 | 5 | 3 carb, 2 fat |
| ***Frappuccino Light Blended Coffee*** | | | | | | | | | | | | |
| Caffè Vanilla | 12 oz | 140 | 0.5 | 5 | 0 | 0 | 0 | 180 | 30 | 2 | 4 | 2 carb |

| | | | | | | | | | | | | |
|---|---|---|---|---|---|---|---|---|---|---|---|---|
| Caramel | 12 oz | 130 | 1 | 10 | 0 | 0 | 5 | 180 | 25 | 2 | 4 | 1 1/2 carb |
| Coffee | 12 oz | 90 | 0.5 | 5 | 0 | 0 | 0 | 160 | 18 | 2 | 4 | 1 carb |
| Mocha | 12 oz | 110 | 1 | 10 | 0 | 0 | 0 | 170 | 23 | 2 | 4 | 1 1/2 carb |
| Pumpkin | 12 oz | 120 | 0.5 | 5 | 0 | 0 | 0 | 190 | 25 | 2 | 5 | 1 1/2 carb |
| ***Frappuccino Blended Crème*** | | | | | | | | | | | | |
| Double Chocolaty Chip with Whipped Cream | 12 oz | 380 | 14 | 120 | 8 | 0 | 35 | 240 | 59 | 2 | 11 | 4 carb, 3 fat |
| Pumpkin Spice with Whipped Cream | 12 oz | 360 | 10 | 90 | 5 | 0 | 35 | 280 | 58 | 0 | 10 | 4 carb, 2 fat |
| Strawberries & Crème with Whipped Cream | 12 oz | 360 | 10 | 90 | 6 | 0 | 30 | 310 | 58 | 1 | 9 | 4 carb, 2 fat |
| Vanilla Bean with Whipped Cream | 12 oz | 470 | 14 | 120 | 7 | 0 | 50 | 320 | 75 | 0 | 12 | 5 carb, 3 fat |
| ***Brownies, Cookies, Bars*** | | | | | | | | | | | | |
| Chocolate Chunk Cookie | 1 | 360 | 17 | 150 | 10 | 0 | 65 | 170 | 50 | 2 | 4 | 3 carb, 3 fat |

| | Serving | Calories | Fat (g) | Cal. from Fat | Sat. Fat (g) | Trans Fat (g) | Chol. (mg) | Sod. (mg) | Carb. (g) | Fiber (g) | Prot. (g) | Servings/Exchanges |
|---|---|---|---|---|---|---|---|---|---|---|---|---|
| Double Chocolate Brownie | 1 | 410 | 24 | 220 | 7 | 0 | 95 | 75 | 46 | 3 | 6 | 3 carb, 5 fat |
| Marshmallow Dream Bar | 1 | 210 | 4 | 35 | 2.5 | 0 | 10 | 250 | 43 | 0 | 1 | 3 carb, 1 fat |
| Outrageous Oatmeal Cookie | 1 | 370 | 14 | 120 | 8 | 0 | 65 | 170 | 56 | 3 | 5 | 3 1/2 carb, 3 fat |
| Starbuck's Indulgent Cookie | 1 | 320 | 19 | 170 | 11 | 0 | 60 | 85 | 40 | 3 | 4 | 2 1/2 carb, 4 fat |
| Rich Toffee Pecan Bar | 1 | 380 | 22 | 200 | 8 | 0 | 85 | 120 | 42 | <1 | 4 | 3 carb, 4 fat |
| ***Cakes, Pies, Tarts*** | | | | | | | | | | | | |
| Cherry Cherry Pie | 1 piece | 370 | 19 | 170 | 11 | 0 | 40 | 410 | 46 | 2 | 4 | 3 carb, 4 fat |
| Luscious Lemon Tart | 1 | 410 | 25 | 220 | 14 | 0.5 | 145 | 25 | 42 | <1 | 5 | 3 carb, 5 fat |
| ***Croissants, Bagels*** | | | | | | | | | | | | |
| Butter Croissant | 1 | 310 | 18 | 160 | 11 | 1 | 45 | 290 | 32 | <1 | 5 | 2 carb, 4 fat |

| | | | | | | | | | | | | |
|---|---|---|---|---|---|---|---|---|---|---|---|---|
| Chonga Bagel | 1 | 310 | 5 | 50 | 2 | 0 | 10 | 540 | 52 | 3 | 12 | 3 1/2 carb, 1 fat |
| ***Doughnuts, Sweet Rolls, Danish*** | | | | | | | | | | | | |
| Apple Fritter | 1 | 420 | 20 | 180 | 9 | 0 | 0 | 360 | 59 | 1 | 5 | 4 carb, 4 fat |
| Cheese Danish | 1 | 420 | 25 | 230 | 16 | 0 | 115 | 370 | 39 | <1 | 7 | 2 1/2 carb, 5 fat |
| Chocolate Old Fashioned Doughnut | 1 | 420 | 21 | 190 | 9 | 0 | 20 | 340 | 57 | 2 | 5 | 4 carb, 4 fat |
| Classic Glazed | 1 | 420 | 21 | 190 | 10 | 0 | 15 | 260 | 57 | <1 | 4 | 4 carb, 4 fat |
| Double Iced Cinnamon Roll | 1 | 490 | 20 | 180 | 12 | 1 | 65 | 480 | 70 | 3 | 7 | 4 1/2 carb, 4 fat |
| Morning Bun | 1 | 350 | 16 | 140 | 9 | 0 | 75 | 330 | 45 | 2 | 6 | 3 carb, 3 fat |
| ***Loaves, Coffee Cakes*** | | | | | | | | | | | | |
| Banana Nut Bread | 1 slice | 480 | 19 | 170 | 2.5 | 0 | 25 | 210 | 73 | 4 | 7 | 5 carb, 4 fat |
| Classic Coffee Cake | 1 slice | 420 | 19 | 170 | 10 | 0 | 90 | 530 | 59 | 1 | 6 | 4 carb, 4 fat |
| Pumpkin Loaf | 1 slice | 320 | 12 | 110 | 2 | 0 | 45 | 400 | 50 | 1 | 5 | 3 carb, 2 fat |
| Reduced-Fat Cinnamon Swirl Coffee Cake | 1 slice | 290 | 7 | 60 | 3.5 | 0 | 10 | 390 | 55 | 2 | 4 | 3 1/2 carb, 1 fat |

| | Serving | Calories | Fat (g) | Cal. from Fat | Sat. Fat (g) | Trans Fat (g) | Chol. (mg) | Sod. (mg) | Carb. (g) | Fiber (g) | Prot. (g) | Servings/Exchanges |
|---|---|---|---|---|---|---|---|---|---|---|---|---|
| Reduced-Fat Very Berry Coffee Cake | 1 slice | 320 | 9 | 90 | 3.5 | 0 | 55 | 470 | 54 | 4 | 6 | 3 1/2 carb, 2 fat |
| ***Muffins, Scones*** | | | | | | | | | | | | |
| Apple Bran Muffin | 1 | 350 | 9 | 80 | 2.5 | 0 | 65 | 520 | 64 | 7 | 6 | 4 carb, 2 fat |
| Blueberry Scone | 1 | 460 | 22 | 190 | 12 | 0.5 | 75 | 420 | 61 | 2 | 7 | 4 carb, 4 fat |
| Blueberry Streusel Muffin | 1 | 360 | 11 | 100 | 6 | 0 | 80 | 390 | 59 | 2 | 7 | 4 carb, 2 fat |
| Petite Vanilla Bean Scone | 1 | 140 | 5 | 45 | 2.5 | 0 | 15 | 90 | 21 | 0 | 0 | 1 1/2 carb, 1 fat |
| **SUBWAY** | | | | | | | | | | | | |
| ***6-Inch Low Fat Sandwiches*** | | | | | | | | | | | | |
| Black Forest Ham | 1 | 290 | 4.5 | 40 | 1 | 0 | 25 | 1200 | 47 | 5 | 18 | 3 carb, 1 med-fat meat |
| Oven Roasted Chicken Breast | 1 | 320 | 4.5 | 40 | 1 | 0 | 25 | 750 | 49 | 5 | 23 | 3 carb, 2 lean meat |

| | | | | | | | | | | | |
|---|---|---|---|---|---|---|---|---|---|---|---|
| Roast Beef | 1 | 310 | 4.5 | 40 | 1.5 | 0 | 25 | 840 | 46 | 5 | 26 | 3 carb, 2 lean meat |
| Subway Club | 1 | 320 | 5 | 45 | 1.5 | 0 | 35 | 1160 | 47 | 5 | 26 | 3 carb, 2 lean meat |
| Sweet Onion Chicken Teriyaki | 1 | 380 | 4.5 | 40 | 1 | 0 | 50 | 1010 | 60 | 5 | 26 | 4 carb, 2 lean meat |
| Turkey Breast | 1 | 280 | 3.5 | 30 | 1 | 0 | 20 | 920 | 47 | 5 | 18 | 3 carb, 1 med-fat meat |
| Veggie Delite | 1 | 230 | 2.5 | 20 | 0.5 | 0 | 0 | 410 | 45 | 5 | 8 | 3 carb, 1 fat |
| ***6-Inch Sandwiches*** | | | | | | | | | | | | |
| Big Philly Cheesesteak | 1 | 520 | 18 | 160 | 9 | 0.5 | 90 | 1570 | 53 | 6 | 39 | 3 1/2 carb, 4 med-fat meat |
| BLT | 1 | 360 | 13 | 120 | 6 | 0 | 30 | 990 | 45 | 5 | 17 | 3 carb, 1 med-fat meat, 2 fat |
| Chicken & Bacon Ranch | 1 | 570 | 28 | 250 | 10 | 0.5 | 95 | 1190 | 49 | 6 | 35 | 3 carb, 4 med-fat meat, 2 fat |
| Cold Cut Combo | 1 | 410 | 16 | 150 | 6 | 0.5 | 60 | 1450 | 48 | 5 | 21 | 3 carb, 2 med-fat meat, 1 fat |
| Italian BMT | 1 | 450 | 20 | 180 | 8 | 0.5 | 55 | 1730 | 48 | 5 | 22 | 3 carb, 2 med-fat meat, 2 fat |

| | Serving | Calories | Fat (g) | Cal. from Fat | Sat. Fat (g) | Trans Fat (g) | Chol. (mg) | Sod. (mg) | Carb. (g) | Fiber (g) | Prot. (g) | Servings/Exchanges |
|---|---|---|---|---|---|---|---|---|---|---|---|---|
| Meatball Marinara | 1 | 580 | 23 | 200 | 9 | 1 | 45 | 1530 | 70 | 9 | 24 | 4 1/2 carb, 2 med-fat meat, 3 fat |
| Spicy Italian | 1 | 520 | 28 | 250 | 11 | 0.5 | 65 | 1830 | 47 | 5 | 22 | 3 carb, 2 med-fat meat, 4 fat |
| Subway Melt | 1 | 380 | 11 | 100 | 5 | 0 | 45 | 1530 | 49 | 5 | 25 | 3 carb, 2 med-fat meat |
| The Feast | 1 | 540 | 22 | 200 | 9 | 0.5 | 85 | 2470 | 50 | 5 | 39 | 3 carb, 4 med-fat meat |
| Tuna | 1 | 530 | 30 | 270 | 6 | 0.5 | 45 | 930 | 46 | 5 | 21 | 3 carb, 2 med-fat meat, 4 fat |
| ***Flatbread Sandwiches*** | | | | | | | | | | | | |
| Black Forest Ham | 1 | 320 | 7 | 60 | 1.5 | 0 | 25 | 1270 | 47 | 3 | 18 | 3 carb, 1 med-fat meat |
| Oven Roasted Chicken Breast | 1 | 350 | 7 | 70 | 1.5 | 0 | 25 | 820 | 48 | 3 | 24 | 3 carb, 2 lean meat |
| Roast Beef | 1 | 340 | 8 | 70 | 2 | 0 | 25 | 920 | 45 | 3 | 27 | 3 carb, 3 lean meat |
| Subway Club | 1 | 350 | 8 | 70 | 1.5 | 0 | 35 | 1230 | 47 | 3 | 26 | 3 carb, 2 med-fat meat |

| | | | | | | | | | | | | |
|---|---|---|---|---|---|---|---|---|---|---|---|---|
| Sweet Onion Teriyaki | 1 | 410 | 7 | 70 | 1.5 | 0 | 50 | 1080 | 59 | 3 | 26 | 4 carb, 2 lean meat |
| Turkey Breast | 1 | 310 | 6 | 60 | 1 | 0 | 20 | 990 | 47 | 3 | 18 | 3 carb, 1 med-fat meat |
| Veggie Delite | 1 | 260 | 5 | 45 | 1 | 0 | 0 | 490 | 44 | 3 | 9 | 3 carb, 1 fat |
| ***Salads (dressing & croutons not included)*** | | | | | | | | | | | | |
| Ham | 1 | 110 | 3 | 25 | 1 | 0 | 25 | 850 | 12 | 4 | 12 | 2 vegetable, 1 lean meat |
| Oven Roasted Chicken Breast | 1 | 130 | 2.5 | 25 | 0.5 | 0 | 50 | 280 | 10 | 4 | 20 | 2 vegetable, 2 lean meat |
| Roast Beef | 1 | 140 | 3.5 | 30 | 1 | 0 | 25 | 500 | 10 | 4 | 21 | 2 vegetable, 2 lean meat |
| Subway Club | 1 | 140 | 3.5 | 30 | 1 | 0 | 35 | 810 | 12 | 4 | 20 | 2 vegetable, 2 lean meat |
| Sweet Onion Chicken Teriyaki | 1 | 200 | 3 | 30 | 1 | 0 | 50 | 660 | 25 | 4 | 20 | 1 1/2 carb, 2 lean meat |
| Turkey Breast | 1 | 110 | 2 | 20 | 0.5 | 0 | 20 | 570 | 12 | 4 | 12 | 2 vegetable, 1 lean meat |

| | Serving | Calories | Fat (g) | Cal. from Fat | Sat. Fat (g) | Trans Fat (g) | Chol. (mg) | Sod. (mg) | Carb. (g) | Fiber (g) | Prot. (g) | Servings/Exchanges |
|---|---|---|---|---|---|---|---|---|---|---|---|---|
| Veggie Delite | 1 | 50 | 1 | 10 | 0 | 0 | 0 | 65 | 10 | 4 | 3 | 2 vegetable |
| ***Salad Dressing*** | | | | | | | | | | | | |
| Fat Free Italian | 1 pkg | 35 | 0 | 0 | 0 | 0 | 0 | 720 | 7 | 0 | 1 | 1/2 carb |
| Ranch | 1 pkg | 290 | 30 | 270 | 4.5 | 0.5 | 15 | 540 | 3 | 0 | 1 | 6 fat |
| ***Breakfast Sandwiches, 6-Inch Bread*** | | | | | | | | | | | | |
| Black Forest Ham & Cheese | 1 | 450 | 19 | 170 | 7 | 0 | 200 | 1450 | 47 | 5 | 27 | 3 carb, 3 med-fat meat, 1 fat |
| Cheese | 1 | 420 | 18 | 160 | 7 | 0 | 190 | 1060 | 46 | 5 | 22 | 3 carb, 2 med-fat meat, 2 fat |
| Double Bacon & Cheese | 1 | 520 | 25 | 220 | 11 | 0 | 210 | 1440 | 47 | 5 | 29 | 3 carb, 3 med-fat meat, 2 fat |
| Mega | 1 | 720 | 45 | 400 | 18 | 0 | 235 | 1580 | 47 | 5 | 33 | 3 carb, 3 med-fat meat, 6 fat |
| Sausage & Cheese | 1 | 670 | 41 | 370 | 16 | 0 | 225 | 1390 | 46 | 5 | 30 | 3 carb, 3 med-fat meat, 5 fat |

| | | | | | | | | | | | | |
|---|---|---|---|---|---|---|---|---|---|---|---|---|
| Western Egg with Cheese | 1 | 450 | 19 | 170 | 7 | 0 | 200 | 1460 | 48 | 5 | 27 | 3 carb, 3 med-fat meat, 1 fat |
| ***Cookies & Desserts*** | | | | | | | | | | | | |
| Apple Pie | 1 | 250 | 10 | 90 | 2 | NA | 0 | 290 | 37 | 1 | 0 | 2 1/2 carb, 2 fat |
| Apple Slices | 1 pkg | 35 | 0 | 0 | 0 | 0 | 0 | 0 | 9 | 2 | 0 | 1/2 fruit |
| Chocolate Chip Cookie | 1 | 210 | 10 | 90 | 6 | 0 | 15 | 150 | 30 | 1 | 2 | 2 carb, 2 fat |
| Chocolate Chunk Cookie | 1 | 220 | 10 | 90 | 5 | 0 | 10 | 100 | 30 | <1 | 2 | 2 carb, 2 fat |
| M&M Cookie | 1 | 210 | 10 | 90 | 5 | 0 | 10 | 100 | 32 | <1 | 2 | 2 carb, 2 fat |
| Oatmeal Raisin Cookie | 1 | 200 | 8 | 70 | 4 | 0 | 15 | 170 | 30 | 1 | 3 | 2 carb, 2 fat |
| Peanut Butter Cookie | 1 | 220 | 12 | 110 | 5 | 0 | 15 | 190 | 26 | 1 | 4 | 2 carb, 2 fat |
| Sugar Cookie | 1 | 220 | 12 | 110 | 6 | 0 | 15 | 140 | 28 | <1 | 2 | 2 carb, 2 fat |
| White Chip Macadamia Nut Cookie | 1 | 220 | 11 | 100 | 5 | 0 | 15 | 160 | 29 | <1 | 2 | 2 carb, 2 fat |
| ***Soup*** | | | | | | | | | | | | |
| Chicken & Dumpling | 10 oz | 170 | 6 | 45 | 2 | 0 | 35 | 810 | 23 | 2 | 8 | 1 1/2 carb, 1 med-fat meat |

FAST FOOD

| | Serving | Calories | Fat (g) | Cal. from Fat | Sat. Fat (g) | Trans Fat (g) | Chol. (mg) | Sod. (mg) | Carb. (g) | Fiber (g) | Prot. (g) | Servings/Exchanges |
|---|---|---|---|---|---|---|---|---|---|---|---|---|
| Chicken Tortilla | 10 oz | 110 | 1.5 | 20 | 0.5 | 0 | 10 | 440 | 11 | 3 | 6 | 1 carb |
| Chili Con Carne | 10 oz | 340 | 11 | 100 | 5 | 0 | 60 | 650 | 35 | 10 | 20 | 2 carb, 2 med-fat meat |
| Chipotle Chicken Corn Chowder | 10 oz | 140 | 3 | 30 | 1.5 | 0 | 15 | 900 | 22 | 2 | 6 | 1 1/2 carb, 1 fat |
| Cream of Potato with Bacon | 10 oz | 240 | 13 | 120 | 5 | 0 | 15 | 870 | 26 | 3 | 5 | 2 carb, 3 fat |
| Golden Broccoli & Cheese | 10 oz | 180 | 11 | 100 | 5 | 0 | 25 | 990 | 16 | 4 | 5 | 1 carb, 2 fat |
| Minestrone | 10 oz | 90 | 1 | 10 | 0 | 0 | <5 | 910 | 17 | 3 | 4 | 1 carb |
| New England Style Clam Chowder | 10 oz | 150 | 5 | 45 | 1 | 0 | 10 | 990 | 20 | 4 | 6 | 1 carb, 1 fat |
| Roasted Chicken Noodle | 10 oz | 80 | 2 | 20 | 0.5 | 0 | 15 | 950 | 12 | 1 | 6 | 1 carb |
| Vegetable Beef | 10 oz | 100 | 2 | 20 | 0.5 | 0 | 10 | 960 | 17 | 3 | 5 | 1 carb |

| TACO BELL | | | | | | | | | | | | |
|---|---|---|---|---|---|---|---|---|---|---|---|---|
| ***Fresco Menu*** | | | | | | | | | | | | |
| Crunchy Taco | 1 | 150 | 7 | 70 | 2.5 | 0 | 20 | 350 | 12 | 3 | 7 | 1 carb, 1 med-fat meat |
| Soft Taco, Beef | 1 | 180 | 7 | 60 | 3 | 0 | 20 | 640 | 22 | 3 | 8 | 1 1/2 carb, 1 med-fat meat |
| Ranchero Chicken Soft Taco | 1 | 170 | 4 | 35 | 1.5 | 0 | 25 | 740 | 22 | 2 | 12 | 1 1/2 carb, 1 med-fat meat |
| Grilled Steak Soft Taco | 1 | 160 | 4.5 | 40 | 1.5 | 0 | 15 | 600 | 21 | 2 | 9 | 1 1/2 carb, 1 med-fat meat |
| Burrito Supreme, Chicken | 1 | 340 | 8 | 70 | 2.5 | 0 | 25 | 1390 | 49 | 6 | 18 | 3 carb, 1 med-fat meat, 1 fat |
| Burrito Supreme, Steak | 1 | 330 | 8 | 70 | 2.5 | 0 | 15 | 1310 | 49 | 6 | 15 | 3 carb, 1 med-fat meat, 1 fat |
| ***Value Menu*** | | | | | | | | | | | | |
| Bean Burrito | 1 | 350 | 9 | 80 | 3.5 | 0.5 | 5 | 1220 | 54 | 9 | 13 | 3 1/2 carb, 1 med-fat meat, 1 fat |

FAST FOOD

| | Serving | Calories | Fat (g) | Cal. from Fat | Sat. Fat (g) | Trans Fat (g) | Chol. (mg) | Sod. (mg) | Carb. (g) | Fiber (g) | Prot. (g) | Servings/Exchanges |
|---|---|---|---|---|---|---|---|---|---|---|---|---|
| Caramel Apple Empanada | 1 | 310 | 15 | 140 | 2.5 | 0 | 0 | 310 | 39 | 2 | 3 | 2 1/2 carb, 3 fat |
| Cheese Roll-Up | 1 | 200 | 10 | 90 | 5 | 0 | 20 | 530 | 19 | 2 | 9 | 1 carb, 1 med-fat meat, 1 fat |
| Cinnamon Twists | 1 order | 170 | 7 | 60 | 0 | 0 | 0 | 200 | 26 | 1 | 1 | 2 carb, 1 fat |
| Crispy Potato Soft Taco | 1 | 260 | 13 | 120 | 3 | 0 | 10 | 690 | 31 | 3 | 6 | 2 carb, 3 fat |
| Crunchy Taco | 1 | 170 | 10 | 90 | 3.5 | 0 | 30 | 330 | 12 | 3 | 8 | 1 carb, 1 med-fat meat, 1 fat |
| Grilled Chicken Soft Taco | 1 | 440 | 20 | 180 | 5 | 0 | 40 | 1260 | 48 | 3 | 16 | 3 carb, 1 med-fat meat, 3 fat |
| Grilled Chicken Soft Taco | 1 | 200 | 8 | 70 | 3 | 0 | 35 | 640 | 19 | 1 | 12 | 1 carb, 1 med-fat meat, 1 fat |
| Soft Taco | 1 | 210 | 9 | 80 | 4 | 0 | 30 | 620 | 21 | 3 | 10 | 1 1/2 carb, 1 med-fat meat, 1 fat |
| Triple Layer Nachos | 1 | 340 | 18 | 160 | 1.5 | 0 | 0 | 720 | 38 | 6 | 7 | 2 1/2 carb, 4 fat |

| | | | | | | | | | | | | |
|---|---|---|---|---|---|---|---|---|---|---|---|---|
| ***Tacos*** | | | | | | | | | | | | |
| Crunchy Taco Supreme | 1 | 200 | 12 | 100 | 5 | 0 | 35 | 350 | 15 | 3 | 9 | 1 carb, 1 med-fat meat, 1 fat |
| Double Decker Taco | 1 | 320 | 13 | 120 | 4.5 | 0.5 | 30 | 800 | 38 | 7 | 14 | 2 1/2 carb, 1 med-fat meat, 2 fat |
| Double Decker Taco Supreme | 1 | 350 | 15 | 140 | 6 | 1 | 35 | 820 | 40 | 7 | 14 | 2 1/2 carb, 1 med-fat meat, 2 fat |
| Grilled Steak Soft Taco | 1 | 250 | 14 | 130 | 4 | 0 | 30 | 710 | 20 | 2 | 11 | 1 carb, 1 med-fat meat, 2 fat |
| Ranchero Chicken Soft Taco | 1 | 270 | 14 | 120 | 4 | 0 | 40 | 840 | 21 | 2 | 14 | 1 1/2 carb, 1 med-fat meat, 2 fat |
| Soft Taco Supreme, Beef | 1 | 240 | 11 | 100 | 5 | 0 | 35 | 650 | 24 | 3 | 11 | 1 1/2 carb, 1 med-fat meat, 1 fat |
| ***Gorditas*** | | | | | | | | | | | | |
| Gordita Baja, Beef | 1 | 360 | 21 | 190 | 5 | 0 | 35 | 800 | 30 | 5 | 13 | 2 carb, 1 med-fat meat, 3 fat |

| | Serving | Calories | Fat (g) | Cal. from Fat | Sat. Fat (g) | Trans Fat (g) | Chol. (mg) | Sod. (mg) | Carb. (g) | Fiber (g) | Prot. (g) | Servings/Exchanges |
|---|---|---|---|---|---|---|---|---|---|---|---|---|
| Gordita Baja, Chicken | 1 | 340 | 18 | 160 | 3.5 | 0 | 40 | 840 | 29 | 3 | 17 | 2 carb, 2 med-fat meat, 2 fat |
| Gordita Baja, Steak | 1 | 330 | 18 | 160 | 4 | 0 | 30 | 760 | 28 | 3 | 14 | 2 carb, 1 med-fat meat, 2 fat |
| Gordita Nacho Cheese, Beef | 1 | 320 | 16 | 150 | 3.5 | 0 | 20 | 780 | 31 | 4 | 12 | 2 carb, 1 med-fat meat, 2 fat |
| Gordita Nacho Cheese, Chicken | 1 | 300 | 13 | 120 | 2 | 0 | 25 | 820 | 30 | 2 | 15 | 2 carb, 1 med-fat meat, 2 fat |
| Gordita Nacho Cheese, Steak | 1 | 290 | 13 | 120 | 2 | 0 | 15 | 740 | 29 | 2 | 13 | 2 carb, 1 med-fat meat, 2 fat |
| Gordita Supreme, Beef | 1 | 320 | 16 | 150 | 5 | 0 | 35 | 640 | 30 | 4 | 13 | 2 carb, 1 med-fat meat, 2 fat |
| Gordita Supreme, Chicken | 1 | 300 | 13 | 120 | 3.5 | 0 | 35 | 680 | 29 | 3 | 17 | 2 carb, 2 med-fat meat, 1 fat |
| Gordita Supreme, Steak | 1 | 290 | 13 | 120 | 4 | 0 | 30 | 610 | 29 | 3 | 14 | 2 carb, 1 med-fat meat, 2 fat |

| | | | | | | | | | | | | |
|---|---|---|---|---|---|---|---|---|---|---|---|---|
| ***Chalupas*** | | | | | | | | | | | | |
| Chalupa Baja, Beef | 1 | 410 | 26 | 230 | 5 | 0 | 35 | 770 | 31 | 4 | 13 | 2 carb, 1 med-fat meat, 4 fat |
| Chalupa Baja, Chicken | 1 | 390 | 23 | 200 | 4 | 0 | 40 | 800 | 29 | 2 | 17 | 2 carb, 2 med-fat meat, 3 fat |
| Chalupa Nacho Cheese, Beef | 1 | 370 | 21 | 190 | 3.5 | 0 | 25 | 750 | 32 | 3 | 12 | 2 carb, 1 med-fat meat, 4 fat |
| Chalupa Nacho Cheese, Chicken | 1 | 350 | 18 | 160 | 2 | 0 | 25 | 780 | 30 | 2 | 16 | 2 carb, 1 med-fat meat, 3 fat |
| Chalupa Supreme, Beef | 1 | 370 | 21 | 190 | 6 | 0.5 | 35 | 310 | 31 | 3 | 14 | 2 carb, 1 med-fat meat, 3 fat |
| Chalupa Supreme, Chicken | 1 | 350 | 18 | 160 | 4 | 0 | 40 | 650 | 30 | 2 | 17 | 2 carb, 2 med-fat meat, 2 fat |
| Chalupa Supreme, Steak | 1 | 340 | 18 | 160 | 4 | 0 | 30 | 580 | 29 | 2 | 15 | 2 carb, 1 med-fat meat, 3 fat |
| ***Burritos*** | | | | | | | | | | | | |
| 1/2 lb Combo Burrito | 1 | 450 | 17 | 160 | 7 | 1 | 50 | 1610 | 51 | 9 | 21 | 3 1/2 carb, 2 med-fat meat, 1 fat |

| | Serving | Calories | Fat (g) | Cal. from Fat | Sat. Fat (g) | Trans Fat (g) | Chol. (mg) | Sod. (mg) | Carb. (g) | Fiber (g) | Prot. (g) | Servings/Exchanges |
|---|---|---|---|---|---|---|---|---|---|---|---|---|
| 1/2 lb Nacho Crunch Burrito | 1 | 520 | 25 | 230 | 8 | 0.5 | 50 | 1400 | 54 | 6 | 19 | 3 1/2 carb, 1 med-fat meat, 4 fat |
| 7-Layer Burrito | 1 | 490 | 17 | 160 | 6 | 1 | 20 | 1360 | 67 | 10 | 17 | 4 1/2 carb, 1 med-fat meat, 2 fat |
| Bean Burrito | 1 | 350 | 9 | 80 | 3.5 | 0.5 | 5 | 1220 | 54 | 9 | 13 | 3 1/2 carb, 1 med-fat meat, 1 fat |
| Burrito Supreme, Chicken | 1 | 390 | 12 | 110 | 5 | 0 | 40 | 1390 | 51 | 6 | 20 | 3 1/2 carb, 2 med-fat meat |
| Burrito Supreme, Steak | 1 | 380 | 12 | 110 | 5 | 0.5 | 30 | 1320 | 50 | 6 | 17 | 3 carb, 1 med-fat meat, 1 fat |
| Cheesy Bean & Rice Burrito | 1 | 470 | 21 | 180 | 5 | 0 | 15 | 1420 | 60 | 6 | 12 | 4 carb, 4 fat |
| Cheesy Double Beef Burrito | 1 | 470 | 20 | 180 | 6 | 0.5 | 40 | 1580 | 54 | 6 | 18 | 3 1/2 carb, 1 med-fat meat, 3 fat |

| | | | | | | | | | | | | |
|---|---|---|---|---|---|---|---|---|---|---|---|---|
| Grilled Stuft Burrito, Beef | 1 | 690 | 30 | 270 | 10 | 1 | 60 | 2110 | 79 | 10 | 26 | 5 carb, 2 med-fat meat, 4 fat |
| Grilled Stuft Burrito, Chicken | 1 | 650 | 23 | 210 | 7 | 0.5 | 70 | 2180 | 76 | 7 | 33 | 5 carb, 3 med-fat meat, 2 fat |
| Grilled Stuft Burrito, Steak | 1 | 630 | 24 | 220 | 8 | 1 | 50 | 2040 | 75 | 7 | 28 | 5 carb, 2 med-fat meat, 3 fat |
| ***Volcano Menu*** | | | | | | | | | | | | |
| Volcano Nachos | 1 order | 990 | 61 | 550 | 9 | 1.5 | 45 | 1880 | 88 | 14 | 20 | 6 carb, 12 fat |
| Volcano Taco | 1 | 240 | 17 | 150 | 5 | 0 | 35 | 470 | 14 | 3 | 8 | 1 carb, 1 med-fat meat, 2 fat |
| Volcano Burrito | 1 | 800 | 42 | 380 | 12 | 1 | 70 | 2010 | 81 | 8 | 24 | 5 1/2 carb, 1 med-fat meat, 7 fat |
| ***Taco Salads*** | | | | | | | | | | | | |
| Chicken Ranch Taco Salad | 1 | 960 | 57 | 510 | 10 | 1 | 70 | 1710 | 78 | 8 | 36 | 5 carb, 3 med-fat meat, 8 fat |
| Chipotle Steak Taco Salad | 1 | 950 | 59 | 530 | 11 | 1 | 65 | 1760 | 76 | 8 | 29 | 5 carb, 2 med-fat meat, 10 fat |

FAST FOOD

| | Serving | Calories | Fat (g) | Cal. from Fat | Sat. Fat (g) | Trans Fat (g) | Chol. (mg) | Sod. (mg) | Carb. (g) | Fiber (g) | Prot. (g) | Servings/Exchanges |
|---|---|---|---|---|---|---|---|---|---|---|---|---|
| Fiesta Taco Salad | 1 | 820 | 43 | 380 | 10 | 1.5 | 60 | 1740 | 81 | 15 | 30 | 5 1/2 carb, 2 med-fat meat, 7 fat |
| Fiesta Taco Salad without Shell | 1 | 460 | 22 | 200 | 8 | 1.5 | 60 | 1470 | 41 | 13 | 24 | 2 1/2 carb, 2 med-fat meat, 2 fat |
| ***Specialties*** | | | | | | | | | | | | |
| Chicken Grilled Taquito | 1 | 320 | 11 | 100 | 4.5 | 0 | 40 | 1000 | 37 | 2 | 18 | 2 1/2 carb, 2 med-fat meat |
| Steak Grilled Taquito | 1 | 310 | 11 | 100 | 5 | 0 | 30 | 930 | 37 | 2 | 15 | 2 1/2 carb, 1 med-fat meat, 1 fat |
| Chicken Quesadilla | 1 | 520 | 27 | 240 | 12 | 0.5 | 80 | 1490 | 41 | 4 | 28 | 2 1/2 carb, 3 med-fat meat, 2 fat |
| Steak Quesadilla | 1 | 510 | 28 | 250 | 12 | 1 | 65 | 1340 | 40 | 4 | 25 | 2 1/2 carb, 2 med-fat meat, 4 fat |
| Crunchwrap Supreme | 1 | 540 | 21 | 190 | 7 | 0 | 30 | 1400 | 71 | 6 | 16 | 4 1/2 carb, 1 med-fat meat, 3 fat |

| | | | | | | | | | | | | |
|---|---|---|---|---|---|---|---|---|---|---|---|---|
| Enchirito, Beef | 1 | 360 | 17 | 150 | 8 | 1 | 45 | 1410 | 35 | 7 | 18 | 2 carb, 2 med-fat meat, 1 fat |
| Enchirito, Chicken | 1 | 340 | 13 | 120 | 7 | 0.5 | 50 | 1450 | 33 | 6 | 22 | 2 carb, 2 med-fat meat, 1 fat |
| Enchirito, Steak | 1 | 330 | 14 | 120 | 7 | 0.5 | 45 | 1370 | 33 | 6 | 19 | 2 carb, 2 med-fat meat, 1 fat |
| Express Taco Salad | 1 | 600 | 30 | 270 | 9 | 1.5 | 60 | 1380 | 57 | 15 | 25 | 4 carb, 2 med-fat meat, 4 fat |
| Mexican Pizza | 1 | 530 | 30 | 270 | 8 | 1 | 45 | 990 | 46 | 7 | 20 | 3 carb, 2 med-fat meat, 4 fat |
| MexiMelt | 1 | 280 | 14 | 130 | 7 | 0.5 | 45 | 870 | 23 | 4 | 15 | 1 1/2 carb, 2 med-fat meat, 1 fat |
| ***Nacho, Sides*** | | | | | | | | | | | | |
| Cheesy Fiesta Potatoes | 1 order | 270 | 16 | 140 | 2.5 | 0 | 5 | 840 | 28 | 3 | 4 | 2 carb, 3 fat |
| Mexican Rice | 1 order | 130 | 3.5 | 35 | 0 | 0 | 0 | 410 | 21 | 1 | 2 | 1 1/2 carb, 1 fat |
| Nachos | 1 order | 330 | 21 | 190 | 2 | 0 | 0 | 520 | 31 | 2 | 4 | 2 carb, 4 fat |

FAST FOOD

| | Serving | Calories | Fat (g) | Cal. from Fat | Sat. Fat (g) | Trans Fat (g) | Chol. (mg) | Sod. (mg) | Carb. (g) | Fiber (g) | Prot. (g) | Servings/Exchanges |
|---|---|---|---|---|---|---|---|---|---|---|---|---|
| Nachos Supreme | 1 order | 430 | 24 | 220 | 4.5 | 0.5 | 30 | 780 | 41 | 7 | 13 | 2 1/2 carb, 1 med-fat meat, 4 fat |
| Nachos BellGrande | 1 order | 760 | 42 | 380 | 6 | 1 | 30 | 1250 | 77 | 12 | 19 | 5 carb, 1 med-fat meat, 7 fat |
| Pintos 'n Cheese | 1 order | 170 | 6 | 60 | 3 | 0.5 | 15 | 670 | 18 | 7 | 9 | 1 carb, 1 med-fat meat |
| **TACO JOHN'S** | | | | | | | | | | | | |
| ***Burritos*** | | | | | | | | | | | | |
| Bean Burrito | 1 | 380 | 9 | 80 | 3 | 0 | 15 | 830 | 58 | 9 | 15 | 4 carb, 2 fat |
| Beefy Burrito | 1 | 440 | 20 | 180 | 7 | 1 | 50 | 860 | 45 | 7 | 22 | 3 carb, 2 med-fat meat, 2 fat |
| Beef Grilled Burrito | 1 | 600 | 32 | 280 | 13 | 1 | 75 | 1230 | 52 | 8 | 27 | 3 1/2 carb, 2 med-fat meat, 4 fat |
| Chicken & Potato Burrito | 1 | 470 | 19 | 170 | 4.5 | 0 | 30 | 1220 | 54 | 7 | 17 | 3 1/2 carb, 1 med-fat meat, 3 fat |

| | | | | | | | | | | | | |
|---|---|---|---|---|---|---|---|---|---|---|---|---|
| Chicken Grilled Burrito | 1 | 590 | 29 | 260 | 11 | 0.5 | 90 | 1510 | 50 | 6 | 32 | 3 carb, 3 med-fat meat, 3 fat |
| Combination Burrito | 1 | 400 | 14 | 130 | 5 | 0.5 | 35 | 830 | 50 | 8 | 18 | 3 carb, 1 med-fat meat, 2 fat |
| Meat & Potato Burrito | 1 | 500 | 23 | 210 | 6 | 0.5 | 30 | 1100 | 58 | 8 | 15 | 4 carb, 5 fat |
| Super Burrito | 1 | 450 | 18 | 160 | 7 | 0.5 | 40 | 920 | 54 | 9 | 19 | 3 1/2 carb, 1 med-fat meat, 3 fat |
| ***Desserts*** | | | | | | | | | | | | |
| Apple Grande | 1 | 270 | 12 | 110 | 3 | 0 | 5 | 420 | 38 | 2 | 5 | 2 1/2 carb, 2 fat |
| Choco Taco | 1 | 390 | 20 | 180 | 15 | 0 | 15 | 160 | 48 | 1 | 5 | 3 carb, 4 fat |
| Churros | 1 | 190 | 7 | 60 | 1.5 | 0 | 20 | 170 | 15 | 4 | 2 | 1 carb, 1 fat |
| ***Local Favorites*** | | | | | | | | | | | | |
| Chili Cheese Potato Oles | 1 | 590 | 36 | 320 | 8 | 0.5 | 25 | 2130 | 55 | 8 | 13 | 3 1/2 carb, 1 med-fat meat, 6 fat |
| Chili Enchilada | 1 | 310 | 16 | 140 | 7 | 1 | 50 | 1000 | 24 | 4 | 18 | 1 1/2 carb, 2 med-fat meat, 1 fat |

| | Serving | Calories | Fat (g) | Cal. from Fat | Sat. Fat (g) | Trans Fat (g) | Chol. (mg) | Sod. (mg) | Carb. (g) | Fiber (g) | Prot. (g) | Servings/Exchanges |
|---|---|---|---|---|---|---|---|---|---|---|---|---|
| Chillito | 1 | 510 | 20 | 180 | 8 | 1 | 45 | 1330 | 60 | 10 | 23 | 4 carb, 2 med-fat meat, 2 fat |
| Mexi Rolls with Nacho Cheese | 4 pieces | 260 | 10 | 90 | 4 | 0.5 | 20 | 370 | 28 | 4 | 13 | 2 carb, 1 med-fat meat, 1 fat |
| Ranch Burrito, Beef | 1 | 440 | 22 | 220 | 6 | 0 | 45 | 850 | 45 | 6 | 17 | 3 carb, 1 med-fat meat, 3 fat |
| Ranch Burrito, Chicken | 1 | 400 | 17 | 160 | 4.5 | 0 | 45 | 970 | 44 | 5 | 19 | 3 carb, 1 med-fat meat, 2 fat |
| Smothered Burrito | 1 | 510 | 20 | 180 | 8 | 1 | 45 | 1330 | 60 | 10 | 23 | 4 carb, 2 med-fat meat, 2 fat |
| ***Sides*** | | | | | | | | | | | | |
| Chili without Crackers | 1 order | 220 | 11 | 100 | 5 | 0 | 35 | 1240 | 17 | 4 | 14 | 1 carb, 2 med-fat meat |
| Mexican Rice | 1 order | 250 | 6 | 50 | 0 | 0 | 0 | 1080 | 45 | 0 | 5 | 3 carb, 1 fat |
| Nachos | 1 order | 380 | 23 | 210 | 6 | 0 | 10 | 750 | 38 | 1 | 6 | 2 1/2 carb, 5 fat |
| Potato Oles, Small | 1 order | 430 | 26 | 230 | 3.5 | 0 | 0 | 1220 | 45 | 6 | 4 | 3 carb, 5 fat |

| | | | | | | | | | | | | |
|---|---|---|---|---|---|---|---|---|---|---|---|---|
| Potato Oles, Medium | 1 order | 600 | 36 | 330 | 5 | 0.5 | 0 | 1710 | 62 | 8 | 6 | 4 carb, 7 fat |
| Potato Oles, Large | 1 order | 770 | 46 | 420 | 6 | 1 | 0 | 2200 | 80 | 11 | 7 | 5 carb, 9 fat |
| Refried Beans | 1 order | 320 | 6 | 60 | 3.5 | 1 | 15 | 1020 | 47 | 11 | 18 | 3 carb, 1 med-fat meat |
| ***Specialties*** | | | | | | | | | | | | |
| Taco Salad, No Dressing | 1 | 520 | 33 | 290 | 11 | 1 | 60 | 860 | 37 | 7 | 21 | 2 1/2 carb, 2 med-fat meat, 5 fat |
| Chicken Taco Salad, No Dressing | 1 | 480 | 27 | 240 | 9 | 0.5 | 65 | 24 | 35 | 6 | 24 | 2 carb, 3 med-fat meat, 2 fat |
| Quesadilla Melt, Cheesy | 1 | 440 | 22 | 220 | 10 | 0.5 | 55 | 1050 | 43 | 5 | 19 | 3 carb, 1 med-fat meat, 3 fat |
| Quesadilla Melt, Fajita Chicken | 1 | 510 | 23 | 210 | 11 | 0.5 | 75 | 1360 | 47 | 6 | 28 | 3 carb, 3 med-fat meat, 2 fat |
| Quesadilla Melt, Fajita Beef | 1 | 540 | 28 | 250 | 12 | 1 | 70 | 1240 | 49 | 7 | 26 | 3 1/2 carb, 2 med-fat meat, 4 fat |
| Super Nachos | Regular order | 810 | 48 | 430 | 16 | 1 | 55 | 1450 | 74 | 5 | 22 | 5 carb, 1 med-fat meat, 9 fat |
| Super Potato Oles | Regular order | 1030 | 65 | 580 | 19 | 1.5 | 55 | 2850 | 87 | 13 | 24 | 5 1/2 carb, 1 med-fat meat, 12 fat |

| | Serving | Calories | Fat (g) | Cal. from Fat | Sat. Fat (g) | Trans Fat (g) | Chol. (mg) | Sod. (mg) | Carb. (g) | Fiber (g) | Prot. (g) | Servings/Exchanges |
|---|---|---|---|---|---|---|---|---|---|---|---|---|
| ***Tacos*** | | | | | | | | | | | | |
| Chicken Softshell Taco | 1 | 190 | 6 | 50 | 3 | 0 | 30 | 700 | 19 | 1 | 13 | 1 carb, 1 med-fat meat |
| Crispy Taco | 1 | 180 | 10 | 90 | 3.5 | 0 | 25 | 270 | 13 | 2 | 9 | 1 carb, 1 med-fat meat, 1 fat |
| Softshell Taco | 1 | 220 | 11 | 90 | 4.5 | 0.5 | 25 | 580 | 21 | 2 | 11 | 1 1/2 carb, 1 med-fat meat, 1 fat |
| Taco Bravo | 1 | 340 | 13 | 120 | 4.5 | 0.5 | 25 | 750 | 40 | 5 | 15 | 2 1/2 carb, 1 med-fat meat, 2 fat |
| Taco Burger | 1 | 270 | 12 | 110 | 4 | 0.5 | 30 | 600 | 28 | 3 | 14 | 2 carb, 1 med-fat meat, 1 fat |
| **WENDY'S** | | | | | | | | | | | | |
| ***Sandwiches*** | | | | | | | | | | | | |
| Hamburger Kid's Meal | 1 | 220 | 8 | 70 | 3 | 0 | 30 | 490 | 25 | 1 | 12 | 1 1/2 carb, 1 med-fat meat, 1 fat |

| | | | | | | | | | | | | |
|---|---|---|---|---|---|---|---|---|---|---|---|---|
| Cheeseburger, Kid's Meal | 1 | 260 | 11 | 100 | 5 | 0.5 | 40 | 700 | 26 | 1 | 15 | 2 carb, 1 med-fat meat, 1 fat |
| Jr. Hamburger | 1 | 230 | 8 | 70 | 3 | 0 | 30 | 490 | 26 | 1 | 13 | 2 carb, 1 med-fat meat, 1 fat |
| Jr. Cheeseburger | 1 | 270 | 11 | 100 | 5 | 0.5 | 40 | 700 | 26 | 1 | 15 | 2 carb, 1 med-fat meat, 2 fat |
| Jr. Cheeseburger Deluxe | 1 | 300 | 14 | 130 | 6 | 0.5 | 45 | 730 | 28 | 2 | 15 | 2 carb, 1 med-fat meat, 2 fat |
| Jr. Bacon Cheeseburger | 1 | 310 | 16 | 140 | 6 | 0.5 | 50 | 670 | 25 | 1 | 17 | 1 1/2 carb, 2 med-fat meat, 1 fat |
| Single with Everything | 1 | 430 | 20 | 180 | 7 | 1 | 75 | 870 | 38 | 2 | 25 | 2 1/2 carb, 3 med-fat meat, 1 fat |
| Double with Everything & Cheese | 1 | 700 | 40 | 360 | 17 | 2 | 160 | 1440 | 38 | 2 | 47 | 2 1/2 carb, 6 med-fat meat, 2 fat |
| Triple with Everything & Cheese | 1 | 970 | 60 | 540 | 27 | 3.5 | 245 | 2010 | 39 | 2 | 69 | 2 1/2 carb, 9 med-fat meat, 3 fat |

FAST FOOD

| | Serving | Calories | Fat (g) | Cal. from Fat | Sat. Fat (g) | Trans Fat (g) | Chol. (mg) | Sod. (mg) | Carb. (g) | Fiber (g) | Prot. (g) | Servings/Exchanges |
|---|---|---|---|---|---|---|---|---|---|---|---|---|
| Double Stack | 1 | 360 | 18 | 160 | 8 | 1 | 70 | 810 | 26 | 1 | 23 | 2 carb, 2 med-fat meat, 2 fat |
| Baconator | 1 | 830 | 51 | 460 | 23 | 2.5 | 195 | 1880 | 35 | 1 | 56 | 2 carb, 7 med-fat meat, 3 fat |
| Crispy Chicken Sandwich | 1 | 360 | 18 | 160 | 3.5 | 0 | 30 | 710 | 36 | 2 | 15 | 2 1/2 carb, 1 med-fat meat, 3 fat |
| Grilled Chicken Go Wrap | 1 | 250 | 10 | 90 | 3 | 0 | 45 | 730 | 24 | 1 | 17 | 1 1/2 carb, 2 med-fat meat |
| Homestyle Chicken Fillet Sandwich | 1 | 440 | 16 | 140 | 3 | 0 | 50 | 1050 | 47 | 2 | 25 | 3 carb, 2 med-fat meat, 1 fat |
| Spicy Chicken Fillet Sandwich | 1 | 440 | 16 | 140 | 3 | 0 | 55 | 1200 | 49 | 2 | 26 | 3 carb, 2 med-fat meat, 1 fat |
| Ultimate Chicken Grill Sandwich | 1 | 320 | 7 | 60 | 1.5 | 0 | 70 | 950 | 36 | 2 | 28 | 2 1/2 carb, 3 lean meat |

| | | | | | | | | | | | | |
|---|---|---|---|---|---|---|---|---|---|---|---|---|
| Chicken Club Sandwich | 1 | 550 | 26 | 230 | 8 | 0 | 75 | 1290 | 48 | 2 | 34 | 3 carb, 4 med-fat meat, 1 fat |
| ***Chicken*** | | | | | | | | | | | | |
| 4-Piece Kid's Chicken Nuggets Meal | 4 pieces | 190 | 13 | 120 | 3 | 0 | 25 | 380 | 9 | 0 | 9 | 1/2 carb, 1 med-fat meat, 2 fat |
| 5-Piece Chicken Nuggets | 5 pieces | 230 | 16 | 50 | 3.5 | 0 | 30 | 480 | 11 | 0 | 12 | 1 carb, 1 med-fat meat, 2 fat |
| Bold Buffalo Boneless Wings | 1 order | 520 | 18 | 160 | 3.5 | 0 | 75 | 2630 | 58 | 2 | 31 | 4 carb, 3 med-fat meat, 1 fat |
| Honey BBQ Boneless Wings | 1 order | 580 | 18 | 160 | 3.5 | 0 | 75 | 1990 | 75 | 2 | 32 | 5 carb, 2 med-fat meat, 2 fat |
| BBQ Nugget Sauce | 1 pkt | 45 | 0 | 0 | 0 | 0 | 0 | 160 | 11 | 0 | 1 | 1 carb |
| Honey Mustard Nugget Sauce | 1 pkt | 130 | 12 | 110 | 2 | 0 | 10 | 220 | 6 | 0 | 0 | 1/2 carb, 2 fat |
| Sweet & Sour Sauce | 1 pkt | 50 | 0 | 0 | 0 | 0 | 0 | 120 | 12 | 0 | 0 | 1 carb |
| ***Salads*** | | | | | | | | | | | | |
| Chicken Caesar | 1 | 370 | 20 | 170 | 4 | 0 | 85 | 1015 | 18 | 3 | 31 | 1 carb, 4 med-fat meat |

| | Serving | Calories | Fat (g) | Cal. from Fat | Sat. Fat (g) | Trans Fat (g) | Chol. (mg) | Sod. (mg) | Carb. (g) | Fiber (g) | Prot. (g) | Servings/Exchanges |
|---|---|---|---|---|---|---|---|---|---|---|---|---|
| Mandarin Chicken | 1 | 550 | 26 | 230 | 3 | 0 | 65 | 1250 | 49 | 4 | 31 | 3 carb, 3 med-fat meat, 2 fat |
| Southwest Taco | 1 | 645 | 39 | 350 | 16 | 1 | 105 | 1565 | 44 | 8 | 31 | 3 carb, 3 med-fat meat, 5 fat |
| ***Sides*** | | | | | | | | | | | | |
| Baked Potato, Plain | 1 | 270 | 0 | 0 | 0 | 0 | 0 | 25 | 61 | 7 | 7 | 4 carb |
| Baked Potato, Sour Cream & Chives | 1 | 320 | 3.5 | 30 | 0 | 0 | 10 | 50 | 63 | 7 | 8 | 4 carb, 1 fat |
| Caesar Side Salad | 1 | 70 | 4 | 40 | 0 | 0 | 10 | 170 | 4 | 2 | 6 | 1 vegetable, 1 fat |
| Chili, Small | 1 | 190 | 6 | 50 | 2.5 | 0 | 40 | 830 | 19 | 5 | 14 | 1 carb, 2 lean meat |
| Chili, Large | 1 | 280 | 9 | 80 | 3.5 | 0.5 | 60 | 1240 | 29 | 7 | 21 | 2 carb, 2 med-fat meat |
| Fries, Small | 1 order | 330 | 16 | 140 | 0 | 0 | 0 | 300 | 44 | 4 | 4 | 3 carb, 3 fat |
| Fries, Medium | 1 order | 420 | 20 | 180 | 4 | 0 | 0 | 380 | 55 | 5 | 5 | 3 1/2 carb, 4 fat |
| Fries, Large | 1 order | 540 | 26 | 230 | 5 | 0 | 0 | 500 | 71 | 7 | 7 | 4 1/2 carb, 5 fat |

| | | | | | | | | | | | | |
|---|---|---|---|---|---|---|---|---|---|---|---|---|
| Mandarin Orange Cup | 1 | 80 | 0 | 0 | 0 | 0 | 0 | 15 | 19 | 1 | 1 | 1 fruit |
| Side Salad | 1 | 35 | 0 | 0 | 0 | 0 | 0 | 25 | 8 | 2 | 1 | 1 vegetable |
| Frosty, Vanilla, Small | 1 | 310 | 8 | 70 | 5 | 0 | 35 | 180 | 52 | 0 | 8 | 3 1/2 carb, 2 fat |
| Frosty, Vanilla, Large | 1 | 500 | 12 | 110 | 8 | 0.5 | 45 | 220 | 88 | 0 | 9 | 5 1/2 carb, 2 fat |

# FROZEN MEALS, MEAT, CHICKEN, FISH

| | Serving | Calories | Fat (g) | Cal. from Fat | Sat. Fat (g) | Trans Fat (g) | Chol. (mg) | Sod. (mg) | Carb (g) | Fiber (g) | Prot. (g) | Servings/Exchanges |
|---|---|---|---|---|---|---|---|---|---|---|---|---|
| **FROZEN MEALS, ENTRÉES** | | | | | | | | | | | | |
| ***Aunt Jemima Entrees*** | | | | | | | | | | | | |
| Eggs & Bacon | 1 | 300 | 20 | 180 | 6 | 0 | 340 | 910 | 14 | 1 | 15 | 1 carb, 2 med-fat meat, 2 fat |
| Ham & Cheese Omelet | 1 | 260 | 13 | 120 | 3.5 | 0 | 195 | 920 | 21 | 2 | 16 | 1 1/2 carb, 2 med-fat meat, 1 fat |
| Pancakes & Bacon | 1 | 450 | 17 | 150 | 4.5 | 0 | 65 | 1100 | 61 | 3 | 14 | 4 carb, 3 fat |
| Sausage & Egg Scramble | 1 | 300 | 18 | 160 | 5 | 0 | 200 | 890 | 21 | 2 | 15 | 1 1/2 carb, 2 med-fat meat, 2 fat |
| ***Banquet Meals*** | | | | | | | | | | | | |
| Beef Pot Pie | 1 | 450 | 27 | 250 | 11 | 0.5 | 30 | 730 | 36 | 2 | 14 | 2 1/2 carb, 1 med-fat meat, 4 fat |
| Chicken Fingers | 1 | 460 | 15 | 130 | 3.5 | 0.5 | 20 | 730 | 69 | 11 | 13 | 4 1/2 carb, 1 med-fat meat, 2 fat |

| | | | | | | | | | | | | |
|---|---|---|---|---|---|---|---|---|---|---|---|---|
| Chicken Pot Pie | 1 | 370 | 21 | 190 | 9 | 0 | 35 | 850 | 34 | 2 | 10 | 2 carb, 1 med-fat meat, 3 fat |
| Corn Dog | 1 | 470 | 18 | 160 | 4 | 4 | 35 | 730 | 68 | 8 | 11 | 4 1/2 carb, 4 fat |
| Country Fried Beefsteak | 1 | 390 | 19 | 170 | 6 | 0.5 | 35 | 1040 | 41 | 3 | 14 | 2 1/2 carb, 1 med-fat meat, 3 fat |
| Country Fried Pork | 1 | 420 | 23 | 210 | 7 | 0 | 20 | 1140 | 40 | 5 | 13 | 2 1/2 carb, 1 med-fat meat, 4 fat |
| Macaroni & Cheese | 1 | 260 | 6 | 60 | 3 | 0 | 15 | 770 | 40 | 4 | 11 | 2 1/2 carb, 1 med-fat meat |
| Meatloaf | 1 | 280 | 13 | 120 | 5 | 0 | 40 | 1000 | 28 | 4 | 12 | 2 carb, med-fat meat, 2 fat |
| Meatloaf | 1 | 300 | 15 | 140 | 6 | 1 | 35 | 820 | 28 | 5 | 14 | 2 carb, 1 med-fat meat, 3 fat |
| Original Fried Chicken | 1 | 380 | 20 | 210 | 5 | 0 | 30 | 930 | 35 | 5 | 14 | 2 carb, 1 med-fat meat, 3 fat |
| Salisbury Steak | 1 | 300 | 16 | 150 | 6 | 1 | 25 | 1090 | 25 | 5 | 14 | 1 1/2 carb, 2 med-fat meat, 2 fat |

| | Serving | Calories | Fat (g) | Cal. from Fat | Sat. Fat (g) | Trans Fat (g) | Chol. (mg) | Sod. (mg) | Carb. (g) | Fiber (g) | Prot. (g) | Servings/Exchanges |
|---|---|---|---|---|---|---|---|---|---|---|---|---|
| Spaghetti & Meatballs | 1 | 380 | 16 | 150 | 6 | 0 | 25 | 650 | 42 | 5 | 17 | 3 carb, 1 med-fat meat, 2 fat |
| Swedish Meatballs | 1 | 430 | 23 | 210 | 10 | 0.5 | 90 | 950 | 35 | 4 | 20 | 2 carb, 2 med-fat meat, 3 fat |
| Turkey | 1 | 200 | 8 | 80 | 2 | 0 | 30 | 980 | 27 | 5 | 14 | 2 carb, 1 med-fat meat, 1 fat |
| ***Boston Market*** | | | | | | | | | | | | |
| Beef Sirloin & Noodles | 14 oz | 460 | 12 | 110 | 5 | 1 | 105 | 960 | 58 | 4 | 29 | 4 carb, 2 med-fat meat |
| Chicken Parmesan | 16.1 oz | 620 | 24 | 220 | 8 | 1 | 50 | 1580 | 69 | 7 | 33 | 4 1/2 carb, 3 med-fat meat, 2 fat |
| Chicken Pot Pie | 8 oz | 560 | 36 | 330 | 13 | 55 | 0 | 930 | 43 | 2 | 16 | 3 carb, 1 med-fat meat, 6 fat |
| Lasagna with Meat Sauce | 12.6 oz | 500 | 23 | 210 | 11 | 1 | 85 | 1290 | 49 | 4 | 22 | 3 carb, 2 med-fat meat, 3 fat |

| | | | | | | | | | | | | |
|---|---|---|---|---|---|---|---|---|---|---|---|---|
| Meatloaf | 16.1 oz | 710 | 42 | 380 | 15 | 3 | 95 | 1590 | 53 | 5 | 30 | 3 1/2 carb, 3 med-fat meat, 5 fat |
| Salisbury Steak | 16 oz | 710 | 40 | 360 | 17 | 3 | 95 | 1760 | 53 | 5 | 34 | 3 1/2 carb, 3 med-fat meat, 5 fat |
| Turkey Breast Medallions | 15.1 oz | 360 | 14 | 130 | 3 | 1 | 55 | 1570 | 35 | 5 | 24 | 2 carb, 3 med-fat meat |
| ***Eating Right*** | | | | | | | | | | | | |
| Beef Portabello | 9 oz | 260 | 7 | 60 | 2 | 0 | 30 | 680 | 42 | 4 | 16 | 3 carb, 1 med-fat meat |
| Cashew Chicken | 9.7 oz | 290 | 4 | 35 | 1 | 0 | 30 | 460 | 44 | 3 | 18 | 3 carb, 1 med-fat meat |
| Cheese Ravioli | 8.5 oz | 280 | 8 | 70 | 4.5 | 0 | 55 | 610 | 38 | 3 | 12 | 2 1/2 carb, 1 med-fat meat, 1 fat |
| Chicken Poblano | 9 oz | 310 | 8 | 70 | 3 | 0 | 40 | 490 | 37 | 2 | 22 | 2 1/2 carb, 2 med-fat meat |
| Chicken Teriyaki | 8.2 oz | 270 | 4 | 35 | 1 | 0 | 20 | 580 | 44 | 3 | 15 | 3 carb, 1 med-fat meat |
| Five Grain Beef & Vegetables | 8.75 oz | 280 | 5 | 45 | 1 | 0 | 25 | 500 | 43 | 4 | 13 | 3 carb, 1 med-fat meat |

| | Serving | Calories | Fat (g) | Cal. from Fat | Sat. Fat (g) | Trans Fat (g) | Chol. (mg) | Sod. (mg) | Carb. (g) | Fiber (g) | Prot. (g) | Servings/Exchanges |
|---|---|---|---|---|---|---|---|---|---|---|---|---|
| Lasagna with Meat Sauce | 10.7 oz | 370 | 8 | 70 | 3.5 | 0 | 25 | 630 | 55 | 3 | 15 | 3 1/2 carb, 1 med-fat meat, 1 fat |
| Lemongrass Chicken | 9.25 oz | 230 | 7 | 60 | 3 | 0 | 40 | 500 | 26 | 3 | 16 | 2 carb, 1 med-fat meat |
| Macaroni & Cheese | 10 oz | 330 | 8 | 70 | 4.5 | 0 | 25 | 770 | 46 | 2 | 18 | 3 carb, 1 med-fat meat, 1 fat |
| Roasted Turkey | 9.75 oz | 320 | 7 | 80 | 2 | 0 | 55 | 790 | 40 | 3 | 21 | 2 1/2 carb, 2 lean meat |
| Sesame Chicken | 9 oz | 370 | 5 | 45 | 0.5 | 0 | 25 | 450 | 67 | 3 | 16 | 4 1/2 carb, 1 med-fat meat |
| Spaghetti with Meat Sauce | 11.5 oz | 330 | 9 | 80 | 3 | 0 | 15 | 800 | 47 | 4 | 14 | 3 carb, 1 med-fat meat, 1 fat |
| Turkey Lasagna | 11.25 oz | 370 | 9 | 90 | 3 | 0 | 60 | 640 | 48 | 5 | 21 | 3 carb, 2 med-fat meat |
| ***Green Giant Complete Skillet Meal*** | | | | | | | | | | | | |
| Cheesy Macaroni & Beef | 1 cup | 370 | 14 | 120 | 6 | 0 | 35 | 1170 | 48 | 2 | 15 | 3 carb, 1 med-fat meat, 2 fat |

| | | | | | | | | | | | | |
|---|---|---|---|---|---|---|---|---|---|---|---|---|
| Chicken Alfredo | 1 1/4 cup | 260 | 5 | 45 | 2.5 | 0 | 30 | 660 | 39 | 3 | 17 | 2 1/2 carb, 2 lean meat |
| Mexican Style Rice & Beef | 1 cup | 280 | 7 | 70 | 3.5 | 0 | 20 | 810 | 42 | 4 | 11 | 3 carb, 1 fat |
| Pasta Primavera | 1 1/2 cup | 300 | 6 | 50 | 3 | 0 | 30 | 730 | 45 | 4 | 19 | 3 carb, 1 med-fat meat |
| ***Healthy Choice Café Steamers*** | | | | | | | | | | | | |
| Cajun Style Chicken & Shrimp | 10.4 oz | 260 | 4 | 40 | 1 | 0 | 50 | 570 | 40 | 3 | 15 | 2 1/2 carb, 1 med-fat meat |
| Chicken Margherita | 10 oz | 320 | 7 | 70 | 1.5 | 0 | 35 | 580 | 45 | 5 | 18 | 3 carb, 1 med-fat meat |
| Chicken Red Pepper Alfredo | 10.3 oz | 250 | 5 | 45 | 2 | 0 | 35 | 520 | 30 | 4 | 20 | 2 carb, 2 lean meat |
| Grilled Chicken Marinara | 10 oz | 270 | 4.5 | 45 | 1.5 | 0 | 30 | 550 | 35 | 5 | 21 | 2 carb, 2 lean meat |
| Grilled Whiskey Steak | 9.5 oz | 250 | 4 | 40 | 1.5 | 0 | 35 | 560 | 37 | 6 | 15 | 2 1/2 carb, 1 med-fat meat |
| Roasted Beef Merlot | 10 oz | 230 | 8 | 80 | 2 | 0 | 35 | 600 | 21 | 5 | 17 | 1 1/2 carb, 2 med-fat meat |

| | Serving | Calories | Fat (g) | Cal. from Fat | Sat. Fat (g) | Trans Fat (g) | Chol. (mg) | Sod. (mg) | Carb. (g) | Fiber (g) | Prot. (g) | Servings/Exchanges |
|---|---|---|---|---|---|---|---|---|---|---|---|---|
| Sweet Sesame Chicken | 10.3 oz | 340 | 6 | 50 | 1 | 0 | 30 | 330 | 53 | 3 | 17 | 3 1/2 carb, 1 med-fat meat |
| ***Healthy Choice Meals*** | | | | | | | | | | | | |
| Beef Pot Roast | 11.1 oz | 310 | 7 | 45 | 3 | 0 | 45 | 500 | 45 | 5 | 15 | 3 carb, 1 med-fat meat |
| Beef Tips Portabella | 11.4 oz | 300 | 8 | 80 | 2.5 | 0 | 35 | 600 | 33 | 7 | 20 | 2 carb, 2 med-fat meat |
| Chicken Alfredo Florentine | 8.5 oz | 230 | 3.5 | 35 | 1.5 | 0 | 25 | 560 | 31 | 4 | 17 | 2 carb, 2 lean meat |
| Chicken Parmigiana | 11.1 oz | 370 | 9 | 90 | 2 | 0 | 15 | 500 | 56 | 6 | 16 | 3 1/2 carb, 1 med-fat meat, 1 fat |
| Classic Meatloaf | 10 oz | 300 | 7 | 70 | 2.5 | 0 | 35 | 530 | 44 | 7 | 15 | 3 carb, 1 med-fat meat |
| Classic Meatloaf | 12 oz | 300 | 7 | 70 | 2.5 | 0 | 35 | 530 | 44 | 7 | 15 | 3 carb, 1 med-fat meat |
| Country Breaded Chicken | 10.8 oz | 370 | 9 | 90 | 2 | 0 | 25 | 560 | 53 | 6 | 15 | 3 1/2 carb, 1 med-fat meat, 1 fat |
| Country Herb Chicken | 11.5 oz | 240 | 5 | 45 | 1.5 | 0 | 30 | 600 | 34 | 5 | 15 | 2 carb, 1 med-fat meat |
| Fajita Steak | 12.5 oz | 360 | 6 | 60 | 6 | 2 | 40 | 590 | 56 | 7 | 20 | 3 1/2 carb, 2 lean meat |

| | | | | | | | | | | | | |
|---|---|---|---|---|---|---|---|---|---|---|---|---|
| Golden Roast Turkey Breast | 8.6 oz | 300 | 4 | 40 | 1 | 0 | 25 | 550 | 42 | 6 | 21 | 3 carb, 2 lean meat |
| Grilled Chicken Teriyaki | 11.1 oz | 300 | 5 | 45 | 1 | 0 | 30 | 590 | 49 | 5 | 14 | 3 carb, 1 med-fat meat |
| Homestyle Salisbury Steak | 12.8 oz | 360 | 9 | 80 | 3.5 | 0 | 40 | 600 | 46 | 7 | 20 | 3 carb, 2 med-fat meat |
| Honey Ginger Chicken | 8.5 oz | 310 | 4.5 | 45 | 1 | 0 | 25 | 310 | 53 | 3 | 14 | 3 1/2 carb, 1 med-fat meat |
| Lemon Pepper Fish | 10.8 oz | 310 | 4.5 | 45 | 1 | 0 | 20 | 440 | 53 | 5 | 13 | 3 1/2 carb, 1 med-fat meat |
| Marina Manicotti Formaggio | 11.1 oz | 380 | 6 | 60 | 3 | 0 | 25 | 600 | 63 | 8 | 16 | 4 carb, 1 med-fat meat |
| Sesame Chicken | 9.1 oz | 230 | 4.5 | 40 | 1 | 0 | 15 | 600 | 34 | 5 | 12 | 2 carb, 1 med-fat meat |
| Sweet & Sour Chicken | 11.1 oz | 430 | 9 | 90 | 1 | 0 | 20 | 600 | 69 | 5 | 16 | 4 1/2 carb, 1 med-fat meat, 1 fat |
| ***Jimmy Dean*** | | | | | | | | | | | | |
| Bacon, Egg, Cheese Biscuit | 1 | 320 | 18 | 160 | 7 | 3 | 100 | 800 | 27 | 1 | 12 | 2 carb, 1 med-fat meat, 3 fat |

FROZEN MEALS, MEAT, CHICKEN, FISH

| | Serving | Calories | Fat (g) | Cal. from Fat | Sat. Fat (g) | Trans Fat (g) | Chol. (mg) | Sod. (mg) | Carb. (g) | Fiber (g) | Prot. (g) | Servings/Exchanges |
|---|---|---|---|---|---|---|---|---|---|---|---|---|
| Eggs, Potato, Ham Breakfast Bowl | 1 | 390 | 23 | 210 | 9 | 0 | 360 | 1170 | 23 | 3 | 24 | 1 1/2 carb, 3 med-fat meat, 2 fat |
| Eggs, Potato, Sausage, Breakfast Bowl | 1 | 490 | 34 | 310 | 13 | 0 | 370 | 1210 | 20 | 3 | 23 | 1 carb, 3 med-fat meat, 4 fat |
| Pancakes & Sausage Links | 1 | 710 | 31 | 280 | 11 | 0 | 45 | 890 | 93 | 3 | 13 | 6 carb, 6 fat |
| Sausage Biscuit | 1 | 360 | 24 | 220 | 8 | 3 | 30 | 600 | 26 | 1 | 8 | 2 carb, 5 fat |
| ***Lean Cuisine Café Classics*** | | | | | | | | | | | | |
| Beef & Broccoli | 9 oz | 260 | 5 | 45 | 1.5 | 0 | 20 | 580 | 39 | 2 | 14 | 2 1/2 carb, 1 med-fat meat |
| Beef Portabello | 9 oz | 220 | 6 | 50 | 2.5 | 0 | 30 | 640 | 25 | 3 | 16 | 1 1/2 carb, 2 lean meat |
| Chicken & Almonds | 8.5 oz | 250 | 4 | 35 | 0.5 | 0 | 30 | 490 | 38 | 4 | 16 | 2 1/2 carb, 1 med-fat meat |
| Chicken Carbonara | 9 oz | 310 | 8 | 70 | 2 | 0 | 30 | 680 | 36 | 4 | 23 | 2 1/2 carb, 2 med-fat meat |

| | | | | | | | | | | | | |
|---|---|---|---|---|---|---|---|---|---|---|---|---|
| Glazed Chicken | 8.5 oz | 220 | 3.5 | 30 | 1 | 0 | 40 | 500 | 25 | 1 | 21 | 1 1/2 carb, 2 lean meat |
| Grilled Chicken Caesar | 8.5 oz | 260 | 6 | 50 | 2 | 0 | 35 | 590 | 33 | 3 | 18 | 2 carb, 2 lean meat |
| Honey Dijon Grilled Chicken | 8 oz | 220 | 7 | 60 | 2.5 | 0 | 50 | 640 | 22 | 2 | 17 | 1 1/2 carb, 2 lean meat |
| Lemon Pepper Fish | 9 oz | 330 | 8 | 70 | 2.5 | 0 | 40 | 590 | 50 | 2 | 15 | 3 carb, 1 med-fat meat, 1 fat |
| Orange Chicken | 9 oz | 300 | 7 | 60 | 1.5 | 0 | 25 | 580 | 46 | 2 | 14 | 3 carb, 1 med-fat meat |
| Roasted Garlic Chicken | 8.9 oz | 180 | 7 | 60 | 2.5 | 0 | 40 | 650 | 9 | 1 | 20 | 1/2 carb, 3 lean meat |
| Sesame Chicken | 9 oz | 330 | 9 | 80 | 1.5 | 0 | 25 | 650 | 47 | 2 | 16 | 3 carb, 1 med-fat meat, 1 fat |
| Shrimp & Angel Hair Pasta | 10 oz | 220 | 4 | 35 | 1 | 0 | 50 | 590 | 32 | 2 | 14 | 2 carb, 1 med-fat meat |
| Shrimp Alfredo | 9 oz | 260 | 5 | 45 | 2 | 0 | 60 | 590 | 36 | 3 | 18 | 2 1/2 carb, 2 lean meat |
| Steak Tips Portabello | 7.5 oz | 160 | 7 | 60 | 2.5 | 0 | 40 | 450 | 10 | 3 | 15 | 1/2 carb, 2 lean meat |
| Sun Dried Tomato Pesto Chicken | 8.6 oz | 290 | 9 | 80 | 2 | 0 | 30 | 570 | 34 | 4 | 18 | 2 carb, 2 med-fat meat |

| | Serving | Calories | Fat (g) | Cal. from Fat | Sat. Fat (g) | Trans Fat (g) | Chol. (mg) | Sod. (mg) | Carb. (g) | Fiber (g) | Prot. (g) | Servings/Exchanges |
|---|---|---|---|---|---|---|---|---|---|---|---|---|
| Sweet & Sour Chicken | 10 oz | 300 | 3 | 25 | 0.5 | 0 | 30 | 560 | 51 | 2 | 18 | 3 1/2 carb, 1 lean meat |
| Thai-Style Chicken | 9 oz | 290 | 7 | 60 | 2 | 0 | 30 | 560 | 39 | 2 | 18 | 2 1/2 carb, 2 lean meat |
| Three Cheese Chicken | 8 oz | 210 | 9 | 90 | 3 | 0 | 40 | 500 | 10 | 3 | 21 | 1/2 carb, 3 lean meat |
| ***Lean Cuisine One Dish Favorites*** | | | | | | | | | | | | |
| Angel Hair Pomodoro | 10 oz | 250 | 5 | 45 | 2 | 0 | 5 | 620 | 42 | 4 | 8 | 3 carb, 1 fat |
| BBQ Chicken Quesadilla | 5 oz | 260 | 7 | 60 | 2.5 | 0 | 15 | 630 | 35 | 2 | 16 | 2 carb, 1 med-fat meat |
| Cheddar Potatoes with Broccoli | 10.25 oz | 230 | 5 | 45 | 3 | 0 | 15 | 640 | 35 | 4 | 12 | 2 carb, 1 med-fat meat |
| Cheese Ravioli | 8.5 oz | 220 | 5 | 45 | 3 | 0 | 35 | 620 | 33 | 3 | 11 | 2 carb, 1 med-fat meat |
| Chicken Chow Mein with Rice | 9 oz | 260 | 4 | 25 | 1 | 0 | 25 | 550 | 41 | 3 | 14 | 2 1/2 carb, 1 med-fat meat |
| Chicken Enchilada Suiza | 9 oz | 270 | 4 | 35 | 1.5 | 0 | 20 | 550 | 47 | 3 | 12 | 3 carb, 1 med-fat meat |
| Chicken Fettucini | 9.3 oz | 270 | 6 | 50 | 3 | 0 | 40 | 690 | 32 | 0 | 22 | 2 carb, 2 lean meat |

| | | | | | | | | | | | | |
|---|---|---|---|---|---|---|---|---|---|---|---|---|
| Classic Five Cheese Lasagna | 11.5 oz | 360 | 8 | 70 | 3.5 | 0 | 20 | 600 | 51 | 3.5 | 21 | 3 1/2 carb, 2 med-fat meat |
| Fettucini Alfredo | 9.3 oz | 330 | 7 | 60 | 3 | 0 | 15 | 600 | 54 | 3 | 12 | 3 1/2 carb, 1 fat |
| Lasagna with Meat Sauce | 10.5 oz | 320 | 8 | 70 | 4 | 0 | 30 | 630 | 45 | 4 | 17 | 3 carb, 1 med-fat meat, 2 fat |
| Linguine Cabrera | 9.25 oz | 300 | 8 | 70 | 2 | 0 | 15 | 590 | 43 | 2 | 14 | 3 carb, 1 med-fat meat, 1 fat |
| Macaroni & Cheese | 10 oz | 290 | 7 | 60 | 4 | 0 | 20 | 630 | 41 | 1 | 15 | 2 1/2 carb, 1 med-fat meat |
| Pasta Romano with Bacon | 10 oz | 280 | 7 | 60 | 2 | 0 | 10 | 650 | 43 | 4 | 12 | 3 carb, 1 med-fat meat |
| Roasted Chicken with Lemon Pepper Fettuccini | 8.1 oz | 260 | 6 | 50 | 1.5 | 0 | 30 | 650 | 36 | 3 | 16 | 2 1/2 carb, 1 med-fat meat |
| Sante Fe-Style Rice & Beans | 10.4 oz | 300 | 5 | 45 | 2.5 | 0 | 15 | 590 | 52 | 5 | 11 | 3 1/2 carb, 1 fat |
| Spaghetti | 9.5 oz | 270 | 5 | 45 | 2 | 0 | 25 | 560 | 38 | 2 | 18 | 2 1/2 carb, 2 lean meat |

FROZEN MEALS, MEAT, CHICKEN, FISH

| | Serving | Calories | Fat (g) | Cal. from Fat | Sat. Fat (g) | Trans Fat (g) | Chol. (mg) | Sod. (mg) | Carb. (g) | Fiber (g) | Prot. (g) | Servings/Exchanges |
|---|---|---|---|---|---|---|---|---|---|---|---|---|
| Stuffed Cabbage with Whipped Potatoes | 9.5 oz | 210 | 6 | 50 | 1.5 | 0 | 15 | 670 | 28 | 3 | 10 | 2 carb, 1 med-fat meat |
| Swedish Meatballs | 9.125 oz | 300 | 8 | 70 | 3 | 0 | 45 | 620 | 34 | 3 | 22 | 2 carb, 2 med-fat meat |
| ***Lean Cuisine Dinnertime Selects*** | | | | | | | | | | | | |
| Balsamic Glazed Chicken | 12 oz | 330 | 7 | 60 | 2.5 | 0 | 40 | 660 | 41 | 4 | 25 | 2 1/2 carb, 3 lean meat |
| Chicken Fettuccini | 12 oz | 400 | 8 | 70 | 4 | 0 | 50 | 850 | 48 | 6 | 33 | 3 carb, 3 lean meat |
| Chicken Florentine | 13.3 oz | 410 | 9 | 80 | 3.5 | 0 | 45 | 840 | 54 | 6 | 28 | 3 1/2 carb, 2 med-fat meat |
| Grilled Chicken & Penne Pasta | 12 oz | 330 | 4.5 | 40 | 1.5 | 0 | 40 | 580 | 52 | 6 | 20 | 3 1/2 carb, 2 lean meat |
| Jumbo Rigatoni with Meatballs | 15.4 oz | 390 | 8 | 70 | 2.5 | 0 | 35 | 830 | 56 | 7 | 23 | 3 1/2 carb, 2 med-fat meat |
| Roasted Turkey Breast | 12 oz | 290 | 7 | 60 | 1 | 0 | 30 | 890 | 38 | 5 | 19 | 2 1/2 carb, 2 lean meat |
| Salisbury Steak | 12.5 oz | 270 | 8 | 70 | 4 | 0 | 45 | 650 | 27 | 10 | 22 | 2 carb, 2 med-fat meat |

| | | | | | | | | | | | | |
|---|---|---|---|---|---|---|---|---|---|---|---|---|
| Steak Tips Dijon | 12 oz | 280 | 7 | 60 | 2.5 | 0 | 30 | 650 | 33 | 5 | 21 | 2 carb, 2 lean meat |
| ***Lean Cuisine Spa Cuisine*** | | | | | | | | | | | | |
| Chicken in Peanut Sauce | 9 oz | 280 | 8 | 70 | 1.5 | 0 | 25 | 560 | 30 | 5 | 22 | 2 carb, 2 med-fat meat |
| Chicken Mediterranean | 10.5 oz | 240 | 4 | 35 | 1 | 0 | 40 | 590 | 32 | 6 | 19 | 2 carb, 2 lean meat |
| Chicken Pecan | 9 oz | 250 | 6 | 50 | 1 | 0 | 30 | 490 | 33 | 3 | 17 | 2 carb, 2 lean meat |
| Lemon Chicken | 9 oz | 300 | 9 | 80 | 2 | 0 | 25 | 550 | 41 | 3 | 13 | 2 1/2 carb, 1 med-fat meat, 1 fat |
| Lemongrass Chicken | 9.4 oz | 250 | 6 | 50 | 3.5 | 0 | 30 | 610 | 30 | 4 | 18 | 2 carb, 2 lean meat |
| Salmon with Basil | 9.6 oz | 220 | 6 | 50 | 2 | 0 | 20 | 660 | 23 | 4 | 19 | 1 1/2 carb, 2 lean meat |
| ***Marie Callender's Meals*** | | | | | | | | | | | | |
| Beef Pot Pie | 1 cup | 540 | 32 | 290 | 12 | 2 | 25 | 700 | 46 | 4 | 16 | 3 carb, 1 med-fat meat, 5 fat |
| Beef Tips | 1 meal | 360 | 12 | 110 | 4.5 | 0 | 70 | 1450 | 35 | 6 | 26 | 2 carb, 2 med-fat meat |
| Cheesy Chicken Breast & Rice | 1 meal | 480 | 18 | 170 | 13 | 0.5 | 80 | 1500 | 47 | 5 | 31 | 3 carb, 3 med-fat meat, 1 fat |

| | Serving | Calories | Fat (g) | Cal. from Fat | Sat. Fat (g) | Trans Fat (g) | Chol. (mg) | Sod. (mg) | Carb. (g) | Fiber (g) | Prot. (g) | Servings/Exchanges |
|---|---|---|---|---|---|---|---|---|---|---|---|---|
| Chicken & Noodles | 1 meal | 610 | 34 | 310 | 14 | 0.5 | 100 | 1500 | 52 | 5 | 24 | 3 1/2 carb, 2 med-fat meat, 5 fat |
| Chicken Parmesan | 1 meal | 650 | 29 | 270 | 8 | 0 | 35 | 1000 | 66 | 5 | 31 | 4 1/2 carb, 3 med-fat meat, 3 fat |
| Chicken Pot Pie | 1 cup | 600 | 37 | 340 | 15 | 2 | 30 | 850 | 46 | 3 | 17 | 3 carb, 1 med-fat meat, 6 fat |
| Chicken Teriyaki | 1 meal | 430 | 4 | 40 | 1 | 0 | 45 | 1230 | 78 | 5 | 19 | 5 carb, 1 med-fat meat |
| Country Fried Beef | 1 meal | 540 | 28 | 260 | 11 | 1 | 45 | 1510 | 51 | 6 | 19 | 3 1/2 carb, 1 med-fat meat, 5 fat |
| Country Fried Chicken & Gravy | 1 meal | 500 | 21 | 190 | 7 | 0 | 30 | 1590 | 52 | 7 | 24 | 3 1/2 carb, 2 med-fat meat, 2 fat |
| Country Fried Pork Chop | 1 meal | 510 | 23 | 210 | 7 | 0 | 45 | 1560 | 53 | 11 | 21 | 3 1/2 carb, 2 med-fat meat, 3 fat |
| Creamy Mushroom Chicken Pot Pie | 1 cup | 560 | 35 | 320 | 13 | 2 | 30 | 700 | 45 | 3 | 15 | 3 carb, 1 med-fat meat,6 fat |

| | | | | | | | | | | | | |
|---|---|---|---|---|---|---|---|---|---|---|---|---|
| Creamy Parmesan Chicken Pot Pie | 1 cup | 530 | 32 | 290 | 12 | 2 | 30 | 720 | 43 | 2 | 17 | 3 carb, 1 med-fat meat, 5 fat |
| Fettuccini with Chicken & Broccoli | 1 meal | 630 | 37 | 340 | 15 | 0.5 | 90 | 900 | 43 | 6 | 30 | 3 carb, 3 med-fat meat, 4 fat |
| Fried Chicken Tenders | 1 meal | 470 | 19 | 180 | 8 | 0 | 40 | 1450 | 52 | 5 | 21 | 3 1/2 carb, 2 med-fat meat, 2 fat |
| Golden Battered Fish Fillet | 1 meal | 450 | 16 | 150 | 4.5 | 0 | 35 | 1170 | 53 | 4 | 22 | 3 1/2 carb, 2 med-fat meat, 1 fat |
| Grilled Chicken Bake | 1 meal | 610 | 35 | 320 | 14 | 0.5 | 75 | 990 | 43 | 5 | 30 | 3 carb, 3 med-fat meat, 4 fat |
| Herb Roasted Chicken | 1 meal | 460 | 25 | 230 | 7 | 0 | 65 | 1030 | 26 | 5 | 30 | 2 carb, 3 med-fat meat, 2 fat |
| Honey Roasted Chicken Pot Pie | 1 | 530 | 30 | 270 | 12 | 2 | 25 | 880 | 47 | 7 | 16 | 3 carb, 1 med-fat meat, 1 fat |
| Lasagna Bake with Meat Sauce | 1 cup | 240 | 8 | 70 | 4 | 0 | 20 | 870 | 28 | 4 | 13 | 2 carb, 1 med-fat meat, 1 fat |
| Meat Lasagna | 1 cup | 240 | 9 | 80 | 5 | 0 | 45 | 950 | 24 | 2 | 14 | 1 1/2 carb, 1 med-fat meat, 1 fat |

FROZEN MEALS, MEAT, CHICKEN, FISH

| | Serving | Calories | Carb. (g) | Fat (g) | Cal from Fat. | Sat. Fat (g) | Trans Fat (g) | Chol. (mg) | Sod. (mg) | Fiber (g) | Prot. (g) | Servings/Exchanges |
|---|---|---|---|---|---|---|---|---|---|---|---|---|
| Meatloaf & Gravy | 1 meal | 480 | 22 | 200 | 9 | 0.5 | 60 | 1080 | 39 | 3 | 31 | 2 1/2 carb, 3 med-fat meat, 1 fat |
| Old Fashioned Beef Pot Roast | 1 meal | 330 | 10 | 90 | 4 | 0 | 45 | 970 | 32 | 9 | 27 | 2 carb, 3 lean meat |
| Salisbury Steak | 1 meal | 400 | 16 | 150 | 6 | 0 | 50 | 820 | 38 | 7 | 27 | 2 1/2 carb, 3 med-fat meat |
| Sweet & Sour Chicken | 1 meal | 600 | 18 | 160 | 20 | 0 | 25 | 860 | 88 | 10 | 22 | 6 carb, 1 med-fat meat, 3 fat |
| Turkey Pot Pie | 1 | 670 | 41 | 370 | 16 | 2.5 | 25 | 1000 | 56 | 4 | 19 | 3 1/2 carb, 1 med-fat meat, 7 fat |
| Turkey with Stuffing | 1 meal | 400 | 9 | 90 | 2.5 | 0 | 65 | 1230 | 45 | 4 | 32 | 3 carb, 3 lean meat |
| ***Michael Angelo's*** | | | | | | | | | | | | |
| Chicken Alfredo | 1 cup | 310 | 10 | 90 | 8 | 0 | 55 | 690 | 34 | 1 | 19 | 2 carb, 2 med-fat meat |
| Eggplant Parmesan | 6 oz | 250 | 15 | 140 | 7 | 0 | 60 | 540 | 16 | 3 | 13 | 1 carb, 1 med-fat meat, 2 fat |

| | | | | | | | | | | | | |
|---|---|---|---|---|---|---|---|---|---|---|---|---|
| Lasagna with Meat Sauce | 1 cup | 300 | 11 | 100 | 6 | 0 | 55 | 560 | 30 | 3 | 20 | 2 carb, 2 med-fat meat |
| Vegetable Lasagna | 1 cup | 230 | 7 | 60 | 3 | 0 | 15 | 720 | 23 | 3 | 20 | 1 1/2 carb, 2 lean meat |
| ***Michelina's Authentico*** | | | | | | | | | | | | |
| Chicken Fried Rice | 8.1 oz | 410 | 11 | 100 | 2 | 0 | 40 | 1100 | 64 | 2 | 12 | 4 carb, 2 fat |
| Chicken Primavera with Spirals | 8.1 oz | 320 | 7 | 60 | 3 | 0 | 25 | 630 | 48 | 3 | 14 | 3 carb, 1 med-fat meat |
| Chicken Primavira with Spirals | 8.1 oz | 320 | 7 | 60 | 3 | 0 | 25 | 630 | 48 | 3 | 14 | 3 carb, 1 med-fat meat |
| Fettucine Alfredo | 9.1 oz | 390 | 16 | 150 | 8 | 0.5 | 40 | 650 | 45 | 2 | 14 | 3 carb, 1 med-fat meat, 2 fat |
| Four Cheese Lasagna | 8.1 oz | 280 | 6 | 60 | 3 | 0 | 15 | 500 | 43 | 3 | 12 | 3 carb, 1 med-fat meat |
| Lasagana Mozarella | 8.1 oz | 260 | 7 | 60 | 3.5 | 0 | 20 | 540 | 39 | 3 | 9 | 2 1/2 carb, 1 med-fat meat |
| Lasagna with Meat Sauce | 9.1 oz | 320 | 10 | 90 | 4 | 0 | 35 | 740 | 40 | 3 | 14 | 2 1/2 carb, 1 med-fat meat, 1 fat |

| | Serving | Calories | Carb. (g) | Fat (g) | Cal from Fat. | Sat. Fat (g) | Trans Fat (g) | Chol. (mg) | Sod. (mg) | Fiber (g) | Prot. (g) | Servings/Exchanges |
|---|---|---|---|---|---|---|---|---|---|---|---|---|
| Macaroni & Cheese Bake | 8.1 oz | 240 | 4 | 35 | 2 | 0 | 10 | 540 | 41 | 2 | 9 | 2 1/2 carb, 1 fat |
| Pasta with Chicken | 8.1 oz | 290 | 10 | 90 | 4 | 0 | 35 | 800 | 38 | 2 | 12 | 2 1/2 carb, 1 med-fat meat, 1 fat |
| Penne with Chicken | 8.6 oz | 330 | 9 | 80 | 4 | 0 | 35 | 610 | 48 | 2 | 14 | 3 carb, 1 med-fat meat, 1 fat |
| Risotto Parmigiano | 8.1 oz | 420 | 18 | 160 | 9 | 0.5 | 45 | 770 | 49 | 1 | 16 | 3 carb, 1 med-fat meat, 2 fat |
| Stroganoff | 8.1 oz | 400 | 18 | 160 | 7 | 0 | 35 | 740 | 38 | 2 | 13 | 2 1/2 carb, 1 med-fat meat, 3 fat |
| Sweet & Sour Chicken | 8.6 oz | 370 | 2.5 | 25 | 0.5 | 0 | 15 | 970 | 68 | 1 | 10 | 4 1/2 carb, 1 fat |
| Wheels & Cheese | 8.1 oz | 350 | 11 | 90 | 4.5 | 0 | 20 | 780 | 48 | 2 | 13 | 3 carb, 1 med-fat meat, 1 fat |
| ***Michelina's Budget Gourmet*** | | | | | | | | | | | | |
| Angel Hair Pasta | 8 oz | 290 | 5 | 50 | 2 | 0 | 10 | 410 | 48 | 4 | 11 | 3 carb, 1 fat |

| | | | | | | | | | | | | |
|---|---|---|---|---|---|---|---|---|---|---|---|---|
| Chinese-Style Vegetables & White Chicken | 8 oz | 310 | 5 | 45 | 0.5 | 0 | 5 | 670 | 57 | 2 | 8 | 4 carb, 1 fat |
| Fettuccine Alfredo | 8 oz | 300 | 9 | 90 | 4.5 | 0 | 25 | 640 | 42 | 2 | 11 | 3 carb, 2 fat |
| Italian-Style Vegetables & White Chicken | 8 oz | 270 | 5 | 45 | 1 | 0 | 10 | 540 | 44 | 4 | 11 | 3 carb, 1 fat |
| Lasagna Alfredo with Broccoli | 8 oz | 300 | 12 | 110 | 6 | 0 | 30 | 560 | 36 | 2 | 10 | 2 1/2 carb, 1 med-fat meat, 1 fat |
| Lasagna with Meat Sauce | 8 oz | 260 | 8 | 70 | 2.5 | 0 | 15 | 680 | 34 | 3 | 10 | 2 carb, 1 med-fat meat, 1 fat |
| Macaroni & Cheese | 8 oz | 310 | 10 | 90 | 4 | 0 | 20 | 730 | 42 | 2 | 12 | 3 carb, 1 med-fat meat, 1 fat |
| Rigatoni in Sauce | 8 oz | 290 | 9 | 70 | 3.5 | 0 | 25 | 570 | 43 | 3 | 11 | 3 carb, 2 fat |
| Spaghetti Marinara | 8 oz | 270 | 3.5 | 30 | 1 | 0 | 0 | 620 | 49 | 3 | 9 | 3 carb, 1 fat |
| Stir Fry Rice & Vegetables | 8 oz | 450 | 20 | 180 | 4 | 0 | 10 | 700 | 60 | 2 | 7 | 4 carb, 4 fat |

| | Serving | Calories | Fat (g) | Cal. from Fat | Sat. Fat (g) | Trans Fat (g) | Chol. (mg) | Sod. (mg) | Carb. (g) | Fiber (g) | Prot. (g) | Servings/Exchanges |
|---|---|---|---|---|---|---|---|---|---|---|---|---|
| Szechwan-Style Vegetables & White Chicken | 8 oz | 280 | 2.5 | 20 | 0 | 0 | 5 | 880 | 51 | 2 | 10 | 3 1/2 carb, 1 fat |
| Wild Rice Pilaf with Vegetables | 8 oz | 320 | 6 | 50 | 2.5 | 0 | 10 | 630 | 59 | 2 | 7 | 4 carb, 1 fat |
| Ziti Parmesano | 8 oz | 250 | 7 | 60 | 3 | 0 | 10 | 500 | 37 | 3 | 10 | 2 1/2 carb, 1 fat |
| ***Michelina's Lean Gourmet*** | | | | | | | | | | | | |
| Beef Pepper Steak & Rice | 8.1 oz | 270 | 4 | 30 | 1 | 0 | 10 | 700 | 47 | 2 | 11 | 3 carb, 1 fat |
| Cheese Stuffed Rigatoni | 8.1 oz | 220 | 6 | 50 | 3 | 0 | 30 | 510 | 33 | 3 | 8 | 2 carb, 1 fat |
| Chicken Alfredo Florentine | 8.1 oz | 250 | 7 | 60 | 3.5 | 0 | 40 | 690 | 34 | 2 | 12 | 2 carb, 1 med-fat meat |
| Creamy Parmesan Chicken | 8.1 oz | 250 | 4.5 | 40 | 2 | 0 | 30 | 580 | 37 | 2 | 13 | 2 1/2 carb, 1 med-fat meat |
| Enchilada Bake | 8.6 oz | 300 | 8 | 70 | 2.5 | 0 | 15 | 750 | 47 | 6 | 11 | 3 carb, 2 fat |

| | | | | | | | | | | | | |
|---|---|---|---|---|---|---|---|---|---|---|---|---|
| Five Cheese Lasagna | 8.1 oz | 290 | 5 | 50 | 2 | 0 | 10 | 560 | 50 | 8 | 13 | 3 carb, 1 med-fat meat |
| Glazed Chicken | 8.1 oz | 250 | 3 | 25 | 0.5 | 0 | 20 | 470 | 46 | 1 | 10 | 3 carb, 1 fat |
| Macaroni & Cheese | 9.1 oz | 270 | 3.5 | 35 | 1.5 | 0 | 10 | 520 | 47 | 2 | 10 | 3 carb, 1 fat |
| Meatloaf | 8.1 oz | 180 | 6 | 60 | 3 | 0 | 35 | 860 | 21 | 2 | 11 | 1 1/2 carb, 1 med-fat meat |
| Penne Primavera | 8.1 oz | 280 | 6 | 60 | 3 | 0 | 15 | 480 | 43 | 3 | 11 | 3 carb, 1 fat |
| Roasted Sirloin Supreme | 8.1 oz | 230 | 5 | 45 | 1.5 | 0 | 15 | 950 | 34 | 2 | 13 | 2 carb, 1 med-fat meat |
| Salisbury Steak | 8.1 oz | 190 | 6 | 60 | 3 | 0 | 35 | 760 | 23 | 2 | 11 | 1 1/2 carb, 1 med-fat meat |
| Sante Fe Style Rice & Beans | 8.6 oz | 330 | 9 | 80 | 4 | 0 | 15 | 710 | 55 | 4 | 8 | 3 1/2 carb, 2 fat |
| Shrimp with Pasta & Vegetables | 8.1 oz | 260 | 6 | 60 | 3 | 0 | 45 | 620 | 39 | 2 | 11 | 2 1/2 carb, 1 med-fat meat |
| Spaghetti & Meat Sauce | 8.6 oz | 330 | 5 | 45 | 1.5 | 0 | 10 | 400 | 55 | 4 | 12 | 3 1/2 carb, 1 fat |
| Swedish Meatballs | 8.6 oz | 310 | 9 | 80 | 4 | 0 | 25 | 620 | 42 | 2 | 14 | 3 carb, 1 med-fat meat, 1 fat |

## FROZEN MEALS, MEAT, CHICKEN, FISH

| | Serving | Calories | Fat (g) | Cal. from Fat | Sat. Fat (g) | Trans Fat (g) | Chol. (mg) | Sod. (mg) | Carb. (g) | Fiber (g) | Prot. (g) | Servings/Exchanges |
|---|---|---|---|---|---|---|---|---|---|---|---|---|
| ***Red Baron*** | | | | | | | | | | | | |
| Biscuit-Style Scrambles, Bacon | 1 | 410 | 21 | 190 | 10 | 0.5 | 65 | 960 | 36 | 2 | 17 | 2 1/2carb, 2 med-fat meat, 2 fat |
| Biscuit-Style Scrambles, Western | 1 | 350 | 16 | 140 | 7 | 0 | 60 | 760 | 36 | 2 | 15 | 2 1/2 carb, 1 med-fat meat, 2 fat |
| ***Stouffer's*** | | | | | | | | | | | | |
| Baked Chicken Breast | 8.9 oz | 250 | 10 | 90 | 3 | 0 | 60 | 730 | 20 | 1 | 20 | 1 carb, 2 med-fat meat |
| Beef Pot Roast | 16 oz | 320 | 8 | 70 | 3 | 0 | 30 | 1570 | 41 | 8 | 20 | 2 1/2 carb, 2 med-fat meat |
| Beef Stroganoff | 9.8 oz | 380 | 17 | 150 | 5 | 0 | 70 | 990 | 34 | 2 | 22 | 2 carb, 2 med-fat meat, 1 fat |
| Chicken à la King | 11.5 oz | 360 | 12 | 110 | 4 | 0 | 35 | 800 | 44 | 0 | 18 | 3 carb, 1 med-fat meat, 1 fat |
| Corn Souffle | 6 oz | 150 | 5 | 45 | 1 | 0 | 65 | 490 | 22 | 2 | 5 | 1 1/2 carb, 1 fat |

| | | | | | | | | | | | | |
|---|---|---|---|---|---|---|---|---|---|---|---|---|
| Creamed Chipped Beef | 5.5 oz | 140 | 7 | 60 | 4 | 0 | 35 | 590 | 9 | 0 | 9 | 1/2 carb, 1 med-fat meat |
| Escalloped Chicken & Noodles | 8 oz | 330 | 18 | 160 | 4 | 0 | 35 | 910 | 28 | 2 | 14 | 2 carb, 1 med-fat meat, 3 fat |
| Fish Filet | 9 oz | 400 | 16 | 140 | 4.5 | 0.5 | 55 | 1050 | 36 | 4 | 27 | 2 1/2 carb, 3 med-fat meat |
| Five Cheese Lasagna | 10.8 oz | 370 | 14 | 130 | 7 | 0 | 35 | 960 | 39 | 4 | 21 | 2 1/2 carb, 2 med-fat meat, 1 fat |
| Fried Chicken Breast | 8.9 oz | 360 | 18 | 160 | 4.5 | 0 | 45 | 880 | 30 | 2 | 20 | 2 carb, 2 med-fat meat, 2 fat |
| Grilled Chicken Teriyaki | 9.4 oz | 300 | 3.5 | 30 | 1 | 0 | 40 | 880 | 45 | 3 | 21 | 3 carb, 2 lean meat |
| Grilled Herb Chicken | 9 oz | 250 | 6 | 50 | 1 | 0 | 35 | 740 | 29 | 3 | 19 | 2 carb, 2 lean meat |
| Grilled Lemon Pepper Chicken | 9 oz | 240 | 8 | 70 | 2 | 0 | 40 | 670 | 24 | 4 | 19 | 1 1/2 carb, 2 med-fat meat |
| Lasagna with Meat Sauce | 10.5 oz | 350 | 11 | 100 | 6 | 0.5 | 40 | 930 | 38 | 3 | 24 | 2 1/2 carb, 2 med-fat meat |

FROZEN MEALS, MEAT, CHICKEN, FISH

| | Serving | Calories | Fat (g) | Cal. from Fat | Sat. Fat (g) | Trans Fat (g) | Chol. (mg) | Sod. (mg) | Carb. (g) | Fiber (g) | Prot. (g) | Servings/Exchanges |
|---|---|---|---|---|---|---|---|---|---|---|---|---|
| Macaroni & Beef | 12.8 oz | 410 | 16 | 140 | 7 | 0 | 40 | 990 | 45 | 4 | 22 | 3 carb, 2 med-fat meat, 1 fat |
| Macaroni & Cheese | 6 oz | 340 | 16 | 140 | 7 | 0 | 25 | 820 | 33 | 3 | 15 | 2 carb, 1 med-fat meat, 2 fat |
| Meatloaf | 16 oz | 600 | 31 | 280 | 12 | 1.5 | 90 | 1310 | 45 | 5 | 35 | 3 carb, 3 med-fat meat, 3 fat |
| Roast Turkey | 9.6 oz | 290 | 12 | 110 | 3.5 | 0 | 45 | 970 | 30 | 2 | 16 | 2 carb, 1 med-fat meat, 1 fat |
| Roasted Chicken | 9.6 oz | 460 | 24 | 220 | 6 | 0 | 80 | 990 | 34 | 5 | 26 | 2 carb, 3 med-fat meat, 2 fat |
| Salisbury Steak | 16 oz | 710 | 39 | 350 | 16 | 1.5 | 100 | 1820 | 48 | 3 | 41 | 3 carb, 4 med-fat meat, 4 fat |
| Spaghetti with Meat Sauce | 12 oz | 350 | 12 | 110 | 4 | 0 | 30 | 660 | 44 | 5 | 17 | 3 carb, 1 med-fat meat, 1 fat |

| | | | | | | | | | | | | |
|---|---|---|---|---|---|---|---|---|---|---|---|---|
| Spaghetti with Meatballs | 12.6 oz | 360 | 12 | 110 | 3.5 | 0 | 35 | 850 | 45 | 6 | 19 | 3 carb, 1 med-fat meat, 1 fat |
| Spinach Souffle | 4 oz | 150 | 10 | 90 | 2 | 0 | 110 | 390 | 9 | 1 | 6 | 1/2 carb, 1 med-fat meat, 1 fat |
| Swedish Meatballs | 11.5 oz | 560 | 27 | 240 | 12 | 1 | 100 | 1250 | 47 | 3 | 32 | 3 carb, 3 med-fat meat, 2 fat |
| Tuna Noodle Casserole | 12 oz | 450 | 20 | 180 | 6 | 0 | 70 | 990 | 45 | 3 | 22 | 3 carb, 2 med-fat meat, 2 fat |
| White Meat Chicken Pot Pie | 10 oz | 660 | 37 | 330 | 14 | 0.5 | 50 | 1060 | 62 | 2 | 19 | 4 carb, 1 med-fat meat, 6 fat |
| ***Stouffer's Easy Express Skillets*** | | | | | | | | | | | | |
| Chicken Alfredo | 12.5 oz | 410 | 10 | 90 | 4 | 0 | 50 | 980 | 48 | 6 | 31 | 3 carb, 3 lean meat |
| Garlic Chicken | 11.5 oz | 320 | 6 | 50 | 2.5 | 0 | 40 | 1440 | 42 | 6 | 24 | 3 carb, 2 lean meat |
| Steak Teriyaki | 11.8 oz | 310 | 5 | 45 | 2 | 0 | 25 | 1390 | 49 | 6 | 17 | 3 carb, 1 med-fat meat |
| ***Swanson Hungry-Man*** | | | | | | | | | | | | |
| Beer Battered Chicken | 16 oz | 900 | 46 | 410 | 10 | 0 | 100 | 2090 | 78 | 7 | 37 | 5 carb, 3 med-fat meat, 6 fat |

FROZEN MEALS, MEAT, CHICKEN, FISH

| | Serving | Calories | Fat (g) | Cal. from Fat | Sat. Fat (g) | Trans Fat (g) | Chol. (mg) | Sod. (mg) | Carb. (g) | Fiber (g) | Prot. (g) | Servings/Exchanges |
|---|---|---|---|---|---|---|---|---|---|---|---|---|
| Boneless Fried Chicken | 16 oz | 860 | 39 | 350 | 9 | 0 | 130 | 1340 | 85 | 6 | 39 | 5 1/2 carb, 3 med-fat meat, 5 fat |
| Classic Fried Chicken | 16 oz | 1040 | 59 | 530 | 13 | 0 | 180 | 1610 | 64 | 4 | 60 | 4 carb, 7 med-fat meat, 5 fat |
| Country Fried Beef Patties | 16 oz | 810 | 50 | 450 | 16 | 0 | 75 | 1850 | 72 | 5 | 23 | 5 carb, 1 med-fat meat, 9 fat |
| Grilled Bourbon Steak Strips | 16 oz | 620 | 15 | 140 | 4 | 0 | 55 | 1990 | 94 | 4 | 26 | 6 carb, 1 med-fat meat, 2 fat |
| Meatloaf | 16 oz | 690 | 29 | 260 | 9 | 0 | 95 | 1510 | 74 | 5 | 34 | 5 carb, 2 med-fat meat, 4 fat |
| Mexican Style Fiesta | 18.1 oz | 600 | 23 | 210 | 8 | 0 | 20 | 1570 | 87 | 10 | 18 | 6 carb, 5 fat |
| Roasted Carved Turkey | 17 oz | 560 | 18 | 160 | 6 | 0 | 55 | 1620 | 78 | 5 | 19 | 5 carb, 1 med-fat meat, 3 fat |
| Salisbury Steak | 16 oz | 580 | 31 | 280 | 11 | 0 | 85 | 1380 | 50 | 5 | 27 | 3 carb, 3 med-fat meat, 3 fat |

| | | | | | | | | | | | | |
|---|---|---|---|---|---|---|---|---|---|---|---|---|
| Southwest Style Fried Chicken | 16 oz | 630 | 19 | 170 | 5 | 0 | 60 | 1630 | 85 | 3 | 29 | 5 1/2 carb, 2 med-fat meat, 2 fat |
| ***Weight Watchers Smart Ones*** | | | | | | | | | | | | |
| Chicken Enchiladas Suiza | 9.1 oz | 290 | 5 | 50 | 2 | 0 | 25 | 640 | 49 | 3 | 11 | 3 carb, 1 fat |
| Chicken Marsala | 9 oz | 180 | 7 | 60 | 1 | 0 | 50 | 530 | 10 | 2 | 20 | 1/2 carb, 3 lean meat |
| Chicken Parmesan | 11.1 oz | 290 | 5 | 50 | 1.5 | 0 | 40 | 630 | 35 | 4 | 26 | 2 carb, 2 lean meat |
| Chicken Sante Fe | 9 oz | 140 | 2.5 | 20 | 0 | 0 | 30 | 800 | 11 | 4 | 20 | 1 carb, 2 lean meat |
| Creamy Parmesan Chicken | 9 oz | 250 | 8 | 70 | 3.5 | 0 | 45 | 570 | 24 | 3 | 21 | 1 1/2 carb, 2 med-fat meat |
| Fettucini Alfredo | 9.3 oz | 240 | 3.5 | 30 | 1.5 | 0 | 5 | 570 | 41 | 4 | 12 | 2 1/2 carb, 1 med-fat meat |
| Ravioli Florentine | 8.5 oz | 250 | 5 | 45 | 2 | 0 | 30 | 720 | 40 | 4 | 11 | 2 1/2 carb, 1 med-fat meat |
| Slow-Roasted Turkey Breast | 10 oz | 210 | 7 | 60 | 2 | 0 | 45 | 770 | 18 | 2 | 18 | 1 carb, 2 lean meat |
| Sweet & Sour Chicken | 9 oz | 210 | 2 | 20 | 0 | 0 | 20 | 510 | 31 | 2 | 16 | 2 carb, 2 lean meat |

| | Serving | Calories | Fat (g) | Cal. from Fat | Sat. Fat (g) | Trans Fat (g) | Chol. (mg) | Sod. (mg) | Carb. (g) | Fiber (g) | Prot. (g) | Servings/Exchanges |
|---|---|---|---|---|---|---|---|---|---|---|---|---|
| Thai Style Chicken & Rice Noodles | 10.2 oz | 260 | 4 | 35 | 0.5 | 0 | 25 | 570 | 43 | 2 | 14 | 3 carb, 1 med-fat meat |
| Traditional Lasagna with Meat Sauce | 10.6 oz | 300 | 6 | 50 | 3 | 0 | 25 | 780 | 43 | 5 | 17 | 3 carb, 1 med-fat meat |
| Tuna Noodle Gratin | 9.6 oz | 240 | 4.5 | 40 | 2 | 0 | 30 | 720 | 37 | 3 | 15 | 2 1/2 carb, 1 med-fat meat |
| **FROZEN CHICKEN** | | | | | | | | | | | | |
| ***Banquet*** | | | | | | | | | | | | |
| Chicken Breast Nuggets | 6 pieces | 240 | 16 | 140 | 2.5 | 0 | 20 | 540 | 12 | 1 | 12 | 1 carb, 1 med-fat meat, 2 fat |
| Chicken Breast Patty | 1 | 200 | 13 | 120 | 2.5 | 0 | 15 | 340 | 11 | 1 | 9 | 1 carb, 1 med-fat meat, 2 fat |
| Chicken Breast Strips | 2 | 190 | 10 | 90 | 1.5 | 0 | 15 | 500 | 14 | 2 | 12 | 1 carb, 1 med-fat meat, 1 fat |

| | | | | | | | | | | | | |
|---|---|---|---|---|---|---|---|---|---|---|---|---|
| Chicken Breast Tenders | 5 pieces | 220 | 14 | 130 | 2 | 0 | 15 | 470 | 12 | <1 | 11 | 1 carb, 1 med-fat meat, 2 fat |
| Chicken Nuggets | 6 pieces | 220 | 13 | 120 | 2.5 | 0 | 25 | 530 | 15 | 2 | 11 | 1 carb, 1 med-fat meat, 2 fat |
| Chicken Wings, Honey BBQ | 3 oz | 270 | 17 | 160 | 4.5 | 1 | 65 | 520 | 12 | 5 | 17 | 1 carb, 2 med-fat meat, 1 fat |
| Chicken, Crispy Fried | 1 piece | 330 | 21 | 190 | 5 | 1.5 | 75 | 890 | 12 | <1 | 24 | 1 carb, 3 med-fat meat, 1 fat |
| Chicken, Popcorn | 11 pieces | 180 | 9 | 80 | 2.5 | 0 | 20 | 510 | 18 | <1 | 8 | 1 carb, 1 med-fat meat, 1 fat |
| ***Foster Farms*** | | | | | | | | | | | | |
| Breast Nuggets | 4 | 160 | 9 | 80 | 2 | 0 | 25 | 360 | 9 | 1 | 13 | 1/2 carb, 2 med-fat meat |
| Buffalo Style Strips | 3 oz | 190 | 8 | 70 | 2 | 0 | 30 | 1100 | 15 | 0 | 14 | 1 carb, 2 med-fat meat |
| Crispy Strips | 3 oz | 200 | 8 | 70 | 1.5 | 0 | 35 | 790 | 14 | 0 | 18 | 1 carb, 2 med-fat meat |
| Honey BBQ Wings | 4 | 170 | 10 | 90 | 3 | 0 | 50 | 390 | 5 | 0 | 13 | 2 med-fat meat |
| Hot & Spicy Wings | 4 | 170 | 13 | 120 | 4 | 0 | 55 | 460 | 1 | 0 | 14 | 2 med-fat meat, 1 fat |

## FROZEN MEALS, MEAT, CHICKEN, FISH

| | Serving | Calories | Fat (g) | Cal. from Fat | Sat. Fat (g) | Trans Fat (g) | Chol. (mg) | Sod. (mg) | Carb. (g) | Fiber (g) | Prot. (g) | Servings/Exchanges |
|---|---|---|---|---|---|---|---|---|---|---|---|---|
| ***Tyson*** | | | | | | | | | | | | |
| Breaded Chicken Breast Fillets | 1 piece | 240 | 9 | 80 | 1.5 | 0 | 45 | 680 | 20 | 0 | 19 | 1 carb, 2 med-fat meat |
| Buffalo Style Hot Wings | 3 pieces | 230 | 15 | 130 | 4 | 0 | 115 | 580 | 1 | 0 | 21 | 3 med-fat meat |
| Chicken Breast Nuggets | 5 pieces | 270 | 17 | 160 | 4 | 0 | 50 | 470 | 15 | 0 | 14 | 1 carb, 2 med-fat meat, 1 fat |
| Chicken Breast Patties | 1 patty | 180 | 11 | 90 | 2.5 | 0 | 25 | 390 | 12 | 1 | 10 | 1 carb, 1 med-fat meat, 1 fat |
| Chicken Breast Strips | 2 pieces | 200 | 10 | 90 | 2 | 0 | 30 | 520 | 13 | 1 | 16 | 1 carb, 2 med-fat meat |
| Chicken Breast Tenderloins | 1 piece | 150 | 7 | 60 | 1.5 | 0 | 20 | 370 | 12 | 1 | 10 | 1 carb, 1 med-fat meat |
| Diced Roasted Chicken Strips | 3 oz | 110 | 2.5 | 20 | 1 | 0 | 65 | 330 | 2 | 0 | 20 | 3 lean meat |
| Fajita Chicken Breast Strips | 3 oz | 110 | 4 | 35 | 1 | 0 | 55 | 540 | 1 | 0 | 17 | 2 lean meat |

| | | | | | | | | | | | | |
|---|---|---|---|---|---|---|---|---|---|---|---|---|
| Fun Shaped Chicken Nuggets | 5 pieces | 280 | 18 | 160 | 4 | 0 | 45 | 490 | 16 | 0 | 14 | 1 carb, 2 med-fat meat, 2 fat |
| Honey BBQ Wings | 3 pieces | 230 | 14 | 130 | 3.5 | 0 | 100 | 470 | 9 | 0 | 15 | 2 med-fat meat, |
| Popcorn Chicken Bites | 7 pieces | 180 | 9 | 80 | 1.5 | 0 | 30 | 560 | 11 | 0 | 13 | 1 carb, 1 med-fat meat, 1 fat |
| **FROZEN FISH** | | | | | | | | | | | | |
| ***Fisher Boy*** | | | | | | | | | | | | |
| Crispy Battered Fish Portions | 1 piece | 170 | 10 | 90 | 2 | 0 | 20 | 320 | 15 | 0 | 7 | 1 carb, 1 med-fat meat, 1 fat |
| Crunchy Breaded Fish Tenders | 4 pieces | 230 | 11 | 100 | 1.5 | 0 | 30 | 450 | 22 | 0 | 11 | 1 1/2 carb, 1 med-fat meat, 1 fat |
| Fish Sticks | 3 oz | 210 | 9 | 80 | 1.5 | 0 | 10 | 520 | 24 | 0 | 10 | 1 1/2 carb, 1 med-fat meat, 1 fat |
| ***Gorton's*** | | | | | | | | | | | | |
| Classic Breaded Fish Sticks | 3.7 oz | 250 | 16 | 140 | 4 | 0 | 25 | 340 | 19 | 1 | 10 | 1 carb, 1 med-fat meat, 2 fat |

FROZEN MEALS, MEAT, CHICKEN, FISH

| | Serving | Calories | Fat (g) | Cal. from Fat | Sat. Fat (g) | Trans Fat (g) | Chol. (mg) | Sod. (mg) | Carb. (g) | Fiber (g) | Prot. (g) | Servings/Exchanges |
|---|---|---|---|---|---|---|---|---|---|---|---|---|
| Classic Crispy Battered Fillets | 3.8 oz | 230 | 12 | 110 | 3 | 0 | 25 | 650 | 22 | 3 | 8 | 1 1/2 carb, 1 med-fat meat, 1 fat |
| Classic Crunchy Golden Fish Fillets | 1 fillet | 170 | 9 | 80 | 1.5 | 0 | 20 | 260 | 16 | 0 | 7 | 1 carb, 1 med-fat meat, 1 fat |
| Crunchy Fish Portions | 1 piece | 200 | 10 | 90 | 1.5 | 0 | 15 | 460 | 19 | 2 | 9 | 1 carb, 1 med-fat meat, 1 fat |
| Crunchy Golden Popcorn Shrimp | 3.2 oz | 240 | 12 | 110 | 3 | 0 | 55 | 630 | 24 | 0 | 8 | 1 1/2 carb, 1 med-fat meat, 1 fat |
| Garlic Butter Grilled Fillets | 3.8 oz | 100 | 3 | 25 | 0 | 0 | 70 | 290 | 1 | 0 | 17 | 2 lean meat |
| Grilled Shrimp Classic | 4 oz | 110 | 1 | 15 | 0 | 0 | 50 | 960 | 5 | 0 | 18 | 3 lean meat |
| Lemon Pepper Grilled Fillets | 3.8 oz | 100 | 3 | 25 | 0 | 0 | 70 | 290 | 1 | 0 | 17 | 2 lean meat |
| Original Batter Fish Tenders | 3.6 oz | 230 | 12 | 110 | 3 | 0 | 20 | 660 | 23 | 2 | 8 | 1 1/2 carb, 1 med-fat meat, 1 fat |

| | | | | | | | | | | | | |
|---|---|---|---|---|---|---|---|---|---|---|---|---|
| Salmon Classic Grilled Fillets | 3.1 oz | 100 | 3 | 25 | 0 | 0 | 35 | 270 | 2 | 0 | 15 | 2 lean meat |
| ***Mrs. Paul's*** | | | | | | | | | | | | |
| Battered Fish Tenders | 4 pieces | 210 | 10 | 90 | 3.5 | 0 | 20 | 700 | 22 | 1 | 9 | 1 1/2 carb, 1 med-fat meat, 1 fat |
| Breaded Fish Sticks | 6 | 250 | 12 | 110 | 4.5 | 0 | 25 | 390 | 25 | 1 | 10 | 1 1/2 carb, 1 med-fat meat, 1 fat |
| Lightly Breaded Cod Fillets | 1 fillet | 220 | 11 | 100 | 5 | 0 | 40 | 430 | 17 | 1 | 12 | 1 carb, 1 med-fat meat, 1 fat |
| Lightly Breaded Flounder Fillets | 1 fillet | 150 | 7 | 60 | 3.5 | 0 | 25 | 290 | 12 | 1 | 8 | 1 carb, 1 med-fat meat |
| ***Van de Kamp's*** | | | | | | | | | | | | |
| Breaded Popcorn Fish | 8 pieces | 220 | 12 | 110 | 5 | 0 | 30 | 480 | 18 | 2 | 11 | 1 carb, 1 med-fat meat, 1 fat |
| Breaded Popcorn Shrimp | 4 oz | 260 | 11 | 100 | 4.5 | 0 | 80 | 750 | 30 | 2 | 11 | 2 carb, 1 med-fat meat, 1 fat |

FROZEN MEALS, MEAT, CHICKEN, FISH

| | Serving | Calories | Fat (g) | Cal. from Fat | Sat. Fat (g) | Trans Fat (g) | Chol. (mg) | Sod. (mg) | Carb. (g) | Fiber (g) | Prot. (g) | Servings/Exchanges |
|---|---|---|---|---|---|---|---|---|---|---|---|---|
| Crisp & Healthy Breaded Fish Fillets | 2 fillets | 150 | 1.5 | 15 | 1 | 0 | 20 | 470 | 25 | 1 | 8 | 1 1/2 carb, 1 lean meat |
| Crisp & Healthy Breaded Fish Stitcks | 6 sticks | 140 | 1 | 10 | 0.5 | 0 | 25 | 380 | 24 | 1 | 9 | 1 1/2 carb, 1 lean meat |
| Crunchy Breaded Fish Fillets | 2 fillets | 230 | 13 | 120 | 4.5 | 0 | 20 | 440 | 21 | <1 | 8 | 1 1/2 carb, 1 med-fat meat, 2 fat |
| Crunchy Breaded Fish Shaped Nuggets | 4 pieces | 260 | 12 | 110 | 1.5 | 0 | 15 | 790 | 29 | 1 | 9 | 2 carb, 1 med-fat meat, 1 fat |
| Crunchy Golden Breaded Fish Sticks | 6 sticks | 230 | 11 | 100 | 4 | 0 | 25 | 370 | 23 | 1 | 10 | 1 1/2 carb, 1 med-fat meat, 1 fat |

# FROZEN PIZZA, SNACKS

| | Serving | Calories | Fat (g) | Cal. from Fat | Sat. Fat (g) | Trans Fat (g) | Chol. (mg) | Sod. (mg) | Carb. (g) | Fiber (g) | Prot. (g) | Servings/Exchanges |
|---|---|---|---|---|---|---|---|---|---|---|---|---|
| **FROZEN PIZZA** | | | | | | | | | | | | |
| ***California Pizza Kitchen*** | | | | | | | | | | | | |
| Crispy Thin Crust, Margherita | 1/3 pizza | 300 | 13 | 120 | 5 | 1 | 20 | 520 | 33 | 2 | 14 | 2 carb, 1 med-fat meat, 2 fat |
| Crispy Thin Crust, Sicilian | 1/3 pizza | 310 | 13 | 120 | 5 | 0.5 | 35 | 810 | 32 | 2 | 17 | 2 carb, 2 med-fat meat, 1 fat |
| Crispy Thin Crust, White Pizza | 1/3 pizza | 300 | 12 | 100 | 6 | 1 | 25 | 540 | 32 | 2 | 16 | 2 carb, 1 med-fat meat, 1 fat |
| Five Cheese & Tomato | 1/3 pizza | 320 | 15 | 140 | 8 | 0.5 | 40 | 700 | 29 | 1 | 18 | 2 carb, 2 med-fat meat, 1 fat |
| Hawaiian | 1/3 pizza | 260 | 9 | 80 | 4 | 0 | 20 | 730 | 31 | 2 | 14 | 2 carb, 2 med-fat meat |
| Rising Crust BBQ Chicken | 1/5 pizza | 320 | 10 | 90 | 4 | 0 | 25 | 750 | 43 | 2 | 16 | 3 carb, 1 med-fat meat, 1 fat |

FROZEN PIZZA, SNACKS

| | Serving | Calories | Fat (g) | Cal. from Fat | Sat. Fat (g) | Trans Fat (g) | Chol. (mg) | Sod. (mg) | Carb. (g) | Fiber (g) | Prot. (g) | Servings/Exchanges |
|---|---|---|---|---|---|---|---|---|---|---|---|---|
| ***DiGiorno*** | | | | | | | | | | | | |
| Cheese Stuffed Crust Pepperoni | 1/5 pizza | 380 | 16 | 150 | 8 | 0 | 40 | 720 | 40 | 3 | 15 | 2 1/2 carb, 2 med-fat meat, 1 fat |
| Cheese Stuffed Crust Supreme | 1/6 pizza | 350 | 16 | 150 | 7 | 0 | 40 | 950 | 35 | 3 | 17 | 2 carb, 2 med-fat meat, 1 fat |
| Cheese Stuffed Crust Three Meat | 1/6 pizza | 350 | 16 | 150 | 7 | 0.5 | 40 | 950 | 34 | 2 | 17 | 2 carb, 2 med-fat meat, 1 fat |
| Rising Crust Four Cheese | 1/2 pizza | 310 | 11 | 100 | 5 | 0 | 25 | 850 | 40 | 2 | 15 | 2 1/2 carb, 1 med-fat meat, 1 fat |
| Rising Crust Pepperoni | 1/2 pizza | 330 | 13 | 110 | 5 | 0 | 30 | 940 | 40 | 2 | 14 | 2 1/2 carb, 1 med-fat meat, 2 fat |
| Rising Crust Supreme | 1/2 pizza | 360 | 15 | 130 | 6 | 0 | 30 | 990 | 41 | 3 | 16 | 2 1/2 carb, 1 med-fat meat, 2 fat |
| Thin Crispy Crust Four Cheese | 1/5 pizza | 310 | 13 | 120 | 7 | 1 | 35 | 660 | 32 | 3 | 18 | 2 carb, 2 med-fat meat, 1 fat |

| | | | | | | | | | | | | |
|---|---|---|---|---|---|---|---|---|---|---|---|---|
| Thin Crispy Crust Four Meat | 1/5 pizza | 320 | 14 | 130 | 6 | 0.5 | 35 | 850 | 32 | 2 | 18 | 2 carb, 2 med-fat meat, 1 fat |
| Thin Crispy Crust Pepperoni | 1/5 pizza | 320 | 15 | 140 | 7 | 0.5 | 35 | 790 | 31 | 2 | 16 | 2 carb, 1 med-fat meat, 2 fat |
| Thin Crispy Crust Supreme | 1/5 pizza | 320 | 15 | 130 | 6 | 0.5 | 30 | 720 | 33 | 3 | 16 | 2 carb, 1 med-fat meat, 1 fat |
| ***Freschetta*** | | | | | | | | | | | | |
| Brick Oven, 5 Italian Cheese | 1/4 pizza | 340 | 15 | 130 | 6 | 0 | 25 | 780 | 37 | 3 | 15 | 2 1/2 carb, 1 med-fat meat, 2 fat |
| Brick Oven, Italian Pepperoni | 1/4 pizza | 410 | 20 | 180 | 20 | 0.5 | 40 | 1120 | 38 | 2 | 19 | 2 1/2 carb, 2 med-fat meat, 2 fat |
| Brick Oven, Spinach and Mushroom | 1/4 pizza | 310 | 11 | 100 | 3.5 | 0 | 15 | 710 | 40 | 3 | 13 | 2 1/2 carb, 1 med-fat meat, 1 fat |
| ***Jenos Crisp 'n Tasty*** | | | | | | | | | | | | |
| Cheese | 6.9 oz | 450 | 21 | 190 | 3.5 | 6 | 0 | 1020 | 51 | 2 | 14 | 3 1/2 carb, 1 med-fat meat, 3 fat |

FROZEN PIZZA, SNACKS

| | Serving | Calories | Fat (g) | Cal. from Fat | Sat. Fat (g) | Trans Fat (g) | Chol. (mg) | Sod. (mg) | Carb. (g) | Fiber (g) | Prot. (g) | Servings/Exchanges |
|---|---|---|---|---|---|---|---|---|---|---|---|---|
| Combination | 7 oz | 480 | 25 | 220 | 6 | 4.5 | 15 | 1140 | 50 | 2 | 15 | 3 carb, 1 med-fat meat, 4 fat |
| Hamburger | 7.3 oz | 500 | 25 | 230 | 6 | 25 | 0 | 1040 | 51 | 2 | 18 | 3 1/2 carb, 1 med-fat meat, 4 fat |
| Pepperoni | 6.8 oz | 490 | 26 | 230 | 7 | 2.5 | 15 | 1060 | 50 | 2 | 15 | 3 carb, 1 med-fat meat, 4 fat |
| Sausage | 7 oz | 480 | 25 | 220 | 6 | 4.5 | 10 | 1110 | 50 | 2 | 15 | 3 carb, 1 med-fat meat, 4 fat |
| Supreme | 7.2 oz | 480 | 24 | 220 | 6 | 4.5 | 15 | 1130 | 49 | 1 | 15 | 3 carb, 1 med-fat meat, 4 fat |
| ***Red Baron*** | | | | | | | | | | | | |
| Classic 4-Cheese | 1/4 pizza | 380 | 16 | 150 | 9 | 0.5 | 30 | 690 | 40 | 2 | 18 | 2 1/2 carb, 1 med-fat meat, 2 fat |
| Classic 4-Meat | 1/4 pizza | 380 | 16 | 150 | 8 | 0 | 30 | 770 | 41 | 2 | 17 | 2 1/2 carb, 1 med-fat meat, 2 fat |

| | | | | | | | | | | | | |
|---|---|---|---|---|---|---|---|---|---|---|---|---|
| Classic Hamburger | 1/4 pizza | 360 | 15 | 130 | 7 | 0.5 | 30 | 770 | 40 | 2 | 17 | 2 1/2 carb, 1 med-fat meat, 1 fat |
| Classic Mexican Style Supreme | 1/5 pizza | 370 | 16 | 150 | 8 | 0 | 25 | 670 | 42 | 3 | 15 | 3 carb, 1 med-fat meat, 1 fat |
| Classic Pepperoni | 1/5 pizza | 370 | 16 | 150 | 8 | 0 | 30 | 740 | 40 | 2 | 16 | 2 1/2 carb, 1 med-fat meat, 1 fat |
| Classic Supreme | 1/5 pizza | 310 | 14 | 130 | 7 | 0 | 25 | 590 | 34 | 2 | 13 | 2 carb, 1 med-fat meat, 2 fat |
| Deep Dish Mini Pizza, Cheese | 4 pieces | 420 | 20 | 180 | 11 | 0 | 25 | 770 | 44 | 2 | 16 | 3 carb, 1 med-fat meat, 3 fat |
| Deep Dish Mini Pizza, Pepperoni | 4 pieces | 460 | 25 | 220 | 12 | 0 | 40 | 990 | 44 | 2 | 16 | 3 carb, 1 med-fat meat, 4 fat |
| Deep Dish Singles, Pepperoni | 1 | 420 | 19 | 170 | 9 | 0 | 25 | 870 | 45 | 2 | 17 | 3 carb, 1 med-fat meat, 3 fat |
| Deep Dish Singles, Supreme | 1 | 420 | 19 | 170 | 9 | 0 | 30 | 770 | 45 | 2 | 17 | 3 carb, 1 med-fat meat, 3 fat |

| | Serving | Calories | Fat (g) | Cal. from Fat | Sat. Fat (g) | Trans Fat (g) | Chol. (mg) | Sod. (mg) | Carb. (g) | Fiber (g) | Prot. (g) | Servings/Exchanges |
|---|---|---|---|---|---|---|---|---|---|---|---|---|
| Fire Baked Pepperoni | 1/4 pizza | 370 | 17 | 150 | 7 | 0 | 30 | 910 | 40 | 3 | 16 | 2 1/2 carb, 1 med-fat meat, 2 fat |
| French Bread 5 Cheese & Garlic | 1 | 410 | 22 | 200 | 8 | 0 | 25 | 880 | 39 | 2 | 14 | 2 1/2 carb, 1 med-fat meat, 3 fat |
| French Bread Pepperoni | 1 | 360 | 15 | 130 | 7 | 0 | 30 | 1070 | 42 | 2 | 16 | 3 carb, 1 med-fat meat, 2 fat |
| Thin & Crispy 5-Cheese | 1/3 pizza | 360 | 16 | 140 | 8 | 0 | 25 | 780 | 39 | 2 | 16 | 2 1/2 carb, 1 med-fat meat, 2 fat |
| Thin & Crispy Pepperoni | 1/3 pizza | 410 | 20 | 180 | 9 | 0.5 | 35 | 970 | 40 | 2 | 17 | 2 1/2 carb, 1 med-fat meat, 3 fat |
| ***Tombstone*** | | | | | | | | | | | | |
| Original Deluxe Cheese | 1/5 pizza | 290 | 12 | 110 | 5 | 0 | 30 | 580 | 31 | 3 | 14 | 2 carb, 1 med-fat meat, 1 fat |
| Original Hamburger | 1/4 pizza | 350 | 15 | 140 | 7 | 0.5 | 35 | 720 | 37 | 4 | 18 | 2 1/2 carb, 2 med-fat meat, 1 fat |

| | | | | | | | | | | | | |
|---|---|---|---|---|---|---|---|---|---|---|---|---|
| Original Pepperoni | 1/3 pizza | 280 | 14 | 120 | 6 | 0 | 30 | 620 | 28 | 3 | 13 | 2 carb, 1 med-fat meat, 2 fat |
| Original Pepperoni & Sausage | 1/3 pizza | 290 | 14 | 130 | 6 | 0 | 30 | 650 | 28 | 3 | 14 | 2 carb, 1 med-fat meat, 2 fat |
| Original Supreme | 1/5 pizza | 300 | 14 | 120 | 6 | 0 | 30 | 640 | 31 | 3 | 14 | 2 carb, 1 med-fat meat, 2 fat |
| Original Xtra Cheese | 1/2 pizza | 360 | 14 | 130 | 7 | 0.5 | 30 | 680 | 42 | 4 | 17 | 3 carb, 1 med-fat meat, 2 fat |
| ***Tony's*** | | | | | | | | | | | | |
| Original Cheese | 1/3 pizza | 290 | 12 | 100 | 5 | 0 | 15 | 570 | 37 | 2 | 11 | 2 1/2 carb, 1 med-fat meat, 1 fat |
| Original Four Cheese | 1/3 pizza | 300 | 13 | 110 | 6 | 0 | 20 | 570 | 36 | 2 | 12 | 3 1/2 carb, 1 med-fat meat, 2 fat |
| Original Meat Trio | 1/3 pizza | 340 | 16 | 140 | 7 | 0 | 15 | 680 | 37 | 2 | 13 | 2 1/2 carb, 1 med-fat meat, 2 fat |
| Original Pepperoni | 1/3 pizza | 310 | 14 | 120 | 7 | 0 | 10 | 620 | 36 | 2 | 11 | 2 1/2 carb, 1 med-fat meat, 2 fat |

| | Serving | Calories | Fat (g) | Cal. from Fat | Sat. Fat (g) | Trans Fat (g) | Chol. (mg) | Sod. (mg) | Carb. (g) | Fiber (g) | Prot. (g) | Servings/Exchanges |
|---|---|---|---|---|---|---|---|---|---|---|---|---|
| Original Sausage & Pepperoni | 1/3 pizza | 340 | 17 | 150 | 8 | 0 | 15 | 660 | 37 | 2 | 12 | 2 1/2 carb, 1 med-fat meat, 2 fat |
| Original Supreme | 1/3 pizza | 330 | 16 | 140 | 7 | 0 | 10 | 630 | 37 | 2 | 12 | 2 1/2 carb, 1 med-fat meat, 2 fat |
| Thin Crust Supreme | 1/3 pizza | 360 | 19 | 170 | 5 | 0 | 15 | 930 | 34 | 2 | 14 | 2 carb, 1 med-fat meat, 3 fat |
| ***Totino's Party Pizza*** | | | | | | | | | | | | |
| Crisp Crust Canadian Style Bacon | 1/2 pizza | 320 | 15 | 130 | 2.5 | 4 | 10 | 890 | 34 | 1 | 13 | 2 carb, 1 med-fat meat, 2 fat |
| Crisp Crust Combination | 1/2 pizza | 370 | 20 | 180 | 4.5 | 4 | 10 | 910 | 35 | 1 | 12 | 2 carb, 1 med-fat meat, 3 fat |
| Crisp Crust Mexican Style | 1/2 pizza | 370 | 19 | 180 | 4.5 | 4 | 15 | 890 | 36 | 2 | 14 | 2 1/2 carb, 1 med-fat meat, 3 fat |
| Crisp Crust Pepperoni | 1/2 pizza | 360 | 20 | 180 | 4.5 | 4 | 10 | 920 | 34 | 1 | 12 | 2 carb, 1 med-fat meat, 3 fat |

| | | | | | | | | | | | | |
|---|---|---|---|---|---|---|---|---|---|---|---|---|
| Crisp Crust Sausage | 1/2 pizza | 370 | 20 | 180 | 4.5 | 4 | 10 | 890 | 35 | 2 | 12 | 2 carb, 1 med-fat meat, 3 fat |
| Crisp Crust Supreme | 1/2 pizza | 360 | 19 | 170 | 4.5 | 4 | 10 | 590 | 35 | 1 | 12 | 2 carb, 1 med-fat meat, 3 fat |
| Crisp Crust Triple Cheese | 1/2 pizza | 320 | 16 | 140 | 5 | 3 | 15 | 720 | 34 | 1 | 12 | 2 carb, 1 med-fat meat, 2 fat |
| Crisp Crust Triple Meat | 1/2 pizza | 350 | 18 | 160 | 4 | 4 | 10 | 900 | 34 | 1 | 12 | 2 carb, 1 med-fat meat, 3 fat |
| **FROZEN SNACKS** | | | | | | | | | | | | |
| ***Bagel Bites*** | | | | | | | | | | | | |
| Cheese & Pepperoni | 4 | 220 | 7 | 60 | 3 | 0 | 15 | 480 | 30 | 2 | 9 | 2 carb, 1 med-fat meat |
| Three Cheese | 4 | 210 | 6 | 60 | 3 | 0 | 15 | 400 | 30 | 2 | 9 | 2 carb, 1 med-fat meat |
| ***Delime*** | | | | | | | | | | | | |
| Taquitos, Beef | 5 | 370 | 15 | 140 | 2 | 0 | 15 | 760 | 46 | 8 | 15 | 3 carb, 1 med-fat meat, 2 fat |
| Taquitos, Chicken | 5 | 370 | 14 | 130 | 3 | 0 | 30 | 480 | 47 | 8 | 15 | 3 carb, 1 med-fat meat, 2 fat |

| | Serving | Calories | Fat (g) | Cal. from Fat | Sat. Fat (g) | Trans Fat (g) | Chol. (mg) | Sod. (mg) | Carb. (g) | Fiber (g) | Prot. (g) | Servings/Exchanges |
|---|---|---|---|---|---|---|---|---|---|---|---|---|
| ***Hot Pockets*** | | | | | | | | | | | | |
| BBQ Beef | 1 | 340 | 14 | 130 | 7 | 0 | 30 | 670 | 44 | 2 | 9 | 3 carb, 3 fat |
| Ham & Cheese | 1 | 290 | 12 | 110 | 5 | 0 | 30 | 640 | 36 | 1 | 10 | 2 1/2 carb, 1 med-fat meat, 1 fat |
| Meatballs & Mozarella | 1 | 340 | 16 | 150 | 7 | 0 | 30 | 570 | 37 | 2 | 10 | 2 1/2 carb, 1 med-fat meat, 2 fat |
| Pizzeria Four Cheese Pizza | 1 | 330 | 13 | 120 | 6 | 0 | 25 | 750 | 39 | 1 | 13 | 2 1/2 carb, 1 med-fat meat, 2 fat |
| Pizzeria Pepperoni | 1 | 340 | 17 | 150 | 8 | 0 | 25 | 730 | 37 | 2 | 10 | 2 1/2 carb, 1 med-fat meat, 2 fat |
| ***Jose Ole Mexi-Minis*** | | | | | | | | | | | | |
| Beef & Cheese Mini Tacos | 4 | 210 | 11 | 100 | 4 | 0 | 20 | 440 | 19 | 5 | 7 | 1 carb, 1 med-fat meat, 1 fat |
| Chicken Taquitos | 3 | 200 | 8 | 70 | 1.5 | 0 | 10 | 390 | 26 | 3 | 7 | 2 carb, 2 fat |

| | | | | | | | | | | | | |
|---|---|---|---|---|---|---|---|---|---|---|---|---|
| Shredded Steak Taquitos | 3 | 210 | 9 | 80 | 2 | 0 | 10 | 420 | 25 | 3 | 6 | 1 1/2 carb, 2 fat |
| ***Lean Pockets*** | | | | | | | | | | | | |
| Barbeque Recipe Beef | 1 | 290 | 7 | 60 | 3.5 | 0 | 25 | 700 | 46 | 3 | 11 | 3 carb, 1 fat |
| Cheeseburger | 1 | 290 | 8 | 70 | 3.5 | 0 | 25 | 550 | 41 | 3 | 12 | 2 1/2 carb, 1 med-fat meat, 1 fat |
| Chicken Parmesan | 1 | 290 | 7 | 60 | 3 | 0 | 25 | 470 | 45 | 3 | 10 | 3 carb, 1 fat |
| Four Cheese Pizza | 1 | 300 | 7 | 60 | 3.5 | 0 | 20 | 680 | 45 | 3 | 15 | 3 carb, 1 med-fat meat |
| Ham & Cheddar | 1 | 270 | 8 | 70 | 4 | 0 | 30 | 540 | 40 | 3 | 12 | 2 1/2 carb, 1 med-fat meat, 1 fat |
| Meatball Mozzarella | 1 | 290 | 9 | 80 | 4 | 0 | 25 | 560 | 40 | 3 | 12 | 2 1/2 carb, 1 med-fat meat, 1 fat |
| Mexican Style Chicken Fiesta | 1 | 240 | 7 | 60 | 3 | 0 | 20 | 660 | 35 | 3 | 10 | 2 carb, 1 med-fat meat |
| Pepperoni Pizza | 1 | 280 | 8 | 70 | 3.5 | 0 | 20 | 630 | 46 | 2 | 13 | 3 carb, 1 med-fat meat, 1 fat |

| | Serving | Calories | Fat (g) | Cal. from Fat | Sat. Fat (g) | Trans Fat (g) | Chol. (mg) | Sod. (mg) | Carb. (g) | Fiber (g) | Prot. (g) | Servings/Exchanges |
|---|---|---|---|---|---|---|---|---|---|---|---|---|
| Philly Steak & Cheese | 1 | 270 | 7 | 70 | 3.5 | 0 | 25 | 640 | 39 | 2 | 11 | 2 1/2 carb, 1 med-fat meat |
| Southwest Style Bacon, Egg & Cheese | 1 | 250 | 8 | 70 | 2.5 | 0 | 50 | 530 | 33 | 1 | 11 | 2 carb, 1 med-fat meat, 1 fat |
| Stuffed Quesadilla Grilled Chicken Fajita | 1 | 360 | 9 | 80 | 4 | 0 | 35 | 670 | 48 | 2 | 19 | 3 carb, 1 med-fat meat, 1 fat |
| ***Ling Ling Potstickers*** | | | | | | | | | | | | |
| Chicken & Vegetable Dumplings | 5 | 260 | 6 | 60 | 1.5 | 0 | 35 | 620 | 39 | 2 | 13 | 2 1/2 carb, 1 med-fat meat |
| Pork & Dumplings | 5 | 280 | 8 | 80 | 2.5 | 0 | 25 | 640 | 38 | 2 | 12 | 2 1/2 carb, 1 med-fat meat, 1 fat |
| ***Michelina's*** | | | | | | | | | | | | |
| Four Melt Pizza Snack Rolls | 6 rolls | 230 | 12 | 100 | 3.5 | 0 | 15 | 410 | 23 | 1 | 9 | 1 1/2 carb, 1 med-fat meat, 1 fat |

| | | | | | | | | | | | | |
|---|---|---|---|---|---|---|---|---|---|---|---|---|
| Pepperoni Pizza Snack Rolls | 6 | 230 | 11 | 100 | 3 | 0 | 10 | 460 | 24 | 1 | 8 | 1 1/2 carb, 1 med-fat meat, 1 fat |
| ***Poppers*** | | | | | | | | | | | | |
| Cream Cheese Jalapeños | 3 | 220 | 15 | 130 | 6 | 0 | 25 | 470 | 15 | 1 | 4 | 1 carb, 3 fat |
| ***Totino's*** | | | | | | | | | | | | |
| Pizza Rolls, Cheese | 6 rolls | 200 | 8 | 70 | 2 | 1 | 5 | 440 | 26 | 1 | 7 | 2 carb, 2 fat |
| Pizza Rolls, Supreme | 6 rolls | 200 | 8 | 80 | 2 | 1.5 | 5 | 390 | 25 | 1 | 7 | 1 1/2 carb, 2 fat |
| Pizza Rolls, Taco | 6 rolls | 200 | 8 | 80 | 3 | 1 | 15 | 470 | 24 | 1 | 7 | 1 1/2 carb, 2 fat |

# FRUIT, FRUIT JUICES, DRINKS

| | Serving | Calories | Fat (g) | Cal. from Fat | Sat. Fat (g) | Trans Fat (g) | Chol. (mg) | Sod. (mg) | Carb. (g) | Fiber (g) | Prot. (g) | Servings/Exchanges |
|---|---|---|---|---|---|---|---|---|---|---|---|---|
| **FRUIT** | | | | | | | | | | | | |
| Apple, Unpeeled | 1 small | 54 | 0 | 0 | 0 | 0 | 0 | 1 | 14 | 3 | 0 | 1 fruit |
| Apple, Unpeeled | 1 large | 125 | 0 | 0 | 0 | 0 | 0 | 0 | 32 | 6 | 0 | 2 fruit |
| Apples, Dried | 4 rings | 63 | 0 | 0 | 0 | 0 | 0 | 23 | 17 | 2 | 0 | 1 fruit |
| Applesauce, Sweetened | 1/2 cup | 97 | 0 | 0 | 0 | 0 | 0 | 35 | 51 | 2 | <1 | 1 fruit, 2 1/2 carb |
| Applesauce, Unsweetened | 1/2 cup | 53 | 0 | 0 | 0 | 0 | 0 | 3 | 14 | 2 | <1 | 1 fruit |
| Apricots, Canned, EXtra Light Syrup | 1/2 cup | 61 | 0 | 0 | 0 | 0 | 0 | 3 | 15 | 2 | <1 | 1 fruit |
| Apricots, Canned, Heavy Syrup | 1/2 cup | 107 | 0 | 0 | 0 | 0 | 0 | 5 | 28 | 2 | <1 | 1 fruit, 1 carb |
| Apricots, Canned, Juice Pack | 1/2 cup | 59 | 0 | 0 | 0 | 0 | 0 | 5 | 15 | 2 | <1 | 1 fruit |

| | | | | | | | | | | | | |
|---|---|---|---|---|---|---|---|---|---|---|---|---|
| Apricots, Canned, Light Syrup | 1/2 cup | 80 | 0 | 0 | 0 | 0 | 0 | 5 | 21 | 2 | <1 | 1 fruit, 1/2 carb |
| Apricots, Canned, Water Pack | 1/2 cup | 33 | 0 | 0 | 0 | 0 | 0 | 4 | 8 | 2 | <1 | 1/2 fruit |
| Apricots, Dried | 8 halves | 67 | 0 | 0 | 0 | 0 | 0 | 3 | 18 | 2 | 0 | 1 fruit |
| Banana | 6 inches | 72 | 0 | 0 | 0 | 0 | 0 | 1 | 19 | 2 | <1 | 1 fruit |
| Blackberries, Canned, Heavy Syrup | 1/2 cup | 118 | 0 | 0 | 0 | 0 | 0 | 4 | 29 | 4 | 2 | 1 fruit, 1 carb |
| Blackberries, Fresh | 3/4 cup | 56 | 0 | 0 | 0 | 0 | 0 | 0 | 14 | 6 | <1 | 1 fruit |
| Blackberries, Frozen, Unsweetened | 1 cup | 97 | 0 | 0 | 0 | 0 | 0 | 2 | 24 | 8 | 2 | 1 1/2 fruit |
| Blueberries, Canned, Heavy Syrup | 1/2 cup | 113 | 0 | 0 | 0 | 0 | 0 | 8 | 28 | 4 | <1 | 1 fruit, 1 carb |
| Blueberries, Dried | 2 Tbsp | 69 | 0 | 0 | 0 | 0 | 0 | 0 | 16 | 1 | <1 | 1 fruit |
| Blueberries, Fresh | 3/4 cup | 62 | 0 | 0 | 0 | 0 | 0 | 1 | 16 | 3 | <1 | 1 fruit |
| Blueberries, Frozen, Sweetened | 1 cup | 186 | 0 | 0 | 0 | 0 | 0 | 2 | 50 | 5 | <1 | 1 fruit, 2 carb |

FRUIT, FRUIT JUICES, DRINKS

| | Serving | Calories | Fat (g) | Cal. from Fat | Sat. Fat (g) | Trans Fat (g) | Chol. (mg) | Sod. (mg) | Carb. (g) | Fiber (g) | Prot. (g) | Servings/Exchanges |
|---|---|---|---|---|---|---|---|---|---|---|---|---|
| Blueberries, Frozen, Unsweetened | 1 cup | 79 | 0 | 0 | 0 | 0 | 0 | 2 | 19 | 4 | <1 | 1 fruit |
| Boysenberries, Canned, Heavy Syrup | 1/2 cup | 113 | 0 | 0 | 0 | 0 | 0 | 4 | 29 | <1 | 2 | 1 fruit, 1 carb |
| Boysenberries, Frozen, Unsweetened | 1 cup | 66 | 0 | 0 | 0 | 0 | 0 | 1 | 16 | 7 | 1 | 1 fruit |
| Cantaloupe, Fresh | 1 cup | 56 | 0 | 0 | 0 | 0 | 0 | 14 | 13 | 1 | 1 | 1 fruit |
| Cheeries, Sour, Frozen, Unsweetened | 1 cup | 71 | 0 | 0 | 0 | 0 | 0 | 2 | 17 | 25 | 1 | 1 fruit |
| Cherries, Dried | 2 Tbsp | 66 | 0 | 0 | 0 | 0 | 0 | 0 | 16 | 1 | 0 | 1 fruit |
| Cherries, Sour, Canned, Extra Heavy Syrup | 1/2 cup | 149 | 0 | 0 | 0 | 0 | 0 | 9 | 38 | 1 | 1 | 1 fruit, 1 1/2 carb |
| Cherries, Sour, Canned, Heavy Syrup | 1/2 cup | 117 | 0 | 0 | 0 | 0 | 0 | 9 | 30 | 1 | 1 | 1 fruit, 1 carb |

| | | | | | | | | | | | | |
|---|---|---|---|---|---|---|---|---|---|---|---|---|
| Cherries, Sour, Canned, Light Syrup | 1/2 cup | 95 | 0 | 0 | 0 | 0 | 0 | 9 | 25 | 1 | 1 | 1 fruit, 1/2 carb |
| Cherries, Sour, Canned, Water Pack | 1/2 cup | 44 | 0 | 0 | 0 | 0 | 0 | 9 | 11 | 1 | 2 | 1 fruit |
| Cherries, Sweet, Canned, Extra Heavy Syrup | 1/2 cup | 133 | 0 | 0 | 0 | 0 | 0 | 4 | 34 | 2 | <1 | 1 fruit, 1 carb |
| Cherries, Sweet, Canned, Heavy Syrup | 1/2 cup | 105 | 0 | 0 | 0 | 0 | 0 | 4 | 27 | 2 | <1 | 1 fruit, 1 carb |
| Cherries, Sweet, Canned, Juice Pack | 1/2 cup | 68 | 0 | 0 | 0 | 0 | 0 | 4 | 18 | 2 | <1 | 1 fruit |
| Cherries, Sweet, Canned, Light Syrup | 1/2 cup | 85 | 0 | 0 | 0 | 0 | 0 | 4 | 22 | 2 | <1 | 1 fruit, 1/2 carb |
| Cherries, Sweet, Canned, Water Pack | 1/2 cup | 57 | 0 | 0 | 0 | 0 | 0 | 1 | 15 | 2 | 1 | 1 fruit |
| Cherries, Sweet, Fresh | 12 | 56 | 0 | 0 | 0 | 0 | 0 | 0 | 14 | 2 | 1 | 1 fruit |

## FRUIT, FRUIT JUICES, DRINKS

| | Serving | Calories | Fat (g) | Cal. from Fat | Sat. Fat (g) | Trans Fat (g) | Chol. (mg) | Sod. (mg) | Carb. (g) | Fiber (g) | Prot. (g) | Servings/Exchanges |
|---|---|---|---|---|---|---|---|---|---|---|---|---|
| Cherries, Sweet, Frozen, Unsweetened | 1 cup | 231 | 0 | 0 | 0 | 0 | 0 | 3 | 17 | 5 | 3 | 1 fruit |
| Cranberries | 1 cup | 47 | <1 | 0 | <1 | 0 | 0 | <1 | 12 | 4 | <1 | 1 fruit |
| Cranberries, Dried | 2 Tbsp | 47 | 0 | 0 | 0 | 0 | 0 | 0 | 13 | <1 | 0 | 1 fruit |
| Cranberry Sauce, Canned, Sweetened | 1/2 cup | 209 | 0 | 0 | 0 | 0 | 0 | 40 | 54 | 1 | <1 | 1 fruit, 2 1/2 carb |
| Currants, Red/White, Fresh | 1 cup | 63 | 0 | 0 | 0 | 0 | 0 | 1 | 15 | 5 | 2 | 1 fruit |
| Figs, Canned, Extra Heavy Syrup | 1/2 cup | 140 | 0 | 0 | 0 | 0 | 0 | 2 | 37 | NA | <1 | 1 fruit, 1 1/2 carb |
| Figs, Canned, Heavy Syrup | 1/2 cup | 114 | 0 | 0 | 0 | 0 | 0 | 2 | 30 | 3 | <1 | 1 fruit, 1 carb |
| Figs, Canned, Light Syrup | 1/2 cup | 87 | 0 | 0 | 0 | 0 | 0 | 2 | 23 | 2 | <1 | 1 fruit, 1/2 carb |

| | | | | | | | | | | | | |
|---|---|---|---|---|---|---|---|---|---|---|---|---|
| Figs, Canned, Water Pack | 1/2 cup | 66 | 0 | 0 | 0 | 0 | 0 | 1 | 18 | 3 | <1 | 1 fruit |
| Figs, Dried | 1 1/2 | 71 | 0 | 0 | 0 | 0 | 0 | 3 | 18 | 3 | <1 | 1 fruit |
| Figs, Fresh | 2 medium | 74 | 0 | 0 | 0 | 0 | 0 | 1 | 19 | 3 | <1 | 1 fruit |
| Fruit Cocktail, Canned, Extra Heavy Syrup | 1/2 cup | 114 | 0 | 0 | 0 | 0 | 0 | 8 | 30 | 1 | <1 | 1 fruit, 1 carb |
| Fruit Cocktail, Canned, Extra Light Syrup | 1/2 cup | 55 | 0 | 0 | 0 | 0 | 0 | 5 | 14 | 1 | <1 | 1 fruit |
| Fruit Cocktail, Canned, Heavy Syrup | 1/2 cup | 91 | 0 | 0 | 0 | 0 | 0 | 15 | 24 | 1 | <1 | 1 fruit, 1/2 carb |
| Fruit Cocktail, Canned, Juice Pack | 1/2 cup | 104 | 0 | 0 | 0 | 0 | 0 | 5 | 14 | 1 | <1 | 1 fruit |
| Fruit Cocktail, Canned, Water Pack | 1/2 cup | 38 | 0 | 0 | 0 | 0 | 0 | 5 | 10 | 1 | <1 | 1 fruit |
| Fruit Coctail, Canned, Light Syrup | 1/2 cup | 69 | 0 | 0 | 0 | 0 | 0 | 8 | 18 | 1 | <1 | 1 fruit |

| | Serving | Calories | Fat (g) | Cal. from Fat | Sat. Fat (g) | Trans Fat (g) | Chol. (mg) | Sod. (mg) | Carb. (g) | Fiber (g) | Prot. (g) | Servings/Exchanges |
|---|---|---|---|---|---|---|---|---|---|---|---|---|
| Fruit Salad, Canned, Extra Heavy Syrup | 1/2 cup | 114 | 0 | 0 | 0 | 0 | 0 | 7 | 30 | 1 | <1 | 1 fruit, 1 carb |
| Fruit Salad, Canned, Heavy Syrup | 1/2 cup | 93 | 0 | 0 | 0 | 0 | 0 | 8 | 25 | 1 | <1 | 1 fruit, 1/2 carb |
| Fruit Salad, Canned, Juice Pack | 1/2 cup | 62 | 0 | 0 | 0 | 0 | 0 | 6 | 16 | 1 | <1 | 1 fruit |
| Fruit Salad, Canned, Light Syrup | 1/2 cup | 73 | 0 | 0 | 0 | 0 | 0 | 8 | 19 | 1 | <1 | 1 fruit |
| Fruit Salad, Canned, Water Pack | 1/2 cup | 37 | 0 | 0 | 0 | 0 | 0 | 4 | 10 | 1 | <1 | 1 fruit |
| Grapefruit Sections, Canned, Juice Pack | 1/2 cup | 46 | 0 | 0 | 0 | 0 | 0 | 9 | 12 | <1 | <1 | 1 fruit |
| Grapefruit Sections, Canned, Light Syrup | 1/2 cup | 76 | 0 | 0 | 0 | 0 | 0 | 3 | 20 | <1 | <1 | 1 fruit |

| | | | | | | | | | | | | |
|---|---|---|---|---|---|---|---|---|---|---|---|---|
| Grapefruit Sections, Canned, Water Pack | 1/2 cup | 44 | 0 | 0 | 0 | 0 | 0 | 3 | 11 | <1 | <1 | 1 fruit |
| Grapefruit, Fresh | 1/2 | 53 | 0 | 0 | 0 | 0 | 0 | 0 | 13 | 2 | 1 | 1 fruit |
| Grapes, Canned, Heavy Syrup | 1/2 cup | 94 | 0 | 0 | 0 | 0 | 0 | 7 | 25 | <1 | <1 | 1 fruit, 1/2 carb |
| Grapes, Canned, Water Pack | 1/2 cup | 49 | 0 | 0 | 0 | 0 | 0 | 8 | 13 | <1 | <1 | 1 fruit |
| Grapes, Fresh, Seedless | 17 | 60 | 0 | 0 | 0 | 0 | 0 | 2 | 15 | <1 | <1 | 1 fruit |
| Guava, Fresh | 1 | 46 | 0 | 0 | 0 | 0 | 0 | 3 | 11 | 5 | 1 | 1 fruit |
| Honeydew Melon, Fresh | 1 cup | 61 | 0 | 0 | 0 | 0 | 0 | 31 | 16 | 1 | <1 | 1 fruit |
| Kiwi | 1 large | 56 | 0 | 0 | 0 | 0 | 0 | 3 | 13 | 3 | 1 | 1 fruit |
| Kumquats, Fresh | 2 | 27 | 0 | 0 | 0 | 0 | 0 | 4 | 6 | 2 | 1 | 1/2 fruit |
| Melon Balls, Mixed, Frozen | 1 cup | 57 | <1 | 0 | <1 | 0 | 0 | 54 | 14 | 1 | 2 | 1 fruit |
| Mixed Fruit, Canned, Heavy Syrup | 1/2 cup | 92 | 0 | 0 | 0 | 0 | 0 | 5 | 24 | 2 | <1 | 1 fruit, 1/2 carb |

FRUIT, FRUIT JUICES, DRINKS

| | Serving | Calories | Fat (g) | Cal. from Fat | Sat. Fat (g) | Trans Fat (g) | Chol. (mg) | Sod. (mg) | Carb. (g) | Fiber (g) | Prot. (g) | Servings/Exchanges |
|---|---|---|---|---|---|---|---|---|---|---|---|---|
| Mixed Fruit, Frozen, Sweetened | 1 cup | 245 | 0 | 0 | 0 | 0 | 0 | 8 | 61 | 5 | 4 | 1 fruit, 3 carb |
| Nectarine, Fresh | 1 small | 60 | 0 | 0 | 0 | 0 | 0 | 0 | 14 | 2 | 1 | 1 fruit |
| Orange, Fresh | 1 | 62 | 0 | 0 | 0 | 0 | 0 | 0 | 15 | 3 | 1 | 1 fruit |
| Oranges, Mandarin, Canned, Juice Pack | 3/4 cup | 69 | <1 | 0 | 0 | 0 | 0 | 9 | 18 | 1 | 1 | 1 fruit |
| Papaya, Fresh | 1 cup | 55 | 0 | 0 | 0 | 0 | 0 | 4 | 14 | 3 | <1 | 1 fruit |
| Peach, Fresh | 1 medium | 57 | 0 | 0 | 0 | 0 | 0 | 0 | 14 | 2 | 1 | 1 fruit |
| Peaches, Canned, Extra Heavy Syrup | 1/2 cup | 126 | 0 | 0 | 0 | 0 | 0 | 11 | 34 | 2 | <1 | 1 fruit, 1 carb |
| Peaches, Canned, Extra Light Syrup | 1/2 cup | 52 | 0 | 0 | 0 | 0 | 0 | 6 | 14 | 1 | <1 | 1 fruit |
| Peaches, Canned, Heavy Syrup | 1/2 cup | 97 | 0 | 0 | 0 | 0 | 0 | 8 | 26 | <1 | <1 | 1 fruit, 1 carb |

| | | | | | | | | | | | | |
|---|---|---|---|---|---|---|---|---|---|---|---|---|
| Peaches, Canned, Juice Pack | 1/2 cup | 55 | 0 | 0 | 0 | 0 | 0 | 5 | 14 | 1 | <1 | 1 fruit |
| Peaches, Canned, Light Syrup | 1/2 cup | 68 | 0 | 0 | 0 | 0 | 0 | 7 | 18 | 1 | <1 | 1 fruit |
| Peaches, Canned, Water Pack | 1/2 cup | 30 | 0 | 0 | 0 | 0 | 0 | 4 | 8 | 1 | <1 | 1/2 fruit |
| Peaches, Frozen, Sweetened | 1 cup | 235 | 0 | 0 | 0 | 0 | 0 | 15 | 60 | 5 | 2 | 1 fruit, 2 carb |
| Pear, Fresh | 1/2 large | 61 | 0 | 0 | 0 | 0 | 0 | 1 | 16 | 3 | <1 | 1 fruit |
| Pears, Canned, Extra Heavy Syrup | 1/2 cup | 129 | 0 | 0 | 0 | 0 | 0 | 7 | 34 | 2 | <1 | 1 fruit, 1 carb |
| Pears, Canned, Extra Light Syrup | 1/2 cup | 58 | 0 | 0 | 0 | 0 | 0 | 3 | 15 | 2 | <1 | 1 fruit |
| Pears, Canned, Heavy Syrup | 1/2 cup | 99 | 0 | 0 | 0 | 0 | 0 | 7 | 25 | 2 | <1 | 1 fruit, 1/2 carb |
| Pears, Canned, Juice Pack | 1/2 cup | 62 | 0 | 0 | 0 | 0 | 0 | 5 | 16 | 2 | <1 | 1 fruit |

FRUIT, FRUIT JUICES, DRINKS

| | Serving | Calories | Fat (g) | Cal. from Fat | Sat. Fat (g) | Trans Fat (g) | Chol. (mg) | Sod. (mg) | Carb. (g) | Fiber (g) | Prot. (g) | Servings/Exchanges |
|---|---|---|---|---|---|---|---|---|---|---|---|---|
| Pears, Canned, Light Syrup | 1/2 cup | 72 | 0 | 0 | 0 | 0 | 0 | 7 | 19 | 2 | <1 | 1 fruit |
| Pears, Canned, Water Pack | 1/2 cup | 36 | 0 | 0 | 0 | 0 | 0 | 3 | 10 | 2 | <1 | 1 fruit |
| Pineapple, Canned, Extra Heavy Syrup | 1/2 cup | 108 | 0 | 0 | 0 | 0 | 0 | 2 | 28 | 1 | <1 | 1 fruit, 1 carb |
| Pineapple, Canned, Heavy Syrup | 1/2 cup | 99 | 0 | 0 | 0 | 0 | 0 | 2 | 26 | 1 | <1 | 1 fruit, 1 carb |
| Pineapple, Canned, Juice Pack | 1/2 cup | 75 | 0 | 0 | 0 | 0 | 0 | 1 | 20 | 1 | <1 | 1 fruit |
| Pineapple, Canned, Light Juice Pack | 1/2 cup | 66 | 0 | 0 | 0 | 0 | 0 | 2 | 17 | 1 | <1 | 1 fruit |
| Pineapple, Canned, Water Pack | 1/2 cup | 40 | 0 | 0 | 0 | 0 | 0 | 1 | 10 | 1 | <1 | 1 fruit |
| Pineapple, Fresh | 3/4 cup | 56 | 0 | 0 | 0 | 0 | 0 | 1 | 15 | 2 | <1 | 1 fruit |

| | | | | | | | | | | | | |
|---|---|---|---|---|---|---|---|---|---|---|---|---|
| Pineapple, Frozen, Sweetened | 1 cup | 211 | 0 | 0 | 0 | 0 | 0 | 5 | 54 | 3 | <1 | 1 fruit, 2 1/2 carb |
| Plum, Fresh | 2 | 61 | 0 | 0 | 0 | 0 | 0 | 0 | 15 | 2 | <1 | 1 fruit |
| Plums, Canned, Extra Heavy Syrup | 1/2 cup | 132 | 0 | 0 | 0 | 0 | 0 | 25 | 35 | 2 | <1 | 1 fruit, 1 carb |
| Plums, Canned, Heavy Syrup | 1/2 cup | 115 | 0 | 0 | 0 | 0 | 0 | 25 | 30 | 1 | <1 | 1 fruit, 1 carb |
| Plums, Canned, Juice Pack | 1/2 cup | 73 | 0 | 0 | 0 | 0 | 0 | 2 | 19 | 1 | <1 | 1 fruit |
| Plums, Canned, Light Syrup | 1/2 cup | 80 | 0 | 0 | 0 | 0 | 0 | 25 | 21 | 1 | <1 | 1 fruit, 1/2 carb |
| Plums, Canned, Water Pack | 1/2 cup | 51 | 0 | 0 | 0 | 0 | 0 | 1 | 14 | 1 | <1 | 1 fruit |
| Plums, Dried | 3 | 60 | 0 | 0 | 0 | 0 | 0 | 1 | 16 | 2 | <1 | 1 fruit |
| Pomegranate, Fresh | 1 | 105 | 0 | 0 | 0 | 0 | 0 | 5 | 26 | 1 | 1 | 2 fruit |
| Raisins, Seedless | 2 Tbsp | 54 | 0 | 0 | 0 | 0 | 0 | 2 | 14 | <1 | <1 | 1 fruit |

FRUIT, FRUIT JUICES, DRINKS

| | Serving | Calories | Fat (g) | Cal. from Fat | Sat. Fat (g) | Trans Fat (g) | Chol. (mg) | Sod. (mg) | Carb. (g) | Fiber (g) | Prot. (g) | Servings/Exchanges |
|---|---|---|---|---|---|---|---|---|---|---|---|---|
| Raspberries, Canned, Heavy Syrup | 1/2 cup | 117 | 0 | 0 | 0 | 0 | 0 | 4 | 30 | 4 | 1 | 1 fruit, 1 carb |
| Raspberries, Fresh | 1 cup | 60 | 0 | 0 | 0 | 0 | 0 | 0 | 14 | 8 | 1 | 1 fruit |
| Raspberries, Frozen, Sweetened | 1 cup | 258 | 0 | 0 | 0 | 0 | 0 | 1 | 65 | 6 | 2 | 1 fruit, 3 carb |
| Rhubarb, Frozen, Unsweetened | 1 cup | 29 | 0 | 0 | 0 | 0 | 0 | 3 | 7 | 3 | <1 | 1/2 fruit |
| Star Fruit (Carambola) | 2 medium | 60 | 0 | 0 | 0 | 0 | 0 | 4 | 14 | 4 | 0 | 1 fruit |
| Strawberries, Canned, Heavy Syrup | 1/2 cup | 117 | 0 | 0 | 0 | 0 | 0 | 10 | 30 | 2 | 1 | 1 fruit, 1 carb |
| Strawberries, Fresh | 1 1/4 cup | 57 | 0 | 0 | 0 | 0 | 0 | 2 | 13 | 4 | 1 | 1 fruit |
| Strawberries, Frozen, Sweetened | 1 cup | 199 | 0 | 0 | 0 | 0 | 0 | 3 | 54 | 5 | 1 | 1 fruit, 2 1/2 carb |

| | | | | | | | | | | | | |
|---|---|---|---|---|---|---|---|---|---|---|---|---|
| Strawberries, Frozen, Unsweetened | 1 cup | 52 | 0 | 0 | 0 | 0 | 0 | 3 | 14 | 3 | <1 | 1 fruit |
| Tangerine, Fresh | 2 small | 81 | 0 | 0 | 0 | 0 | 0 | 3 | 20 | 3 | 1 | 1 fruit |
| Tangerines, Juice Pack | 1/2 cup | 36 | 0 | 0 | 0 | 0 | 0 | 5 | 9 | 1 | <1 | 1/2 fruit |
| Tangerines, Light Syrup | 1/2 cup | 77 | 0 | 0 | 0 | 0 | 0 | 8 | 20 | 1 | <1 | 1 fruit |
| Watermelon, Fresh | 1 1/4 cup | 57 | 0 | 0 | 0 | 0 | 0 | 2 | 14 | <1 | 1 | 1 fruit |
| **FRUIT JUICES** | | | | | | | | | | | | |
| Apple Juice/Cider, Canned/Bottled | 1/2 cup | 58 | 0 | 0 | 0 | 0 | 0 | 4 | 15 | 0 | 0 | 1 fruit |
| Apricot Nectar, Canned | 1/2 cup | 71 | 0 | 0 | 0 | 0 | 0 | 4 | 18 | 0 | 0 | 1 fruit |
| Cranberry Juice Cocktail, Bottled | 1/3 cup | 48 | 0 | 0 | 0 | 0 | 0 | 2 | 12 | 0 | 0 | 1 fruit |
| Cranberry Juice Cocktail, Reduced Calorie | 1 cup | 50 | 0 | 0 | 0 | 0 | 0 | 7 | 11 | 0 | 0 | 1 fruit |
| Fruit Juice Blends, 100% Juice | 1/3 cup | 50 | 0 | 0 | 0 | 0 | 0 | 10 | 12 | 0 | 0 | 1 fruit |

FRUIT, FRUIT JUICES, DRINKS

| | Serving | Calories | Fat (g) | Cal. from Fat | Sat. Fat (g) | Trans Fat (g) | Chol. (mg) | Sod. (mg) | Carb. (g) | Fiber (g) | Prot. (g) | Servings/Exchanges |
|---|---|---|---|---|---|---|---|---|---|---|---|---|
| Grape Juice | 1/3 cup | 50 | 0 | 0 | 0 | 0 | 0 | 3 | 13 | 0 | 0 | 1 fruit |
| Grapefruit Juice, Canned | 1/2 cup | 47 | 0 | 0 | 0 | 0 | 0 | 1 | 11 | 0 | <1 | 1 fruit |
| Orange Juice, Canned | 1/2 cup | 52 | 0 | 0 | 0 | 0 | 0 | 3 | 12 | 0 | <1 | 1 fruit |
| Orange Juice, Fresh | 1/2 cup | 56 | 0 | 0 | 0 | 0 | 0 | 1 | 13 | 0 | <1 | 1 fruit |
| Orange Juice, Frozen | 1/2 cup | 56 | 0 | 0 | 0 | 0 | 0 | 1 | 13 | <1 | <1 | 1 fruit |
| Pineapple Juice, Canned | 1/2 cup | 70 | 0 | 0 | 0 | 0 | 0 | 1 | 17 | <1 | <1 | 1 fruit |
| Prune Juice, Bottled | 1/3 cup | 60 | 0 | 0 | 0 | 0 | 0 | 3 | 15 | <1 | <1 | 1 fruit |
| **FRUIT JUICES** | | | | | | | | | | | | |
| ***Capri Sun (Single Serving Pouch)*** | | | | | | | | | | | | |
| Juice Drink, Lemonade | 6.6 oz | 70 | 0 | 0 | 0 | 0 | 0 | 15 | 19 | 0 | 0 | 1 carb |
| Juice Drink, Strawberry Kiwi | 6.7 oz | 70 | 0 | 0 | 0 | 0 | 0 | 15 | 19 | 0 | 0 | 1 carb |

| | | | | | | | | | | | | |
|---|---|---|---|---|---|---|---|---|---|---|---|---|
| Roarin' Waters, Fruit-Flavored Water | 6.7 oz | 35 | 0 | 0 | 0 | 0 | 0 | 15 | 9 | 0 | 0 | 1/2 carb |
| Sports Drink, Assorted Flavors | 6.75 oz | 60 | 0 | 0 | 0 | 0 | 0 | 55 | 16 | 0 | 0 | 1 carb |
| ***Dole*** | | | | | | | | | | | | |
| Juice Blend, Orange Peach Mango | 8 oz | 120 | 0 | 0 | 0 | 0 | 0 | 25 | 29 | 0 | <1 | 2 fruit |
| Juice Blend, Orange Strawberry Banana | 8 oz | 120 | 0 | 0 | 0 | 0 | 0 | 10 | 30 | 0 | 1 | 2 fruit |
| Juice Blend, Paradise Blend | 8 oz | 120 | 0 | 0 | 0 | 0 | 0 | 40 | 29 | 0 | <1 | 2 fruit |
| Juice Blend, Piña Colada | 8 oz | 120 | 0 | 0 | 0 | 0 | 0 | 10 | 29 | 0 | 0 | 2 fruit |
| Juice Blend, Pineapple Peach Mango | 8 oz | 130 | 0 | 0 | 0 | 0 | 0 | 10 | 31 | 0 | <1 | 2 fruit |
| Juice Blend, Strawberry Kiwi | 8 oz | 120 | 0 | 0 | 0 | 0 | 0 | 25 | 31 | 0 | 0 | 2 fruit |

FRUIT, FRUIT JUICES, DRINKS

| | Serving | Calories | Fat (g) | Cal. from Fat | Sat. Fat (g) | Trans Fat (g) | Chol. (mg) | Sod. (mg) | Carb. (g) | Fiber (g) | Prot. (g) | Servings/Exchanges |
|---|---|---|---|---|---|---|---|---|---|---|---|---|
| Pineapple Juice | 8 oz | 130 | 0 | 0 | 0 | 0 | 0 | 10 | 30 | 0 | 0 | 2 fruit |
| ***Donald Duck*** | | | | | | | | | | | | |
| Orange Juice, No Pulp Plus Calcium | 8 oz | 110 | 0 | 0 | 0 | 0 | 0 | 20 | 27 | 0 | 2 | 2 fruit |
| Orange Juice, Original No Pulp | 8 oz | 110 | 0 | 0 | 0 | 0 | 0 | 20 | 27 | 0 | 2 | 2 fruit |
| ***Florida's Natural*** | | | | | | | | | | | | |
| Orange Juice, Original | 8 oz | 110 | 0 | 0 | 0 | 0 | 0 | 0 | 26 | 0 | 2 | 2 fruit |
| Orange Juice, Calcium & Vitamin D | 8 oz | 110 | 0 | 0 | 0 | 0 | 0 | 0 | 26 | 0 | 2 | 2 fruit |
| Ruby Red Grapefruit Juice, Original | 8 oz | 90 | 0 | 0 | 0 | 0 | 0 | 0 | 22 | 0 | 1 | 1 1/2 fruit |
| ***Hansen's*** | | | | | | | | | | | | |
| Smoothie, Assorted Flavors | 11.5 oz | 170–180 | 0 | 0 | 0 | 0 | 0 | 50 | 43–45 | 0 | 0 | 3 carb |

| | | | | | | | | | | | | |
|---|---|---|---|---|---|---|---|---|---|---|---|---|
| ***Hawaiian Punch*** | | | | | | | | | | | | |
| Fruit Punch, Assorted Flavors | 8 oz | 120 | 0 | 0 | 0 | 0 | 0 | 115–120 | 29–30 | 0 | 0 | 2 carb |
| ***Hollywood*** | | | | | | | | | | | | |
| Carrot Juice | 11 oz can | 100 | 0 | 0 | 0 | 0 | 0 | 170 | 22 | 2 | 2 | 1 1/2 fruit |
| ***Kool-Aid (Single Serving)*** | | | | | | | | | | | | |
| Bursts, Soft Drink, Assorted Flavors | 6.8 oz | 35 | 0 | 0 | 0 | 0 | 0 | 30 | 9 | 0 | 0 | 1/2 carb |
| Jammers, Juice Drink, Cherry | 5.9 oz | 80 | 0 | 0 | 0 | 0 | 0 | 15 | 20 | 0 | 0 | 1 carb |
| Jammers, Juice Drink, Tropical | 6.7 oz | 10 | 0 | 0 | 0 | 0 | 0 | 25 | 2 | 0 | 0 | free |
| ***Juicy Juice 100% Juice*** | | | | | | | | | | | | |
| Apple Juice | 8 oz | 110 | 0 | 0 | 0 | 0 | 0 | 20 | 28 | 0 | 0 | 2 fruit |
| ***Kern's*** | | | | | | | | | | | | |
| Aguas Frescas Limon Juice Drink | 8 oz | 120 | 0 | 0 | 0 | 0 | 0 | 5 | 31 | 0 | 0 | 2 carb |

FRUIT, FRUIT JUICES, DRINKS

| | Serving | Calories | Fat (g) | Cal. from Fat | Sat. Fat (g) | Trans Fat (g) | Chol. (mg) | Sod. (mg) | Carb. (g) | Fiber (g) | Prot. (g) | Servings/Exchanges |
|---|---|---|---|---|---|---|---|---|---|---|---|---|
| Apricot Nectar | 8 oz | 140 | 0 | 0 | 0 | 0 | 0 | 5 | 35 | 0 | 0 | 2 carb |
| Guava Nectar | 8 oz | 150 | 0 | 0 | 0 | 0 | 0 | 10 | 37 | 0 | 0 | 2 1/2 carb |
| Pear Nectar | 8 oz | 150 | 0 | 0 | 0 | 0 | 0 | 10 | 37 | 0 | 0 | 2 1/2 carb |
| Mango Nectar, Single Serving | 11.5 oz can | 210 | 0 | 0 | 0 | 0 | 0 | 25 | 52 | 0 | 0 | 3 1/2 carb |
| Peach Nectar, Single Serving | 11.5 oz can | 200 | 0 | 0 | 0 | 0 | 0 | 10 | 46 | 0 | 0 | 3 carb |
| Strawberry Banana | 8 oz | 220 | 0 | 0 | 0 | 0 | 0 | 10 | 52 | 0 | 0 | 3 1/2 carb |
| ***Langer's*** | | | | | | | | | | | | |
| Apple Cider | 8 oz | 120 | 0 | 0 | 0 | 0 | 0 | 0 | 28 | 0 | 0 | 2 fruit |
| Apple Juice | 8 oz | 120 | 0 | 0 | 0 | 0 | 0 | 0 | 28 | 0 | 0 | 2 fruit |
| Cranberry Grape Blend | 8 oz | 165 | 0 | 0 | 0 | 0 | 0 | 10 | 41 | 0 | 0 | 2 1/2 fruit |
| Cranberry Juice Cocktail | 8 oz | 140 | 0 | 0 | 0 | 0 | 0 | 10 | 35 | 0 | 0 | 2 carb |

| | | | | | | | | | | | | |
|---|---|---|---|---|---|---|---|---|---|---|---|---|
| Cranberry Raspberry | 8 oz | 150 | 0 | 0 | 0 | 0 | 0 | 10 | 36 | 0 | 0 | 2 1/2 fruit |
| Diet Low Carb Apple Juice Cocktail | 8 oz | 60 | 0 | 0 | 0 | 0 | 0 | 10 | 14 | 0 | 0 | 1 carb |
| Diet Low Carb Cranberry Cocktail | 8 oz | 30 | 0 | 0 | 0 | 0 | 0 | 10 | 8 | 0 | 0 | 1/2 carb |
| Diet Low Carb Ruby Red Grapefruit Juice Cocktail | 8 oz | 30 | 0 | 0 | 0 | 0 | 0 | 10 | 40 | 0 | 0 | 2 1/2 carb |
| Ruby Red Grapefruit Juice Cocktail | 8 oz | 130 | 0 | 0 | 0 | 0 | 0 | 10 | 33 | 0 | 0 | 2 carb |
| ***Martinelli's*** | | | | | | | | | | | | |
| Apple Juice | 8 oz | 140 | 0 | 0 | 0 | 0 | 0 | 0 | 35 | 0 | 0 | 2 fruit |
| Apple Pomegranate Juice | 8 oz | 150 | 0 | 0 | 0 | 0 | 0 | 10 | 38 | 0 | 0 | 2 1/2 fruit |
| ***Minute Maid*** | | | | | | | | | | | | |
| Apple Juice, Single Serving | 10 oz | 140 | 0 | 0 | 0 | 0 | 0 | 25 | 35 | 0 | 0 | 2 fruit |

FRUIT, FRUIT JUICES, DRINKS

| | Serving | Calories | Fat (g) | Cal. from Fat | Sat. Fat (g) | Trans Fat (g) | Chol. (mg) | Sod. (mg) | Carb. (g) | Fiber (g) | Prot. (g) | Servings/Exchanges |
|---|---|---|---|---|---|---|---|---|---|---|---|---|
| Apple Strawberry | 6.75 oz box | 100 | 0 | 0 | 0 | 0 | 0 | 15 | 25 | 0 | 0 | 1 1/2 carb |
| Berry Punch | 8 oz | 120 | 0 | 0 | 0 | 0 | 0 | 15 | 32 | 0 | 0 | 2 carb |
| Cherry Limeade | 8 oz | 120 | 0 | 0 | 0 | 0 | 0 | 15 | 34 | 0 | 0 | 2 carb |
| Fruit Punch | 8 oz | 120 | 0 | 0 | 0 | 0 | 0 | 15 | 31 | 0 | 0 | 2 carb |
| Lemonade | 8 oz | 110 | 0 | 0 | 0 | 0 | 0 | 15 | 31 | 0 | 0 | 2 carb |
| Light Orange Juice Beverage | 8 oz | 50 | 0 | 0 | 0 | 0 | 0 | 15 | 13 | 0 | 0 | 1 carb |
| Light Raspberry Passion | 8 oz | 10 | 0 | 0 | 0 | 0 | 0 | 50 | 2 | 0 | 0 | free |
| Limeade | 8 oz | 90 | 0 | 0 | 0 | 0 | 0 | 0 | 25 | 0 | 0 | 1 1/2 carb |
| Mixed Berry, Single Serving | 6.75 oz box | 100 | 0 | 0 | 0 | 0 | 0 | 15 | 25 | 0 | 0 | 1 1/2 fruit |
| Orange Juice, Country Style | 8 oz | 110 | 0 | 0 | 0 | 0 | 0 | 15 | 27 | 0 | 2 | 2 fruit |

| | | | | | | | | | | | | |
|---|---|---|---|---|---|---|---|---|---|---|---|---|
| Orange Juice, Heart Wise | 8 oz | 110 | 0 | 0 | 0 | 0 | 0 | 20 | 27 | 0 | 2 | 2 fruit |
| Orange Juice, Home Squeezed, Calcium & Vitamin D | 8 oz | 110 | 0 | 0 | 0 | 0 | 0 | 15 | 27 | 0 | 2 | 2 fruit |
| Orange Juice, Kid's + | 8 oz | 100 | 0 | 0 | 0 | 0 | 0 | 15 | 23 | 0 | 2 | 1 1/2 fruit |
| Orange Juice, Multi-Vitamin | 8 oz | 120 | 0 | 0 | 0 | 0 | 0 | 20 | 27 | 0 | 0 | 2 fruit |
| Orange Juice, Original | 8 oz | 110 | 0 | 0 | 0 | 0 | 0 | 15 | 27 | 0 | 2 | 2 fruit |
| Orange Juice, Original with Calcium | 8 oz | 110 | 0 | 0 | 0 | 0 | 0 | 15 | 27 | 0 | 0 | 2 fruit |
| Orange Juice, Original, Single Serve | 8 oz | 110 | 0 | 0 | 0 | 0 | 0 | 20 | 27 | 0 | 2 | 2 fruit |
| Pink Lemonade, Single Serving | 8 oz | 100 | 0 | 0 | 0 | 0 | 0 | 35 | 28 | 0 | 0 | 2 carb |
| ***Mott's*** | | | | | | | | | | | | |
| Plus Light Juice | 8 oz | 130 | 0 | 0 | 0 | 0 | 0 | 35 | 15 | 0 | 0 | 1 carb |

FRUIT, FRUIT JUICES, DRINKS

| | Serving | Calories | Fat (g) | Cal. from Fat | Sat. Fat (g) | Trans Fat (g) | Chol. (mg) | Sod. (mg) | Carb. (g) | Fiber (g) | Prot. (g) | Servings/Exchanges |
|---|---|---|---|---|---|---|---|---|---|---|---|---|
| ***Naked*** | | | | | | | | | | | | |
| Berry Blast | 8 oz | 130 | 0 | 0 | 0 | 0 | 0 | 10 | 29 | 0 | 1 | 2 fruit |
| Mighty Mango | 8 oz | 150 | 0 | 0 | 0 | 0 | 0 | 10 | 36 | 0 | 1 | 2 1/2 fruit |
| Power-C | 8 oz | 120 | 0 | 0 | 0 | 0 | 0 | 15 | 29 | 3 | 1 | 2 fruit |
| Protein Zone | 8 oz | 220 | 2 | 20 | 1 | 0 | 30 | 140 | 34 | 0 | 16 | 2 carb, 2 lean meat |
| Strawberry Banana | 8 oz | 120 | 0 | 0 | 0 | 0 | 0 | 20 | 29 | 0 | 1 | 2 fruit |
| Superfood Green Machine | 8 oz | 140 | 0 | 0 | 0 | 0 | 0 | 15 | 33 | 0 | 2 | 2 fruit |
| ***Ocean Spray*** | | | | | | | | | | | | |
| Cran-Apple Juice Drink | 8 oz | 130 | 0 | 0 | 0 | 0 | 0 | 80 | 32 | 0 | 0 | 2 carb |
| Cranberry Juice Cocktail | 8 oz | 120 | 0 | 0 | 0 | 0 | 0 | 35 | 30 | 0 | 0 | 2 carb |
| Cranergy Juice Drink | 8 oz | 35 | 0 | 0 | 0 | 0 | 0 | 50 | 8 | 0 | 0 | 1/2 carb |
| Cran-Grape Juice Drink | 8 oz | 120 | 0 | 0 | 0 | 0 | 0 | 31 | 80 | 0 | 0 | 2 carb |

| | | | | | | | | | | | | |
|---|---|---|---|---|---|---|---|---|---|---|---|---|
| Cran-Pomegranate | 8 oz | 120 | 0 | 0 | 0 | 0 | 0 | 35 | 30 | 0 | 0 | 2 carb |
| Cran-Raspberry Juice Drink | 8 oz | 110 | 0 | 0 | 0 | 0 | 0 | 70 | 28 | 0 | 0 | 2 carb |
| Diet Cranberry | 8 oz | 5 | 0 | 0 | 0 | 0 | 0 | 50 | 2 | 0 | 0 | free |
| Diet Grape | 8 oz | 5 | 0 | 0 | 0 | 0 | 0 | 50 | 2 | 0 | 0 | free |
| Light Cranberry Juice Cocktail | 8 oz | 40 | 0 | 0 | 0 | 0 | 0 | 75 | 10 | 0 | 0 | 1/2 carb |
| Light Cran-Grape Juice Drink | 8 oz | 40 | 0 | 0 | 0 | 0 | 0 | 75 | 10 | 0 | 0 | 1/2 carb |
| Light Ruby Grapefruit Juice Drink | 8 oz | 40 | 0 | 0 | 0 | 0 | 0 | 65 | 10 | 0 | 0 | 1/2 carb |
| No Sugar Added 100% Cranberry Juice Blend | 8 oz | 140 | 0 | 0 | 0 | 0 | 0 | 35 | 36 | 0 | 0 | 2 1/2 fruit |
| No Sugar Added Pink Grapefruit 100% Juice | 8 oz | 130 | 0 | 0 | 0 | 0 | 0 | 35 | 32 | 0 | 1 | 2 fruit |
| No Sugar Added White Grapefruit 100% Juice | 8 oz | 90 | 0 | 0 | 0 | 0 | 0 | 35 | 21 | 0 | 2 | 1 1/2 fruit |

FRUIT, FRUIT JUICES, DRINKS

| | Serving | Calories | Fat (g) | Cal. from Fat | Sat. Fat (g) | Trans Fat (g) | Chol. (mg) | Sod. (mg) | Carb. (g) | Fiber (g) | Prot. (g) | Servings/Exchanges |
|---|---|---|---|---|---|---|---|---|---|---|---|---|
| ***Old Orchard*** | | | | | | | | | | | | |
| Apple Cherry Juice Cocktail | 8 oz | 91 | 0 | 0 | 0 | 0 | 0 | 9 | 21 | 0 | 0 | 1 1/2 carb |
| Apple Cranberry Juice | 8 oz | 130 | 0 | 0 | 0 | 0 | 0 | 25 | 29 | 0 | 0 | 2 fruit |
| Apple Kiwi Strawberry Juice Cocktail | 8 oz | 91 | 0 | 0 | 0 | 0 | 0 | 9 | 21 | 0 | 0 | 1 1/2 carb |
| Healthy Balance Grape Juice Cocktail | 8 oz | 35 | 0 | 0 | 0 | 0 | 0 | 6 | 9 | 0 | 0 | 1/2 carb |
| Peach Mango 100% Juice Blend | 8 oz | 120 | 0 | 0 | 0 | 0 | 0 | 25 | 29 | 0 | 0 | 2 fruit |
| ***SunnyD*** | | | | | | | | | | | | |
| Fruit Punch | 8 oz | 80 | 0 | 0 | 0 | 0 | 0 | 160 | 21 | 0 | 0 | 1 1/2 carb |
| Reduced Sugar | 8 oz | 60 | 0 | 0 | 0 | 0 | 0 | 170 | 15 | 0 | 0 | 1 carb |
| Tangy Original | 8 oz | 90 | 0 | 0 | 0 | 0 | 0 | 170 | 22 | 0 | 0 | 1 1/2 carb |

| | | | | | | | | | | | | |
|---|---|---|---|---|---|---|---|---|---|---|---|---|
| ***Sunsweet*** | | | | | | | | | | | | |
| Prune Juice | 8 oz | 180 | 0 | 0 | 0 | 0 | 0 | 30 | 43 | 3 | 2 | 3 fruit |
| Prune Juice with Pulp | 8 oz | 180 | 0 | 0 | 0 | 0 | 0 | 30 | 43 | 3 | 2 | 3 fruit |
| ***Tree Top*** | | | | | | | | | | | | |
| Apple Juice | 8 oz | 120 | 0 | 0 | 0 | 0 | 0 | 25 | 29 | 0 | 0 | 2 fruit |
| Fiber Rich, Apple Orange Banana | 8 oz | 160 | 0 | 0 | 0 | 0 | 0 | 30 | 38 | 6 | <1 | 2 1/2 carb |
| ***Tropicana*** | | | | | | | | | | | | |
| Light 'n Healthy Juice Beverage | 8 oz | 50 | 0 | 0 | 0 | 0 | 0 | 10 | 13 | 0 | <1 | 1 carb |
| Orange Juice, Antioxidant Advantage | 8 oz | 110 | 0 | 0 | 0 | 0 | 0 | 0 | 26 | 0 | 2 | 2 fruit |
| Orange Juice, Calcium & Vitamin D | 8 oz | 110 | 0 | 0 | 0 | 0 | 0 | 0 | 26 | 0 | 2 | 2 fruit |
| Orange Juice, Healthy Heart | 8 oz | 120 | 0.5 | 5 | 0 | 0 | 0 | 0 | 26 | 0 | 2 | 2 fruit |
| Orange Juice, Low Acid | 8 oz | 110 | 0 | 0 | 0 | 0 | 0 | 0 | 26 | 0 | 2 | 2 fruit |

FRUIT, FRUIT JUICES, DRINKS

| | Serving | Calories | Fat (g) | Cal. from Fat | Sat. Fat (g) | Trans Fat (g) | Chol. (mg) | Sod. (mg) | Carb. (g) | Fiber (g) | Prot. (g) | Servings/Exchanges |
|---|---|---|---|---|---|---|---|---|---|---|---|---|
| Orange Juice, Original | 8 oz | 110 | 0 | 0 | 0 | 0 | 0 | 0 | 26 | 0 | 2 | 2 fruit |
| Orange Strawberry Banana Juice | 8 oz | 130 | 0 | 0 | 0 | 0 | 0 | 0 | 30 | 0 | 2 | 2 fruit |
| Orange Tangerine Juice | 8 oz | 110 | 0 | 0 | 0 | 0 | 0 | 0 | 25 | 0 | 2 | 1 1/2 fruit |
| Ruby Red Grapefruit Juice | 8 oz | 90 | 0 | 0 | 0 | 0 | 0 | 0 | 22 | 0 | 1 | 1 1/2 fruit |
| Tropics, Orange Peach Mango | 8 oz | 120 | 0 | 0 | 0 | 0 | 0 | 10 | 29 | 0 | 1 | 2 fruit |
| Twister Juice Drink, Assorted Flavors | 8 oz | 120 | 0 | 0 | 0 | 0 | 0 | 25 | 30 | 0 | 0 | 2 carb |
| ***V8 Splash*** | | | | | | | | | | | | |
| Berry Blend | 8 oz | 70 | 0 | 0 | 0 | 0 | 0 | 50 | 18 | 0 | 0 | 1 carb |
| Mango Peach | 8 oz | 80 | 0 | 0 | 0 | 0 | 0 | 40 | 19 | 0 | 0 | 1 carb |
| Tropical Blend | 8 oz | 70 | 0 | 0 | 0 | 0 | 0 | 30 | 18 | 0 | 0 | 1 carb |

***Welch's***

| | | | | | | | | | | | | |
|---|---|---|---|---|---|---|---|---|---|---|---|---|
| 100% Grape Juice | 8 oz | 170 | 0 | 0 | 0 | 0 | 0 | 20 | 42 | 0 | 0 | 3 fruit |
| 100% White Grape Juice | 8 oz | 160 | 0 | 0 | 0 | 0 | 0 | 20 | 39 | 0 | 0 | 2 1/2 fruit |
| Blueberry Kiwi Blast Juice Drink | 8 oz | 160 | 0 | 0 | 0 | 0 | 0 | 20 | 40 | 0 | 0 | 2 1/2 carb |
| Concord Grape Juice Cocktail | 8 oz | 140 | 0 | 0 | 0 | 0 | 0 | 20 | 34 | 0 | 0 | 2 carb |
| Cranberry Juice Cocktail | 8 oz | 140 | 0 | 0 | 0 | 0 | 0 | 5 | 35 | 0 | 0 | 2 carb |
| Diet Berry Pomegranate | 8 oz | 10 | 0 | 0 | 0 | 0 | 0 | 20 | 3 | 0 | 0 | free |
| Guava Pineapple Juice Cocktail | 8 oz | 140 | 0 | 0 | 0 | 0 | 0 | 5 | 36 | 0 | 0 | 2 1/2 carb |
| Light Grape Juice Cocktail | 8 oz | 50 | 0 | 0 | 0 | 0 | 0 | 80 | 13 | 0 | 0 | 1 carb |
| Mango Twist Juice Cocktail | 8 oz | 150 | 0 | 0 | 0 | 0 | 0 | 5 | 38 | 0 | 0 | 2 1/2 carb |

FRUIT, FRUIT JUICES, DRINKS

| | Serving | Calories | Fat (g) | Cal. from Fat | Sat. Fat (g) | Trans Fat (g) | Chol. (mg) | Sod. (mg) | Carb. (g) | Fiber (g) | Prot. (g) | Servings/Exchanges |
|---|---|---|---|---|---|---|---|---|---|---|---|---|
| Mountain Berry Juice Cocktail | 8 oz | 140 | 0 | 0 | 0 | 0 | 0 | 5 | 34 | 0 | 0 | 2 carb |
| Orange Pineapple Juice Drink | 8 oz | 120 | 0 | 0 | 0 | 0 | 0 | 50 | 31 | 0 | 0 | 2 carb |
| Passion Fruit Juice Cocktail | 8 oz | 150 | 0 | 0 | 0 | 0 | 0 | 5 | 38 | 0 | 0 | 2 1/2 carb |
| Strawberry Breeze Juice Cocktail | 8 oz | 130 | 0 | 0 | 0 | 0 | 0 | 5 | 33 | 0 | 0 | 2 carb |
| Tropical Cherry Juice Cocktail | 8 oz | 140 | 0 | 0 | 0 | 0 | 0 | 5 | 36 | 0 | 0 | 2 1/2 carb |

# GLUTEN-FREE FOODS

| | Serving | Calories | Fat (g) | Cal. from Fat | Sat. Fat (g) | Trans Fat (g) | Chol. (mg) | Sod. (mg) | Carb. (mg) | Fiber (g) | Prot. (g) | Servings/Exchanges |
|---|---|---|---|---|---|---|---|---|---|---|---|---|
| ***Ancient Quinoa Harvest*** | | | | | | | | | | | | |
| Spaghetti, Elbows, or Rotelle Pasta | 2 oz | 205 | 1 | 7 | 0 | 0 | 0 | 4 | 46 | 4 | 4 | 3 carb |
| ***Bakery On Main*** | | | | | | | | | | | | |
| Granola, Extreme Fruit & Nut | 2 oz | 270 | 13 | 120 | 2 | 0 | 0 | 45 | 34 | 3 | 4 | 2 carb, 3 fat |
| Granola, Nutty Maple Cranberry | 2 oz | 260 | 12 | 100 | 1 | 0 | 0 | 45 | 35 | 3 | 4 | 2 carb, 2 fat |
| Granola, Rainforest | 2 oz | 290 | 14 | 120 | 0.5 | 0 | 0 | 50 | 38 | 2 | 4 | 2 1/2 carb, 3 fat |
| ***Betty Crocker (Gluten Free)*** | | | | | | | | | | | | |
| Chocolate Chip Cookie Mix | 2 cookies | 150 | 7 | 60 | 4 | 0 | 25 | 160 | 23 | <1 | 1 | 1 1/2 carb, 1 fat |
| Yellow Cake Mix | 1/10 cake | 260 | 11 | 100 | 6 | 0 | 90 | 310 | 37 | 0 | 3 | 2 1/2 carb, 2 fat |

| | Serving | Calories | Fat (g) | Cal. from Fat | Sat. Fat (g) | Trans Fat (g) | Chol. (mg) | Sod. (mg) | Carb. (g) | Fiber (g) | Prot. (g) | Servings/Exchanges |
|---|---|---|---|---|---|---|---|---|---|---|---|---|
| ***DeBoles*** | | | | | | | | | | | | |
| Rice Angel Hair Pasta | 2 oz | 210 | 0.5 | 5 | 0 | 0 | 0 | 15 | 46 | <1 | 4 | 3 carb |
| Rice Angel Hair Pasta Plus Golden Flax | 2 oz | 210 | 1.5 | 15 | 0 | 0 | 0 | 10 | 44 | 1 | 4 | 3 carb |
| Rice Fettucini | 2 oz | 210 | 0.5 | 5 | 0 | 0 | 0 | 15 | 46 | 1 | 4 | 3 carb |
| Rice Lasagna | 2.5 oz | 260 | 0.5 | 5 | 0 | 0 | 0 | 15 | 56 | <1 | 5 | 3 carb |
| Rice Spaghetti Style Pasta | 2 oz | 210 | 0.5 | 5 | 0 | 0 | 0 | 15 | 46 | <1 | 4 | 3 carb |
| Rice Spirals | 2 oz | 210 | 0.5 | 5 | 0 | 0 | 0 | 15 | 46 | <1 | 4 | 3 carb |
| Wheat Free Corn Spaghetti Style Pasta | 2 oz | 200 | 2 | 20 | 0 | 0 | 0 | 15 | 43 | 5 | 4 | 3 carb |
| ***Divine Foods*** | | | | | | | | | | | | |
| Apricot Cashew Boomi Bar | 1 | 190 | 7 | 60 | 1 | 0 | 0 | 75 | 28 | 3 | 4 | 2 carb, 1 fat |

| | | | | | | | | | | | | |
|---|---|---|---|---|---|---|---|---|---|---|---|---|
| Cashew Almond Boomi Bar | 1 | 260 | 17 | 150 | 2 | 0 | 0 | 55 | 23 | 4 | 8 | 1 1/2 carb, 3 fat |
| Fruit 'n Nut Boomi Bar | 1 | 210 | 9 | 90 | 1 | 0 | 0 | 55 | 27 | 3 | 6 | 2 carb, 2 fat |
| Macadamia Paradise Boomi Bar | 1 | 240 | 15 | 140 | 3 | 0 | 0 | 25 | 28 | 3 | 3 | 2 carb, 3 fat |
| Perfect Pumpkin Boomi Bar | 1 | 230 | 10 | 100 | 2 | 0 | 0 | 45 | 23 | 1 | 9 | 1 1/2 carb, 2 fat |
| Walnut Date Boomi Bar | 1 | 200 | 9 | 80 | 1 | 0 | 0 | 20 | 29 | 2 | 4 | 2 carb, 2 fat |
| ***Ener-G Foods*** | | | | | | | | | | | | |
| Brown Rice English Muffins with Flax | 1 | 180 | 5 | 45 | 0 | 0 | 0 | 250 | 35 | 7 | 2 | 2 carb, 1 fat |
| Cinnamon Crackers | 10 | 70 | 5 | 45 | 0 | 0 | 0 | 85 | 12 | 5 | 0 | 1 carb, 1 fat |
| Cinnamon Rolls | 1 roll | 220 | 5 | 45 | 0.5 | 0 | 0 | 230 | 33 | 8 | 2 | 2 carb, 1 fat |
| Corn Loaf | 1 slice | 40 | 1.5 | 15 | 0 | 0 | 0 | 50 | 8 | 3 | 0 | 1/2 carb |
| Doughnut Holes, Plain | 1 | 50 | 2.5 | 25 | 1 | 0 | 5 | 105 | 5 | <1 | 1 | 1 fat |
| Four Flour Loaf | 1 slice | 80 | 2.5 | 20 | 0 | 0 | 0 | 100 | 17 | 3 | 1 | 1 carb, 1 fat |
| Gourmet Crackers | 3 | 160 | 7 | 60 | 3 | 0 | 0 | 330 | 23 | <1 | 1 | 1 1/2 carb, 1 fat |

GLUTEN-FREE FOODS

| | Serving | Calories | Fat (g) | Cal. from Fat | Sat. Fat (g) | Trans Fat (g) | Chol. (mg) | Sod. (mg) | Carb. (g) | Fiber (g) | Prot. (g) | Servings/Exchanges |
|---|---|---|---|---|---|---|---|---|---|---|---|---|
| Light White Rice Flax Loaf | 1 slice | 50 | 2 | 20 | 0 | 0 | 0 | 60 | 7 | 1 | 0 | 1/2 carb |
| Plain Croutons | 1 Tbsp | 25 | 1 | 10 | 0 | 0 | 0 | 25 | 3 | 0 | 0 | free |
| Seattle Brown Hamburger Buns | 1 bun | 160 | 4.5 | 40 | 0 | 0 | 0 | 190 | 34 | 8 | 2 | 2 carb, 1 fat |
| Seattle Brown Hot Dog Buns | 1 bun | 160 | 4.5 | 40 | 0 | 0 | 0 | 190 | 34 | 8 | 2 | 2 carb, 1 fat |
| Seattle Crackers | 16 | 80 | 4.5 | 40 | 0 | 0 | 0 | 190 | 9 | 5 | 0 | 1/2 carb, 1 fat |
| Tapioca Hamburger Buns | 1 bun | 120 | 3 | 30 | 0 | 0 | 0 | 150 | 21 | 4 | 1 | 1 1/2 carb, 1 fat |
| Tapioca Hot Dog Buns | 1 bun | 120 | 3 | 30 | 0 | 0 | 0 | 150 | 21 | 4 | 1 | 1 1/2 carb, 1 fat |
| Tapioca Loaf, Thin Sliced | 1 slice | 80 | 3 | 30 | 0 | 0 | 0 | 95 | 11 | 2 | 1 | 1 carb, 1 fat |
| Wylde Pretzels | 40 | 130 | 3 | 30 | 1.5 | 0 | 0 | 230 | 24 | 3 | <1 | 1 1/2 carb, 1 fat |

| **_Enjoy Life Foods_** | | | | | | | | | | | | |
|---|---|---|---|---|---|---|---|---|---|---|---|---|
| Caramel Apple Snack Bar | 1 | 110 | 2.5 | 25 | 0 | 0 | 0 | 95 | 21 | 2 | 2 | 1 1/2 carb, 1 fat |
| Chewy Chocolate Chip Cookies | 2 | 130 | 5 | 45 | 1 | 0 | 0 | 105 | 21 | 2 | 1 | 1 1/2 carb, 1 fat |
| Cinnamon Crunch Granola | 1/2 cup | 170 | 3 | 30 | 1 | 0 | 0 | 10 | 32 | 5 | 3 | 2 carb, 1 fat |
| Cinnamon Raisin Bagels | 1 | 280 | 7 | 60 | 0 | 0 | 0 | 430 | 53 | 4 | 4 | 3 1/2 carb, 1 fat |
| Classic Original Bagels | 1 | 270 | 7 | 60 | 0 | 0 | 0 | 380 | 46 | 3 | 5 | 3 carb, 1 fat |
| Crunchy Flax Cereal | 3/4 cup | 200 | 3 | 25 | 0 | 0 | 0 | 115 | 42 | 6 | 7 | 3 carb, 1 fat |
| Crunchy Rice Cereal | 3/4 cup | 210 | 1 | 20 | 0 | 0 | 0 | 110 | 46 | 2 | 4 | 3 carb |
| Gingerbread Spice Cookies | 2 | 120 | 4 | 35 | 0 | 0 | 0 | 120 | 19 | 2 | 1 | 1 carb, 1 fat |
| No-Oats Oatmeal Cookies | 2 | 120 | 3.5 | 30 | 0 | 0 | 0 | 50 | 21 | 1 | 1 | 1 1/2 carb, 1 fat |
| Perky's Nutty Flax Cereal | 3/4 cup | 220 | 3 | 30 | 0 | 0 | 0 | 115 | 44 | 7 | 5 | 3 carb, 1 fat |

## GLUTEN-FREE FOODS

| | Serving | Calories | Fat (g) | Cal. from Fat | Sat. Fat (g) | Trans Fat (g) | Chol. (mg) | Sod. (mg) | Carb. (g) | Fiber (g) | Prot. (g) | Servings/Exchanges |
|---|---|---|---|---|---|---|---|---|---|---|---|---|
| Perky's Nutty Rice Cereal | 3/4 cup | 210 | 1.5 | 15 | 0 | 0 | 0 | 110 | 46 | 2 | 4 | 3 carb |
| Very Berry Snack Bar | 1 | 120 | 2.5 | 20 | 0 | 0 | 0 | 95 | 23 | 2 | 1 | 1 1/2 carb, 1 fat |
| ***General Mills Gluten Free*** | | | | | | | | | | | | |
| Corn Chex | 1 cup | 120 | 0.5 | 5 | 0 | 0 | 0 | 290 | 26 | 1 | 2 | 2 carb |
| Rice Chex | 1 cup | 100 | 0 | 0 | 0 | 0 | 0 | 250 | 23 | 0 | 2 | 1 1/2 carb |
| ***Gillian's Foods*** | | | | | | | | | | | | |
| Cinnamon Raisin Rolls | 1/2 roll | 130 | 0.5 | 5 | 0 | 0 | 0 | 330 | 25 | 2 | 5 | 1 1/2 carb |
| Sesame Seed Rolls | 1/2 roll | 130 | 0.5 | 5 | 0 | 0 | 0 | 330 | 25 | 2 | 5 | 1 1/2 carb |
| French Rolls | 1/2 roll | 130 | 4 | 35 | 0.5 | 0 | 0 | 160 | 20 | 1 | 3 | 1 carb, 1 fat |
| ***Foods By George*** | | | | | | | | | | | | |
| Biscotti | 1 | 90 | 4.5 | 40 | 1 | 0 | 0 | 25 | 11 | 1 | 2 | 1 carb, 1 fat |
| Blueberry Muffins | 1 | 220 | 8 | 70 | 1 | 0 | 25 | 450 | 33 | 1 | 3 | 2 carb, 2 fat |
| Brownies | 1/9 tray | 180 | 9 | 80 | 1 | 0 | 40 | 45 | 24 | 1 | 2 | 1 1/2 carb, 2 fat |

| | | | | | | | | | | | | |
|---|---|---|---|---|---|---|---|---|---|---|---|---|
| Corn Muffins | 1 | 240 | 9 | 80 | 1 | 0 | 30 | 480 | 36 | 1 | 4 | 2 1/2 carb, 2 fat |
| English Muffins | 1 | 210 | 3.5 | 30 | 0 | 0 | 0 | 270 | 39 | 1 | 4 | 2 1/2 carb, 1 fat |
| No-Rye Rye English Muffins | 1 | 210 | 4 | 35 | 0 | 0 | 0 | 270 | 40 | 2 | 4 | 2 1/2 carb |
| Pecan Tarts | 1 | 470 | 28 | 250 | 7 | 0 | 95 | 160 | 51 | 3 | 6 | 3 1/2 carb, 6 fat |
| ***French Meadow Bakery*** | | | | | | | | | | | | |
| Chocolate Chip Cookie | 1 | 320 | 16 | 150 | 8 | 0 | 25 | 260 | 43 | 1 | 1 | 3 carb, 3 fat |
| Cinnamon Raisin Bread | 1 slice | 150 | 5 | 45 | 3 | 0 | 0 | 270 | 22 | 2 | 2 | 1 1/2 carb, 1 fat |
| Fudge Brownie | 1 | 170 | 7 | 60 | 1 | 0 | 15 | 25 | 25 | 1 | 2 | 1 1/2 carb, 1 fat |
| Italian Rolls | 1 | 340 | 9 | 80 | 1 | 0 | 40 | 470 | 63 | 8 | 3 | 4 carb, 2 fat |
| Muffins | 1 | 210 | 8 | 80 | 1.5 | 0.5 | 45 | 110 | 31 | 1 | 2 | 2 carb, 2 fat |
| Multigrain Bread | 1 slice | 150 | 4.5 | 40 | 2 | 0 | 0 | 230 | 23 | 3 | 4 | 1 1/2 carb, 1 fat |
| Sandwich Bread | 1 slice | 120 | 4 | 35 | 2.5 | 0 | 0 | 310 | 20 | 1 | 2 | 1 carb, 1 fat |
| Tortilla | 1 | 120 | 1 | 5 | 0 | 0 | 0 | 290 | 24 | 1 | 1 | 1 1/2 carb |
| ***Glutinos*** | | | | | | | | | | | | |
| Apple Breakfast Bar | 1 | 130 | 2 | 20 | 0 | 0 | 0 | 5 | 28 | 3 | 2 | 2 carb |

GLUTEN-FREE FOODS

| | Serving | Calories | Fat (g) | Cal. from Fat | Sat. Fat (g) | Trans Fat (g) | Chol. (mg) | Sod. (mg) | Carb. (g) | Fiber (g) | Prot. (g) | Servings/Exchanges |
|---|---|---|---|---|---|---|---|---|---|---|---|---|
| Breadsticks, Sesame Flavored | 9 | 60 | 1.5 | 15 | 1 | 0 | 0 | 100 | 12 | 0 | 0 | 1 carb |
| Cheddar Crackers | 8 | 140 | 5 | 45 | 2.5 | 0 | 10 | 180 | 21 | <1 | 2 | 1 1/2 carb, 1 fat |
| Honey Nut Cereal | 1/2 cup | 120 | 1.5 | 15 | 0 | 0 | 0 | 120 | 26 | 1 | 1 | 2 carb |
| Lemon Wafers | 3 | 150 | 6 | 55 | 4 | 0 | 0 | 25 | 24 | 0 | 0 | 1 1/2 carb, 1 fat |
| Pretzels, Sticks | 33 | 140 | 6 | 50 | 2.5 | 0 | 0 | 420 | 21 | 0 | 0 | 1 1/2 carb, 1 fat |
| Vanilla Wafers | 4 | 160 | 8 | 70 | 5 | 0 | 5 | 25 | 19 | 0 | 1 | 1 carb, 2 fat |
| ***Heartland's Finest*** | | | | | | | | | | | | |
| All Natural Macaroni & Cheese | 3 oz | 340 | 7 | 65 | 4.5 | 0 | 20 | 800 | 53 | 6 | 14 | 3 1/2 carb, 1 fat |
| CerO's Cereal, Original | 1 cup | 120 | 0 | 0 | 0 | 0 | 0 | 125 | 24 | 3 | 5 | 1 1/2 carb |
| CerO's Cereal, Raspberry | 1 cup | 110 | 0 | 0 | 0 | 0 | 0 | 115 | 23 | 2 | 4 | 1 1/2 carb |
| Elbow Macaroni Pasta | 3/4 oz | 210 | 1.5 | 15 | 0.5 | 0 | 0 | 0 | 41 | 5 | 7 | 2 1/2 carb |
| Lasagna Pasta | 2 oz | 210 | 1.5 | 15 | 0.5 | 0 | 0 | 0 | 41 | 5 | 7 | 2 1/2 carb |

| | | | | | | | | | | | | |
|---|---|---|---|---|---|---|---|---|---|---|---|---|
| Linguini Pasta | 2 oz | 210 | 1.5 | 15 | 0.5 | 0 | 0 | 0 | 41 | 5 | 7 | 2 1/2 carb |
| Spaghetti Pasta | 2 oz | 210 | 1.5 | 15 | 0.5 | 0 | 0 | 0 | 41 | 5 | 7 | 2 1/2 carb |
| ***Hodgson Mill Brown Rice Pasta*** | | | | | | | | | | | | |
| Elbows, Penne, Spaghetti, Angel Hair, Linguine | 2 oz | 209 | 1 | 12 | 0 | 0 | 0 | 0 | 44 | 2 | 5 | 3 carb |
| ***Kay's Naturals Better Balance*** | | | | | | | | | | | | |
| Almond Delight Crisps | 1 oz | 120 | 3.5 | 30 | 0 | 0 | 0 | 250 | 14 | 2 | 10 | 1 carb, 1 lean meat |
| Apple Cinnamon Cereal | 1 oz | 100 | 1.5 | 10 | 0 | 0 | 0 | 140 | 15 | 3 | 9 | 1 carb, 1 lean meat |
| Chili Nacho Cheese Protein Chips | 1 oz | 110 | 3.5 | 30 | 0 | 0 | 0 | 230 | 14 | 3 | 10 | 1 carb, 1 lean meat |
| Crispy Parmesan Protein Chips | 1 oz | 110 | 3.5 | 30 | 0 | 0 | 0 | 230 | 14 | 3 | 10 | 1 carb, 1 lean meat |
| French Vanilla Cereal | 1 oz | 100 | 1.5 | 10 | 0 | 0 | 0 | 140 | 15 | 3 | 9 | 1 carb, 1 lean meat |
| Golden Butter Pretzels | 1 oz | 110 | 5 | 30 | 1.5 | 0 | 0 | 220 | 12 | 2 | 10 | 1 carb, 1 med-fat meat |
| Lemon Herb Protein Chips | 1 oz | 110 | 3.5 | 30 | 0 | 0 | 0 | 230 | 14 | 3 | 10 | 1 carb, 1 lean meat |

| | Serving | Calories | Fat (g) | Cal. from Fat | Sat. Fat (g) | Trans Fat (g) | Chol. (mg) | Sod. (mg) | Carb. (g) | Fiber (g) | Prot. (g) | Servings/Exchanges |
|---|---|---|---|---|---|---|---|---|---|---|---|---|
| White Cheddar Kruncheeze | 1 oz | 130 | 6 | 60 | 0.5 | 0 | 0 | 200 | 10 | 2 | 9 | 1/2 carb, 1 med-fat meat |
| ***Kinnikinnick Foods*** | | | | | | | | | | | | |
| Blueberry Muffin | 1 | 190 | 7 | 65 | 2 | 0 | 10 | 320 | 32 | 3 | 1 | 2 carb, 1 fat |
| Brown Sandwich Bread | 1 slice | 70 | 2 | 20 | <1 | 0 | 15 | 180 | 14 | 2 | 2 | 1 carb |
| Chocolate Chip Muffin | 1 | 170 | 9 | 80 | 2 | 0 | 20 | 170 | 28 | 2 | 1 | 2 carb, 2 fat |
| Chocolate Dipped Donuts | 1 | 220 | 6 | 55 | 3 | 0 | 0 | 200 | 41 | 2 | 2 | 2 1/2 carb, 1 fat |
| Cinnamon Sugar Donuts | 1 | 170 | 4.5 | 40 | 2.5 | 0 | 0 | 230 | 30 | 1 | 2 | 2 carb, 1 fat |
| Ginger Snap Cookies | 2 | 25 | 1 | 10 | 0.5 | 0 | 0 | 40 | 5 | 0 | 0 | 1/2 carb |
| Italian White Tapioca Rice Bread | 1 slice | 90 | 2.5 | 25 | <1 | 0 | 20 | 190 | 20 | 1 | 2 | 1 carb, 1 fat |
| KinniToos Vanilla Sandwich Cookies | 1 | 60 | 2.5 | 20 | 1 | 0 | 0 | 50 | 9 | 1 | 0 | 1/2 carb, 1 fat |
| Many Wonder Multigrain Rice Bread | 1 slice | 90 | 3.5 | 30 | <1 | 0 | 20 | 120 | 18 | 3 | 2 | 1 carb, 1 fat |

| | | | | | | | | | | | | |
|---|---|---|---|---|---|---|---|---|---|---|---|---|
| Montanas Chocolate Chip Cookies | 2 | 115 | 5 | 45 | 1.5 | 0 | 15 | 90 | 15 | 0 | 1 | 1 carb, 1 fat |
| Tapioca Rice English Muffins | 1 | 240 | 3.5 | 30 | <1 | 0 | 0 | 260 | 41 | 2 | 3 | 2 1/2 carb, 1 fat |
| Tapioca Rice Hamburger Bun | 1 | 230 | 7 | 65 | 0.5 | 0 | 5 | 330 | 36 | 4 | 5 | 2 1/2 carb, 1 fat |
| Tapioca Rice Hot Dog Bun | 1 | 250 | 8 | 70 | 0.5 | 0 | 5 | 360 | 39 | 4 | 5 | 2 1/2 carb, 2 fat |
| Tapioca Rice New York Style Plain Bagel | 1 | 210 | 7 | 65 | 2.5 | 0 | 35 | 430 | 48 | 3 | 4 | 3 carb, 1 fat |
| White Sandwich Bread | 1 slice | 70 | 2 | 20 | <1 | 0 | 15 | 150 | 15 | 2 | 1 | 1 carb |
| ***La Tortilla Factory*** | | | | | | | | | | | | |
| Dark Teff Wraps | 1 wrap | 180 | 5 | 45 | 0.5 | 0 | 0 | 320 | 31 | 3 | 2 | 2 carb, 1 fat |
| Ivory Teff Wraps | 1 wrap | 180 | 5 | 45 | 0.5 | 0 | 0 | 320 | 30 | 3 | 2 | 2 carb, 1 fat |
| ***Lundberg Organic Brown Rice Pasta*** | | | | | | | | | | | | |
| Rotini, Penne, Spaghetti | 2 oz | 190 | 3 | 30 | 0.5 | 0 | 0 | 0 | 40 | 4 | 4 | 2 1/2 carb |

| GLUTEN-FREE FOODS | Serving | Calories | Fat (g) | Cal. from Fat | Sat. Fat (g) | Trans Fat (g) | Chol. (mg) | Sod. (mg) | Carb. (g) | Fiber (g) | Prot. (g) | Servings/Exchanges |
|---|---|---|---|---|---|---|---|---|---|---|---|---|
| ***Mary's Gone Crackers*** | | | | | | | | | | | | |
| Black Pepper Crackers | 13 | 140 | 5 | 45 | 0.5 | 0 | 0 | 180 | 21 | 3 | 3 | 1 1/2 carb, 1 fat |
| Original Crackers | 13 | 140 | 5 | 45 | 0.5 | 0 | 0 | 190 | 21 | 3 | 3 | 1 1/2 carb, 1 fat |
| Sticks & Twigs, Chipotle Tomato | 15 | 150 | 5 | 45 | 0.5 | 0 | 0 | 160 | 20 | 4 | 4 | 1 carb, 1 fat |
| Sticks & Twigs, Sea Salt Crackers | 15 | 150 | 5 | 45 | 0.5 | 0 | 0 | 300 | 21 | 4 | 4 | 1 1/2 carb, 1 fat |
| ***Mi-Del*** | | | | | | | | | | | | |
| Arrowroot Cookies | 10 | 130 | 6 | 35 | 1 | NA | 10 | 85 | 23 | 2 | 2 | 1 1/2 carb, 1 fat |
| Chocolate Chip Cookies | 5 | 130 | 4.5 | 40 | 1.5 | 0 | 0 | 130 | 21 | 1 | 2 | 1 1/2 carb, 1 fat |
| Ginger Snaps | 5 | 140 | 6 | 50 | 0 | 0 | 0 | 85 | 21 | 1 | 2 | 1 1/2 carb, 1 fat |
| Pecan Cookies | 5 | 140 | 6 | 60 | 1.5 | 0 | 5 | 150 | 19 | 1 | 2 | 1 carb, 1 fat |
| Royal Vanilla Sandwich Cookies | 3 | 170 | 8 | 70 | 0.5 | 0 | 5 | 85 | 24 | 1 | 2 | 1 1/2 carb, 2 fat |

| | | | | | | | | | | | | |
|---|---|---|---|---|---|---|---|---|---|---|---|---|
| ***Nature's Path*** | | | | | | | | | | | | |
| Crunchy Maple Sunrise | 2/3 cup | 110 | 1 | 10 | 0 | 0 | 0 | 130 | 25 | 3 | 2 | 1 1/2 carb |
| Crunchy Vanilla Sunrise | 2/3 cup | 110 | 1 | 10 | 0 | 0 | 0 | 130 | 25 | 3 | 2 | 1 1/2 carb |
| EnviroKidz Panda Puffs | 3/4 cup | 130 | 2.5 | 25 | 0 | 0 | 0 | 130 | 24 | 2 | 2 | 1 1/2 carb, 1 fat |
| Whole O's Cereal | 2/3 cup | 110 | 1.5 | 10 | 0 | 0 | 0 | 115 | 25 | 3 | 2 | 1 1/2 carb |
| ***Nu-World Foods*** | | | | | | | | | | | | |
| Amaranth Berry Delicious Hot Cereal | 1 cup | 90 | 1 | 10 | <1 | 0 | 0 | 10 | 16 | 3 | 4 | 1 carb |
| Flatbread, Amaranth-Garbanzo | 1 piece | 165 | 4 | 35 | 0.5 | 0 | 0 | 100 | 28 | 6 | 8 | 2 carb, 1 fat |
| Puffed Amaranth Cereal | 1 cup | 120 | 1 | 15 | 0 | 0 | 0 | 1 | 15 | 3 | 6 | 1 carb |
| ***Pamela's Products*** | | | | | | | | | | | | |
| Almond Anise Biscotti | 1 | 120 | 6 | 50 | 2.5 | 0 | 10 | 150 | 18 | 1 | 1 | 1 carb, 1 fat |
| Butter Shortbread Cookies | 1 | 110 | 7 | 60 | 4 | 0 | 15 | 70 | 13 | 1 | 1 | 1 carb, 1 fat |
| Chocolate Chip Walnut Cookies | 1 | 120 | 7 | 70 | 1 | 0 | 10 | 80 | 13 | 0.5 | 1 | 1 carb, 1 fat |

GLUTEN-FREE FOODS

| | Serving | Calories | Fat (g) | Cal. from Fat | Sat. Fat (g) | Trans Fat (g) | Chol. (mg) | Sod. (mg) | Carb. (g) | Fiber (g) | Prot. (g) | Servings/Exchanges |
|---|---|---|---|---|---|---|---|---|---|---|---|---|
| Chunky Chocolate Chip Cookies | 1 | 120 | 6 | 60 | 1 | 0 | 10 | 80 | 14 | 0.5 | 1 | 1 carb, 2 fat |
| Lemon Shortbread Cookies | 1 | 120 | 6 | 50 | 4 | 0 | 15 | 50 | 15 | 0 | 0.5 | 1 carb, 1 fat |
| Peanut Butter Cookies | 1 | 100 | 5 | 45 | 1 | 0 | 15 | 120 | 11 | 0.5 | 3 | 1 carb, 1 fat |
| Shortbread Swirl Cookies | 1 | 120 | 7 | 60 | 4 | 0 | 15 | 70 | 14 | 0.5 | 0 | 1 carb, 1 fat |
| ***Schèr*** | | | | | | | | | | | | |
| Chocolate-Dipped Cookies | 3 | 150 | 7 | 70 | 3.5 | 0 | 0 | 60 | 21 | 1 | 1 | 1 1/2 carb, 1 fat |
| Classic White Bread | 1 slice | 70 | 1.5 | 15 | 1 | 0 | 0 | 130 | 12 | 1 | <1 | 1 carb |
| Classic White Rolls | 1 | 170 | 5 | 45 | 1 | 0 | 0 | 370 | 30 | 0 | 2 | 2 carb, 1 fat |
| Crispbread | 4 slices | 100 | 0.5 | 5 | 0 | 0 | 0 | 250 | 22 | <1 | 2 | 1 1/2 carb |
| Italian Breadsticks | 7 | 120 | 2.5 | 25 | 0.5 | 0 | 0 | 310 | 24 | 1 | <1 | 1 1/2 carb, 1 fat |
| Ladyfingers | 3 | 110 | 2 | 20 | 0.5 | 0 | 40 | 40 | 22 | 1 | 2 | 1 1/2 carb |

| | | | | | | | | | | | | |
|---|---|---|---|---|---|---|---|---|---|---|---|---|
| Multigrain Bread | 1 slice | 70 | 1.5 | 15 | 0.5 | 0 | 0 | 140 | 12 | 2 | 2 | 1 carb |
| Shortbread Cookies | 4 | 130 | 5 | 45 | 2.5 | 0 | 10 | 20 | 20 | <1 | <1 | 1 carb, 1 fat |
| Table Crackers | 3 | 120 | 3.5 | 35 | 1.5 | 0 | 0 | 220 | 21 | 1 | <1 | 1 1/2 carb, 1 fat |
| Vanilla Wafers | 4 | 160 | 8 | 70 | 7 | 0 | 0 | 160 | 20 | 1 | 1 | 1 carb, 2 fat |
| ***Tinkyada Brown Rice Pasta*** | | | | | | | | | | | | |
| Fettucini, Lasagne, Penne, Spaghetti, Shells, Spirals | 2 oz | 210 | 2 | 15 | 0 | 0 | 0 | 15 | 43 | 2 | 4 | 3 carb |
| ***Trader Joe's*** | | | | | | | | | | | | |
| Brown Rice Tortillas | 1 tortilla | 130 | 2.5 | 25 | 0 | 0 | 0 | 160 | 24 | 2 | 2 | 1 1/2 carb, 1 fat |
| Organic Brown Rice Penne Pasta | 2 oz | 200 | 0 | 0 | 0 | 0 | 0 | 0 | 45 | 1 | 5 | 3 carb |
| Rice Sticks | 1/4 cup | 210 | 0.5 | 5 | 0 | 0 | 0 | 10 | 46 | 1 | 4 | 3 carb |
| ***Whole Foods Gluten Free Bakehouse*** | | | | | | | | | | | | |
| Almond Cookies | 1 | 270 | 12 | 110 | 1 | 0 | 0 | 20 | 34 | <1 | 6 | 2 carb, 2 fat |
| Apple Pie | 2 oz | 120 | 5 | 45 | 3 | 0 | 20 | 70 | 20 | 1 | 1 | 1 carb, 1 fat |

GLUTEN-FREE FOODS

| | Serving | Calories | Fat (g) | Cal. from Fat | Sat. Fat (g) | Trans Fat (g) | Chol. (mg) | Sod. (mg) | Carb. (g) | Fiber (g) | Prot. (g) | Servings/Exchanges |
|---|---|---|---|---|---|---|---|---|---|---|---|---|
| Banana Bread | 2 oz | 220 | 11 | 100 | 4.5 | 0 | 55 | 170 | 28 | 0 | 3 | 2 carb, 2 fat |
| Blueberry Muffins | 1 | 330 | 13 | 110 | 1 | 0 | 60 | 380 | 53 | 1 | 4 | 3 1/2 carb, 3 fat |
| Chocolate Chip Cookies | 1 | 160 | 8 | 80 | 4.5 | 0 | 30 | 95 | 22 | 0 | 2 | 1 1/2 carb, 2 fat |
| Cornbread | 2 oz | 160 | 7 | 70 | 1 | 0 | 50 | 320 | 21 | 2 | 3 | 1 1/2 carb, 1 fat |
| Cream Biscuits | 1 | 220 | 13 | 120 | 8 | 0 | 50 | 400 | 24 | <1 | 2 | 1 1/2 carb, 1 fat |
| Hamburger Buns | 1 | 330 | 10 | 90 | 6 | 0 | 65 | 300 | 55 | 1 | 4 | 3 1/2 carb, 2 fat |
| Honey Oat Bread | 2 oz | 140 | 3.5 | 35 | 0 | 0 | 35 | 200 | 24 | 1 | 2 | 1 1/2 carb, 1 fat |
| Lemon Poppy Seed Muffin | 1 | 390 | 20 | 180 | 0 | 0 | 120 | 300 | 48 | <1 | 5 | 3 carb, 4 fat |
| Morning Glory Muffin | 1 | 310 | 18 | 160 | 1.5 | 0 | 70 | 310 | 36 | 1 | 4 | 2 1/2 carb, 4 fat |
| Prairie Bread | 1 slice | 150 | 5 | 45 | 0 | 0 | 35 | 180 | 23 | <1 | 3 | 1 1/2 carb, 1 fat |
| Sandwich Bread | 1 slice | 150 | 4.5 | 40 | 0 | 0 | 40 | 190 | 24 | 0 | 3 | 1 1/2 carb, 1 fat |
| Walnut Brownies | 2 oz | 270 | 16 | 140 | 6 | 0 | 65 | 150 | 31 | <1 | 5 | 2 carb, 3 fat |

| | Serving | Calories | Fat (g) | Cal. from Fat | Sat. Fat (g) | Trans Fat (g) | Chol. (mg) | Sod. (mg) | Carb. (g) | Fiber (g) | Prot. (g) | Servings/Exchanges |
|---|---|---|---|---|---|---|---|---|---|---|---|---|
| **ICE CREAM, FROZEN YOGURT, PUDDING, GELATIN** | | | | | | | | | | | | |
| Frozen Yogurt, Fat Free | 1/3 cup | 66 | 0 | 0 | 0 | 0 | 0 | 43 | 13 | 0 | 3 | 1 carb |
| Frozen Yogurt, Regular | 1/2 cup | 110 | 3 | 30 | 2 | 0 | 10 | 40 | 19 | 0 | 3 | 1 carb, 1 fat |
| Fruit Juice Bar, Frozen, 100% Juice | 3 oz | 75 | <1 | 0 | 0 | 0 | 0 | 4 | 19 | 0 | 1 | 1 carb |
| Gelatin, Dessert | 1/2 cup | 84 | 0 | 0 | 0 | 0 | 0 | 101 | 19 | 0 | 2 | 1 carb |
| Ice Cream | 1/2 cup | 165 | 10 | 90 | 5 | 0 | 23 | 102 | 15 | 0 | 3 | 1 carb, 2 fat |
| Ice Cream, Fat Free | 1/2 cup | 90 | 0 | 0 | 0 | 0 | 0 | 55 | 22 | 4 | 3 | 1 1/2 carb |
| Ice Cream, Light | 1/2 cup | 120 | 5 | 45 | 2 | 0 | 15 | 90 | 16 | 0 | 3 | 1 carb, 1 fat |
| Ice Cream, No Sugar Added | 1/2 cup | 115 | 6 | 55 | 2 | 0 | 10 | 93 | 15 | 3 | 3 | 1 carb, 1 fat |
| Ice Pops | 1 | 27 | 0 | 0 | 0 | 0 | 0 | 4 | 7 | 0 | 0 | 1/2 carb |
| Pudding, Chocolate | 1/2 cup | 153 | 5 | 45 | 1 | 0 | 1 | 164 | 25 | 0 | 2 | 1 1/2 carb, 1 fat |
| Pudding, Fat Free | 3.5 oz | 88 | 0 | 0 | 0 | 0 | 0 | 189 | 20 | 0 | 2 | 1 carb |

| | Serving | Calories | Carb. (g) | Fat (g) | % Cal. Fat | Sat. Fat (g) | Trans Fat (g) | Chol. (mg) | Sod. (mg) | Fiber (g) | Prot. (g) | Servings/Exchanges |
|---|---|---|---|---|---|---|---|---|---|---|---|---|
| Pudding, Tapioca | 1/2 cup | 143 | 4 | 35 | 1 | 0 | 1 | 160 | 24 | 0 | 2 | 1 1/2 carb, 1 fat |
| Pudding, Vanilla | 1/2 cup | 143 | 4 | 35 | 1 | 0 | 1 | 156 | 25 | 0 | 2 | 1 1/2 carb, 1 fat |
| Sherbet, Orange | 1/2 cup | 138 | 2 | 20 | 1 | 0 | 0 | 44 | 29 | 3 | 1 | 2 carb |
| Sorbet | 1/2 cup | 130 | 0 | 0 | 0 | 0 | 0 | 21 | 31 | 1 | <1 | 2 carb |
| Topping, Butterscotch | 2 Tbsp | 103 | 0 | 0 | 0 | 0 | <1 | 143 | 27 | <1 | <1 | 2 carb |
| Topping, Hot Fudge | 2 Tbsp | 147 | 6 | 55 | 2 | 0 | 5 | 28 | 25 | <1 | 2 | 1 1/2 carb, 1 fat |
| Topping, Marshmallow | 2 Tbsp | 118 | 0 | 0 | 0 | 0 | 0 | 18 | 30 | <1 | <1 | 2 carb |
| Topping, Whipped | 2 Tbsp | 24 | 2 | 20 | 1 | 0 | 0 | 0 | 2 | 0 | 0 | free |
| Topping, Whipped, Light | 2 Tbsp | 19 | 1 | 10 | <1 | 0 | 0 | 0 | 2 | 0 | 0 | free |
| **ICE CREAM/FROZEN YOGURT** | | | | | | | | | | | | |
| **BRANDS** | | | | | | | | | | | | |
| ***Ben & Jerry's*** | | | | | | | | | | | | |
| Frozen Yogurt, Cherry Garcia | 1/2 cup | 160 | 3 | 30 | 2 | 0 | 15 | 15 | 31 | 1 | 4 | 2 carb, 1 fat |

| | | | | | | | | | | | | |
|---|---|---|---|---|---|---|---|---|---|---|---|---|
| Frozen Yogurt, Chocolate Fudge Brownie | 1/2 cup | 170 | 2.5 | 25 | 0.5 | 0 | 15 | 95 | 34 | 1 | 5 | 2 carb, 1 fat |
| Frozen Yogurt, Half Baked | 1/2 cup | 180 | 3 | 25 | 1.5 | 0 | 20 | 95 | 35 | 1 | 4 | 2 carb, 1 fat |
| Ice Cream, Cherry Garcia | 1/2 cup | 200 | 14 | 100 | 8 | 0 | 45 | 50 | 23 | 0 | 3 | 1 1/2 carb, 3 fat |
| Ice Cream, Chocolate Chip Cookie Dough | 1/2 cup | 220 | 12 | 110 | 7 | 0 | 55 | 70 | 26 | 0 | 4 | 2 carb, 2 fat |
| Ice Cream, Chocolate Fudge Brownie | 1/2 cup | 220 | 11 | 100 | 6 | 0 | 25 | 70 | 27 | 1 | 3 | 2 carb, 2 fat |
| Ice Cream, Chubby Hubby | 1/2 cup | 330 | 20 | 180 | 11 | 0 | 55 | 150 | 31 | 1 | 7 | 2 carb, 4 fat |
| Ice Cream, Chunky Monkey | 1/2 cup | 240 | 14 | 130 | 8 | 0 | 45 | 35 | 24 | 0 | 4 | 1 1/2 carb, 3 fat |
| Ice Cream, Coffee Heath Bar Crunch | 1/2 cup | 280 | 16 | 150 | 10 | 1 | 60 | 115 | 29 | 0 | 4 | 2 carb, 3 fat |

ICE CREAM, FROZEN YOGURT, PUDDING, GELATIN

| | Serving | Calories | Fat (g) | Cal. from Fat | Sat. Fat (g) | Trans Fat (g) | Chol. (mg) | Sod. (mg) | Carb. (g) | Fiber (g) | Prot. (g) | Servings/Exchanges |
|---|---|---|---|---|---|---|---|---|---|---|---|---|
| Ice Cream, Light, Chocolate Chip Cookie Dough | 1/2 cup | 200 | 6 | 50 | 3.5 | 0 | 35 | 80 | 35 | 2 | 4 | 2 carb, 1 fat |
| Ice Cream, Light, Phish Food | 1/2 cup | 210 | 6 | 60 | 4.5 | 0 | 25 | 90 | 37 | 1 | 4 | 2 1/2 carb, 1 fat |
| Ice Cream, Light, Raspberry Chocolate | 1/2 cup | 180 | 5 | 50 | 4 | 0 | 25 | 60 | 32 | 2 | 3 | 2 carb, 1 fat |
| Ice Cream, Mint Chocolate Cookie | 1/2 cup | 250 | 14 | 130 | 8 | 0 | 60 | 100 | 26 | 0 | 4 | 2 carb, 3 fat |
| Ice Cream, No Sugar Added, Vanilla Fudge Chip | 1/2 cup | 180 | 13 | 120 | 10 | 0 | 45 | 40 | 20 | 3 | 3 | 1 carb, 3 fat |
| Ice Cream, Original Butter Pecan | 1/2 cup | 260 | 20 | 180 | 8 | 0 | 50 | 105 | 17 | 0 | 4 | 1 carb, 4 fat |

| | | | | | | | | | | | | |
|---|---|---|---|---|---|---|---|---|---|---|---|---|
| Ice Cream, Original Vanilla | 1/2 cup | 230 | 14 | 130 | 9 | 0 | 70 | 60 | 22 | 0 | 4 | 1 1/2 carb, 3 fat |
| Ice Cream, Peanut Butter Cup | 1/2 cup | 340 | 24 | 220 | 12 | 0 | 55 | 125 | 28 | 1 | 6 | 2 carb, 5 fat |
| Ice Cream, Vanilla Caramel Fudge | 1/2 cup | 270 | 14 | 130 | 10 | 0 | 65 | 100 | 31 | 0 | 4 | 2 carb, 3 fat |
| Sorbet, Berried Treasure | 1/2 cup | 110 | 0 | 0 | 0 | 0 | 0 | 5 | 29 | 1 | 0 | 2 carb |
| Sorbet, Jamaican Me Crazy | 1/2 cup | 130 | 0 | 0 | 0 | 0 | 0 | 10 | 33 | 1 | 0 | 2 carb |
| ***Blue Bunny*** | | | | | | | | | | | | |
| Sweet Freedom No Sugar Added, Lite Chocolate Ice Cream | 1 bar | 100 | 7 | 60 | 5 | 0 | <5 | 25 | 12 | 2 | 2 | 1 carb, 1 fat |
| ***Breyers*** | | | | | | | | | | | | |
| Carb Smart, Chocolate | 1/2 cup | 90 | 6 | 50 | 3.5 | 0 | 15 | 75 | 13 | 4 | 2 | 1 carb, 1 fat |
| Carb Smart, Vanilla | 1/2 cup | 90 | 6 | 50 | 3.5 | 0 | 15 | 45 | 13 | 4 | 2 | 1 carb, 1 fat |
| Ice Cream, Chocolate | 1/2 cup | 140 | 7 | 60 | 4.5 | 0 | 20 | 45 | 17 | 1 | 2 | 1 carb, 1 fat |

ICE CREAM, FROZEN YOGURT, PUDDING, GELATIN

| | Serving | Calories | Fat (g) | Cal. from Fat | Sat. Fat (g) | Trans Fat (g) | Chol. (mg) | Sod. (mg) | Carb. (g) | Fiber (g) | Prot. (g) | Servings/Exchanges |
|---|---|---|---|---|---|---|---|---|---|---|---|---|
| Ice Cream, Heath English Toffee | 1/2 cup | 160 | 6 | 50 | 3.5 | 0 | 10 | 130 | 25 | 0 | 2 | 1 1/2 carb, 1 fat |
| Ice Cream, Natural Vanilla | 1/2 cup | 130 | 7 | 60 | 4 | 0 | 20 | 35 | 14 | 0 | 3 | 1 carb, 1 fat |
| Ice Cream, Reese's Peanut Butter Cup | 1/2 cup | 160 | 6 | 50 | 2.5 | 0 | 10 | 110 | 25 | 1 | 3 | 1 1/2 carb, 1 fat |
| Ice Cream, Smooth & Dreamy | 1/2 cup | 110 | 3.5 | 30 | 2 | 0 | 10 | 50 | 16 | 0 | 3 | 1 carb, 1 fat |
| Ice Cream, Smooth & Dreamy, 1/2 Fat Creamy Chocolate | 1 | 110 | 3.5 | 35 | 2 | 0 | 10 | 55 | 17 | 1 | 3 | 1 carb, 1 fat |
| Ice Cream, Smooth & Dreamy, Chocolate Cookies & Cream | 1/2 cup | 110 | 0 | 0 | 0 | 0 | 0 | 70 | 25 | 3 | 3 | 1 1/2 carb |

| | | | | | | | | | | | | |
|---|---|---|---|---|---|---|---|---|---|---|---|---|
| Ice Cream, Smooth & Dreamy, French Chocolate | 1/2 cup | 90 | 0 | 0 | 0 | 0 | 0 | 55 | 22 | 4 | 3 | 1 1/2 carb |
| Ice Cream, No Sugar Added, Chocolate Fudge Brownie | 1/2 cup | 90 | 1.5 | 15 | 1 | 0 | 5 | 85 | 20 | 4 | 3 | 1 carb |
| Ice Cream, Smooth & Dreamy, No Sugar Added, French Vanilla | 1/2 cup | 90 | 4.5 | 40 | 2.5 | 0 | 30 | 45 | 14 | 4 | 2 | 1 carb, 1 fat |
| Ice Cream, Snickers | 1/2 cup | 170 | 8 | 70 | 4.5 | 0 | 20 | 80 | 20 | 0 | 3 | 1 carb, 2 fat |
| Ice Cream, Strawberry | 1/2 cup | 120 | 5 | 45 | 3 | 0 | 15 | 35 | 15 | 0 | 2 | 1 carb, 1 fat |
| ***Häagen-Dazs*** | | | | | | | | | | | | |
| Frozen Yogurt, Coffee | 1/2 cup | 200 | 4.5 | 40 | 2.5 | 0 | 65 | 50 | 31 | 0 | 8 | 2 carb, 1 fat |
| Frozen Yogurt, Dulce de Leche | 1/2 cup | 190 | 2.5 | 25 | 2 | 0 | 5 | 75 | 35 | 2 | 6 | 2 carb, 1 fat |
| Frozen Yogurt, Vanilla | 1/2 cup | 200 | 4.5 | 40 | 2.5 | 0 | 65 | 55 | 31 | 0 | 9 | 2 carb, 1 fat |

| | Serving | Calories | Fat (g) | Cal. from Fat | Sat. Fat (g) | Trans Fat (g) | Chol. (mg) | Sod. (mg) | Carb. (g) | Fiber (g) | Prot. (g) | Servings/Exchanges |
|---|---|---|---|---|---|---|---|---|---|---|---|---|
| Frozen Yogurt, Vanilla Raspberry Swirl | 1/2 cup | 170 | 2.5 | 25 | 1.5 | 0 | 25 | 35 | 32 | 0 | 4 | 2 carb, 1 fat |
| Ice Cream, Butter Pecan | 1/2 cup | 310 | 23 | 210 | 11 | 0.5 | 110 | 110 | 21 | <1 | 5 | 1 1/2 carb, 5 fat |
| Ice Cream, Chocolate | 1/2 cup | 270 | 18 | 160 | 11 | 0.5 | 115 | 60 | 22 | 1 | 5 | 1 1/2 carb, 4 fat |
| Ice Cream, Chocolate Chocolate Chip | 1/2 cup | 300 | 20 | 180 | 12 | 0.5 | 105 | 55 | 26 | 2 | 5 | 2 carb, 4 fat |
| Ice Cream, Rocky Road | 1/2 cup | 300 | 18 | 160 | 9 | 0 | 90 | 75 | 29 | 1 | 5 | 2 carb, 4 fat |
| Sorbet, Mango | 1/2 cup | 120 | 0 | 0 | 0 | 0 | 0 | 10 | 37 | 0 | 0 | 2 1/2 carb |
| ***Kraft*** | | | | | | | | | | | | |
| Cool Whip Free Whipped Topping | 2 Tbsp | 15 | 0 | 0 | 0 | 0 | 0 | 5 | 3 | 0 | 0 | free |
| Cool Whip Lite Whipped Topping | 2 Tbsp | 15 | 1 | 10 | 1 | 0 | 0 | 0 | 2 | 0 | 0 | free |
| Cool Whip Sugar Free Whipped Topping | 2 Tbsp | 20 | 1 | 10 | 1 | 0 | 0 | 0 | 3 | 0 | 0 | free |

| | | | | | | | | | | | | |
|---|---|---|---|---|---|---|---|---|---|---|---|---|
| Cool Whip Whipped Topping, Regular | 2 Tbsp | 25 | 1.5 | 15 | 1.5 | 0 | 0 | 0 | 2 | 0 | 0 | free |
| Dream Whip Whipped Topping Mix | 2 Tbsp | 15 | 0 | 0 | 0 | 0 | 0 | 0 | 2 | 0 | 0 | free |
| Marshmallow Creme, Jet Puffed | 2 Tbsp | 40 | 0 | 0 | 0 | 0 | 0 | 10 | 11 | 0 | 0 | 1 carb |
| Marshmallows, Jet Puffed | 4 | 100 | 0 | 0 | 0 | 0 | 0 | 25 | 24 | 0 | 1 | 1 1/2 carb |
| Marshmallows, Miniature | 2/3 cup | 100 | 0 | 0 | 0 | 0 | 0 | 25 | 24 | 0 | 1 | 1 1/2 carb |
| ***Smuckers*** | | | | | | | | | | | | |
| Topping, Butterscotch | 2 Tbsp | 120 | 2 | 20 | 1 | 0 | 0 | 105 | 30 | 0 | 0 | 2 carb |
| Topping, Hot Fudge | 2 Tbsp | 130 | 4.5 | 40 | 1.5 | 0 | 0 | 45 | 22 | <1 | 2 | 1 1/2 carb, 1 fat |
| Topping, Magic Shell, Chocolate Fudge | 2 Tbsp | 210 | 16 | 140 | 7 | 0 | 0 | 45 | 17 | 0 | 1 | 1 carb, 3 fat |
| Topping, Strawberry | 2 Tbsp | 100 | 0 | 0 | 0 | 0 | 0 | 15 | 26 | 0 | 0 | 2 carb |

ICE CREAM, FROZEN YOGURT, PUDDING, GELATIN

| | Serving | Calories | Fat (g) | Cal. from Fat | Sat. Fat (g) | Trans Fat (g) | Chol. (mg) | Sod. (mg) | Carb. (g) | Fiber (g) | Prot. (g) | Servings/Exchanges |
|---|---|---|---|---|---|---|---|---|---|---|---|---|
| Topping, Sugar Free Caramel | 2 Tbsp | 90 | 0 | 0 | 0 | 0 | 0 | 65 | 24 | 0 | 2 | 1 1/2 carb |
| Topping, Sugar Free Hot Fudge | 2 Tbsp | 90 | 0.5 | 5 | 0 | 0 | 0 | 40 | 23 | 1 | 1 | 1 1/2 carb |
| **FROZEN NOVELTIES** | | | | | | | | | | | | |
| ***Blue Bunny*** | | | | | | | | | | | | |
| Banana Pop | 1 | 35 | 0 | 0 | 0 | 0 | 0 | 5 | 9 | 0 | 0 | 1/2 carb |
| Big Star Bar | 1 | 130 | 8 | 70 | 7 | 0 | 5 | 40 | 13 | 0 | 2 | 1 carb, 2 fat |
| Champ! Banana Split Ice Cream Cone | 1 | 220 | 8 | 80 | 6 | 0 | 10 | 65 | 33 | <1 | 3 | 2 carb, 2 fat |
| Champ! Caramel Lovers Ice Cream Cone | 1 | 350 | 19 | 170 | 12 | 0 | 35 | 140 | 40 | 1 | 7 | 2 1/2 carb, 4 fat |
| Champ! Chocolate Lovers Ice Cream | 1 | 290 | 15 | 130 | 10 | 0.5 | 30 | 110 | 37 | 2 | 4 | 2 1/2 carb, 3 fat |

| | | | | | | | | | | | | |
|---|---|---|---|---|---|---|---|---|---|---|---|---|
| Chips Galore! Ice Cream Sandwich | 1 | 310 | 16 | 150 | 8 | 0 | 35 | 170 | 40 | 1 | 3 | 2 1/2 carb, 3 fat |
| Chips Galore! Ice Cream Sandwich | 1 | 310 | 16 | 150 | 8 | 0 | 35 | 170 | 40 | 1 | 3 | 2 1/2 carb, 3 fat |
| Chocolate Raspberry Ice Cream Bar | 1 | 270 | 18 | 160 | 12 | 0 | 35 | 45 | 25 | 1 | 3 | 1 1/2 carb, 4 fat |
| Classic Sundae Cone | 1 | 270 | 14 | 130 | 9 | 0 | 25 | 105 | 32 | 1 | 4 | 2 carb, 3 fat |
| Cookies 'N Cream Ice Cream Sandwich | 1 | 250 | 10 | 90 | 5 | 0 | 20 | 310 | 36 | 2 | 4 | 2 1/2 carb, 2 fat |
| Health Smart FrozFruit Chunky Strawberry Bar | 1 | 35 | 0 | 0 | 0 | 0 | 0 | 10 | 15 | 3 | 0 | 1 carb |
| Hot Fudge Bar | 1 | 370 | 25 | 220 | 14 | 0 | 30 | 90 | 33 | 2 | 7 | 2 carb, 5 fat |
| Jolly Rancher Bomb Pop | 1 | 40 | 0 | 0 | 0 | 0 | 0 | 15 | 11 | 0 | 0 | 1 carb |
| Krunch Bar | 1 | 190 | 13 | 120 | 10 | 0 | 20 | 55 | 17 | 0 | 2 | 1 carb, 3 fat |
| Malt Cup | 1 | 330 | 11 | 100 | 7 | 0 | 45 | 160 | 52 | 0 | 6 | 3 1/2 carb, 2 fat |

ICE CREAM, FROZEN YOGURT, PUDDING, GELATIN

| | Serving | Calories | Fat (g) | Cal. from Fat | Sat. Fat (g) | Trans Fat (g) | Chol. (mg) | Sod. (mg) | Carb. (g) | Fiber (g) | Prot. (g) | Servings/Exchanges |
|---|---|---|---|---|---|---|---|---|---|---|---|---|
| Neapolitan Sandwich | 1 | 150 | 3.5 | 30 | 1.5 | 0 | 10 | 170 | 27 | <1 | 3 | 2 carb, 1 fat |
| Orange Dream Bar | 1 | 80 | 1.5 | 15 | 1 | 0 | 5 | 35 | 16 | 0 | 1 | 1 carb |
| Original Bomb Pop | 1 | 50 | 0 | 0 | 0 | 0 | 0 | 5 | 11 | 0 | 0 | 1 carb |
| Root Beer Float Bar | 1 | 80 | 2 | 20 | 1.5 | 0 | 10 | 25 | 14 | 0 | <1 | 1 carb |
| Slush Pop | 1 | 45 | 0 | 0 | 0 | 0 | 0 | 10 | 11 | 0 | 0 | 1 carb |
| Sour Power Bomb Pop | 1 | 50 | 0 | 0 | 0 | 0 | 0 | 5 | 12 | 0 | 0 | 1 carb |
| Star Bar | 1 | 110 | 7 | 60 | 6 | 0 | 5 | 30 | 11 | 0 | 1 | 1 carb, 1 fat |
| Sugar Free Bomb Pop | 1 | 25 | 0 | 0 | 0 | 0 | 0 | 5 | 8 | 2 | 0 | 1/2 carb |
| Sweet Freedom No Sugar Added Ice Cream Bar, Almond | 1 | 150 | 11 | 100 | 7 | 0 | 5 | 45 | 16 | 2 | 3 | 1 carb, 2 fat |
| Sweet Freedom No Sugar Added Krunch Lites | 1 | 100 | 7 | 70 | 6 | 0 | <5 | 30 | 11 | 1 | 2 | 1 carb, 1 fat |

| | | | | | | | | | | | | |
|---|---|---|---|---|---|---|---|---|---|---|---|---|
| Sweet Freedom No Sugar Added, Ice Cream Bar, Lites | 1 | 100 | 8 | 70 | 6 | 0 | 5 | 30 | 11 | 1 | 2 | 1 carb, 2 fat |
| Sweet Freedom Sugar Free Pops | 1 | 20 | 0 | 0 | 0 | 0 | 0 | 15 | 7 | <1 | 0 | 1/2 carb |
| Turtle Bar | 1 | 360 | 24 | 220 | 14 | 0 | 30 | 80 | 33 | <1 | 5 | 2 carb, 5 fat |
| Twin Pops | 1 | 70 | 0 | 0 | 0 | 0 | 0 | 10 | 18 | 0 | 0 | 1 carb |
| Vanilla Ice Cream Sandwich | 1 | 140 | 3 | 30 | 1.5 | 0 | 5 | 170 | 25 | <1 | 3 | 1 1/2 carb, 1 fat |
| ***Breyers*** | | | | | | | | | | | | |
| All Natural No Sugar Added Pure Fruit Bar | 1 | 25 | 0 | 0 | 0 | 0 | 0 | 0 | 5 | 0 | 0 | free |
| All Natural Pure Fruit Bar, All Varieties | 1 | 40 | 0 | 0 | 0 | 0 | 0 | 0 | 10 | 0 | 0 | 1 carb |
| Carb Smart Fudge Ice Cream Bar | 1 | 100 | 7 | 60 | 4.5 | 0 | 20 | 50 | 9 | 1 | 2 | 1/2 carb, 1 fat |

| | Serving | Calories | Fat (g) | Cal. from Fat | Sat. Fat (g) | Trans Fat (g) | Chol. (mg) | Sod. (mg) | Carb. (g) | Fiber (g) | Prot. (g) | Servings/Exchanges |
|---|---|---|---|---|---|---|---|---|---|---|---|---|
| Carb Smart Vanilla Ice Cream Bar | 1 | 170 | 15 | 130 | 11 | 0 | 15 | 45 | 9 | 2 | 2 | 1/2 carb, 3 fat |
| Double Churn Creamy Vanilla Ice Cream Bar | 1 | 160 | 8 | 70 | 5 | 0 | 5 | 45 | 21 | 3 | 3 | 1 1/2 carb, 2 fat |
| Double Churn Rocky Road Ice Cream Bar | 1 | 180 | 9 | 90 | 5 | 0 | 5 | 80 | 23 | 3 | 4 | 1 1/2 carb, 2 fat |
| Oreo Ice Cream Sandwich | 1 | 170 | 6 | 60 | 2.5 | 0 | 10 | 190 | 26 | 1 | 2 | 2 carb, 1 fat |
| ***Dole*** | | | | | | | | | | | | |
| Fruit Juice Bar, All Varieties | 1 | 70 | 0 | 0 | 0 | 0 | 0 | 15 | 17 | 0 | 0 | 1 carb |
| ***Dove*** | | | | | | | | | | | | |
| Dove Bar, Dark Chocolate with Vanilla | 1 | 330 | 21 | 190 | 14 | 0 | 35 | 40 | 31 | 2 | 4 | 2 carb, 4 fat |

| | | | | | | | | | | | | |
|---|---|---|---|---|---|---|---|---|---|---|---|---|
| Dove Bar, Milk Chocolate with Almonds | 1 | 340 | 23 | 200 | 13 | 0 | 35 | 135 | 28 | 1 | 6 | 2 carb, 5 fat |
| Dove Bar, Milk Chocolate with Vanilla | 1 | 330 | 21 | 190 | 14 | 0 | 35 | 40 | 31 | 2 | 4 | 2 carb, 4 fat |
| ***Dreyer's*** | | | | | | | | | | | | |
| Fruit Bar, Creamy Coconut | 1 | 120 | 3 | 25 | 2 | 0 | 0 | 40 | 21 | 1 | 3 | 1 1/2 carb, 1 fat |
| Fruit Bar, Strawberry | 1 | 80 | 0 | 0 | 0 | 0 | 0 | 0 | 21 | 1 | 0 | 1 1/2 carb |
| ***Eskimo Pie*** | | | | | | | | | | | | |
| No Sugar Added Vanilla with Dark Chocolatey Coating | 1 | 150 | 10 | 90 | 7 | NA | 5 | 45 | 13 | 2 | 2 | 1 carb, 2 fat |
| Vanilla with Dark Chocolatey Coating | 1 | 150 | 10 | 90 | 7 | NA | 10 | 40 | 15 | 1 | 1 | 1 carb, 2 fat |
| Vanilla with Nestlé Crunch Coating | 1 | 200 | 13 | 120 | 9 | NA | 10 | 55 | 19 | 0 | 1 | 1 carb, 3 fat |

ICE CREAM, FROZEN YOGURT, PUDDING, GELATIN

| | Serving | Calories | Fat (g) | Cal. from Fat | Sat. Fat (g) | Trans Fat (g) | Chol. (mg) | Sod. (mg) | Carb. (g) | Fiber (g) | Prot. (g) | Servings/Exchanges |
|---|---|---|---|---|---|---|---|---|---|---|---|---|
| ***Good Humor*** | | | | | | | | | | | | |
| Chocolate Chip Cookie Sandwich | 1 | 270 | 10 | 90 | 6 | 0 | 5 | 200 | 44 | 1 | 3 | 3 carb, 2 fat |
| Chocolate Eclair Bar | 1 | 220 | 10 | 90 | 5 | 0 | 10 | 55 | 30 | 1 | 2 | 2 carb, 2 fat |
| Cookies & Cream Bar | 1 | 90 | 1.5 | 15 | 1 | 0 | 5 | 55 | 18 | 2 | 2 | 1 carb |
| Premium Sundae Cone | 1 | 260 | 15 | 140 | 9 | 0 | 15 | 80 | 29 | 1 | 4 | 2 carb, 3 fat |
| Strawberry Shortcake Bar | 1 | 230 | 12 | 110 | 5 | 0 | 10 | 55 | 31 | 1 | 2 | 2 carb, 2 fat |
| Toasted Almond Bar | 1 | 240 | 12 | 110 | 4 | 0.5 | 10 | 40 | 30 | 1 | 2 | 2 carb, 2 fat |
| Vanilla Ice Cream Sandwich | 1 | 160 | 5 | 45 | 3 | 0 | 10 | 90 | 26 | 0 | 2 | 2 carb, 1 fat |
| ***Häagen-Dazs*** | | | | | | | | | | | | |
| Chocolate & Dark Chocolate Ice Cream Bar | 1 | 290 | 20 | 180 | 12 | 0 | 65 | 30 | 24 | 2 | 4 | 1 1/2 carb, 4 fat |

| | | | | | | | | | | | | |
|---|---|---|---|---|---|---|---|---|---|---|---|---|
| Vanilla & Almonds Ice Cream Bar | 1 | 310 | 22 | 200 | 13 | 0 | 65 | 40 | 22 | <1 | 5 | 1 1/2 carb, 4 fat |
| Vanilla & Dark Chocolate Ice Cream Bar | 1 | 300 | 21 | 190 | 13 | 0 | 70 | 45 | 23 | <1 | 4 | 1 1/2 carb, 4 fat |
| Vanilla & Milk Chocolate Ice Cream Bar | 1 | 290 | 21 | 190 | 14 | 0 | 75 | 55 | 22 | 0 | 4 | 1 1/2 carb, 4 fat |
| ***Healthy Choice*** | | | | | | | | | | | | |
| Caramel Swirl Sandwich | 1 | 150 | 2 | 20 | 1 | 0 | 10 | 115 | 30 | 1 | 3 | 2 carb |
| Fudge Bar | 1 | 80 | 1 | 10 | 0.5 | 0 | 5 | 60 | 13 | 0 | 4 | 1 carb |
| Ice Cream Sandwich | 1 | 130 | 2 | 20 | 1 | 0 | 5 | 115 | 25 | 2 | 3 | 1 1/2 carb |
| Mocha Swirl Bar | 1 | 90 | 1.5 | 15 | 1 | 0 | 5 | 50 | 17 | 1 | 2 | 1 carb |
| Sorbet & Cream Bar | 1 | 90 | 1 | 10 | 0.5 | 0 | 5 | 35 | 17 | 1 | 1 | 1 carb |
| ***Klondike*** | | | | | | | | | | | | |
| Caramel Pretzel Bar | 1 | 260 | 15 | 130 | 12 | 0 | 10 | 170 | 29 | 1 | 3 | 2 carb, 3 fat |

ICE CREAM, FROZEN YOGURT, PUDDING, GELATIN

| | Serving | Calories | Fat (g) | Cal. from Fat | Sat. Fat (g) | Trans Fat (g) | Chol. (mg) | Sod. (mg) | Carb. (g) | Fiber (g) | Prot. (g) | Servings/Exchanges |
|---|---|---|---|---|---|---|---|---|---|---|---|---|
| Choco Taco | 1 | 290 | 15 | 140 | 11 | 0 | 10 | 120 | 36 | 1 | 4 | 2 1/2 carb, 3 fat |
| Dark Chocolate Bar | 1 | 250 | 14 | 130 | 11 | 0 | 10 | 55 | 29 | 1 | 3 | 2 carb, 3 fat |
| Double Chocolate Bar | 1 | 240 | 14 | 130 | 11 | 0 | 10 | 75 | 27 | 1 | 3 | 2 carb, 3 fat |
| Heath Bar | 1 | 230 | 15 | 130 | 11 | 0 | 10 | 70 | 24 | 1 | 3 | 1 1/2 carb, 3 fat |
| Krunch Bar | 1 | 250 | 14 | 130 | 11 | 0 | 10 | 55 | 30 | 1 | 3 | 2 carb, 3 fat |
| Neapolitan Bar | 1 | 250 | 14 | 120 | 11 | 0 | 10 | 75 | 29 | 1 | 3 | 2 carb, 3 fat |
| Oreo Cookie Sandwich | 1 | 260 | 17 | 150 | 12 | 0 | 15 | 115 | 26 | 1 | 2 | 2 carb, 3 fat |
| Reese's Bar | 1 | 260 | 16 | 150 | 11 | 0 | 10 | 90 | 26 | 1 | 3 | 2 carb, 3 fat |
| Slim-a-Bear 100 Calorie Chocolate Fudge Bar | 1 | 100 | 3 | 25 | 2 | 0 | 5 | 90 | 20 | 4 | 3 | 1 carb, 1 fat |
| Slim-a-Bear 100 Calorie English Toffee Bar | 1 | 100 | 6 | 60 | 5 | 0 | 5 | 30 | 12 | 2 | 1 | 1 carb, 1 fat |
| Slim-a-Bear 100 Calorie Vanilla Sandwich | 1 | 100 | 1.5 | 15 | 1 | 0 | 0 | 65 | 21 | 2 | 2 | 1 1/2 carb |

| | | | | | | | | | | | | |
|---|---|---|---|---|---|---|---|---|---|---|---|---|
| Slim-a-Bear No Sugar Added Krunch Bar | 1 | 170 | 10 | 90 | 8 | 0 | 5 | 85 | 22 | 4 | 4 | 1 1/2 carb, 2 fat |
| Slim-a-Bear No Sugar Added Vanilla Bar | 1 | 170 | 9 | 90 | 8 | 0 | 5 | 65 | 21 | 4 | 4 | 1 1/2 carb, 2 fat |
| Triple Chocolate Bar | 1 | 230 | 14 | 120 | 11 | 0 | 10 | 55 | 26 | 1 | 3 | 2 carb, 3 fat |
| Vanilla Cone | 1 | 280 | 14 | 130 | 9 | 0 | 0 | 95 | 35 | 1 | 5 | 2 carb, 3 fat |
| Whitehouse Cherry Bar | 1 | 250 | 14 | 120 | 15 | 0 | 10 | 75 | 31 | 1 | 3 | 2 carb, 3 fat |
| ***Luigi's*** | | | | | | | | | | | | |
| Italian Ice, All Varieties | 6 oz cup | 120 | 0 | 0 | 0 | 0 | 0 | 10 | 31–32 | <1 | 0 | 2 carb |
| Italian Ice, No Sugar Added | 6 oz cup | 60 | 0 | 0 | 0 | 0 | 0 | 10 | 20 | 0 | 0 | 1 carb |
| ***Nestlé*** | | | | | | | | | | | | |
| Drumstick, Classic, Vanilla | 1 | 290 | 16 | 140 | 9 | 0 | 15 | 100 | 33 | 2 | 4 | 2 carb, 3 fat |
| Drumstick, Classic, Vanilla Caramel | 1 | 320 | 17 | 150 | 9 | 0 | 15 | 125 | 37 | 2 | 4 | 2 1/2 carb, 3 fat |

ICE CREAM, FROZEN YOGURT, PUDDING, GELATIN

| | Serving | Calories | Fat (g) | Cal. from Fat | Sat. Fat (g) | Trans Fat (g) | Chol. (mg) | Sod. (mg) | Carb. (g) | Fiber (g) | Prot. (g) | Servings/Exchanges |
|---|---|---|---|---|---|---|---|---|---|---|---|---|
| Drumstick, Simply Dipped, Cookies & Cream | 1 | 300 | 14 | 130 | 10 | 0 | 15 | 115 | 39 | 1 | 3 | 2 1/2 carb, 3 fat |
| Drumstick, Simply Dipped, Vanilla | 1 | 270 | 13 | 120 | 9 | 0 | 15 | 115 | 37 | 1 | 2 | 2 1/2 carb, 3 fat |
| Lil' Drums Cone, Cookie Dough | 1 | 140 | 7 | 80 | 4 | 0 | 5 | 60 | 18 | 0 | 1 | 1 carb, 1 fat |
| Popsicle All Natural Ice Pop | 1.8 oz pop | 50 | 0 | 0 | 0 | 0 | 0 | 5 | 12 | 0 | 0 | 1 carb |
| Big Stick Cherry Pineapple Ice Pop | 1 | 70 | 0 | 0 | 0 | 0 | 0 | 5 | 17 | 0 | 0 | 1 carb |
| Cotton Candy Swirl Bar | 1 | 45 | 0 | 0 | 0 | 0 | 0 | 5 | 12 | 0 | 0 | 1 carb |
| Creamsicle 100 Calorie | 1 | 100 | 2 | 20 | 0.5 | 0 | <5 | 30 | 20 | 0 | 1 | 1 carb |
| Fat Free Fudgsicle | 1 | 60 | 0 | 0 | 0 | 0 | 0 | 60 | 13 | 1 | 2 | 1 carb |

| | | | | | | | | | | | | |
|---|---|---|---|---|---|---|---|---|---|---|---|---|
| Firecracker Ice Pop | 1 | 35 | 0 | 0 | 0 | 0 | 0 | 0 | 9 | 0 | 0 | 1/2 carb |
| Fudgsicle 100 Calorie Pop | 1 | 100 | 2 | 20 | 1 | 0 | 0 | 80 | 17 | <1 | 2 | 1 carb |
| Fudgsicle Triple Chocolate Bar | 1 | 60 | 1.5 | 15 | 1 | 0 | 0 | 60 | 11 | 0 | 1 | 1 carb |
| Lemon Lime Shots | 1 | 80 | 1 | 10 | 1 | 0 | 0 | 0 | 17 | 0 | 0 | 1 carb |
| Lick-A-Color Ice Pop | 1 | 90 | 0 | 0 | 0 | 0 | 0 | 10 | 22 | 0 | 0 | 1 1/2 carb |
| Lowfat Creamsicle Bar | 1 | 70 | 1 | 10 | 0 | 0 | <5 | 20 | 13 | 0 | <1 | 1 carb |
| No Sugar Added Creamsicle Pop | 1 | 25 | 0 | 0 | 0 | 0 | 0 | 10 | 5 | <1 | <1 | free |
| Orange Burst Pop-Ups | 1 | 90 | 1 | 10 | 1 | 0 | 5 | 20 | 18 | 0 | 1 | 1 carb |
| Rainbow Ice Pops | 1 | 45 | 0 | 0 | 0 | 0 | 0 | 0 | 11 | 0 | 0 | 1 carb |
| Root Beer, Banana & Lemon Lime Ice Pop | 1 | 45 | 0 | 0 | 0 | 0 | 0 | 0 | 11 | 0 | 0 | 1 carb |
| Scribblers Ice Pop | 1 | 30 | 0 | 0 | 0 | 0 | 0 | 0 | 8 | 0 | 0 | 1/2 carb |
| Slow Melt Ice Age | 1 | 40 | 0 | 0 | 0 | 0 | 0 | 0 | 10 | 0 | 2 | 1/2 carb |

ICE CREAM, FROZEN YOGURT, PUDDING, GELATIN

| | Serving | Calories | Fat (g) | Cal. from Fat | Sat. Fat (g) | Trans Fat (g) | Chol. (mg) | Sod. (mg) | Carb. (g) | Fiber (g) | Prot. (g) | Servings/Exchanges |
|---|---|---|---|---|---|---|---|---|---|---|---|---|
| Slow Melt Swirlwinds | 1 | 40 | 0 | 0 | 0 | 0 | 0 | 0 | 10 | 0 | 0 | 1/2 carb |
| Snow Cone | 1 | 30 | 0 | 0 | 0 | 0 | 0 | 0 | 8 | 0 | 0 | 1/2 carb |
| Spider Man Bar | 1 | 100 | 0 | 0 | 0 | 0 | 0 | 20 | 25 | 0 | 0 | 1 1/2 carb |
| SpongeBob SquarePants Pop Ups | 1 | 80 | 1 | 10 | 0 | 0 | 5 | 10 | 16 | 0 | <1 | 1 carb |
| Sugar Free Fudgsicle | 1 | 40 | 1 | 10 | 0 | 0 | 0 | 50 | 10 | 2 | 2 | 1/2 carb |
| Sugar Free Ice Pop, All Varieties | 1 | 15 | 0 | 0 | 0 | 0 | 0 | 0 | 4 | 0 | 0 | free |
| Super Heroes Ice Pop | 1 | 40 | 0 | 0 | 0 | 0 | 0 | 0 | 11 | 0 | 0 | 1 carb |
| ***The Skinny Cow/Silhouette*** | | | | | | | | | | | | |
| Chocolate With Fudge Cone | 1 | 150 | 3 | 25 | 2 | 0 | 4 | 95 | 28 | 3 | 4 | 2 carb, 1 fat |
| Fudge Bar | 1 | 100 | 1 | 10 | 0.5 | 0 | 3 | 45 | 22 | 4 | 4 | 1 1/2 carb |
| Ice Cream Sandwich, Vanilla | 1 | 140 | 2 | 15 | 1 | 0 | 1 | 95 | 30 | 3 | 4 | 2 carb |

| | | | | | | | | | | | | |
|---|---|---|---|---|---|---|---|---|---|---|---|---|
| Ice Cream Sandwich, Vanilla, No Sugar Added | 1 | 140 | 2 | 20 | 1 | 0 | 0 | 95 | 28 | 4 | 4 | 2 carb |
| ***Snickers*** | | | | | | | | | | | | |
| Snickers Ice Cream Bar | 1 | 180 | 11 | 100 | 6 | 0 | 10 | 60 | 18 | 1 | 3 | 1 carb, 2 fat |
| ***Weight Watchers*** | | | | | | | | | | | | |
| Smart Ones Chocolate Chip Cookie Dough | 1 | 170 | 3 | 30 | 1.5 | 0 | 5 | 100 | 32 | 1 | 3 | 2 carb, 1 fat |
| Smart Ones Mocha Fudge Sundae | 1 | 160 | 4 | 35 | 2 | 0 | 5 | 85 | 27 | 1 | 3 | 2 carb, 1 fat |
| Smart Ones Peanut Butter Cup Sundae | 1 | 170 | 5 | 50 | 2.5 | 0 | 5 | 90 | 28 | 3 | 4 | 2 carb, 1 fat |
| **PUDDING & GELATIN** | | | | | | | | | | | | |
| ***Jell-O Gelatin*** | | | | | | | | | | | | |
| Gelatin Desserts, Dry Mix, All Varieties | 1/2 cup | 80 | 0 | 0 | 0 | 0 | 0 | 80–120 | 19 | 0 | 2 | 1 carb |

| | Serving | Calories | Fat (g) | Cal. from Fat | Sat. Fat (g) | Trans Fat (g) | Chol. (mg) | Sod. (mg) | Carb. (g) | Fiber (g) | Prot. (g) | Servings/Exchanges |
|---|---|---|---|---|---|---|---|---|---|---|---|---|
| Gelatin Desserts, Dry Mix, Sugar Free | 1/2 cup | 55 | 0 | 0 | 0 | 0 | 0 | 45–80 | 0 | 0 | 1 | free |
| Gelatin Snacks, All Flavors | 3.5 oz | 70 | 0 | 0 | 0 | 0 | 0 | 40 | 17 | 0 | 1 | 1 carb |
| Sugar-Free Snacks, All Flavors | 3.5 oz | 10 | 0 | 0 | 0 | 0 | 0 | 45–80 | 0 | 0 | 1 | free |
| ***Jell-O Pudding Snacks*** | | | | | | | | | | | | |
| Cheesecake | 3.5 oz | 130 | 2 | 20 | 1.5 | 0 | 5 | 120 | 26 | 0 | 2 | 2 carb |
| Chocolate | 4 oz | 140 | 4 | 35 | 1.5 | 0 | 0 | 170 | 26 | 1 | 2 | 2 carb, 1 fat |
| Chocolate Fudge Sundae | 4 oz | 140 | 3.5 | 30 | 1.5 | 0 | 0 | 170 | 25 | 0 | 2 | 1 1/2 carb, 1 fat |
| Chocolate Vanilla Swirl | 4 oz | 140 | 4 | 35 | 1.5 | 0 | 0 | 170 | 26 | 1 | 2 | 2 carb, 1 fat |
| Fat Free Chocolate | 4 oz | 100 | 0 | 0 | 0 | 0 | 0 | 180 | 23 | 1 | 2 | 1 1/2 carb |
| Fat Free Chocolate Vanilla Swirl | 4 oz | 100 | 0 | 0 | 0 | 0 | 0 | 200 | 23 | 1 | 2 | 1 1/2 carb |

| | | | | | | | | | | | | |
|---|---|---|---|---|---|---|---|---|---|---|---|---|
| Fat Free Devil's Food | 4 oz | 100 | 0 | 0 | 0 | 0 | 0 | 190 | 22 | 1 | 2 | 1 1/2 carb |
| Fat Free Tapioca | 4 oz | 100 | 0 | 0 | 0 | 0 | 0 | 230 | 23 | 0 | 1 | 1 1/2 carb |
| Oreo | 4 oz | 120 | 1.5 | 15 | 1.5 | 0 | 0 | 200 | 25 | 1 | 2 | 1 1/2 carb |
| Sugar Free Double Chocolate | 3.8 oz | 60 | 1.5 | 10 | 1 | 0 | 0 | 170 | 14 | 1 | 2 | 1 carb |
| Sugar Free Vanilla | 3.8 oz | 60 | 1 | 10 | 1 | 0 | 0 | 190 | 13 | 0 | 1 | 1 carb |
| Tapioca | 4 oz | 130 | 3 | 25 | 1 | 0 | 0 | 150 | 25 | 0 | 1 | 1 1/2 carb, 1 fat |
| Vanilla | 4 oz | 130 | 3.5 | 30 | 1.5 | 0 | 0 | 160 | 24 | 0 | 1 | 1 1/2 carb, 1 fat |
| ***Jell-O Smoothie Snacks*** | | | | | | | | | | | | |
| Mixed Berry | 4 oz | 100 | 2.5 | 25 | 1.5 | 0 | 10 | 40 | 18 | 0 | 1 | 1 carb, 1 fat |
| Strawberry Banana | 4 oz | 100 | 2.5 | 25 | 1.5 | 0 | 10 | 40 | 18 | 0 | 1 | 1 carb, 1 fat |
| ***Kozy Shack*** | | | | | | | | | | | | |
| Chocolate Pudding | 1/2 cup | 140 | 3.5 | 30 | 2 | 0 | 15 | 140 | 24 | <1 | 4 | 1 1/2 carb, 1 fat |
| Cinnamon Raisin Rice Pudding | 1/2 cup | 140 | 3 | 30 | 2 | 0 | 20 | 130 | 24 | 0 | 4 | 1 1/2 carb, 1 fat |
| Créme Caramel Flan | 1/2 cup | 150 | 3.5 | 35 | 2 | 0 | 35 | 85 | 27 | 0 | 4 | 2 carb, 1 fat |

ICE CREAM, FROZEN YOGURT, PUDDING, GELATIN

| | Serving | Calories | Fat (g) | Cal. from Fat | Sat. Fat (g) | Trans Fat (g) | Chol. (mg) | Sod. (mg) | Carb. (g) | Fiber (g) | Prot. (g) | Servings/Exchanges |
|---|---|---|---|---|---|---|---|---|---|---|---|---|
| Dulce De Leche Flan | 1 cup | 190 | 6 | 50 | 3 | 0 | 50 | 135 | 28 | 0 | 5 | 2 carb, 1 fat |
| European Style Rice Pudding | 1/2 cup | 130 | 3.5 | 30 | 2 | 0 | 25 | 130 | 22 | 0 | 4 | 1 1/2 carb, 1 fat |
| No Sugar Added Chocolate Pudding | 1/2 cup | 90 | 3 | 30 | 1.5 | 0 | 10 | 120 | 10 | 4 | 3 | 1/2 carb, 1 fat |
| No Sugar Added Rice Pudding | 1/2 cup | 90 | 3 | 30 | 2 | 0 | 15 | 115 | 14 | 3 | 4 | 1 carb, 1 fat |
| No Sugar Added Tapioca Pudding | 1/2 cup | 90 | 3 | 30 | 2 | 0 | 15 | 140 | 11 | 4 | 3 | 1 carb, 1 fat |
| Original Rice Pudding | 1/2 cup | 130 | 3 | 30 | 2 | 0 | 20 | 135 | 22 | 0 | 4 | 1 1/2 carb, 1 fat |
| Tapioca Pudding | 1/2 cup | 130 | 3 | 25 | 2 | 0 | 15 | 140 | 23 | 0 | 3 | 1 1/2 carb, 1 fat |
| ***Kraft Handi-Snacks Pudding Cups*** | | | | | | | | | | | | |
| Butterscotch | 3.5 oz | 90 | 1 | 10 | 1 | 0 | 0 | 160 | 21 | 0 | 1 | 1 1/2 carb |
| Chocolate | 3.5 oz | 100 | 1 | 10 | 1 | 0 | 0 | 150 | 23 | 1 | 1 | 1 1/2 carb |

| | | | | | | | | | | | | |
|---|---|---|---|---|---|---|---|---|---|---|---|---|
| Fat Free Chocolate | 3.5 oz | 90 | 0 | 0 | 0 | 0 | 0 | 170 | 21 | 0 | 2 | 1 1/2 carb |
| Rice | 3.5 oz | 140 | 6 | 50 | 1 | 0 | 0 | 130 | 19 | 0 | 3 | 1 carb, 1 fat |
| Vanilla | 3.5 oz | 90 | 0 | 0 | 0 | 0 | 0 | 160 | 20 | 0 | 1 | 1 carb |
| ***Snack Pack*** | | | | | | | | | | | | |
| Gel Snack | 3.5 oz | 100 | 0 | 0 | 0 | 0 | 0 | 45 | 25 | 0 | 0 | 1 1/2 carb |
| Gel Snack, Sugar Free | 3.5 oz | 10 | 0 | 0 | 0 | 0 | 0 | 65 | 2 | <1 | 0 | free |
| Pudding Cups, Banana | 3.5 oz | 110 | 3.5 | 30 | 2 | 0 | 0 | 150 | 19 | 0 | 1 | 1 carb, 1 fat |
| Pudding Cups, Banana Creme Pie | 3.5 oz | 110 | 3.5 | 30 | 2 | 0 | 0 | 150 | 19 | 0 | 1 | 1 carb, 1 fat |
| Pudding Cups, Butterscotch | 3.5 oz | 120 | 3.5 | 30 | 1.5 | 0 | 0 | 150 | 21 | 0 | 1 | 1 1/2 carb, 1 fat |
| Pudding Cups, Caramel Creme | 3.5 oz | 120 | 3.5 | 30 | 1.5 | 0 | 0 | 160 | 21 | 0 | 1 | 1 1/2 carb, 1 fat |
| Pudding Cups, Chocolate | 3.5 oz | 120 | 3.5 | 30 | 2 | 0 | 0 | 135 | 21 | <1 | 2 | 1 1/2 carb, 1 fat |
| Pudding Cups, Chocolate Fudge | 3.5 oz | 120 | 3.5 | 30 | 2 | 0 | 0 | 135 | 22 | <1 | 2 | 1 1/2 carb, 1 fat |

ICE CREAM, FROZEN YOGURT, PUDDING, GELATIN

| | Serving | Calories | Fat (g) | Cal. from Fat | Sat. Fat (g) | Trans Fat (g) | Chol. (mg) | Sod. (mg) | Carb. (g) | Fiber (g) | Prot. (g) | Servings/Exchanges |
|---|---|---|---|---|---|---|---|---|---|---|---|---|
| Pudding Cups, Chocolate Lover's | 3.5 oz | 120 | 3.5 | 30 | 2 | 0 | 0 | 135 | 22 | 0 | 2 | 1 1/2 carb, 1 fat |
| Pudding Cups, Fat Free Chocolate | 3.5 oz | 90 | 0 | 0 | 0 | 0 | 0 | 140 | 20 | 0 | 2 | 1 carb |
| Pudding Cups, Fat Free Tapioca | 3.5 oz | 80 | 0 | 0 | 0 | 0 | 0 | 150 | 19 | 0 | 1 | 1 carb |
| Pudding Cups, Fat Free Vanilla | 3.5 oz | 80 | 0 | 0 | 0 | 0 | 0 | 140 | 18 | 0 | 1 | 1 carb |
| Pudding Cups, Ice Cream Sandwich | 3.5 oz | 120 | 3.5 | 30 | 2 | 0 | 0 | 135 | 21 | 0 | 2 | 1 1/2 carb, 1 fat |
| Pudding Cups, Lemon Meringue | 3.5 oz | 120 | 2.5 | 25 | 1.5 | 0 | 0 | 60 | 25 | 0 | 0 | 1 1/2 carb, 1 fat |
| Pudding Cups, No Sugar Added Chocolate | 3.5 oz | 60 | 3 | 30 | 1 | 0 | 0 | 110 | 8 | <1 | 1 | 1/2 carb, 1 fat |

| | | | | | | | | | | | | |
|---|---|---|---|---|---|---|---|---|---|---|---|---|
| Pudding Cups, No Sugar Added Vanilla | 3.5 oz | 60 | 3.5 | 30 | 1.5 | 0 | 0 | 115 | 8 | 0 | <1 | 1/2 carb, 1 fat |
| Pudding Cups, Tapioca | 3.5 oz | 120 | 3.5 | 30 | 2 | 0 | 0 | 140 | 20 | 0 | 2 | 1 carb, 1 fat |
| Pudding Cups, Vanilla | 3.5 oz | 120 | 3.5 | 30 | 2 | 0 | 0 | 130 | 20 | 0 | 1 | 1 carb, 1 fat |
| ***Swiss Miss Pudding Cups*** | | | | | | | | | | | | |
| Banana Cream | 1 | 130 | 3.5 | 30 | 3.5 | 0 | <5 | 170 | 23 | 0 | 2 | 1 1/2 carb, 1 fat |
| Chocolate Cream | 1 | 150 | 4 | 35 | 3.5 | 0 | <5 | 170 | 26 | <1 | 3 | 2 carb, 1 fat |
| Chocolate Dream | 1 | 150 | 4 | 35 | 3.5 | 0 | <5 | 170 | 26 | <1 | 3 | 2 carb, 1 fat |
| Chocolate Vanilla | 1 | 140 | 3.5 | 30 | 3 | 0 | 0 | 160 | 27 | 0 | 2 | 2 carb, 1 fat |
| Classic Butterscotch | 1 | 130 | 3.5 | 30 | 3 | 0 | 0 | 180 | 22 | 0 | 2 | 1 1/2 carb, 1 fat |
| Creamy Milk Chocolate | 1 | 150 | 3.5 | 30 | 3 | 0 | 0 | 190 | 27 | 0 | 3 | 2 carb, 1 fat |
| Creamy Vanilla | 1 | 140 | 3.5 | 30 | 3 | 0 | 0 | 180 | 24 | 0 | 2 | 1 1/2 carb, 1 fat |
| Lemon Meringue | 1 | 140 | 3 | 30 | 3.5 | 0 | 0 | 600 | 28 | 0 | 0 | 2 carb, 1 fat |
| Low Fat Creamy Chocolate | 1 | 130 | 2 | 20 | 2 | 0 | 0 | 180 | 26 | 0 | 3 | 2 carb |
| Old Fashioned Tapioca | 1 | 140 | 3.5 | 30 | 3 | 0 | 0 | 180 | 24 | 0 | 2 | 1 1/2 carb, 1 fat |

# MEAT, POULTRY, FISH, SEAFOOD (FRESH, COOKED)

| | Serving | Calories | Fat (g) | Cal. from Fat | Sat. Fat (g) | Trans Fat (g) | Chol. (mg) | Sod. (mg) | Carb. (g) | Fiber (g) | Prot. (g) | Servings/Exchanges |
|---|---|---|---|---|---|---|---|---|---|---|---|---|
| **BEEF (Trimmed)** | | | | | | | | | | | | |
| ***Brisket*** | | | | | | | | | | | | |
| Brisket, Flat Cut | 3 oz | 181 | 7 | 63 | 3 | 0 | 34 | 46 | 0 | 0 | 28 | 4 lean meat |
| Brisket, Whole | 3 oz | 247 | 17 | 153 | 6 | 0 | 79 | 55 | 0 | 0 | 23 | 3 med-fat meat |
| ***Chuck*** | | | | | | | | | | | | |
| Arm Pot Roast | 3 oz | 238 | 14 | 126 | 6 | 0 | 85 | 53 | 0 | 0 | 25 | 3 med-fat meat |
| Blade Roast | 3 oz | 284 | 21 | 189 | 8 | 0 | 88 | 55 | 0 | 0 | 23 | 3 high-fat meat |
| Clod Roast | 3 oz | 176 | 9 | 81 | 3 | 0 | 59 | 60 | 0 | 0 | 22 | 3 lean meat |
| Flank Steak | 3 oz | 160 | 7 | 63 | 3 | 0 | 38 | 48 | 0 | 0 | 24 | 3 lean meat |
| Mock Tender Steak | 3 oz | 136 | 5 | 45 | 2 | 0 | 54 | 60 | 0 | 0 | 22 | 3 lean meat |
| Top Blade Steak | 3 oz | 184 | 10 | 90 | 3 | 0 | 52 | 57 | 0 | 0 | 22 | 3 lean meat |
| ***Ground Beef*** | | | | | | | | | | | | |
| 80% Lean Ground Beef | 3 oz | 230 | 15 | 135 | 6 | 0 | 77 | 64 | 0 | 0 | 22 | 3 med-fat meat |

| | | | | | | | | | | | | |
|---|---|---|---|---|---|---|---|---|---|---|---|---|
| 85% Lean Ground Beef | 3 oz | 213 | 13 | 117 | 5 | 0 | 77 | 61 | 0 | 0 | 22 | 3 med-fat meat |
| 90% Lean Ground Beef | 3 oz | 184 | 10 | 90 | 4 | 0 | 72 | 58 | 0 | 0 | 22 | 3 lean meat |
| 95% Lean Ground Beef | 3 oz | 145 | 6 | 54 | 3 | 0 | 65 | 55 | 0 | 0 | 22 | 3 lean meat |
| ***Plate*** | | | | | | | | | | | | |
| Inside Skirt Steak | 3 oz | 187 | 10 | 90 | 4 | 0 | 51 | 64 | 0 | 0 | 22 | 3 lean meat |
| ***Round*** | | | | | | | | | | | | |
| Bottom Round | 3 oz | 159 | 7 | 63 | 2 | 0 | 73 | 31 | 0 | 0 | 23 | 3 lean meat |
| Eye of Round | 3 oz | 145 | 5 | 45 | 2 | 0 | 59 | 53 | 0 | 0 | 24 | 3 lean meat |
| Tip Round | 3 oz | 162 | 7 | 63 | 2 | 0 | 69 | 54 | 0 | 0 | 24 | 3 lean meat |
| Top Round | 3 oz | 178 | 5 | 45 | 2 | 0 | 77 | 38 | 0 | 0 | 30 | 4 lean meat |
| ***Ribs*** | | | | | | | | | | | | |
| Rib Eye | 3 oz | 210 | 13 | 117 | 5 | 0 | 94 | 48 | 0 | 0 | 23 | 3 med-fat meat |
| Short Ribs | 3 oz | 400 | 36 | 324 | 15 | 0 | 80 | 45 | 0 | 0 | 18 | 3 high-fat meat |
| ***Shank*** | | | | | | | | | | | | |
| Shank Crosscuts, Trimmed to 1/4 inch | 3 oz | 224 | 12 | 108 | 5 | 0 | 68 | 52 | 0 | 0 | 26 | 3 med-fat meat |

## MEAT, POULTRY, FISH, SEAFOOD

| | Serving | Calories | Fat (g) | Cal. from Fat | Sat. Fat (g) | Trans Fat (g) | Chol. (mg) | Sod. (mg) | Carb. (g) | Fiber (g) | Prot. (g) | Servings/Exchanges |
|---|---|---|---|---|---|---|---|---|---|---|---|---|
| ***Short Loin*** | | | | | | | | | | | | |
| Porterhouse Steak | 3 oz | 235 | 16 | 144 | 6 | 0 | 57 | 55 | 0 | 0 | 20 | 3 med-fat meat |
| T-bone Steak | 3 oz | 210 | 14 | 126 | 5 | 0 | 51 | 57 | 0 | 0 | 21 | 3 med-fat meat |
| Tenderloin | 3 oz | 200 | 11 | 99 | 4 | 0 | 72 | 53 | 0 | 0 | 23 | 3 med-fat meat |
| Top Loin | 3 oz | 180 | 9 | 81 | 3 | 0 | 65 | 57 | 0 | 0 | 24 | 3 lean meat |
| ***Sirloin*** | | | | | | | | | | | | |
| Bottom Sirloin Roast | 3 oz | 177 | 9 | 81 | 3 | 0 | 71 | 45 | 0 | 0 | 22 | 3 lean meat |
| Top Sirloin | 3 oz | 183 | 8 | 72 | 3 | 0 | 76 | 55 | 0 | 0 | 25 | 3 lean meat |
| ***Variety Cuts*** | | | | | | | | | | | | |
| Liver | 3 oz | 162 | 4 | 36 | 1 | 0 | 337 | 67 | 0 | 0 | 25 | 3 lean meat |
| Tongue | 3 oz | 236 | 19 | 171 | 7 | 0 | 112 | 55 | 0 | 0 | 16 | 2 high-fat meat |
| **BUFFALO** | 3 oz | 120 | 2 | 18 | <2 | 0 | 69 | 48 | 0 | 0 | 24 | 3 lean meat |
| **LAMB** | | | | | | | | | | | | |
| Ground, Broiled | 3 oz | 240 | 17 | 153 | 7 | 0 | 81 | 69 | 0 | 0 | 21 | 3 med-fat meat |

| | | | | | | | | | | | | |
|---|---|---|---|---|---|---|---|---|---|---|---|---|
| Leg, Sirloin, Roast, Lean | 3 oz | 174 | 8 | 70 | 3 | 0 | 78 | 60 | 0 | 0 | 24 | 3 lean meat |
| Rib, Roasted | 3 oz | 198 | 11 | 99 | 3 | 0 | 75 | 69 | 0 | 0 | 22 | 3 med-fat meat |
| Loin, Roast/Chop, Cooked | 3 oz | 183 | 8 | 72 | 3 | 0 | 81 | 72 | 0 | 0 | 26 | 4 lean meat |
| **VEAL** | | | | | | | | | | | | |
| Breast | 3 oz | 226 | 14 | 126 | 6 | 0 | 96 | 55 | 0 | 0 | 23 | 3 med-fat meat |
| Ground Veal | 3 oz | 146 | 6 | 54 | 3 | 0 | 88 | 71 | 0 | 0 | 21 | 3 lean meat |
| Leg (Top Round) | 3 oz | 136 | 4 | 36 | 2 | 0 | 88 | 58 | 0 | 0 | 24 | 3 lean meat |
| Loin | 3 oz | 184 | 10 | 90 | 4 | 0 | 88 | 79 | 0 | 0 | 21 | 3 lean meat |
| Rib | 3 oz | 194 | 12 | 108 | 5 | 0 | 94 | 78 | 0 | 0 | 20 | 3 med-fat meat |
| Shank | 3 oz | 162 | 5 | 45 | 2 | 0 | 105 | 79 | 0 | 0 | 27 | 4 lean meat |
| Shoulder | 3 oz | 156 | 7 | 63 | 3 | 0 | 96 | 82 | 0 | 0 | 22 | 3 lean meat |
| Sirloin | 3 oz | 172 | 9 | 81 | 4 | 0 | 87 | 71 | 0 | 0 | 21 | 3 lean meat |
| **PORK** | | | | | | | | | | | | |
| Ground Pork | 3 oz | 252 | 18 | 162 | 7 | 0 | 80 | 62 | 0 | 0 | 22 | 3 high-fat meat |
| Leg (Ham) | 3 oz | 232 | 15 | 135 | 5 | 0 | 80 | 51 | 0 | 0 | 23 | 3 med-fat meat |

MEAT, POULTRY, FISH, SEAFOOD

| | Serving | Calories | Fat (g) | Cal. from Fat | Sat. Fat (g) | Trans Fat (g) | Chol. (mg) | Sod. (mg) | Carb. (g) | Fiber (g) | Prot. (g) | Servings/Exchanges |
|---|---|---|---|---|---|---|---|---|---|---|---|---|
| ***Loin*** | | | | | | | | | | | | |
| Back Ribs | 3 oz | 315 | 25 | 225 | 9 | 0 | 100 | 86 | 0 | 0 | 21 | 3 high-fat meat |
| Blade Chops | 3 oz | 272 | 21 | 189 | 8 | 0 | 73 | 60 | 0 | 0 | 19 | 3 high-fat meat |
| Center Loin Chops | 3 oz | 210 | 12 | 108 | 5 | 0 | 73 | 50 | 0 | 0 | 24 | 3 med-fat meat |
| Center Rib Roast | 3 oz | 214 | 13 | 117 | 5 | 0 | 69 | 41 | 0 | 0 | 23 | 3 med-fat meat |
| Country-Style Ribs | 3 oz | 279 | 22 | 198 | 8 | 0 | 78 | 44 | 0 | 0 | 20 | 3 high-fat meat |
| Sirloin Roast | 3 oz | 222 | 14 | 126 | 5 | 0 | 74 | 51 | 0 | 0 | 23 | 3 med-fat meat |
| Tenderloin | 3 oz | 147 | 5 | 45 | 2 | 0 | 67 | 47 | 0 | 0 | 24 | 3 lean meat |
| Top Loin Roast | 3 oz | 192 | 10 | 90 | 4 | 0 | 66 | 37 | 0 | 0 | 24 | 3 lean meat |
| Whole Loin | 3 oz | 211 | 12 | 108 | 5 | 0 | 70 | 50 | 0 | 0 | 23 | 3 med-fat meat |
| ***Shoulder*** | | | | | | | | | | | | |
| Arm Picnic | 3 oz | 269 | 20 | 180 | 7 | 0 | 80 | 60 | 0 | 0 | 20 | 3 high-fat meat |
| Blade Boston Roast | 3 oz | 229 | 16 | 144 | 6 | 0 | 73 | 57 | 0 | 0 | 20 | 3 med-fat meat |
| Whole Shoulder | 3 oz | 248 | 18 | 162 | 7 | 0 | 77 | 58 | 0 | 0 | 20 | 3 med-fat meat |

**POULTRY**

| | | | | | | | | | | | | |
|---|---|---|---|---|---|---|---|---|---|---|---|---|
| Chicken Back, No Skin, Roasted | 3 oz | 203 | 11 | 99 | 3 | 0 | 76 | 82 | 0 | 0 | 24 | 3 med-fat meat |
| Chicken Breast, No Skin, Roasted | 3 oz | 141 | 3 | 27 | 1 | 0 | 72 | 63 | 0 | 0 | 26 | 3 lean meat |
| Chicken Drumstick, No Skin, Roasted | 3 oz | 146 | 5 | 45 | 1 | 0 | 79 | 81 | 0 | 0 | 24 | 3 lean meat |
| Chicken Leg, No Skin, Roasted | 3 oz | 162 | 7 | 63 | 2 | 0 | 80 | 77 | 0 | 0 | 23 | 3 lean meat |
| Chicken Thigh, No Skin, Roasted | 3 oz | 178 | 9 | 81 | 3 | 0 | 81 | 75 | 0 | 0 | 22 | 3 lean meat |
| Chicken Wing, No Skin, Roasted | 3 oz | 173 | 7 | 63 | 2 | 0 | 72 | 78 | 0 | 0 | 26 | 4 lean meat |
| Chicken, Capon | 3 oz | 195 | 10 | 90 | 3 | 0 | 73 | 42 | 0 | 0 | 25 | 3 lean meat |
| Chicken, Dark Meat with Skin, Roasted | 3 oz | 216 | 14 | 126 | 3.6 | 0 | 78 | 75 | 0 | 0 | 22 | 3 med-fat meat |

MEAT, POULTRY, FISH, SEAFOOD

| | Serving | Calories | Fat (g) | Cal. from Fat | Sat. Fat (g) | Trans Fat (g) | Chol. (mg) | Sod. (mg) | Carb. (g) | Fiber (g) | Prot. (g) | Servings/Exchanges |
|---|---|---|---|---|---|---|---|---|---|---|---|---|
| Chicken, Dark Meat, No Skin, Roasted | 3 oz | 174 | 8 | 76 | 2 | 0 | 78 | 78 | 0 | 0 | 23 | 3 lean meat |
| Chicken, Light Meat with Skin, Roasted | 3 oz | 189 | 9 | 81 | 3 | 0 | 72 | 63 | 0 | 0 | 25 | 3 lean meat |
| Cornish Game Hen, Whole Bird, Cooked, No Skin | 3 oz | 114 | 3 | 27 | 1 | 0 | 90 | 54 | 0 | 0 | 20 | 3 lean meat |
| Duck, Domestic, No Skin, Roasted | 3 oz | 171 | 10 | 86 | 3 | 0 | 75 | 54 | 0 | 0 | 20 | 3 lean meat |
| Goose, No Skin, Roasted | 3 oz | 201 | 11 | 97 | 3 | 0 | 81 | 66 | 0 | 0 | 25 | 3 med-fat meat |
| Ostrich, cooked | 3 oz | 120 | 2 | 18 | 0 | 0 | 81 | 66 | 0 | 0 | 23 | 3 lean meat |
| Pheasant, No Skin | 3 oz | 114 | 3 | 27 | 0 | 0 | 57 | 30 | 0 | 0 | 20 | 3 lean meat |

| | | | | | | | | | | | | |
|---|---|---|---|---|---|---|---|---|---|---|---|---|
| Turkey Back, No Skin, Roasted | 3 oz | 144 | 5 | 45 | 2 | 0 | 81 | 62 | 0 | 0 | 24 | 3 lean meat |
| Turkey Breast, Roasted | 3 oz | 114 | 1 | 9 | 0 | 0 | 69 | 45 | 0 | 0 | 26 | 3 lean meat |
| Turkey Dark Meat, No Skin, cooked | 3 oz | 159 | 6 | 54 | 3 | 0 | 72 | 66 | 0 | 0 | 24 | 3 lean meat |
| Turkey Leg, No Skin, Roasted | 3 oz | 135 | 3 | 27 | 1 | 0 | 101 | 69 | 0 | 0 | 25 | 3 lean meat |
| Turkey Wing, No Skin, Roasted | 3 oz | 139 | 3 | 27 | 1 | 0 | 87 | 66 | 0 | 0 | 26 | 4 lean meat |
| Turkey, Ground, Cooked | 3 oz | 201 | 11 | 99 | 3 | 0 | 87 | 90 | 0 | 0 | 23 | 3 med-fat meat |
| **FISH/SEAFOOD** | | | | | | | | | | | | |
| Bluefish, Baked | 3 oz | 130 | 5 | 35 | 1 | 0 | 65 | 65 | 0 | 0 | 22 | 3 lean meat |
| Carfish, Baked | 3 oz | 129 | 7 | 63 | 2 | 0 | 54 | 68 | 0 | 0 | 16 | 2 lean meat |
| Catfish, Baked | 3 oz | 129 | 6 | 54 | 2 | 0 | 54 | 69 | 0 | 0 | 15 | 3 lean meat |
| Caviar, Black/Red, Granular | 2 Tbsp | 81 | 6 | 54 | 1 | 0 | 188 | 480 | 1 | 0 | 8 | 1 med-fat meat |

MEAT, POULTRY, FISH, SEAFOOD

| | Serving | Calories | Fat (g) | Cal. from Fat | Sat. Fat (g) | Trans Fat (g) | Chol. (mg) | Sod. (mg) | Carb. (g) | Fiber (g) | Prot. (g) | Servings/Exchanges |
|---|---|---|---|---|---|---|---|---|---|---|---|---|
| Clams, Fresh, Steamed | 1 oz | 42 | <1 | 5 | <1 | 0 | 19 | 32 | 1 | 0 | 7 | 1 lean meat |
| Cod, Baked | 3 oz | 89 | 1 | 9 | 0 | 0 | 47 | 66 | 0 | 0 | 19 | 3 lean meat |
| Crab | 3 oz | 114 | 6 | 54 | 2 | 0 | 81 | 453 | 2 | 0 | 15 | 3 lean meat |
| Escargot/Snails | 1 oz | 51 | <1 | 5 | <1 | 0 | 28 | 34 | 1 | 0 | 9 | 1 lean meat |
| Flounder/Sole, Baked | 3 oz | 99 | 1 | 14 | 0 | 0 | 58 | 89 | 0 | 0 | 21 | 3 lean meat |
| Haddock, Baked | 3 oz | 95 | 1 | 7 | 0 | 0 | 63 | 74 | 0 | 0 | 21 | 3 lean meat |
| Halibut, Baked | 3 oz | 119 | 2 | 22 | 0 | 0 | 35 | 59 | 0 | 0 | 23 | 3 lean meat |
| Herring, Atlantic, Baked | 3 oz | 173 | 10 | 89 | 2 | 0 | 65 | 98 | 0 | 0 | 20 | 3 lean meat |
| Imitation Shellfish, from Surimi | 1 oz | 29 | <1 | 0 | <1 | 0 | 6 | 238 | 3 | 0 | 3 | 1 lean meat |
| Lobster, Fresh, Steamed | 1 oz | 28 | <1 | 0 | <1 | 0 | 20 | 108 | <1 | 0 | 6 | 1 lean meat |
| Mackerel, Atlantic/ Pacific, Baked | 3 oz | 223 | 15 | 120 | 4 | 0 | 64 | 71 | 0 | 0 | 20 | 3 med-fat meat |
| Mackerel, King, Baked | 3 oz | 114 | 2 | 20 | 0 | 0 | 58 | 173 | 0 | 0 | 22 | 3 lean meat |

| | | | | | | | | | | | | |
|---|---|---|---|---|---|---|---|---|---|---|---|---|
| Ocean Perch, Baked | 3 oz | 102 | 2 | 16 | 0 | 0 | 46 | 82 | 0 | 0 | 20 | 3 lean meat |
| Octopus | 1 oz | 46 | <1 | 0 | <1 | 0 | 27 | 130 | 1 | 0 | 9 | 1 lean meat |
| Orange Roughy, Baked | 3 oz | 76 | 1 | 7 | 0 | 0 | 22 | 69 | 0 | 0 | 16 | 2 lean meat |
| Oyster, Medium | 6 | 58 | 2 | 18 | <1 | 0 | 44 | 177 | 3 | 0 | 6 | 1 lean meat |
| Pollock, Baked | 3 oz | 100 | 1 | 9 | 0 | 0 | 77 | 94 | 0 | 0 | 21 | 3 lean meat |
| Rainbow Trout, Baked | 3 oz | 144 | 6 | 55 | 2 | 0 | 58 | 36 | 0 | 0 | 21 | 3 lean meat |
| Rockfish, Baked | 3 oz | 103 | 2 | 15 | 0 | 0 | 37 | 65 | 0 | 0 | 20 | 3 lean meat |
| Sablefish, Baked | 3 oz | 212 | 17 | 152 | 3 | 0 | 54 | 61 | 0 | 0 | 15 | 2 high-fat meat |
| Salmon, Atlantic/Coho, Baked | 3 oz | 175 | 10 | 94 | 2 | 0 | 54 | 52 | 0 | 0 | 19 | 3 lean meat |
| Salmon, Chum/Pink, Baked | 3 oz | 130 | 4 | 32 | 0 | 0 | 81 | 54 | 0 | 0 | 22 | 3 lean meat |
| Salmon, Sockeye, Baked | 3 oz | 184 | 9 | 84 | 2 | 0 | 75 | 55 | 0 | 0 | 23 | 3 lean meat |
| Scallops, Fresh, Steamed | 1 oz | 32 | <1 | 0 | <1 | 0 | 15 | 78 | 0 | 0 | 7 | 1 lean meat |

MEAT, POULTRY, FISH, SEAFOOD

| | Serving | Calories | Fat (g) | Cal. from Fat | Sat. Fat (g) | Trans Fat (g) | Chol. (mg) | Sod. (mg) | Carb. (g) | Fiber (g) | Prot. (g) | Servings/Exchanges |
|---|---|---|---|---|---|---|---|---|---|---|---|---|
| Sea Bass, Baked | 3 oz | 105 | 2 | 20 | 0 | 0 | 45 | 74 | 0 | 0 | 20 | 3 lean meat |
| Shark, Baked | 3 oz | 140 | 5 | 22 | 1 | 0 | 50 | 85 | 0 | 0 | 22 | 3 lean meat |
| Shrimp, Fresh, Cooked in Water | 1 oz | 28 | <1 | 0 | <1 | 0 | 56 | 64 | 0 | 0 | 6 | 1 lean meat |
| Swordfish, Baked | 3 oz | 130 | 4 | 39 | 1 | 0 | 43 | 98 | 0 | 0 | 22 | 3 lean meat |
| Tilefish, Baked | 3 oz | 125 | 4 | 36 | 1 | 0 | 54 | 50 | 0 | 0 | 20 | 3 lean meat |
| Trout | 3 oz | 162 | 6 | 54 | 2 | 0 | 63 | 57 | 0 | 0 | 24 | 3 lean meat |
| Tuna, Yellowfin, Baked | 3 oz | 118 | 1 | 9 | 0 | 0 | 49 | 40 | 0 | 0 | 25 | 3 lean meat |
| Whiting, Baked | 3 oz | 98 | 1 | 13 | 0 | 0 | 71 | 112 | 0 | 0 | 20 | 3 lean meat |
| **RABBIT** | 3 oz | 174 | 6 | 54 | 2 | 0 | 72 | 30 | 0 | 0 | 27 | 3 lean meat |
| **VENISON** | 3 oz | 135 | 2 | 18 | 2 | 0 | 96 | 45 | 0 | 0 | 27 | 3 lean meat |

## MILK, YOGURT, NON-DAIRY MILK

| | Serving | Calories | Fat (g) | Cal. from Fat | Sat. Fat (g) | Trans Fat (g) | Chol. (mg) | Sod. (mg) | Carb. (g) | Fiber (g) | Prot. (g) | Servings/Exchanges |
|---|---|---|---|---|---|---|---|---|---|---|---|---|
| Buttermilk, 1%, Low Fat | 1 cup | 98 | 2 | 20 | 1 | 0 | 10 | 257 | 12 | 0 | 8 | 1 low-fat milk |
| Buttermilk, Fat Free | 1 cup | 98 | 0 | 0 | 0 | 0 | 0 | 257 | 12 | 0 | 8 | 1 fat-free milk |
| Eggnog, Whole | 1/2 cup | 171 | 10 | 90 | 6 | 0 | 75 | 69 | 17 | 0 | 5 | 1 whole milk |
| Kefir, 2% | 1 cup | 120 | 5 | 45 | 3 | 0 | 19 | 70 | 13 | 2 | 9 | 1 reduced-fat milk |
| Milk, 1%, Low Fat | 1 cup | 110 | 2.5 | 23 | 1.5 | 0 | 15 | 125 | 13 | 0 | 8 | 1 lowfat milk |
| Milk, 2% Reduced Fat, Lactaid | 1 cup | 130 | 5 | 45 | 3 | 0 | 19 | 125 | 13 | 0 | 8 | 1 reduced-fat milk |
| Milk, 2%, Low Fat, Acidophilus | 1 cup | 128 | 5 | 45 | 3 | 0 | 19 | 123 | 11 | 0 | 8 | 1 reduced-fat milk |
| Milk, 2%, Reduced Fat | 1 cup | 130 | 5 | 45 | 3 | 0 | 20 | 130 | 12 | 0 | 8 | 1 reduced-fat milk |
| Milk, Evaporated, Fat Free | 1 cup | 100 | 0 | 0 | 0 | 0 | 5 | 147 | 15 | 0 | 10 | 1 fat-free milk |
| Milk, Evaporated, Whole | 1/2 cup | 169 | 10 | 90 | 6 | 0 | 37 | 134 | 13 | 0 | 8 | 1 whole milk |

MILK, YOGURT, NON-DAIRY MILK

| | Serving | Calories | Fat (g) | Cal. from Fat | Sat. Fat (g) | Trans Fat (g) | Chol. (mg) | Sod. (mg) | Carb. (g) | Fiber (g) | Prot. (g) | Servings/Exchanges |
|---|---|---|---|---|---|---|---|---|---|---|---|---|
| Milk, Fat Free, Chocolate | 1 cup | 160 | 0 | 0 | 0 | 0 | 5 | 220 | 31 | 0 | 9 | 1 fat-free milk, 1 carb |
| Milk, Fat Free, Lactaid | 1 cup | 80 | 0 | 0 | 0 | 0 | 0 | 125 | 13 | 0 | 8 | 1 fat-free milk |
| Milk, Fat Free, Nonfat, Skim | 1 cup | 90 | 0 | 0 | 0 | 0 | 4 | 130 | 13 | 0 | 9 | 1 fat-free milk |
| Milk, Goat, Whole | 1 cup | 168 | 10 | 90 | 7 | 0 | 27 | 122 | 11 | 0 | 9 | 1 whole milk |
| Milk, Whole | 1 cup | 150 | 8 | 70 | 5 | 0 | 33 | 120 | 12 | 0 | 8 | 1 whole milk |
| Milk, Whole, Chocolate | 1 cup | 208 | 9 | 81 | 5 | 0 | 30 | 150 | 26 | 2 | 8 | 1 whole milk, 1 carb |
| Rice Drink, Fat Free or 1%, Plain | 1 cup | 90 | 1.5 | 14 | 0 | 0 | 0 | 70 | 18 | 0 | 1 | 1 carb |
| Rice Drink, Low Fat, Flavored | 1 cup | 122 | 2 | 20 | 0 | 0 | 0 | 70 | 25 | 0 | 1 | 1 1/2 carb |
| Smoothie, Regular, Yogurt Based, Flavored | 10 oz | 260 | 3 | 25 | 2 | 0 | 12 | 130 | 50 | 0 | 8 | 1 reduced-fat milk, 2 1/2 carb |

| | | | | | | | | | | | | |
|---|---|---|---|---|---|---|---|---|---|---|---|---|
| Soy Milk, Light | 1 cup | 100 | 2 | 20 | 0 | 0 | 0 | 90 | 15 | 0 | 5 | 1 low-fat milk |
| Soy Milk, Regular, Plain | 1 cup | 115 | 4 | 35 | 0.5 | 0 | 0 | 107 | 11 | 1.5 | 8 | 1 reduced-fat milk |
| Yogurt & Juice Blend | 1 cup | 150 | 0 | 0 | 0 | 0 | 0 | 55 | 34 | 0 | 3 | 2 carb |
| Yogurt with Fruit, Low Fat | 6 oz | 150 | 1.5 | 14 | 1 | 0 | 5 | 100 | 28 | 0 | 6 | 1 low-fat milk, 1 carb |
| Yogurt, Low Fat, Plain | 1 cup | 107 | 2.5 | 23 | 1.5 | 0 | 10 | 119 | 12 | 0 | 9 | 1 low-fat milk |
| Yogurt, Nonfat, Plain | 6 oz | 82 | <1 | 0 | <1 | 0 | 12 | 112 | 12 | 0 | 8 | 1 fat-free milk |
| Yogurt, Whole Milk, Plain | 1 cup | 160 | 8 | 70 | 5 | 0 | 20 | 120 | 12 | 0 | 9 | 1 whole milk |
| **YOGURT** | | | | | | | | | | | | |
| ***Breyers Yogurt*** | | | | | | | | | | | | |
| Creme Savers, Strawberry & Creme | 6 oz | 170 | 1.5 | 15 | 1 | 0 | 10 | 180 | 33 | 0 | 6 | 1 low-fat milk, 1 1/2 carb |
| Fruit on the Bottom, Strawberry | 6 oz | 170 | 1.5 | 15 | 1 | 0 | 10 | 85 | 33 | <1 | 6 | 1 low-fat milk, 1 1/2 carb |
| Inspirations, Natural Strawberry | 4 oz | 110 | 1 | 10 | 0.5 | 0 | 5 | 55 | 22 | <1 | 4 | 1 low-fat milk, 1/2 carb |

| | Serving | Calories | Fat (g) | Cal. from Fat | Sat. Fat (g) | Trans Fat (g) | Chol. (mg) | Sod. (mg) | Carb. (g) | Fiber (g) | Prot. (g) | Servings/Exchanges |
|---|---|---|---|---|---|---|---|---|---|---|---|---|
| Light, Nonfat, Strawberry | 6 oz | 80 | 0 | 0 | 0 | 0 | <5 | 105 | 12 | <1 | 6 | 1 fat-free milk |
| Smooth & Creamy, Strawberry | 6 oz | 170 | 1.5 | 15 | 1 | 0 | 10 | 90 | 34 | 0 | 6 | 1 low-fat milk, 1 1/2 carb |
| ***Dannon Yogurt*** | | | | | | | | | | | | |
| Activia Fiber, Strawberry & Cereal | 4 oz | 110 | 2 | 15 | 1 | 0 | 5 | 80 | 19 | 3 | 5 | 1 low-fat milk, 1/2 carb |
| Activia Light, Strawberry | 4 oz | 70 | 0 | 0 | 0 | 0 | <5 | 80 | 13 | 3 | 5 | 1 fat-free milk |
| Activia, Strawberry | 4 oz | 110 | 2 | 20 | 1 | 0 | 5 | 75 | 19 | 0 | 5 | 1 low-fat milk, 1/2 carb |
| All Natural, Blended, Strawberry | 4 oz | 120 | 1 | 10 | 1 | 0 | 5 | 70 | 21 | 0 | 5 | 1 low-fat milk, 1/2 carb |
| All Natural, Lowfat, Plain | 6 oz | 100 | 2.5 | 25 | 1.5 | 0 | 10 | 115 | 12 | 0 | 8 | 1 low-fat milk |

| | | | | | | | | | | | | |
|---|---|---|---|---|---|---|---|---|---|---|---|---|
| All Natural, Nonfat, Plain | 6 oz | 80 | 0 | 0 | 0 | 0 | 5 | 120 | 12 | 0 | 9 | 1 fat-free milk |
| All Natural, Plain | 8 oz | 160 | 8 | 70 | 5 | 0 | 20 | 120 | 12 | 0 | 9 | 1 whole milk |
| DanActive, Strawberry | 3.1-oz bottle | 80 | 1.5 | 15 | 1 | 0 | 5 | 40 | 13 | 0 | 3 | 1 carb |
| Danimals Drinkable, Swingin' Strawberry/ Banana | 3.1 oz | 70 | 0.5 | 5 | 0 | 0 | <5 | 30 | 15 | 0 | 2 | 1 carb |
| Fruit on the Bottom, Strawberry | 6 oz | 150 | 1.5 | 15 | 1 | 0 | 5 | 110 | 28 | <1 | 6 | 1 low-fat milk, 1 carb |
| Light & Fit 0% Plus, Assorted Flavors | 4 oz | 60 | 0 | 0 | 0 | 0 | <5 | 55 | 10 | 0 | 3 | 1/2 fat-free milk |
| Light & Fit 0% Plus, Strawberry | 6 oz | 80 | 0 | 0 | 0 | 0 | <5 | 80 | 16 | 0 | 5 | 1 fat-free milk |
| Light & Fit Cup, Carb & Sugar Control | 4 oz | 50 | 1.5 | 15 | 1 | 0 | 5 | 25 | 3 | 0 | 5 | 1/2 low-fat milk |
| Light & Fit Smoothie, Carb & Sugar Control | 7 oz | 60 | 2.5 | 25 | 1.5 | 0 | 15 | 35 | 4 | 0 | 6 | 1/2 low-fat milk |

MILK, YOGURT, NON-DAIRY MILK

| | Serving | Calories | Fat (g) | Cal. from Fat | Sat. Fat (g) | Trans Fat (g) | Chol. (mg) | Sod. (mg) | Carb. (g) | Fiber (g) | Prot. (g) | Servings/Exchanges |
|---|---|---|---|---|---|---|---|---|---|---|---|---|
| ***Yoplait Yogurt*** | | | | | | | | | | | | |
| Delights | 4 oz | 100 | 1.5 | 10 | 1 | 0 | 5 | 90 | 18 | 0 | 5 | 1 low-fat milk, 1/2 carb |
| Fiber One, Fat Free | 4 oz | 50 | 0 | 0 | 0 | 0 | <5 | 55 | 13 | 5 | 3 | 1 carb |
| GoGurt, Fruit Flavors | 2.25-oz tube | 70 | 0.5 | 5 | 0 | 0 | <5 | 30 | 13 | 0 | 2 | 1 carb |
| Light, Fruit Flavors | 6 oz | 100 | 0 | 0 | 0 | 0 | <5 | 85 | 19 | 0 | 5 | 1 low-fat milk |
| Original, Fruit Flavors | 6 oz | 170 | 1.5 | 15 | 1 | 0 | 10 | 80 | 33 | 0 | 5 | 1 low-fat milk, 1 1/2 carb |
| Smoothie, Prepared | 8 oz | 110 | 1.5 | 15 | 0.5 | 0 | <5 | 20 | 14 | 2 | 1 | 1 carb |
| Thick & Creamy, Fruit Flavors | 6 oz | 190 | 3.5 | 30 | 2 | 0 | 10 | 100 | 32 | 0 | 7 | 1 reduced-fat milk, 1 carb |
| Tri Yogurt, Fruit Flavors | 4 oz | 90 | 0.5 | 5 | 0.5 | 0 | <5 | 50 | 18 | 0 | 4 | 1 low-fat milk, 1/2 carb |
| Yoplait Kids, Strawberry | 4 oz | 100 | 2 | 20 | 1.5 | 0 | 10 | 75 | 17 | 1 | 5 | 1 low-fat milk |
| Yo-Plus | 4 oz | 110 | 1.5 | 10 | 1 | 0 | 10 | 70 | 21 | 3 | 4 | 1 low-fat milk, 1/2 carb |

| | | | | | | | | | | | | |
|---|---|---|---|---|---|---|---|---|---|---|---|---|
| Yo-Plus Light | 4 oz | 70 | 0 | 0 | 0 | 0 | 5 | 65 | 15 | 3 | 4 | 1 low-fat milk |
| **NON-DAIRY MILK** | | | | | | | | | | | | |
| **Almond Milk** | | | | | | | | | | | | |
| ***Blue Diamond Almond Breeze (Shelf Stable)*** | | | | | | | | | | | | |
| Chocolate | 1 cup | 110 | 3 | 25 | 0 | 0 | 0 | 150 | 22 | 1 | 1 | 1 1/2 carb, 1 fat |
| Chocolate, Unsweetened | 1 cup | 45 | 3.5 | 30 | 0 | 0 | 0 | 180 | 3 | 1 | 2 | 1 fat |
| Original | 1 cup | 60 | 2.5 | 25 | 0 | 0 | 0 | 150 | 8 | <1 | 1 | 1/2 carb, 1 fat |
| Original, Unsweetened | 1 cup | 40 | 3 | 30 | 0 | 0 | 0 | 150 | 2 | 1 | 1 | 1 fat |
| Vanilla | 1 cup | 90 | 2.5 | 25 | 0 | 0 | 0 | 150 | 16 | <1 | 1 | 1 carb, 1 fat |
| Vanilla, Unsweetened | 1 cup | 45 | 3.5 | 30 | 0 | 0 | 0 | 180 | 3 | 1 | 2 | 1 fat |
| ***Pacific (Shelf Stable)*** | | | | | | | | | | | | |
| Original, Unsweetened | 1 cup | 35 | 2.5 | 25 | 0 | 0 | 0 | 180 | 2 | 0 | 1 | 1 fat |
| **Grain Milk** | | | | | | | | | | | | |
| ***Pacific (Shelf Stable)*** | | | | | | | | | | | | |
| Organic Oat, Low Fat, Vanilla | 1 cup | 130 | 2.5 | 20 | 0 | 0 | 0 | 110 | 24 | 2 | 4 | 1 1/2 carb, 1 fat |

| | Serving | Calories | Fat (g) | Cal. from Fat | Sat. Fat (g) | Trans Fat (g) | Chol. (mg) | Sod. (mg) | Carb. (g) | Fiber (g) | Prot. (g) | Servings/Exchanges |
|---|---|---|---|---|---|---|---|---|---|---|---|---|
| **Hazelnut Milk** | | | | | | | | | | | | |
| ***Pacific (Shelf Stable)*** | | | | | | | | | | | | |
| Original | 1 cup | 110 | 3.5 | 30 | 0 | 0 | 0 | 120 | 18 | <1 | 2 | 1 carb, 1 fat |
| **Rice Milk** | | | | | | | | | | | | |
| ***Pacific (Shelf Stable)*** | | | | | | | | | | | | |
| Plain, Low Fat | 1 cup | 130 | 2 | 20 | 0 | 0 | 0 | 60 | 27 | 0 | 1 | 2 carb |
| ***Rice Dream (Refrigerated)*** | | | | | | | | | | | | |
| Original, Enriched | 1 cup | 120 | 2.5 | 20 | 0 | 0 | 0 | 80 | 23 | 0 | 1 | 1 1/2 carb, 1 fat |
| Vanilla, Enriched | 1 cup | 130 | 2.5 | 20 | 0 | 0 | 0 | 80 | 26 | 0 | 1 | 2 carb, 1 fat |
| ***Rice Dream (Shelf Stable)*** | | | | | | | | | | | | |
| Carob | 1 cup | 150 | 2.5 | 25 | 0 | 0 | 0 | 80 | 30 | <1 | 1 | 2 carb, 1 fat |
| Chocolate, Enriched | 1 cup | 160 | 3 | 25 | 0 | 0 | 0 | 90 | 34 | <1 | 2 | 2 carb, 1 fat |
| Horchata | 1 cup | 160 | 2.5 | 25 | 0 | 0 | 0 | 150 | 32 | 0 | 1 | 2 carb, 1 fat |
| Original | 1 cup | 120 | 2.5 | 20 | 0 | 0 | 0 | 100 | 24 | 0 | 1 | 1 1/2 carb, 1 fat |

| | | | | | | | | | | | | |
|---|---|---|---|---|---|---|---|---|---|---|---|---|
| Original, Enriched | 1 cup | 120 | 2.5 | 20 | 0 | 0 | 0 | 100 | 23 | 0 | 1 | 1 1/2 carb, 1 fat |
| Original, Heartwise | 1 cup | 130 | 2 | 20 | 0 | 0 | 0 | 80 | 27 | 3 | 1 | 2 carb |
| Vanilla | 1 cup | 130 | 2.5 | 25 | 0 | 0 | 0 | 105 | 27 | 0 | 1 | 2 carb, 1 fat |
| Vanilla, Enriched | 1 cup | 130 | 2.5 | 20 | 0 | 0 | 0 | 105 | 26 | 0 | 1 | 2 carb, 1 fat |
| Vanilla, Heartwise | 1 cup | 140 | 2 | 20 | 0 | 0 | 0 | 80 | 30 | 3 | 1 | 2 carb |
| ***WestSoy (Shelf Stable)*** | | | | | | | | | | | | |
| Rice Beverage, Plain | 1 cup | 110 | 2.5 | 25 | 0 | 0 | 0 | 105 | 20 | 0 | 1 | 1 carb, 1 fat |
| Rice Beverage, Vanilla | 1 cup | 110 | 2.5 | 25 | 0 | 0 | 0 | 105 | 20 | 0 | 1 | 1 carb, 1 fat |
| **Soy Milk** | | | | | | | | | | | | |
| ***Pacific (Shelf Stable)*** | | | | | | | | | | | | |
| Organic Soy, Unsweetened, Original | 1 cup | 90 | 4.5 | 40 | 0.5 | 0 | 0 | 15 | 4 | 2 | 9 | 1 med-fat meat |
| Select Soy, Low Fat, Plain | 1 cup | 70 | 2.5 | 20 | 0 | 0 | 0 | 115 | 9 | <1 | 5 | 1/2 carb, 1 lean meat |
| Select Soy, Low Fat, Vanilla | 1 cup | 80 | 2.5 | 20 | 0 | 0 | 0 | 115 | 11 | 1 | 5 | 1 carb, 1 fat |

| | Serving | Calories | Fat (g) | Cal. from Fat | Sat. Fat (g) | Trans Fat (g) | Chol. (mg) | Sod. (mg) | Carb. (g) | Fiber (g) | Prot. (g) | Servings/Exchanges |
|---|---|---|---|---|---|---|---|---|---|---|---|---|
| Ultra Soy, Plain | 1 cup | 120 | 4 | 35 | 0.5 | 0 | 0 | 150 | 12 | <1 | 10 | 1 carb, 1 med-fat meat |
| Ultra Soy, Vanilla | 1 cup | 130 | 4 | 35 | 0.5 | 0 | 0 | 150 | 14 | <1 | 10 | 1 carb, 1 med-fat meat |
| ***Silk (Refrigerated)*** | | | | | | | | | | | | |
| Silk Light, Chocolate | 1 cup | 120 | 1.5 | 15 | 0 | 0 | 0 | 100 | 22 | 2 | 5 | 1 1/2 carb |
| Silk Light, Original | 1 cup | 70 | 2 | 20 | 0 | 0 | 0 | 120 | 8 | 1 | 6 | 1/2 carb, 1 lean meat |
| Silk Light, Vanilla | 1 cup | 80 | 2 | 20 | 0 | 0 | 0 | 95 | 10 | 1 | 6 | 1/2 carb, 1 lean meat |
| Simply Silk, Chocolate | 1 cup | 140 | 3.5 | 30 | 0.5 | 0 | 0 | 100 | 23 | 2 | 5 | 1 1/2 carb, 1 med-fat meat |
| Simply Silk, Original | 1 cup | 100 | 4 | 35 | 0.5 | 0 | 0 | 120 | 8 | 1 | 7 | 1/2 carb, 1 med-fat meat |
| Simply Silk, Unsweetened | 1 cup | 80 | 4 | 35 | 0.5 | 0 | 0 | 85 | 4 | 1 | 7 | 1 med-fat meat |
| Simply Silk, Vanilla | 1 cup | 100 | 3.5 | 30 | 0.5 | 0 | 0 | 95 | 10 | 1 | 6 | 1/2 carb, 1 med-fat meat |

| | | | | | | | | | | | | |
|---|---|---|---|---|---|---|---|---|---|---|---|---|
| Simply Silk, Very Vanilla | 1 cup | 130 | 4 | 35 | 0.5 | 0 | 0 | 140 | 19 | 1 | 6 | 1 carb, 1 med-fat meat |
| ***Silk (Shelf Stable)*** | | | | | | | | | | | | |
| Plain Original | 1 cup | 100 | 4 | 35 | 0.5 | 0 | 0 | 120 | 8 | 1 | 7 | 1/2 carb, 1 med-fat meat |
| Unsweetened | 1 cup | 80 | 4 | 35 | 0.5 | 0 | 0 | 85 | 4 | 1 | 7 | 1 med-fat meat |
| Vanilla | 1 cup | 100 | 3.5 | 30 | 0.5 | 0 | 0 | 95 | 10 | 1 | 6 | 1/2 carb, 1 lean meat |
| ***Soy Dream (Refrigerated)*** | | | | | | | | | | | | |
| Classic Original | 1 cup | 130 | 4 | 35 | 0.5 | 0 | 0 | 150 | 16 | 2 | 7 | 1 carb, 1 med-fat meat |
| Vanilla, Enriched | 1 cup | 120 | 3.5 | 30 | 0.5 | 0 | 0 | 130 | 14 | 2 | 8 | 1 carb, 1 med-fat meat |
| ***Soy Dream (Shelf Stable)*** | | | | | | | | | | | | |
| Chocolate, Enriched | 1 cup | 150 | 4 | 40 | 0.5 | 0 | 0 | 125 | 21 | 3 | 7 | 1 1/2 carb, 1 med-fat meat |
| Classic Vanilla | 1 cup | 140 | 4 | 25 | 0.5 | 0 | 0 | 135 | 18 | 2 | 7 | 1 carb, 1 med-fat meat |
| Original, Enriched | 1 cup | 100 | 4 | 35 | 0.5 | 0 | 0 | 135 | 8 | 2 | 7 | 1/2 carb, 1 med-fat meat |
| Vanilla, Enriched | 1 cup | 120 | 4 | 35 | 0.5 | 0 | 0 | 135 | 14 | 2 | 7 | 1 carb, 1 med-fat meat |

| | Serving | Calories | Fat (g) | Cal. from Fat | Sat. Fat (g) | Trans Fat (g) | Chol. (mg) | Sod. (mg) | Carb. (g) | Fiber (g) | Prot. (g) | Servings/Exchanges |
|---|---|---|---|---|---|---|---|---|---|---|---|---|
| ***WestSoy (Shelf Stable)*** | | | | | | | | | | | | |
| Lite, Plain | 1 cup | 60 | 2 | 20 | 0 | 0 | 0 | 85 | 6 | <1 | 4 | 1/2 carb |
| Lite, Vanilla | 1 cup | 70 | 2 | 20 | 0 | 0 | 0 | 75 | 8 | <1 | 5 | 1/2 carb, 1 lean meat |
| Low Fat, Plain | 1 cup | 90 | 1.5 | 15 | 0 | 0 | 0 | 90 | 14 | 2 | 4 | 1 carb |
| Low Fat, Vanilla | 1 cup | 120 | 1.5 | 15 | 0 | 0 | 0 | 90 | 21 | 2 | 4 | 1 1/2 carb |
| Non Fat, Plain | 1 cup | 70 | 0 | 0 | 0 | 0 | 0 | 105 | 10 | <1 | 6 | 1/2 carb, 1 lean meat |
| Non Fat, Vanilla | 1 cup | 80 | 0 | 0 | 0 | 0 | 0 | 105 | 12 | <1 | 6 | 1 carb, 1 lean meat |
| Organic Plus, Plain | 1 cup | 90 | 3.5 | 30 | 0.5 | 0 | 0 | 125 | 7 | <1 | 7 | 1/2 carb, 1 lean meat |
| Organic Plus, Vanilla | 1 cup | 100 | 3.5 | 30 | 0.5 | 0 | 0 | 125 | 10 | <1 | 7 | 1/2 carb, 1 lean meat |
| Organic, Unsweetened Original | 1 cup | 90 | 4.5 | 40 | 0.5 | 0 | 0 | 30 | 5 | 4 | 9 | 1 med-fat meat |
| Organic, Unsweetened, Vanilla | 1 cup | 100 | 4.5 | 40 | 0.5 | 0 | 0 | 30 | 5 | 4 | 9 | 1 med-fat meat |

## NUTS, SEEDS, NUT/SEED PRODUCTS

| | Serving | Calories | Fat (g) | Cal. from Fat | Sat. Fat (g) | Trans Fat (g) | Chol. (mg) | Sod. (mg) | Carb. (g) | Fiber (g) | Prot. (g) | Servings/Exchanges |
|---|---|---|---|---|---|---|---|---|---|---|---|---|
| Almond Butter, Plain | 1 Tbsp | 91 | 10 | 90 | <1 | 0 | 0 | 17 | 3 | <1 | 2 | 2 fat |
| Almond Butter, Salted | 1 Tbsp | 98 | 9 | 80 | <1 | 0 | 0 | 70 | 3 | <1 | 2 | 2 fat |
| Almonds, Dried, Whole | 1 oz | 165 | 15 | 135 | 1 | 0 | 0 | 3 | 6 | 4 | 5 | 1 med-fat meat, 2 fat |
| Almonds, Dry Roasted, Salted | 1 oz | 166 | 15 | 135 | 1 | 0 | 0 | 221 | 7 | 4 | 5 | 1 med-fat meat, 2 fat |
| Almonds, Dry Roasted, Whole, Unsalted | 1 oz | 166 | 15 | 135 | 1 | 0 | 0 | 3 | 7 | 4 | 5 | 1 med-fat meat, 2 fat |
| Almonds, Oil Roasted | 1 oz | 175 | 16 | 145 | 2 | 0 | 0 | 221 | 5 | 3 | 6 | 1 med-fat meat, 2 fat |
| Almonds, Toasted | 1 oz | 167 | 14 | 125 | 1 | 0 | 0 | 3 | 7 | 3 | 6 | 1 med-fat meat, 2 fat |
| Beechnuts, Dried | 1 oz | 164 | 14 | 125 | 2 | 0 | 0 | 11 | 10 | <1 | 2 | 1/2 starch, 3 fat |
| Brazil Nuts, Dried | 1 oz | 186 | 19 | 170 | 5 | 0 | 0 | <1 | 4 | 2 | 4 | 1 med-fat meat, 3 fat |
| Cashew Butter, Plain | 1 Tbsp | 86 | 7 | 65 | 2 | 0 | 0 | 2 | 4 | <1 | 3 | 1 fat |
| Cashews, Dry Roasted | 1 oz | 161 | 13 | 115 | 3 | 0 | 0 | 179 | 9 | <1 | 5 | 1/2 starch, 3 fat |

## NUTS, SEEDS, NUT/SEED PRODUCTS

| | Serving | Calories | Fat (g) | Cal. from Fat | Sat. Fat (g) | Trans Fat (g) | Chol. (mg) | Sod. (mg) | Carb. (g) | Fiber (g) | Prot. (g) | Servings/Exchanges |
|---|---|---|---|---|---|---|---|---|---|---|---|---|
| Cashews, Oil Roasted | 1 oz | 163 | 14 | 125 | 3 | 0 | 0 | 178 | 8 | 1 | 5 | 1/2 starch, 3 fat |
| Chinese Chestnuts, Dried | 1 oz | 103 | <1 | 0 | <1 | 0 | 0 | 1 | 23 | <1 | 2 | 1 1/2 starch |
| Chinese Chestnuts, Roasted | 1 oz | 68 | <1 | 0 | <1 | 0 | 0 | 1 | 15 | <1 | 1 | 1 starch |
| Coconut Milk, Raw | 1 cup | 552 | 57 | 515 | 51 | 0 | 0 | 36 | 13 | 5 | 6 | 1 starch, 11 fat |
| Coconut, Dried, Shredded, Sweetened | 1/4 cup | 117 | 8 | 60 | 7 | 0 | 0 | 61 | 11 | 1 | <1 | 1 starch, 2 fat |
| Coconut, Fresh | 2.52-inch piece | 159 | 15 | 135 | 13 | 0 | 0 | 9 | 7 | 4 | 2 | 1/2 starch, 3 fat |
| Coconut, Toasted | 1 oz | 168 | 13 | 115 | 12 | 0 | 0 | 11 | 13 | 2 | 2 | 1 starch, 3 fat |
| English Walnut Halves, Dried | 1 oz | 182 | 18 | 160 | 2 | 0 | 0 | 3 | 5 | 1 | 4 | 1 med-fat meat, 3 fat |
| European Chestnuts, Roasted | 1 oz | 69 | <1 | 0 | <1 | 0 | 0 | <1 | 15 | 2 | <1 | 1 starch |

| | | | | | | | | | | | | |
|---|---|---|---|---|---|---|---|---|---|---|---|---|
| Filberts/Hazelnuts, Dried, Whole | 1 oz | 177 | 18 | 160 | 1 | 0 | 0 | <1 | 4 | 2 | 4 | 1 med-fat meat, 3 fat |
| Filberts/Hazelnuts, Dry Roasted, Salted | 1 oz | 188 | 18 | 160 | 1 | 0 | 0 | 221 | 5 | 2 | 3 | 3 fat |
| Filberts/Hazelnuts, Oil Roasted, Salted | 1 oz | 187 | 18 | 160 | 1 | 0 | 0 | 223 | 6 | 2 | 4 | 1/2 starch, 3 fat |
| Flaxseed, Whole | 1 Tbsp | 55 | 4 | 35 | <1 | 0 | 0 | 3 | 3 | 3 | 2 | 1 fat |
| Ginkgo Nuts | 1 oz | 52 | 0 | 0 | 0 | 0 | 0 | 2 | 11 | NA | 1 | 1 carb |
| Hickory Nuts, Dried | 1 oz | 186 | 18 | 160 | 2 | 0 | 0 | <1 | 5 | 2 | 4 | 4 fat |
| Japanese Chestnuts, Dried | 1 oz | 101 | <1 | 0 | <1 | 0 | 0 | 10 | 23 | <1 | 2 | 1 1/2 starch |
| Japanese Chestnuts, Roasted | 1 oz | 57 | <1 | 0 | <1 | 0 | 0 | 5 | 13 | <1 | <1 | 1 starch |
| Macadamia Nuts | 1 oz | 199 | 21 | 190 | 3 | 0 | 0 | 1 | 4 | 3 | 2 | 4 fat |
| Macadamia Nuts, Oil Roasted | 1 oz | 204 | 22 | 200 | 3 | 0 | 0 | 74 | 4 | 3 | 2 | 4 fat |

NUTS, SEEDS, NUT/SEED PRODUCTS

| | Serving | Calories | Fat (g) | Cal. from Fat | Sat. Fat (g) | Trans Fat (g) | Chol. (mg) | Sod. (mg) | Carb. (g) | Fiber (g) | Prot. (g) | Servings/Exchanges |
|---|---|---|---|---|---|---|---|---|---|---|---|---|
| Mixed Nuts, Dry Roasted | 1 oz | 168 | 15 | 135 | 2 | 0 | 0 | 190 | 7 | 3 | 5 | 1/2 starch, 3 fat |
| Mixed Nuts, Oil Roasted | 1 oz | 175 | 16 | 145 | 4 | 0 | 0 | 185 | 6 | 3 | 5 | 1/2 starch, 3 fat |
| Mixed Nuts, Oil Roasted, No Peanuts | 1 oz | 172 | 16 | 145 | 3 | 0 | 0 | 196 | 6 | 2 | 4 | 1/2 starch, 3 fat |
| Mixed Nuts, Oil Roasted, Unsalted | 1 oz | 173 | 16 | 145 | 2 | 0 | 0 | 3 | 6 | 2 | 4 | 1 med-fat meat, 2 fat |
| Peanut Butter, Chunky or Creamy | 1 Tbsp | 96 | 8 | 70 | 2 | 0 | 0 | 80 | 3 | <1 | 4 | 1 med-fat meat, 1 fat |
| Peanut Butter, Natural, Salted | 1 Tbsp | 94 | 8 | 70 | 1 | 0 | 0 | 40 | 3 | 1 | 4 | 1 high-fat meat |
| Peanut Butter, Natural, Unsalted | 1 Tbsp | 94 | 8 | 70 | 1 | 0 | 0 | <1 | 3 | 1 | 4 | 1 high-fat meat |
| Peanuts, Dry Roasted, Unsalted | 1 oz | 166 | 14 | 125 | 2 | 0 | 0 | 2 | 6 | 2 | 7 | 1 high-fat meat, 1 fat |

| | | | | | | | | | | | | |
|---|---|---|---|---|---|---|---|---|---|---|---|---|
| Peanuts, Oil Roasted | 1 oz | 165 | 14 | 125 | 2 | 0 | 0 | 123 | 5 | 3 | 8 | 1 high-fat meat, 1 fat |
| Peanuts, Spanish, Raw | 1 oz | 167 | 14 | 125 | 2 | 0 | 0 | 6 | 5 | 3 | 8 | 1 high-fat meat, 1 fat |
| Pecans, Dried Halves | 1 oz | 189 | 19 | 170 | 2 | 0 | 0 | <1 | 5 | 2 | 2 | 4 fat |
| Pecans, Dry Roasted | 1 oz | 187 | 18 | 160 | 2 | 0 | 0 | 222 | 6 | 3 | 2 | 3 fat |
| Pecans, Oil Roasted | 1 oz | 194 | 20 | 180 | 2 | 0 | 0 | 214 | 5 | 2 | 2 | 4 fat |
| Pine Nuts (Pignoli), Dried | 1 oz | 178 | 17 | 155 | 3 | 0 | 0 | 20 | 6 | 3 | 3 | 1/2 carb, 1 high-fat meat, 1 fat |
| Pistachio Nuts, Dry Roasted | 1 oz | 170 | 15 | 135 | 2 | 0 | 0 | 218 | 8 | 3 | 4 | 1/2 starch, 3 fat |
| Pumpkin Kernels, Roasted | 1 oz | 148 | 12 | 110 | 2 | 0 | 0 | 163 | 4 | 1 | 9 | 1 med-fat meat, 1 fat |
| Pumpkin Seeds, Roasted | 1 oz | 126 | 6 | 55 | 1 | 0 | 0 | 163 | 15 | 2 | 5 | 1 starch, 1 fat |
| Sesame Seeds, Dried, Whole | 1 Tbsp | 52 | 5 | 45 | 1 | 0 | 0 | 1 | 2 | 1 | 2 | 1 fat |
| Soy Nut Butter | 1 Tbsp | 96 | 8 | 70 | 1 | 0 | 0 | 70 | 3 | 2 | 4 | 1 high-fat meat |

NUTS, SEEDS, NUT/SEED PRODUCTS

| | Serving | Calories | Fat (g) | Cal. from Fat | Sat. Fat (g) | Trans Fat (g) | Chol. (mg) | Sod. (mg) | Carb. (g) | Fiber (g) | Prot. (g) | Servings/Exchanges |
|---|---|---|---|---|---|---|---|---|---|---|---|---|
| Soy Nuts, Dry Roasted, No Salt | 3/4 oz | 96 | 5 | 45 | <1 | 0 | 0 | 0 | 7 | 2 | 8 | 1/2 carb, 1 med-fat meat |
| Sunflower Seeds, Dry | 1 oz | 162 | 14 | 125 | 2 | 0 | 0 | <1 | 5 | 3 | 7 | 1 high-fat meat, 1 fat |
| Sunflower Seeds, Dry Roasted | 1 oz | 163 | 14 | 125 | 2 | 0 | 0 | <1 | 7 | 3 | 6 | 1 high-fat meat, 1 fat |
| Sunflower Seeds, Oil Roasted | 1 oz | 174 | 16 | 145 | 2 | 0 | 0 | 171 | 4 | 2 | 6 | 1 high-fat meat, 1 fat |
| Tahini/Sesame Butter | 2 Tbsp | 60 | 5 | 45 | <1 | 0 | 0 | 12 | 2 | <1 | 2 | 1 fat |
| **BRANDS** | | | | | | | | | | | | |
| ***Fifty50*** | | | | | | | | | | | | |
| Peanut Butter, Creamy, No Added Sugar | 2 Tbsp | 190 | 16 | 140 | 2 | 0 | 0 | 0 | 7 | 3 | 7 | 1 high-fat meat, 1 fat |
| Peanut Butter, Crunchy, No Added Sugar | 2 Tbsp | 190 | 16 | 140 | 2 | 0 | 0 | 0 | 7 | 3 | 7 | 1 high-fat meat, 1 fat |

| | | | | | | | | | | | | |
|---|---|---|---|---|---|---|---|---|---|---|---|---|
| ***Jif*** | | | | | | | | | | | | |
| Creamy | 2 Tbsp | 190 | 16 | 145 | 3 | 0 | 0 | 150 | 7 | 2 | 7 | 1 high-fat meat, 1 fat |
| Extra Crunchy | 2 Tbsp | 190 | 16 | 145 | 3 | 0 | 0 | 130 | 7 | 2 | 7 | 1 high-fat meat, 1 fat |
| Omega-3 | 2 Tbsp | 190 | 16 | 140 | 2.5 | 0 | 0 | 160 | 8 | 2 | 7 | 1/2 carb, 1 high-fat meat, 1 fat |
| Peanut Butter & Honey | 2 Tbsp | 180 | 14 | 130 | 2.5 | 0 | 0 | 120 | 10 | 2 | 6 | 1/2 carb, 1 high-fat meat, 1 fat |
| Reduced Fat, Creamy | 2 Tbsp | 190 | 12 | 111 | 2.5 | 0 | 0 | 250 | 15 | 2 | 8 | 1 carb, 1 high-fat meat, 1 fat |
| Reduced Fat, Crunchy | 2 Tbsp | 190 | 12 | 110 | 2.5 | 0 | 0 | 210 | 15 | 2 | 8 | 1 carb, 1 high-fat meat, 1 fat |
| Simply Jif, Creamy | 2 Tbsp | 190 | 16 | 130 | 3 | 0 | 0 | 65 | 6 | 2 | 8 | 1/2 carb, 1 high-fat meat, 1 fat |
| ***Laura Scudder's*** | | | | | | | | | | | | |
| Peanut Butter, Nutty | 2 Tbsp | 210 | 16 | 144 | 2.5 | 0 | 0 | 120 | 6 | 2 | 8 | 1 high-fat meat, 2 fat |
| Peanut Butter, Smooth | 2 Tbsp | 210 | 16 | 144 | 2.5 | 0 | 0 | 120 | 6 | 2 | 8 | 1 high-fat meat, 2 fat |

| | Serving | Calories | Fat (g) | Cal. from Fat | Sat. Fat (g) | Trans Fat (g) | Chol. (mg) | Sod. (mg) | Carb. (g) | Fiber (g) | Prot. (g) | Servings/Exchanges |
|---|---|---|---|---|---|---|---|---|---|---|---|---|
| ***Peter Pan*** | | | | | | | | | | | | |
| Creamy | 2 Tbsp | 210 | 17 | 150 | 3 | 0 | 0 | 140 | 6 | 2 | 8 | 1/2 carb, 1 high-fat meat, 1 fat |
| Crunchy | 2 Tbsp | 190 | 16 | 140 | 3 | 0 | 0 | 110 | 6 | 3 | 8 | 1/2 carb, 1 high-fat meat, 1 fat |
| Creamy Spread, Reduced Fat | 2 Tbsp | 200 | 13 | 120 | 2 | 0 | 0 | 150 | 14 | 2 | 8 | 1 carb, 1 high-fat meat, 1 fat |
| Creamy Honey Roast | 2 Tbsp | 200 | 15 | 140 | 3 | 0 | 0 | 125 | 10 | 2 | 8 | 1/2 carb, 1 high-fat meat, 1 fat |
| Creamy Plus | 2 Tbsp | 210 | 17 | 150 | 3 | 0 | 0 | 140 | 7 | 2 | 7 | 1/2 carb, 1 high-fat meat, 1 fat |
| Creamy Whipped | 2 Tbsp | 150 | 12 | 110 | 2.5 | 0 | 0 | 105 | 5 | 2 | 6 | 1 high-fat meat |
| Chunky Reduced Fat | 2 Tbsp | 200 | 13 | 120 | 2.5 | 0 | 0 | 150 | 14 | 2 | 8 | 1 carb, 1 high-fat meat, 1 fat |

| | | | | | | | | | | | | |
|---|---|---|---|---|---|---|---|---|---|---|---|---|
| ***Skippy*** | | | | | | | | | | | | |
| Creamy | 2 Tbsp | 190 | 16 | 140 | 3 | 0 | 3 | 150 | 7 | 2 | 7 | 1/2 carb, 1 high-fat meat, 1 fat |
| Natural Creamy | 2 Tbsp | 180 | 17 | 150 | 3.5 | 0 | 0 | 125 | 6 | 2 | 7 | 1/2 carb, 1 high-fat meat, 1 fat |
| Reduced Fat Creamy | 2 Tbsp | 180 | 12 | 110 | 2 | 0 | 0 | 170 | 15 | 2 | 7 | 1 carb, 1 high-fat meat, 1 fat |
| Reduced Fat Super Chunk | 2 Tbsp | 180 | 12 | 110 | 2 | 0 | 0 | 160 | 15 | 2 | 7 | 1 carb, 1 high-fat meat, 1 fat |
| Roasted Honey Nut | 2 Tbsp | 190 | 16 | 140 | 3 | 0 | 0 | 125 | 7 | 2 | 7 | 1/2 carb, 1 high-fat meat, 1 fat |
| Roasted Honey Nut Super Chunk | 2 Tbsp | 190 | 16 | 140 | 3 | 0 | 0 | 105 | 6 | 2 | 7 | 1/2 carb, 1 high-fat meat, 1 fat |
| ***Smart Balance*** | | | | | | | | | | | | |
| Chunky | 2 Tbsp | 200 | 18 | 160 | 3 | 0 | 0 | 110 | 6 | 2 | 7 | 1/2 carb, 1 high-fat meat, 2 fat |

# PASTA, PASTA MIXES, PASTA SAUCE

| | Serving | Calories | Fat. (g) | Cal. from Fat | Sat. Fat (g) | Trans Fat (g) | Chol. (mg) | Sod. (mg) | Carb. (g) | Fiber (g) | Prot. (g) | Servings/Exchanges |
|---|---|---|---|---|---|---|---|---|---|---|---|---|
| Lasagna, Cut, Cooked | 1/2 cup | 99 | <1 | 0 | <1 | 0 | 0 | <1 | 20 | <1 | 3 | 1 starch |
| Linguine, Cooked | 1/2 cup | 99 | <1 | 0 | <1 | 0 | 0 | <1 | 20 | 2 | 3 | 1 starch |
| Macaroni, Cooked | 1/2 cup | 99 | <1 | 0 | <1 | 0 | 0 | <1 | 20 | <1 | 3 | 1 starch |
| Macaroni, Vegetable, Cooked | 1/2 cup | 86 | <1 | 0 | <1 | 0 | 0 | 4 | 18 | 1 | 3 | 1 starch |
| Macaroni, Whole Wheat, Cooked | 1/2 cup | 87 | <1 | 0 | <1 | 0 | 0 | 2 | 19 | 2 | 4 | 1 starch |
| Noodles, Chow Mein | 1/2 cup | 119 | 7 | 63 | 1 | 0 | 0 | 99 | 13 | <1 | 2 | 1 starch, 1 fat |
| Noodles, Egg, Cooked | 1/2 cup | 107 | 1 | 9 | <1 | 0 | 26 | 6 | 20 | <1 | 4 | 1 starch |
| Noodles, Ramen, Cooked | 1 cup | 156 | 2 | 18 | <1 | 0 | 38 | 1349 | 29 | 3 | 6 | 2 starch |
| Noodles, Rice, Cooked | 1/2 cup | 80 | <1 | 0 | <1 | 0 | 0 | 5 | 20 | <1 | <1 | 1 starch |
| Noodles, Spinach Egg, Cooked | 1/2 cup | 106 | 1 | 9 | <1 | 0 | 27 | 10 | 20 | 2 | 4 | 1 starch |

| | | | | | | | | | | | | |
|---|---|---|---|---|---|---|---|---|---|---|---|---|
| Pasta/Noodles, Fresh, Cooked | 2 oz | 74 | <1 | 0 | <1 | 0 | 19 | 3 | 14 | <1 | 3 | 1 starch |
| Pasta/Noodles, Homemade, No Egg, Cooked | 2 oz | 70 | <1 | 0 | <1 | 0 | 0 | 42 | 14 | <1 | 3 | 1 starch |
| Pasta/Noodles, Homemade, with Egg, Cooked | 2 oz | 74 | <1 | 0 | <1 | 0 | 23 | 47 | 13 | 2 | 3 | 1 starch |
| Pasta/Noodles, Spinach, Fresh, Cooked | 2 oz | 74 | <1 | 0 | <1 | 0 | 19 | 3 | 14 | 1 | 3 | 1 starch |
| Rotini, Cooked | 1/2 cup | 99 | <1 | 0 | <1 | 0 | 0 | <1 | 20 | <1 | 3 | 2 starch |
| Shells, Jumbo, Cooked | 2 | 65 | <1 | 0 | <1 | 0 | 0 | <1 | 13 | <1 | 2 | 1 starch |
| Shells, Small, Cooked | 1/2 cup | 81 | <1 | 0 | <1 | 0 | 0 | <1 | 17 | <1 | 3 | 1 starch |
| Shells, Whole Wheat, Cooked | 1/2 cup | 87 | <1 | 0 | <1 | 0 | 0 | 2 | 19 | 2 | 4 | 1 starch |
| Spaghetti, Cooked | 1/2 cup | 99 | <1 | 0 | <1 | 0 | 0 | <1 | 20 | 3 | 3 | 1 starch |

PASTA, PASTA MIXES, PASTA SAUCE

| | Serving | Calories | Fat (g) | Cal. from Fat | Sat. Fat (g) | Trans Fat (g) | Chol. (mg) | Sod. (mg) | Carb. (g) | Fiber (g) | Prot. (g) | Servings/Exchanges |
|---|---|---|---|---|---|---|---|---|---|---|---|---|
| Spaghetti, Whole Wheat, Cooked | 1/2 cup | 87 | <1 | 0 | <1 | 0 | 0 | 2 | 19 | 3 | 4 | 1 starch |
| Spirals Pasta, Cooked | 1/2 cup | 95 | <1 | 0 | <1 | 0 | 0 | <1 | 19 | <1 | 3 | 1 starch |
| Vermicelli, Cooked | 1/2 cup | 99 | <1 | 0 | <1 | 0 | 0 | <1 | 20 | 2 | 3 | 1 starch |
| Wagon Wheels Pasta, Cooked | 1/2 cup | 99 | <1 | 0 | <1 | 0 | 0 | <1 | 20 | <1 | 3 | 1 starch |
| **BRANDS** | | | | | | | | | | | | |
| **Pasta Mixes** | | | | | | | | | | | | |
| ***Knorr/Lipton*** | | | | | | | | | | | | |
| Pasta Sides, Alfredo | 1 cup | 310 | 12 | 90 | 4.5 | 0 | 15 | 890 | 43 | 1 | 11 | 3 starch, 2 fat |
| Pasta Sides, Chicken | 1 cup | 250 | 6 | 50 | 1 | 0 | <5 | 720 | 43 | 1 | 8 | 3 starch, 1 fat |
| Pasta Sides, Parmesan | 1 cup | 280 | 12 | 80 | 4.5 | 0 | 15 | 760 | 42 | 1 | 10 | 3 starch, 2 fat |
| ***Kraft*** | | | | | | | | | | | | |
| Macaroni & Cheese | 1 cup | 410 | 19 | 170 | 5 | 4 | 15 | 710 | 49 | 1 | 9 | 3 starch, 4 fat |

| | | | | | | | | | | | | |
|---|---|---|---|---|---|---|---|---|---|---|---|---|
| Macaroni & Cheese, Deluxe Original | 1 cup | 320 | 10 | 90 | 3 | 0 | 15 | 930 | 45 | 1 | 12 | 3 starch, 2 fat |
| Macaroni & Cheese, Easy Mac, Original | 1 pouch | 230 | 4 | 35 | 2.5 | 0 | 5 | 550 | 42 | 1 | 7 | 3 starch, 1 fat |
| Macaroni & Cheese, Thick 'n Creamy | 1 cup | 380 | 15 | 140 | 4 | 3 | 5 | 740 | 52 | 2 | 10 | 3 1/2 starch, 3 fat |
| Macaroni & Cheese, Three Cheese | 1 cup | 380 | 15 | 130 | 4 | 3 | 5 | 760 | 51 | 2 | 9 | 3 1/2 starch, 3 fat |
| Velveeta Shells & Cheese, Original | 1 cup | 360 | 12 | 110 | 4 | 0 | 20 | 940 | 49 | 2 | 13 | 3 starch, 1 med-fat meat, 1 fat |
| **Asian Pasta** | | | | | | | | | | | | |
| ***Dynasty*** | | | | | | | | | | | | |
| Maifun Rice Sticks | 2 oz | 200 | 0.5 | 5 | 0 | 0 | 0 | 130 | 48 | 1 | 0 | 3 starch |
| Saifun Bean Threads | 1 bundle | 170 | 0 | 0 | 0 | 0 | 0 | 10 | 42 | 0 | 0 | 3 starch |
| ***Eden*** | | | | | | | | | | | | |
| 100% Buckwheat Soba | 2 oz | 200 | 1 | 10 | 0 | 0 | 0 | 5 | 43 | 3 | 6 | 3 starch |

| | Serving | Calories | Fat (g) | Cal. from Fat | Sat. Fat (g) | Trans Fat (g) | Chol. (mg) | Sod. (mg) | Carb. (g) | Fiber (g) | Prot. (g) | Servings/Exchanges |
|---|---|---|---|---|---|---|---|---|---|---|---|---|
| 40% Buckwheat Soba | 2 oz | 190 | 1 | 5 | 0 | 0 | 0 | 490 | 37 | 3 | 8 | 2 1/2 starch |
| Bifun (Rice) Pasta | 2 oz | 200 | 0.5 | 0 | 0 | 0 | 5 | 5 | 44 | 0 | 5 | 3 starch |
| Brown Rice Udon | 2 oz | 190 | 1 | 5 | 0 | 0 | 0 | 510 | 38 | 2 | 8 | 2 1/2 starch |
| Kamut Soba, Organic | 1/2 cup | 200 | 1 | 10 | 0 | 0 | 0 | 60 | 38 | 3 | 7 | 2 1/2 starch |
| Kamut Udon, Organic | 1/2 cup | 200 | 1.5 | 15 | 0 | 0 | 0 | 55 | 37 | 3 | 10 | 2 1/2 starch |
| Kuzu Pasta | 2 oz | 200 | 0 | 0 | 0 | 0 | 0 | 0 | 48 | 2 | 0 | 3 starch |
| Lotus Root Soba | 2 oz | 190 | 1 | 5 | 0 | 0 | 0 | 470 | 37 | 4 | 9 | 2 1/2 starch |
| Mugwort Soba | 2 oz | 190 | 0.5 | 5 | 0 | 0 | 0 | 550 | 37 | 2 | 8 | 2 1/2 starch |
| Mung Bean Pasta | 2 oz | 190 | 0 | 0 | 0 | 0 | 0 | 5 | 47 | 0 | 0 | 3 starch |
| Soba, Organic | 1/2 cup | 200 | 1.5 | 15 | 0 | 0 | 0 | 70 | 38 | 2 | 8 | 2 1/2 starch |
| Spelt Soba, Organic | 1/2 cup | 200 | 1.5 | 15 | 0 | 0 | 0 | 50 | 37 | 2 | 9 | 2 1/2 starch |
| Udon | 2 oz | 190 | 1.5 | 15 | 0 | 0 | 0 | 660 | 37 | 3 | 8 | 2 1/2 starch |
| ***La Choy*** | | | | | | | | | | | | |
| Chow Mein Noodles | 1/2 cup | 130 | 5 | 50 | 1.5 | NA | 0 | 230 | 19 | 0 | 3 | 1 starch, 1 fat |

| | | | | | | | | | | | | |
|---|---|---|---|---|---|---|---|---|---|---|---|---|
| Rice Noodles | 1/2 cup | 130 | 4 | 36 | 1 | NA | 0 | 350 | 21 | 0 | 2 | 1 1/2 starch, 1 fat |
| ***Thai Kitchen*** | | | | | | | | | | | | |
| Stir-Fry Rice Noodles | 2 oz | 195 | 0 | 0 | 0 | 0 | 0 | 0 | 46 | 2 | 3 | 3 starch |
| Thin Rice Noodles | 2 oz | 196 | 0 | 0 | 0 | 0 | 0 | 0 | 46 | 2 | 3 | 3 starch |
| ***Wel-Pac*** | | | | | | | | | | | | |
| Chinese Noodles | 2 oz | 200 | 0 | 0 | 0 | 0 | 0 | 400 | 42 | 1 | 7 | 3 starch |
| Chow Mein Stir-Fry Noodles | 2 oz | 200 | 1 | 5 | 0 | 0 | 0 | 125 | 42 | 0 | 7 | 3 starch |
| Japanese Udon Noodles | 2 oz | 180 | 0.5 | 0 | 0 | 0 | 0 | 115 | 40 | 1 | 5 | 2 1/2 starch |
| **Dry Pasta** | | | | | | | | | | | | |
| ***Al Dente*** | | | | | | | | | | | | |
| Carba-Nada | 1 1/2 cup | 140 | 1 | 10 | 0 | 0 | 10 | 20 | 24 | 6 | 12 | 1 1/2 starch |
| Garlic Parsley Fettucini | 2 oz | 220 | 2 | 20 | 0.5 | 0 | 33 | 15 | 41 | 2 | 8 | 2 1/2 starch |
| ***American Beauty*** | | | | | | | | | | | | |
| Angel Hair | 2 oz | 210 | 1 | 10 | 0 | 0 | 0 | 0 | 42 | 2 | 7 | 3 starch |
| Ditalini | 2 oz | 210 | 1 | 10 | 0 | 0 | 0 | 0 | 42 | 2 | 7 | 3 starch |

PASTA, PASTA MIXES, PASTA SAUCE

| | Serving | Calories | Fat (g) | Cal. from Fat | Sat. Fat (g) | Trans Fat (g) | Chol. (mg) | Sod. (mg) | Carb. (g) | Fiber (g) | Prot. (g) | Servings/Exchanges |
|---|---|---|---|---|---|---|---|---|---|---|---|---|
| Elbow Macaroni | 2 oz | 210 | 1 | 10 | 0 | 0 | 0 | 0 | 42 | 2 | 7 | 3 starch |
| Extra Wide Egg Noodles | 2 oz | 210 | 2.5 | 25 | 1 | 0 | 70 | 15 | 40 | 2 | 8 | 2 1/2 starch |
| Fettuccine | 2 oz | 210 | 1 | 10 | 0 | 0 | 0 | 0 | 42 | 2 | 7 | 3 starch |
| Fideo Cortado (Fino) | 2 oz | 210 | 1 | 10 | 0 | 0 | 0 | 0 | 42 | 2 | 7 | 3 starch |
| Jumbo Shells | 2 oz | 210 | 1 | 10 | 0 | 0 | 0 | 0 | 42 | 2 | 7 | 3 starch |
| Large Elbows | 2 oz | 210 | 1 | 10 | 0 | 0 | 0 | 0 | 42 | 2 | 7 | 3 starch |
| Large Shells | 2 oz | 210 | 1 | 10 | 0 | 0 | 0 | 0 | 42 | 2 | 7 | 3 starch |
| Manicotti | 2 oz | 210 | 1 | 10 | 0 | 0 | 0 | 0 | 42 | 2 | 7 | 3 starch |
| Oven Ready Lasagna | 2 oz | 210 | 1 | 10 | 0 | 0 | 0 | 0 | 42 | 2 | 7 | 3 starch |
| Penne Rigate | 2 oz | 210 | 1 | 10 | 0 | 0 | 0 | 0 | 42 | 2 | 7 | 3 starch |
| Rainbow Twirls | 2 oz | 210 | 1 | 10 | 0 | 0 | 0 | 30 | 42 | 2 | 7 | 3 starch |
| Rice & Spinach Tortelloni | 2 oz | 220 | 5 | 45 | 2.5 | 0 | 30 | 560 | 35 | 2 | 8 | 2 starch, 1 fat |
| Rotini | 2 oz | 210 | 1 | 10 | 0 | 0 | 0 | 0 | 42 | 2 | 7 | 3 starch |

| | | | | | | | | | | | | |
|---|---|---|---|---|---|---|---|---|---|---|---|---|
| Sea Shells | 2 oz | 210 | 1 | 10 | 0 | 0 | 0 | 0 | 42 | 2 | 7 | 3 starch |
| Small Shells | 2 oz | 210 | 1 | 10 | 0 | 0 | 0 | 0 | 42 | 2 | 7 | 3 starch |
| Spaghetti | 2 oz | 210 | 1 | 10 | 0 | 0 | 0 | 0 | 42 | 2 | 7 | 3 starch |
| Thin Spaghetti | 2 oz | 210 | 1 | 10 | 0 | 0 | 0 | 0 | 42 | 2 | 7 | 3 starch |
| Three Cheese Tortelloni | 2 oz | 210 | 4 | 40 | 2 | 0 | 30 | 620 | 35 | 2 | 7 | 2 starch, 1 fat |
| Vermicelli | 2 oz | 210 | 1 | 10 | 0 | 0 | 0 | 0 | 42 | 2 | 7 | 3 starch |
| Wide Egg Noodles | 2 oz | 210 | 2.5 | 25 | 1 | 0 | 70 | 15 | 40 | 2 | 8 | 2 1/2 starch, 1 fat |
| ***Barilla*** | | | | | | | | | | | | |
| Angel Hair | 2 oz | 200 | 1 | 10 | 0 | 0 | 0 | 0 | 42 | 2 | 7 | 3 starch |
| Elbows | 2 oz | 200 | 1 | 10 | 0 | 0 | 0 | 0 | 42 | 2 | 7 | 3 starch |
| Farfalle | 2 oz | 200 | 1 | 10 | 0 | 0 | 0 | 0 | 42 | 2 | 7 | 3 starch |
| Fetuccine | 2 oz | 200 | 1 | 10 | 0 | 0 | 0 | 0 | 42 | 2 | 7 | 3 starch |
| Lasagna | 2 pieces | 180 | 1 | 10 | 0 | 0 | 0 | 0 | 38 | 2 | 6 | 2 1/2 starch |
| Lasagna, No Boil | 3 pieces | 190 | 2 | 20 | 0.5 | 0 | 50 | 20 | 36 | 2 | 7 | 2 starch |
| Linguine | 2 oz | 200 | 1 | 10 | 0 | 0 | 0 | 0 | 42 | 2 | 7 | 3 starch |
| Medium Shells | 2 oz | 200 | 1 | 10 | 0 | 0 | 0 | 0 | 42 | 2 | 7 | 3 starch |

| | Serving | Calories | Fat (g) | Cal. from Fat | Sat. Fat (g) | Trans Fat (g) | Chol. (mg) | Sod. (mg) | Carb. (g) | Fiber (g) | Prot. (g) | Servings/Exchanges |
|---|---|---|---|---|---|---|---|---|---|---|---|---|
| Mini Penne | 2 oz | 200 | 1 | 10 | 0 | 0 | 0 | 0 | 42 | 2 | 7 | 3 starch |
| Mostaccioli | 2 oz | 200 | 1 | 10 | 0 | 0 | 0 | 0 | 42 | 2 | 7 | 3 starch |
| Penne | 2 oz | 200 | 1 | 10 | 0 | 0 | 0 | 0 | 42 | 2 | 7 | 3 starch |
| Rigatoni | 2 oz | 200 | 1 | 10 | 0 | 0 | 0 | 0 | 42 | 2 | 7 | 3 starch |
| Rotini | 2 oz | 200 | 1 | 10 | 0 | 0 | 0 | 0 | 42 | 2 | 7 | 3 starch |
| Spaghetti | 2 oz | 200 | 1 | 10 | 0 | 0 | 0 | 0 | 42 | 2 | 7 | 3 starch |
| Spaghetti Rigati | 2 oz | 200 | 1 | 10 | 0 | 0 | 0 | 0 | 42 | 2 | 7 | 3 starch |
| Thin Spaghetti | 2 oz | 200 | 1 | 10 | 0 | 0 | 0 | 0 | 42 | 2 | 7 | 3 starch |
| Tortellini Ricotta & Spinach | 3/4 cup | 230 | 8 | 70 | 2.5 | 0 | 60 | 340 | 32 | 5 | 8 | 2 starch |
| Tortellini Three Cheese | 2/3 cup | 230 | 8 | 70 | 2.5 | 0 | 40 | 475 | 33 | 3 | 8 | 2 starch |
| Tri-Color Rotini | 2 oz | 200 | 1 | 10 | 0 | 0 | 0 | 15 | 42 | 2 | 7 | 3 starch |
| ***Barilla Plus*** | | | | | | | | | | | | |
| Angel Hair | 2 oz | 200 | 1 | 10 | 0 | 0 | 0 | 25 | 38 | 4 | 10 | 2 1/2 starch |

| | | | | | | | | | | | | |
|---|---|---|---|---|---|---|---|---|---|---|---|---|
| Elbows | 2 oz | 200 | 1 | 10 | 0 | 0 | 0 | 25 | 38 | 4 | 10 | 2 1/2 starch |
| Penne | 2 oz | 200 | 1 | 10 | 0 | 0 | 0 | 25 | 38 | 4 | 10 | 2 1/2 starch |
| Spaghetti | 2 oz | 200 | 1 | 10 | 0 | 0 | 0 | 25 | 38 | 4 | 10 | 2 1/2 starch |
| Thin Spaghetti | 2 oz | 210 | 1 | 10 | 0 | 0 | 0 | 25 | 38 | 4 | 10 | 2 1/2 starch |
| ***Buitoni (Refrigerated)*** | | | | | | | | | | | | |
| Chicken & Prosciutto Tortelloni | 1 cup | 330 | 9 | 80 | 3 | 0 | 40 | 610 | 46 | 2 | 15 | 3 carb, 2 fat |
| Four Cheese Ravioli | 1 1/4 cup | 340 | 12 | 110 | 4 | 0 | 55 | 650 | 42 | 3 | 15 | 3 carb, 2 fat |
| Linguine | 1 1/4 cup | 240 | 2.5 | 25 | 1 | 0 | 50 | 20 | 45 | 2 | 10 | 3 carb, 1 fat |
| Mixed Cheese Tortellini | 1 cup | 320 | 7 | 60 | 3.5 | 0 | 40 | 490 | 50 | 1 | 15 | 3 carb, 1 fat |
| Spinach Cheese Tortellini | 1 cup | 320 | 7 | 60 | 3.5 | 0 | 55 | 510 | 49 | 3 | 15 | 3 carb, 1 fat |
| ***Colavita*** | | | | | | | | | | | | |
| Angel Hair | 2 oz | 210 | 1 | 10 | 0 | 0 | 0 | 0 | 44 | 2 | 7 | 3 starch |
| Bow Ties | 3/4 cup | 210 | 1 | 10 | 0 | 0 | 0 | 0 | 44 | 2 | 7 | 3 starch |
| Fettuccine Nests | 2 nests | 210 | 1 | 10 | 0 | 0 | 0 | 0 | 44 | 2 | 7 | 3 starch |

PASTA, PASTA MIXES, PASTA SAUCE

| | Serving | Calories | Fat (g) | Cal. from Fat | Sat. Fat (g) | Trans Fat (g) | Chol. (mg) | Sod. (mg) | Carb. (g) | Fiber (g) | Prot. (g) | Servings/Exchanges |
|---|---|---|---|---|---|---|---|---|---|---|---|---|
| Linguine | 2 oz | 210 | 1 | 10 | 0 | 0 | 0 | 0 | 44 | 2 | 7 | 3 starch |
| Long Fusill | 2 oz | 210 | 1 | 10 | 0 | 0 | 0 | 0 | 44 | 2 | 7 | 3 starch |
| ***Creamette*** | | | | | | | | | | | | |
| Angel Hair | 2 oz | 210 | 1 | 10 | 0 | 0 | 0 | 0 | 42 | 2 | 7 | 3 starch |
| Elbow Macaroni | 2 oz | 210 | 1 | 10 | 0 | 0 | 0 | 0 | 42 | 2 | 7 | 3 starch |
| Extra Wide Egg Noodles | 2 oz | 210 | 2.5 | 25 | 1 | 0 | 70 | 15 | 40 | 2 | 8 | 2 1/2 starch |
| Lasagna | 2 oz | 210 | 1 | 10 | 0 | 0 | 0 | 0 | 42 | 2 | 7 | 3 starch |
| Spaghetti | 2 oz | 210 | 1 | 10 | 0 | 0 | 0 | 0 | 42 | 2 | 7 | 3 starch |
| ***Da Vinci*** | | | | | | | | | | | | |
| 100% Whole Wheat Elbows | 1/2 cup | 180 | 1.5 | 10 | 0 | 0 | <5 | 0 | 44 | 5 | 7 | 3 starch |
| 100% Whole Wheat Penne | 3/4 cup | 170 | 1 | 10 | 0 | 0 | <5 | 0 | 42 | 5 | 7 | 3 starch |
| Angel Hair | 2 oz | 210 | 1 | 5 | 0 | 0 | 0 | 0 | 43 | 2 | 6 | 3 starch |

| | | | | | | | | | | | | |
|---|---|---|---|---|---|---|---|---|---|---|---|---|
| Bowties | 1 cup | 210 | 1 | 10 | 0 | 0 | 0 | 0 | 41 | 2 | 7 | 2 1/2 starch |
| Cut Ziti | 3/4 cup | 210 | 1 | 5 | 0 | 0 | 0 | 0 | 43 | 2 | 6 | 3 starch |
| Fettuccine | 2 oz | 210 | 1 | 10 | 0 | 0 | 0 | 0 | 43 | 2 | 6 | 3 starch |
| Fusilli Springs | 3/4 cup | 210 | 1 | 10 | 0 | 0 | 0 | 0 | 43 | 2 | 6 | 3 starch |
| Penne Rigate | 3/4 cup | 210 | 1 | 10 | 0 | 0 | 0 | 0 | 41 | 2 | 7 | 2 1/2 starch |
| Potato Gnocchi | 3/4 cup | 200 | 0 | 0 | 0 | 0 | 0 | 440 | 44 | 2 | 4 | 3 starch |
| Rotini | 1 cup | 210 | 1 | 10 | 0 | 0 | 0 | 0 | 41 | 2 | 6 | 2 1/2 starch |
| Spaghetti | 2 oz | 210 | 1 | 10 | 0 | 0 | 0 | 0 | 41 | 2 | 6 | 2 1/2 starch |
| ***DeBoles*** | | | | | | | | | | | | |
| Organic Whole Wheat Spaghetti Style Pasta | 2 oz | 210 | 1.5 | 10 | 0 | 0 | 0 | 10 | 42 | 5 | 7 | 3 carb |
| Rice Spaghetti Style Pasta | 2 oz | 210 | 0.5 | 5 | 0 | 0 | 0 | 15 | 46 | <1 | 4 | 3 carb |
| Rice Spirals | 2 oz | 210 | 0.5 | 5 | 0 | 0 | 0 | 15 | 46 | <1 | 4 | 3 carb |
| Tomato & Basil Angel Hair Pasta | 2 oz | 210 | 1 | 10 | 0 | 0 | 0 | 0 | 41 | 2 | 7 | 2 1/2 carb |

| | Serving | Calories | Fat (g) | Cal. from Fat | Sat. Fat (g) | Trans Fat (g) | Chol. (mg) | Sod. (mg) | Carb. (g) | Fiber (g) | Prot. (g) | Servings/Exchanges |
|---|---|---|---|---|---|---|---|---|---|---|---|---|
| ***DeCecco*** | | | | | | | | | | | | |
| Farfalle | 1 cup | 200 | 1 | 10 | 0 | 0 | 0 | 0 | 41 | 2 | 7 | 2 1/2 starch |
| Fusilli | 3/4 cup | 200 | 1 | 10 | 0 | 0 | 0 | 0 | 41 | 2 | 7 | 2 1/2 starch |
| Linguine | 2 oz | 200 | 1 | 10 | 0 | 0 | 0 | 0 | 41 | 2 | 7 | 2 1/2 starch |
| Penne Rigate | 1/2 cup | 200 | 1 | 10 | 0 | 0 | 0 | 0 | 41 | 2 | 7 | 2 1/2 starch |
| Spaghetti | 2 oz | 200 | 1 | 10 | 0 | 0 | 0 | 0 | 41 | 2 | 7 | 2 1/2 starch |
| Zita Cut | 2/3 cup | 200 | 1 | 10 | 0 | 0 | 0 | 0 | 41 | 2 | 7 | 2 1/2 starch |
| ***Dreamfields*** | | | | | | | | | | | | |
| Elbows | 2 oz | 190 | 1 | 10 | 0 | 0 | 0 | 10 | 41 | 4 | 7 | 2 1/2 starch |
| Lasagna | 2 oz | 190 | 1 | 10 | 0 | 0 | 0 | 10 | 41 | 5 | 7 | 2 1/2 starch |
| Linguine | 2 oz | 190 | 1 | 10 | 0 | 0 | 0 | 10 | 41 | 2 | 7 | 2 1/2 starch |
| Penne Rigate | 2 oz | 190 | 1 | 10 | 0 | 0 | 0 | 10 | 41 | 4 | 7 | 2 1/2 starch |
| Spaghetti | 2 oz | 190 | 1 | 10 | 0 | 0 | 0 | 10 | 41 | 5 | 7 | 2 1/2 starch |
| ***Fiber Wise*** | | | | | | | | | | | | |

| | | | | | | | | | | | | |
|---|---|---|---|---|---|---|---|---|---|---|---|---|
| High Fiber Elbows | 2 oz | 170 | 1 | 10 | 0 | 0 | 0 | 25 | 41 | 12 | 8 | 2 1/2 starch |
| High Fiber Penne | 2 oz | 170 | 1 | 10 | 0 | 0 | 0 | 25 | 41 | 12 | 8 | 2 1/2 starch |
| High Fiber Spaghetti | 2 oz | 170 | 1 | 10 | 0 | 0 | 0 | 25 | 41 | 12 | 8 | 2 1/2 starch |
| ***Hodgson Mill*** | | | | | | | | | | | | |
| Organic Whole Wheat Fettuccine with Milled Flax Seed | 2 oz | 200 | 2 | 20 | 0 | 0 | 0 | 10 | 40 | 6 | 9 | 2 1/2 starch |
| Organic Whole Wheat Penne with Milled Flax Seed | 2 oz | 215 | 2 | 20 | 0 | 0 | 0 | 0 | 40 | 6 | 9 | 2 1/2 starch |
| Organic Whole Wheat Spaghetti with Milled FlaX Seed | 2 oz | 200 | 2 | 20 | 0 | 0 | 0 | 10 | 40 | 6 | 9 | 2 1/2 starch |
| Organic Whole Wheat Spirals with Milled Flax Seed | 2 oz | 200 | 2 | 20 | 0 | 0 | 0 | 10 | 40 | 6 | 9 | 2 1/2 starch |
| Veggie Rotini | 2 oz | 200 | 1 | 5 | 0 | 0 | 0 | 15 | 41 | 1 | 8 | 2 1/2 starch |

PASTA, PASTA MIXES, PASTA SAUCE

| | Serving | Calories | Fat (g) | Cal. from Fat | Sat. Fat (g) | Trans Fat (g) | Chol. (mg) | Sod. (mg) | Carb. (g) | Fiber (g) | Prot. (g) | Servings/Exchanges |
|---|---|---|---|---|---|---|---|---|---|---|---|---|
| Whole Wheat Fettuccine | 2 oz | 210 | 1 | 15 | 0 | 0 | 0 | 0 | 41 | 6 | 9 | 2 1/2 starch |
| Whole Wheat Spaghetti | 2 oz | 210 | 1 | 15 | 0 | 0 | 0 | 0 | 41 | 6 | 9 | 2 1/2 starch |
| Whole Wheat Spirals | 2 oz | 190 | 1 | 15 | 1 | 0 | 0 | 10 | 34 | 6 | 9 | 2 starch |
| ***No Yolks (Cholesterol Free)*** | | | | | | | | | | | | |
| Dumplings | 2 oz | 210 | 0.5 | 5 | 0 | 0 | 0 | 30 | 41 | 3 | 8 | 2 1/2 starch |
| Extra Broad Noodles | 2 oz | 210 | 0.5 | 5 | 0 | 0 | 0 | 30 | 41 | 3 | 8 | 2 1/2 starch |
| ***Rao's*** | | | | | | | | | | | | |
| Fusilli | 1/2 cup | 200 | 1 | 10 | 0 | 0 | 0 | 10 | 41 | 2 | 7 | 2 1/2 starch |
| Penne Rigate | 1/2 cup | 200 | 1 | 10 | 0 | 0 | 0 | 10 | 41 | 2 | 7 | 2 1/2 starch |
| ***Ronzoni*** | | | | | | | | | | | | |
| Healthy Harvest Whole-Grain Thin Spaghetti | 2 oz | 180 | 2 | 15 | 0 | 0 | 0 | 0 | 41 | 6 | 7 | 2 1/2 starch |
| Healthy Harvest 7 Grain Fusilli | 2 oz | 180 | 2 | 20 | 0 | 0 | 0 | 0 | 40 | 5 | 8 | 2 1/2 starch |

| | | | | | | | | | | | |
|---|---|---|---|---|---|---|---|---|---|---|---|
| **Pasta Sauce** | | | | | | | | | | | |
| ***Amy's Organic*** | | | | | | | | | | | |
| Family Marinara | 1/2 cup | 80 | 4.5 | 40 | 0.5 | 0 | 0 | 590 | 10 | 3 | 1 | 1/2 carb, 1 fat |
| Low Sodium Marinara | 1/2 cup | 40 | 1 | 10 | 0 | 0 | 0 | 100 | 7 | 1 | 1 | 1/2 carb |
| Puttanesca | 1/2 cup | 45 | 2 | 20 | 0 | 0 | 0 | 680 | 6 | 1 | 2 | 1/2 carb |
| Roasted Garlic | 1/2 cup | 130 | 8 | 70 | 1 | 0 | 0 | 470 | 13 | 3 | 2 | 1 carb, 2 fat |
| Tomato Basil | 1/2 cup | 110 | 6 | 50 | 1 | 0 | 0 | 580 | 11 | 3 | 2 | 1 carb, 1 fat |
| ***Barilla*** | | | | | | | | | | | |
| Marinara | 1/2 cup | 70 | 1.5 | 15 | 0 | 0 | 0 | 460 | 12 | 2 | 2 | 1 carb |
| Roasted Garlic | 1/2 cup | 60 | 1 | 10 | 0 | 0 | 0 | 460 | 12 | 2 | 2 | 1/2 carb |
| Tomato & Basil | 1/2 cup | 60 | 1 | 10 | 0 | 0 | 0 | 460 | 12 | 2 | 2 | 1/2 carb |
| ***Bertolli*** | | | | | | | | | | | |
| Alfredo | 1/4 cup | 110 | 10 | 90 | 5 | 0 | 40 | 460 | 3 | 0 | 2 | 2 fat |
| Marinara | 1/2 cup | 80 | 2 | 20 | 0 | 0 | 0 | 530 | 13 | 1 | 2 | 1 carb |
| Mushroom Alfredo | 1/2 cup | 80 | 6 | 50 | 3 | 0 | 30 | 420 | 3 | 0 | 2 | 1 fat |
| Olive Oil & Garlic | 1/2 cup | 90 | 3 | 25 | 0 | 0 | 0 | 500 | 14 | 3 | 3 | 1 carb, 1 fat |

| | Serving | Calories | Fat (g) | Cal. from Fat | Sat. Fat (g) | Trans Fat (g) | Chol. (mg) | Sod. (mg) | Carb. (g) | Fiber (g) | Prot. (g) | Servings/Exchanges |
|---|---|---|---|---|---|---|---|---|---|---|---|---|
| Portobello Mushroom | 1/2 cup | 80 | 2.5 | 25 | 0 | 0 | 0 | 470 | 12 | 1 | 2 | 1 carb, 1 fat |
| ***Buitoni*** | | | | | | | | | | | | |
| Alfredo Sauce | 1/4 cup | 130 | 11 | 100 | 7 | 0 | 35 | 390 | 4 | 0 | 4 | 2 fat |
| Arrabbiata Sauce | 1/2 cup | 90 | 6 | 50 | 1 | 0 | 0 | 610 | 8 | 2 | 1 | 1/2 carb, 1 fat |
| Light Alfredo Sauce | 1/4 cup | 90 | 6 | 50 | 3.5 | 0 | 15 | 350 | 5 | 0 | 4 | 1 fat |
| Marinara | 1/2 cup | 70 | 3 | 25 | 0.5 | 0 | 0 | 560 | 10 | 2 | 1 | 1/2 carb, 1 fat |
| Pesto with Basil | 1/4 cup | 300 | 28 | 250 | 5 | 0 | 20 | 540 | 6 | 2 | 7 | 1/2 carb, 6 fat |
| Reduced Fat Pesto with Basil | 1/4 cup | 240 | 19 | 170 | 4 | 0 | 15 | 540 | 9 | 2 | 7 | 1/2 carb, 4 fat |
| Roasted Garlic Marinara | 1/2 cup | 60 | 1.5 | 15 | 0.5 | 0 | 0 | 530 | 10 | 2 | 2 | 1/2 carb |
| Tomato Herb Parmesan | 1/2 cup | 130 | 8 | 70 | 2.5 | 0 | 10 | 740 | 10 | 2 | 4 | 1/2 carb, 2 fat |
| Vodka Sauce | 1/2 cup | 100 | 7 | 60 | 4 | 0 | 20 | 610 | 7 | 1 | 2 | 1/2 carb, 1 fat |
| ***Classico*** | | | | | | | | | | | | |
| Creamy Alfredo | 1/4 cup | 100 | 9 | 80 | 5 | 0 | 50 | 410 | 3 | 0 | 2 | 2 fat |

| | | | | | | | | | | | | |
|---|---|---|---|---|---|---|---|---|---|---|---|---|
| Florentine Spinach & Cheese | 1/2 cup | 80 | 5 | 45 | 1 | 0 | 5 | 560 | 7 | 2 | 3 | 1/2 carb, 1 fat |
| Four Cheese | 1/2 cup | 90 | 3.5 | 30 | 1 | 0 | 0 | 490 | 11 | 3 | 3 | 1 carb, 1 fat |
| Four Cheese Alfredo | 1/4 cup | 80 | 7 | 60 | 4 | 0 | 35 | 350 | 3 | 0 | 2 | 1 fat |
| Mushroom & Olives | 1/2 cup | 60 | 1 | 10 | 0.5 | 0 | 0 | 390 | 11 | 2 | 2 | 1 carb |
| Organic Tomato, Herbs & Spices | 1/2 cup | 70 | 1 | 10 | 0 | 0 | 0 | 350 | 12 | 2 | 2 | 1 carb |
| Roasted Garlic | 1/2 cup | 60 | 1 | 10 | 0 | 0 | 0 | 220 | 11 | 2 | 2 | 1 carb |
| Spicy Red Pepper | 1/2 cup | 60 | 1.5 | 15 | 0 | 0 | 0 | 300 | 7 | 2 | 2 | 1/2 carb |
| Sun-Dried Tomato | 1/2 cup | 80 | 3 | 25 | 1 | 0 | 0 | 390 | 11 | 2 | 2 | 1 carb, 1 fat |
| Sun-Dried Tomato & Pesto | 1/4 cup | 90 | 5 | 45 | 1 | 0 | 0 | 630 | 8 | 1 | 3 | 1/2 carb |
| Tomato & Basil | 1/2 cup | 60 | 1 | 10 | 0 | 0 | 0 | 310 | 11 | 2 | 2 | 1 carb |
| Vodka Sauce | 1/2 cup | 150 | 10 | 90 | 3.5 | 0 | 10 | 500 | 12 | 3 | 3 | 1 carb, 2 fat |
| ***Eden Organic*** | | | | | | | | | | | | |
| No Salt Added Spaghetti Sauce | 1/2 cup | 70 | 2.5 | 25 | 0 | 0 | 0 | 10 | 9 | 5 | 2 | 1/2 carb, 1 fat |

PASTA, PASTA MIXES, PASTA SAUCE

| | Serving | Calories | Fat (g) | Cal. from Fat | Sat. Fat (g) | Trans Fat (g) | Chol. (mg) | Sod. (mg) | Carb. (g) | Fiber (g) | Prot. (g) | Servings/Exchanges |
|---|---|---|---|---|---|---|---|---|---|---|---|---|
| Spaghetti Sauce | 1/2 cup | 70 | 2.5 | 25 | 0 | 0 | 0 | 300 | 9 | 5 | 2 | 1/2 carb, 1 fat |
| ***Emeril's*** | | | | | | | | | | | | |
| Eggplant Gaaahlic | 1/2 cup | 90 | 4.5 | 40 | 0 | 0 | 0 | 510 | 12 | 2 | 2 | 1 carb, 1 fat |
| Home Style Marinara | 1/2 cup | 90 | 3 | 25 | 0 | 0 | 0 | 640 | 12 | 1 | 2 | 1 carb, 1 fat |
| Tomato & Basil | 1/2 cup | 80 | 2.5 | 25 | 0 | 0 | 0 | 640 | 13 | 1 | 2 | 1 carb, 1 fat |
| ***Healthy Choice*** | | | | | | | | | | | | |
| Garlic & Herb Sauce | 1/2 cup | 60 | 0 | 0 | 0 | 0 | 0 | 370 | 12 | 3 | 2 | 1 carb |
| Traditional | 1/2 cup | 60 | 0 | 0 | 0 | 0 | 0 | 400 | 13 | 3 | 2 | 1 carb |
| ***Hunt's*** | | | | | | | | | | | | |
| Four Cheese Spaghetti Sauce | 1/2 cup | 50 | 1 | 10 | 0 | 0 | 0 | 580 | 10 | 3 | 3 | 1/2 carb |
| Meat Sauce | 1/2 cup | 60 | 1 | 10 | 0 | 0 | 0 | 610 | 11 | 3 | 3 | 1 carb |
| Traditional Spaghetti Sauce | 1/2 cup | 60 | 1 | 1 | 0 | 0 | 0 | 580 | 10 | 2 | 2 | 1/2 carb |

| | | | | | | | | | | | | |
|---|---|---|---|---|---|---|---|---|---|---|---|---|
| Traditional Spaghetti Sauce (Pouch) | 1/2 cup | 50 | 1 | 10 | 0 | 0 | 0 | 580 | 10 | 2 | 2 | 1/2 carb |
| Zesty & Spicy Spaghetti Sauce | 1/2 cup | 60 | 2 | 15 | 0 | 0 | 0 | 700 | 10 | 3 | 1 | 1/2 carb |
| ***Maruchan*** | | | | | | | | | | | | |
| Instant Lunch, Beef | 1 container | 290 | 12 | 110 | 6 | 0 | 0 | 1200 | 38 | 2 | 7 | 2 1/2 carb, 2 fat |
| Ramen Noodle Soup, Chicken | 1/2 pkg | 190 | 7 | 70 | 3.5 | 0 | 0 | 830 | 26 | 1 | 5 | 2 carb, 1 fat |
| ***Muir Glen Organic*** | | | | | | | | | | | | |
| Beef Bolognese | 1/2 cup | 70 | 2 | 20 | 0.5 | 0 | <5 | 410 | 10 | 2 | 3 | 1/2 carb |
| Cabernet Marinara | 1/2 cup | 60 | 1 | 10 | 0 | 0 | 0 | 360 | 11 | 2 | 2 | 1 carb |
| Chunky Tomato & Herb | 1/2 cup | 60 | 0.5 | 5 | 0 | 0 | 0 | 350 | 11 | 2 | 2 | 1 carb |
| Fire Roasted Tomato | 1/2 cup | 70 | 2 | 0 | 0 | 0 | 0 | 390 | 12 | 2 | 2 | 1 carb |
| Four Cheese | 1/2 cup | 80 | 2.5 | 20 | 1 | 0 | 5 | 380 | 11 | 2 | 4 | 1 carb |
| Garden Vegetable | 1/2 cup | 60 | 1 | 5 | 0 | 0 | 0 | 350 | 10 | 2 | 2 | 1/2 carb |

| | Serving | Calories | Fat (g) | Cal. from Fat | Sat. Fat (g) | Trans Fat (g) | Chol. (mg) | Sod. (mg) | Carb. (g) | Fiber (g) | Prot. (g) | Servings/Exchanges |
|---|---|---|---|---|---|---|---|---|---|---|---|---|
| Garlic Roasted Garlic | 1/2 cup | 60 | 0.5 | 5 | 0 | 0 | 0 | 380 | 12 | 2 | 2 | 1 carb |
| Italian Herb | 1/2 cup | 60 | 0.5 | 5 | 0 | 0 | 0 | 350 | 11 | 2 | 2 | 1 carb |
| Italian Sausage with Peppers | 1/2 cup | 80 | 3 | 25 | 1 | 0 | <5 | 420 | 10 | 2 | 3 | 1/2 carb, 1 fat |
| Portabello Mushroom | 1/2 cup | 50 | 0 | 0 | 0 | 0 | 0 | 350 | 10 | 2 | 2 | 1/2 carb |
| Tomato Basil | 1/2 cup | 60 | 1 | 10 | 0 | 0 | 0 | 370 | 12 | 2 | 2 | 1 carb |
| ***Newman's Own*** | | | | | | | | | | | | |
| Five Cheese | 1/2 cup | 80 | 3 | 30 | 1.5 | 0 | 5 | 610 | 10 | <1 | 3 | 1/2 carb, 1 fat |
| Italian Sausage & Peppers | 1/2 cup | 90 | 4 | 35 | 1 | 0 | 10 | 630 | 11 | <1 | 4 | 1 carb, 1 fat |
| Marinara | 1/2 cup | 70 | 2 | 20 | 0 | 0 | 0 | 510 | 12 | <1 | 2 | 1 carb |
| Marinara with Mushrooms | 1/2 cup | 70 | 2 | 20 | 0 | 0 | 0 | 520 | 12 | <1 | 2 | 1 carb |
| Sockarooni | 1/2 cup | 70 | 2 | 20 | 0 | 0 | 0 | 520 | 12 | <1 | 2 | 1 carb |

| | | | | | | | | | | | | |
|---|---|---|---|---|---|---|---|---|---|---|---|---|
| ***Nissin*** | | | | | | | | | | | | |
| Top Ramen, Chicken | 1/2 pkg | 190 | 7 | 60 | 3.5 | 0 | 0 | 910 | 26 | 2 | 5 | 2 carb, 1 fat |
| ***Prego*** | | | | | | | | | | | | |
| Flavored with Meat | 1/2 cup | 130 | 5 | 45 | 1 | 0 | 5 | 570 | 19 | 3 | 2 | 1 carb, 1 fat |
| Garden Combo | 1/2 cup | 70 | 1.5 | 15 | 0.5 | 0 | 0 | 470 | 13 | 3 | 2 | 1 carb |
| Heart Smart Mushroom Italian | 1/2 cup | 100 | 3 | 30 | 0.5 | 0 | 0 | 410 | 15 | 3 | 2 | 1 carb, 1 fat |
| Heart Smart Traditional Italian | 1/2 cup | 90 | 3 | 30 | 1 | 0 | 0 | 430 | 13 | 3 | 2 | 1 carb, 1 fat |
| Marinara | 1/2 cup | 100 | 5 | 45 | 1 | 0 | 0 | 550 | 11 | 4 | 2 | 1 carb, 1 fat |
| Mini Meatball | 1/2 cup | 110 | 5 | 45 | 1.5 | 0 | 5 | 650 | 13 | 3 | 4 | 1 carb, 1 fat |
| Mushroom & Garlic | 1/2 cup | 80 | 2.5 | 25 | 0.5 | 0 | 0 | 470 | 13 | 3 | 2 | 1 carb, 1 fat |
| Organic Mushroom Italian | 1/2 cup | 70 | 2.5 | 25 | 0.5 | 0 | 0 | 470 | 13 | 4 | 2 | 1 carb, 1 fat |
| Organic Tomato & Basil Italian | 1/2 cup | 80 | 2.5 | 25 | 0.5 | 0 | 0 | 470 | 13 | 4 | 2 | 1 carb, 1 fat |

PASTA, PASTA MIXES, PASTA SAUCE

| | Serving | Calories | Fat (g) | Cal. from Fat | Sat. Fat (g) | Trans Fat (g) | Chol. (mg) | Sod. (mg) | Carb. (g) | Fiber (g) | Prot. (g) | Servings/Exchanges |
|---|---|---|---|---|---|---|---|---|---|---|---|---|
| Three Cheese | 1/2 cup | 80 | 1.5 | 15 | 0.5 | 0 | <5 | 430 | 14 | 3 | 3 | 1 carb |
| Traditional | 1/2 cup | 80 | 3 | 30 | 0 | 0 | 0 | 580 | 13 | 3 | 2 | 1 carb, 1 fat |
| ***Ragu*** | | | | | | | | | | | | |
| Cheesy, Classic Alfredo | 1/4 cup | 110 | 10 | 90 | 3.5 | 0 | 30 | 350 | 2 | 0 | 1 | 2 fat |
| Chunky, Garden Combination | 1/2 cup | 80 | 2.5 | 25 | 0 | 0 | 0 | 530 | 12 | 2 | 2 | 1 carb, 1 fat |
| Chunky, Sundried Tomato & Sweet Basil | 1/2 cup | 90 | 2.5 | 25 | 0 | 0 | 0 | 580 | 14 | 3 | 2 | 1 carb, 1 fat |
| Chunky, Super Chunk Mushroom | 1/2 cup | 80 | 2.5 | 25 | 0 | 0 | 0 | 620 | 13 | 2 | 2 | 1 carb, 1 fat |
| Chunky, Super Vegetable Primavera | 1/2 cup | 80 | 2.5 | 25 | 0 | 0 | 0 | 490 | 13 | 3 | 2 | 1 carb, 1 fat |
| Chunky, Tomato, Garlic & Onion | 1/2 cup | 80 | 2.5 | 25 | 0 | 0 | 0 | 510 | 13 | 2 | 2 | 1 carb, 1 fat |
| Old World Style, Meat | 1/2 cup | 70 | 3 | 25 | 0.5 | 0 | 0 | 570 | 10 | 2 | 2 | 1/2 carb, 1 fat |

| | | | | | | | | | | | | |
|---|---|---|---|---|---|---|---|---|---|---|---|---|
| Old World Style, Mushroom | 1/2 cup | 70 | 2.5 | 25 | 0 | 0 | 0 | 580 | 10 | 2 | 2 | 1/2 carb, 1 fat |
| Old World Style, Traditional | 1/2 cup | 70 | 2.5 | 25 | 0 | 0 | 0 | 580 | 10 | 2 | 2 | 1/2 carb, 1 fat |
| Organic, Traditional | 1/2 cup | 80 | 3 | 25 | 0 | 0 | 0 | 510 | 11 | 2 | 2 | 1 carb, 1 fat |
| Robusto, 7-Herb Tomato | 1/2 cup | 80 | 3 | 25 | 0 | 0 | 0 | 550 | 12 | 2 | 2 | 1 carb, 1 fat |
| Robusto, Roasted Garlic | 1/2 cup | 80 | 2.5 | 25 | 0 | 0 | 0 | 550 | 13 | 3 | 2 | 1 carb, 1 fat |
| Robusto, Si Cheese | 1/2 cup | 90 | 3 | 25 | 1 | 0 | <5 | 580 | 12 | 2 | 3 | 1 carb, 1 fat |
| ***Rao's Homemade*** | | | | | | | | | | | | |
| Arrabbiata | 1/2 cup | 70 | 5 | 45 | 0.5 | 0 | 0 | 350 | 6 | 2 | 1 | 1/2 carb, 1 fat |
| Filetto Sauce with Tomato, Prosciutto & Onion | 1/2 cup | 90 | 6 | 60 | 1 | 0 | 5 | 390 | 5 | 2 | 2 | 1 fat |
| Marinara | 1/2 cup | 70 | 4.5 | 40 | 0.5 | 0 | 0 | 350 | 6 | 2 | 1 | 1/2 carb, 1 fat |
| Puttanesca | 1/2 cup | 80 | 5 | 50 | 0.5 | 0 | 0 | 250 | 6 | 2 | 2 | 1/2 carb, 1 fat |
| Roasted Eggplant Siciliana Sauce | 1/2 cup | 70 | 5 | 45 | 0.5 | 0 | 0 | 320 | 6 | 1 | 1 | 1/2 carb, 1 fat |

| | Serving | Calories | Fat (g) | Cal. from Fat | Sat. Fat (g) | Trans Fat (g) | Chol. (mg) | Sod. (mg) | Carb. (g) | Fiber (g) | Prot. (g) | Servings/Exchanges |
|---|---|---|---|---|---|---|---|---|---|---|---|---|
| Southern Italian Pepper & Mushroom | 1/2 cup | 70 | 5 | 45 | 0.5 | 0 | 0 | 430 | 6 | 2 | 1 | 1/2 carb, 1 fat |
| Tomato & Basil | 1/2 cup | 70 | 4.5 | 40 | 0.5 | 0 | 0 | 350 | 6 | 2 | 1 | 1/2 carb, 1 fat |
| Vodka Sauce | 1/2 cup | 80 | 5 | 45 | 1 | 0 | 5 | 450 | 6 | 2 | 2 | 1/2 carb, 1 fat |
| ***Trader Joe's*** | | | | | | | | | | | | |
| Alfredo | 1/4 cup | 90 | 8 | 70 | 4.5 | 0 | 0 | 320 | 2 | 0 | 4 | 2 fat |
| Bolognese Meat Pasta Sauce | 1/2 cup | 80 | 4.5 | 40 | 1 | 0 | 5 | 490 | 8 | 2 | 3 | 1/2 carb, 1 fat |
| Italian Sausage | 1/2 cup | 50 | 2.5 | 20 | 0.5 | 0 | 0 | 570 | 6 | <1 | 3 | 1/2 carb, 1 fat |
| Organic Marinara | 1/2 cup | 50 | 2 | 20 | 0 | 0 | 0 | 490 | 8 | 2 | 1 | 1/2 carb |
| Organic Marinara No Added Salt | 1/2 cup | 50 | 0.5 | 5 | 0 | 0 | 0 | 25 | 11 | <1 | 2 | 1 carb |
| Organic Spaghetti with Mushrooms | 1/2 cup | 45 | 0 | 0 | 0 | 0 | 0 | 350 | 10 | 2 | 1 | 1/2 carb |

| | | | | | | | | | | | | |
|---|---|---|---|---|---|---|---|---|---|---|---|---|
| Organic Tomato Basil Marinara | 1/2 cup | 60 | 3 | 25 | 0 | 0 | 0 | 440 | 8 | 2 | 1 | 1/2 carb, 1 fat |
| Roasted Garlic Spaghetti Sauce | 1/2 cup | 70 | 2.5 | 20 | 0 | 0 | 0 | 450 | 10 | 1 | 2 | 1/2 carb, 1 fat |
| Rustico Pasta Sauce | 1/2 cup | 45 | 1.5 | 15 | 0 | 0 | 0 | 360 | 6 | 2 | 1 | 1/2 carb |
| Tomato Basil Marinara | 1/2 cup | 80 | 4.5 | 40 | 0.5 | 0 | 0 | 540 | 10 | 2 | 2 | 1/2 carb, 1 fat |
| Traditional Marinara | 1/2 cup | 50 | 1 | 10 | 0 | 0 | 0 | 530 | 9 | 2 | 1 | 1/2 carb |
| Walnut Acres Organic | | | | | | | | | | | | |
| Garlic-Garlic | 1/2 cup | 50 | 1 | 10 | 0 | 0 | 0 | 280 | 10 | 1 | 2 | 1/2 carb |
| Low Sodium Tomato & Basil, Fat Free | 1/2 cup | 40 | 0 | 0 | 0 | 0 | 0 | 20 | 9 | <1 | 2 | 1/2 carb |
| Marinara with Herbs | 1/2 cup | 50 | 1 | 10 | 0 | 0 | 0 | 330 | 9 | 1 | 2 | 1/2 carb |
| Roasted Garlic | 1/2 cup | 60 | 1 | 10 | 0 | 0 | 0 | 280 | 11 | 1 | 2 | 1 carb |
| Sweet Pepper & Onion | 1/2 cup | 50 | 1 | 10 | 0 | 0 | 0 | 280 | 9 | 1 | 2 | 1/2 carb |
| Tomato & Basil | 1/2 cup | 50 | 1 | 10 | 0 | 0 | 0 | 330 | 9 | 1 | 2 | 1/2 carb |
| Zesty Basil | 1/2 cup | 50 | 1 | 10 | 0 | 0 | 0 | 330 | 9 | 1 | 2 | 1/2 carb |

| | Serving | Calories | Fat (g) | Cal. from Fat | Sat. Fat (g) | Trans Fat (g) | Chol. (mg) | Sod. (mg) | Carb. (g) | Fiber (g) | Prot. (g) | Servings/Exchanges |
|---|---|---|---|---|---|---|---|---|---|---|---|---|
| ***Whole Foods 365 Everyday*** | | | | | | | | | | | | |
| Marinara | 1/2 cup | 50 | 1.5 | 10 | 0 | 0 | 0 | 430 | 9 | 2 | 2 | 1/2 carb |
| Pesto & Sundried Tomato | 1/2 cup | 60 | 1.5 | 15 | 0.5 | 0 | 0 | 460 | 10 | 3 | 2 | 1/2 carb |
| Roasted Garlic | 1/2 cup | 60 | 1.5 | 15 | 0 | 0 | 0 | 480 | 10 | 2 | 2 | 1/2 carb |
| Roasted Red Pepper | 1/2 cup | 50 | 1 | 10 | 0 | 0 | 0 | 420 | 10 | 2 | 1 | 1/2 carb |
| Roasted Vegetable | 1/2 cup | 25 | 1 | 10 | 0 | 0 | 0 | 490 | 3 | <1 | 0 | free |
| ***Whole Foods 365 Everyday Organic*** | | | | | | | | | | | | |
| Classic Pasta Sauce | 1/2 cup | 70 | 4 | 35 | 0.5 | 0 | 0 | 500 | 9 | 2 | 1 | 1/2 carb, 1 fat |
| Eggplant Marinara | 1/2 cup | 40 | 1 | 10 | 0 | 0 | 0 | 470 | 7 | 2 | 1 | 1/2 carb |
| Fat Free Pasta Sauce | 1/2 cup | 35 | 0 | 0 | 0 | 0 | 0 | 470 | 7 | 2 | 1 | 1/2 carb |
| Four Cheese | 1/2 cup | 70 | 4 | 35 | 1.5 | 0 | <5 | 480 | 7 | <1 | 3 | 1/2 carb, 1 fat |
| Italian Herb | 1/2 cup | 50 | 1 | 10 | 0 | 0 | 0 | 480 | 8 | <1 | 2 | 1/2 carb |
| Mushroon Marinara | 1/2 cup | 45 | 1.5 | 15 | 0 | 0 | 0 | 450 | 6 | <1 | 2 | 1/2 carb |

| | Serving | Calories | Fat (g) | Cal. from Fat | Sat. Fat (g) | Trans Fat (g) | Chol. (mg) | Sod. (mg) | Carb. (g) | Fiber (g) | Prot. (g) | Servings/Exchanges |
|---|---|---|---|---|---|---|---|---|---|---|---|---|

## PROCESSED MEAT, BREAKFAST MEAT, LUNCH MEAT, HOT DOGS, CANNED TUNA AND CHICKEN

| | Serving | Calories | Fat (g) | Cal. from Fat | Sat. Fat (g) | Trans Fat (g) | Chol. (mg) | Sod. (mg) | Carb. (g) | Fiber (g) | Prot. (g) | Servings/Exchanges |
|---|---|---|---|---|---|---|---|---|---|---|---|---|
| Applegate Farms | 1 Tbsp | 98 | 9 | 80 | <1 | 0 | 0 | 70 | 3 | <1 | 2 | 2 fat |
| Chicken & Apple Sausage | 1 link | 140 | 6 | 60 | 1.5 | 0 | 65 | 500 | 6 | 1 | 14 | 2 lean meat |
| Fire Roasted Red Pepper Sausage | 1 link | 120 | 6 | 60 | 1.5 | 0 | 65 | 500 | 2 | 1 | 14 | 2 lean meat |
| Natural Canadian Bacon | 2 slices | 90 | 4 | 35 | 1.5 | 0 | 35 | 500 | 1 | 0 | 12 | 2 lean meat |
| Natural Dry Cured Bacon | 2 slices | 60 | 5 | 45 | 2 | 0 | 10 | 290 | 0 | 0 | 4 | 1 med-fat meat |
| Natural Sunday Bacon | 2 slices | 60 | 5 | 45 | 2 | 0 | 10 | 290 | 0 | 0 | 4 | 1 med-fat meat |
| Natural Turkey Bacon | 2 slices | 35 | 1.5 | 15 | 0 | 0 | 25 | 200 | 0 | 0 | 6 | 1 lean meat |
| Organic Sunday Bacon | 2 slices | 60 | 5 | 45 | 2 | 0 | 10 | 290 | 0 | 0 | 4 | 1 med-fat meat |
| Organic Turkey Bacon | 1 slice | 35 | 1.5 | 15 | 0 | 0 | 25 | 200 | 0 | 0 | 6 | 1 lean meat |

| | Serving | Calories | Fat (g) | Cal. from Fat | Sat. Fat (g) | Trans Fat (g) | Chol. (mg) | Sod. (mg) | Carb. (g) | Fiber (g) | Prot. (g) | Servings/Exchanges |
|---|---|---|---|---|---|---|---|---|---|---|---|---|
| Pork Andouille Sausage | 1 link | 200 | 15 | 140 | 5 | 0 | 50 | 510 | 2 | 1 | 12 | 2 high-fat meat |
| Pork Bratwurst Sausage | 1 link | 170 | 12 | 110 | 4 | 0 | 45 | 660 | 2 | 0 | 12 | 2 med-fat meat |
| Pork Kielbasa Sausage | 1 link | 190 | 14 | 130 | 5 | 0 | 50 | 600 | 2 | 0 | 12 | 2 med-fat meat, 1 fat |
| Spinach & Feta Sausage | 1 link | 120 | 7 | 60 | 2.5 | 0 | 60 | 470 | 2 | 0 | 13 | 2 lean meat |
| Sweet Italian Sausage | 1 link | 130 | 7 | 60 | 2 | 0 | 70 | 500 | 2 | 1 | 15 | 2 lean meat |
| Banquet Brown 'N Serve | | | | | | | | | | | | |
| Beef Fully Cooked Sausage Links | 3 | 190 | 17 | 160 | 8 | 1 | 15 | 420 | 1 | 0 | 7 | 1 high-fat meat, 1 fat |
| Original Fully Cooked Sausage Links | 3 | 200 | 18 | 160 | 6 | 0 | 30 | 490 | 2 | 1 | 8 | 1 high-fat meat, 1 fat |
| Turkey Fully Cooked Sausage Links | 3 | 110 | 7 | 60 | 2 | 0 | 40 | 390 | 2 | 0 | 9 | 1 med-fat meat |
| ***Bob Evans*** | | | | | | | | | | | | |

| | | | | | | | | | | | | |
|---|---|---|---|---|---|---|---|---|---|---|---|---|
| Brown Sugar and Honey Links | 3 | 140 | 11 | 100 | NA | 0 | 25 | 290 | 4 | 0 | 9 | 1 high-fat meat |
| Canadian Bacon | 4 slices | 60 | 1.5 | 14 | NA | 0 | 20 | 700 | 1 | 0 | 11 | 2 lean meat |
| Country Pepper Bacon | 2 slices | 100 | 8 | 72 | NA | 0 | 20 | 510 | 0 | 0 | 6 | 1 high-fat meat |
| Express Fully Cooked Bacon | 3 slices | 80 | 6 | 55 | NA | 0 | 15 | 280 | 1 | 0 | 5 | 1 med-fat meat |
| Express Fully Cooked Lite | 2 | 80 | 5 | 45 | NA | 0 | 15 | 220 | 0 | 0 | 8 | 1 med-fat meat |
| Express Fully Cooked Original LInks | 2 | 130 | 10 | 90 | NA | 0 | 25 | 290 | 0 | 0 | 8 | 1 high-fat meat |
| Hickory Smoked Bacon | 2 slices | 80 | 7 | 63 | NA | 0 | 15 | 270 | 0 | 0 | 5 | 1 med-fat meat |
| Original Sausage Links | 3 | 140 | 11 | 100 | NA | 0 | 25 | 330 | 0 | 0 | 9 | 1 high-fat meat |
| Original Sausage Patties | 2 | 160 | 13 | 117 | NA | 0 | 30 | 380 | 0 | 0 | 11 | 2 med-fat meat, 1 fat |
| ***Celebrity*** | | | | | | | | | | | | |
| Healthy Canadian Style Bacon | 3 slices | 60 | 1 | 15 | 0.5 | 0 | 30 | 350 | 1 | 0 | 10 | 1 lean meat |

PROCESSED MEAT, BREAKFAST MEAT, LUNCH MEAT

| | Serving | Calories | Fat (g) | Cal. from Fat | Sat. Fat (g) | Trans Fat (g) | Chol. (mg) | Sod. (mg) | Carb. (g) | Fiber (g) | Prot. (g) | Servings/Exchanges |
|---|---|---|---|---|---|---|---|---|---|---|---|---|
| ***Farmer John*** | | | | | | | | | | | | |
| Premium Bacon Links | 2 | 70 | 5 | 45 | 3 | 0 | 15 | 280 | 0 | 0 | 6 | 1 med-fat meat |
| Premium Pork Links | 2 | 140 | 12 | 110 | 4 | 0 | 30 | 400 | <1 | 0 | 6 | 1 high-fat meat, 1 fat |
| ***Farmland*** | | | | | | | | | | | | |
| Hickory Smoked Bacon | 2 slices | 80 | 7 | 60 | 3 | 0 | 15 | 260 | 0 | 0 | 4 | 1 med-fat meat |
| Original Pork Sausage Links | 3 | 250 | 23 | 210 | 9 | 0 | 60 | 510 | 1 | 0 | 10 | 1 high-fat meat, 3 fat |
| Pork & Bacon Sausage Links | 3 | 270 | 25 | 220 | 9 | 0 | 60 | 640 | 1 | 0 | 10 | 1 high-fat meat, 3 fat |
| Thick Sliced Bacon | 1 slice | 70 | 6 | 50 | 2.5 | 0 | 10 | 230 | 0 | 0 | 3 | 1 med-fat meat |
| ***Hormel*** | | | | | | | | | | | | |
| Little Sizzlers Pork Sausage | 3 | 200 | 19 | 170 | 7 | 0 | 40 | 580 | 0 | 0 | 8 | 1 high-fat meat, 2 fat |
| ***Jennie-O Turkey Store*** | | | | | | | | | | | | |

| | | | | | | | | | | | | |
|---|---|---|---|---|---|---|---|---|---|---|---|---|
| Breakfast Bacon | 1/2 oz | 35 | 3 | 25 | 1 | 0 | 13 | 150 | 1 | 0 | 2 | 1 fat |
| Breakfast Lover's Turkey Sausage | 2 oz | 130 | 10 | 100 | 3 | 0 | 45 | 310 | 0 | 0 | 8 | 1 high-fat meat |
| Breakfast Sausage Rolls | 4 oz | 270 | 21 | 190 | 6 | 0.5 | 80 | 720 | 0 | 0 | 16 | 2 high-fat meat |
| Extra Lean Turkey Bacon | 1/2 oz | 20 | 0.5 | 5 | 0 | 0 | 10 | 140 | 0 | 0 | 3 | 1 lean meat |
| Fully Cooked Turkey Breakfast Sausage Patties | 1.2 oz | 65 | 4 | 35 | 1 | 0 | 30 | 250 | 0 | 0 | 6 | 1 med-fat meat |
| Fully Cooked Turkey Sausage Breakfast Links | 2.1 oz | 110 | 7 | 60 | 2 | 0 | 50 | 430 | 0 | 0 | 11 | 2 lean meat |
| Maple Turkey Breakfast Sausage Links | 2 oz | 140 | 11 | 100 | 3 | 0 | 40 | 340 | 3 | 0 | 8 | 1 high-fat meat |
| Turkey Breakfast Sausage Links | 2 oz | 140 | 11 | 100 | 3 | 0 | 45 | 360 | 0 | 0 | 9 | 1 high-fat meat |

PROCESSED MEAT, BREAKFAST MEAT, LUNCH MEAT

| | Serving | Calories | Fat (g) | Cal. from Fat | Sat. Fat (g) | Trans Fat (g) | Chol. (mg) | Sod. (mg) | Carb. (g) | Fiber (g) | Prot. (g) | Servings/Exchanges |
|---|---|---|---|---|---|---|---|---|---|---|---|---|
| ***Jimmy Dean (Uncooked)*** | | | | | | | | | | | | |
| All Natural Regular Pork Sausage | 2 oz | 190 | 15 | 130 | 5 | 0 | 55 | 520 | 1 | 0 | 12 | 2 high-fat meat |
| Hardwood Smoked Turkey Premium Bacon | 1 slice | 25 | 2 | 20 | 1 | 0 | 15 | 200 | 0 | 0 | 2 | 1 fat |
| Lower Sodium Premium Bacon | 1 slice | 50 | 4 | 40 | 1.5 | 0 | 10 | 105 | 0 | 0 | 4 | 1 med-fat meat |
| Maple Sausage Links | 2 oz | 170 | 14 | 130 | 5 | 0 | 35 | 400 | 2 | 0 | 7 | 1 high-fat meat, 1 fat |
| Maple Sausage Patties | 2 patties | 170 | 14 | 130 | 5 | 0 | 35 | 410 | 2 | 0 | 7 | 1 high-fat meat, 1 fat |
| Original Premium Bacon | 1 slice | 50 | 4 | 40 | 1.5 | 0 | 10 | 230 | 0 | 0 | 4 | 1 med-fat meat |
| Original Sausage Links | 3 | 170 | 14 | 130 | 5 | 0 | 35 | 350 | 1 | 0 | 7 | 1 high-fat meat, 1 fat |
| Original Sausage Patties | 2 patties | 240 | 23 | 200 | 8 | 0 | 50 | 610 | 1 | 0 | 9 | 1 high-fat meat, 3 fat |

| | | | | | | | | | | | | |
|---|---|---|---|---|---|---|---|---|---|---|---|---|
| Premium Pork Bold Country Sausage | 2 oz | 190 | 17 | 150 | 6 | 0 | 40 | 340 | 2 | 0 | 8 | 1 high-fat meat, 1 fat |
| Premium Pork Maple Sausage | 2 oz | 180 | 16 | 140 | 5 | 0 | 40 | 450 | 1 | 1 | 8 | 1 high-fat meat, 1 fat |
| Premium Pork Regular Sausage | 2 oz | 180 | 16 | 140 | 5 | 0 | 40 | 450 | 1 | 0 | 8 | 1 high-fat meat, 1 fat |
| Thick Sliced Premium Bacon | 1 slice | 80 | 6 | 50 | 2 | 0 | 15 | 320 | 0 | 0 | 5 | 1 med-fat meat |
| ***Jimmy Dean (Fully Cooked)*** | | | | | | | | | | | | |
| Maple Bacon Links | 3 | 80 | 7 | 60 | 3 | 0 | 15 | 105 | 0 | 0 | 4 | 1 med-fat meat |
| Maple Sausage Patties | 2 | 250 | 22 | 200 | 8 | 0 | 45 | 510 | 3 | 0 | 8 | 1 high-fat meat, 2 fat |
| Original Sausage Links | 3 | 240 | 22 | 200 | 8 | 0 | 45 | 450 | 1 | 0 | 9 | 1 high-fat meat, 2 fat |
| Original Sausage Patties | 2 | 240 | 23 | 200 | 8 | 0 | 50 | 610 | 1 | 0 | 9 | 1 high-fat meat, 3 fat |
| Turkey Sausage Patties | 2 | 120 | 7 | 70 | 2 | 0 | 55 | 490 | 1 | 0 | 13 | 2 lean meat |
| ***Jimmy Dean (Heat 'N Serve)*** | | | | | | | | | | | | |
| Sausage Links | 3 | 250 | 24 | 220 | 8 | 0 | 45 | 200 | 2 | 0 | 7 | 1 high-fat meat, 3 fat |

PROCESSED MEAT, BREAKFAST MEAT, LUNCH MEAT

| | Serving | Calories | Fat (g) | Cal. from Fat | Sat. Fat (g) | Trans Fat (g) | Chol. (mg) | Sod. (mg) | Carb. (g) | Fiber (g) | Prot. (g) | Servings/Exchanges |
|---|---|---|---|---|---|---|---|---|---|---|---|---|
| Sausage Patties | 2 | 190 | 18 | 160 | 6 | 0 | 30 | 250 | 1 | 0 | 6 | 1 high-fat meat, 2 fat |
| ***Jones*** | | | | | | | | | | | | |
| Light Pork Sausage & Rice Links | 2 | 110 | 7 | 60 | 2.5 | 0 | 30 | 440 | 4 | 0 | 8 | 1 med-fat meat |
| Little Pork Sausages | 3 | 190 | 17 | 150 | 7 | 0 | 45 | 420 | 1 | 0 | 8 | 1 high-fat meat, 1 fat |
| Pork Sausage Patties | 1 | 120 | 11 | 100 | 4 | 0 | 30 | 250 | 0 | 0 | 6 | 1 high-fat meat |
| ***Land O'Frost*** | | | | | | | | | | | | |
| Canadian Bacon | 5 slices | 60 | 1.5 | 10 | 0 | 0 | 30 | 750 | 1 | 0 | 10 | 1 lean meat |
| ***Oscar Mayer*** | | | | | | | | | | | | |
| Bacon | 2 slices | 60 | 5 | 45 | 1.5 | 0 | 10 | 250 | 0 | 0 | 4 | 1 med-fat meat |
| Bacon, Center Cut | 2 slices | 50 | 4 | 35 | 2 | 0 | 15 | 270 | 0 | 0 | 4 | 1 med-fat meat |
| Bacon, Lower Sodium | 2 slices | 70 | 6 | 50 | 2.5 | 0 | 10 | 170 | 0 | 0 | 4 | 1 med-fat meat |
| Bacon, Smoked, Uncured | 2 slices | 70 | 5 | 50 | 2 | 15 | 15 | 250 | 0 | 0 | 6 | 1 med-fat meat |

| | | | | | | | | | | | | |
|---|---|---|---|---|---|---|---|---|---|---|---|---|
| ***Trader Joe's*** | | | | | | | | | | | | |
| Uncured Apple Smoked Bacon | 1 slice | 90 | 7 | 70 | 2.5 | 0 | 15 | 240 | 0 | 0 | 5 | 1 med-fat meat |
| Uncured Turkey Bacon | 1 slice | 30 | 0.5 | 5 | 0 | 0 | 25 | 180 | 0 | 0 | 6 | 1 lean meat |
| **LUNCH MEAT & HOT DOGS** | | | | | | | | | | | | |
| ***Applegate Farms*** | | | | | | | | | | | | |
| Honey & Maple Turkey Breast | 2 oz | 60 | 1 | 10 | 0 | 0 | 20 | 450 | 0 | 0 | 11 | 2 lean meat |
| Organic Herb Turkey Breast | 2 oz | 50 | 0.5 | 5 | 0 | 0 | 30 | 420 | 0 | 0 | 11 | 2 lean meat |
| Organic Roasted Chicken Breast | 2 oz | 60 | 1.5 | 15 | 0.5 | 0 | 30 | 580 | 0 | 1 | 10 | 1 lean meat |
| Organic Roasted Turkey Breast | 2 oz | 50 | 0 | 0 | 0 | 0 | 30 | 360 | 0 | 0 | 12 | 2 lean meat |
| Organic Uncured Ham | 2 oz | 50 | 1.5 | 15 | 0.5 | 0 | 35 | 530 | 0 | 0 | 10 | 1 lean meat |
| Roasted Turkey Breast | 2 oz | 50 | 0 | 0 | 0 | 0 | 30 | 360 | 0 | 0 | 12 | 2 lean meat |

PROCESSED MEAT, BREAKFAST MEAT, LUNCH MEAT

| | Serving | Calories | Fat (g) | Cal. from Fat | Sat. Fat (g) | Trans Fat (g) | Chol. (mg) | Sod. (mg) | Carb. (g) | Fiber (g) | Prot. (g) | Servings/Exchanges |
|---|---|---|---|---|---|---|---|---|---|---|---|---|
| Slow Cooked Ham | 2 oz | 60 | 1.5 | 15 | 0.5 | 0 | 35 | 480 | 0 | 0 | 11 | 2 lean meat |
| Uncured Black Forest Ham | 2 oz | 50 | 1.5 | 10 | 0.5 | 0 | 35 | 480 | 0 | 0 | 10 | 1 lean meat |
| Uncured Turkey Bologna | 2 oz | 90 | 5.5 | 50 | 1.5 | 0 | 30 | 400 | 0 | 0 | 9 | 1 med-fat meat |
| ***Armour Healthy Ones 97% Fat Free*** | | | | | | | | | | | | |
| ***Deli Thin-Sliced*** | | | | | | | | | | | | |
| Honey Ham | 1.9 oz | 60 | 1.5 | 15 | 0.5 | 0 | 25 | 450 | 0 | 3 | 9 | 1 lean meat |
| Oven Roasted Turkey Breast | 1.9 oz | 60 | 1.5 | 15 | 0.5 | 0 | 25 | 450 | 0 | 2 | 9 | 1 lean meat |
| Smoked Ham | 1.9 oz | 60 | 1.5 | 15 | 0.5 | 0 | 25 | 450 | 0 | 2 | 9 | 1 lean meat |
| ***Deluxe Thin-Sliced*** | | | | | | | | | | | | |
| Honey Ham | 2 oz | 60 | 1.5 | 15 | 0.5 | 0 | 25 | 470 | 0 | 4 | 10 | 1 lean meat |
| Turkey Breast | 2 oz | 60 | 1.5 | 15 | 0.5 | 0 | 25 | 470 | 0 | 2 | 10 | 1 lean meat |
| ***Ball Park Franks*** | | | | | | | | | | | | |

| | | | | | | | | | | | | |
|---|---|---|---|---|---|---|---|---|---|---|---|---|
| Beef Franks | 1 | 190 | 16 | 150 | 7 | 1 | 35 | 550 | 4 | 0 | 6 | 1 high-fat meat, 1 fat |
| Bun Size Beef Franks | 1 | 180 | 16 | 140 | 6 | 0 | 45 | 550 | 4 | 0 | 6 | 1 high-fat meat, 1 fat |
| Meat Franks | 1 | 180 | 16 | 140 | 6 | 0 | 45 | 550 | 4 | 0 | 6 | 1 high-fat meat, 1 fat |
| ***Bar-S*** | | | | | | | | | | | | |
| Beef Bologna | 1 oz | 110 | 9 | 80 | 3.5 | 0 | 20 | 350 | 0 | 2 | 4 | 1 high-fat meat |
| Bologna | 1 oz | 100 | 8 | 70 | 2.5 | 0 | 35 | 350 | 0 | 2 | 3 | 1 high-fat meat |
| Chicken Bologna | 1 oz | 80 | 7 | 60 | 2 | 0 | 35 | 360 | 0 | 3 | 3 | 1 med-fat meat |
| Cooked Ham | 1.3 oz | 45 | 1.5 | 15 | 0 | 0 | 15 | 510 | 0 | 2 | 5 | 1 lean meat |
| Cotto Salami | 1 oz | 90 | 8 | 70 | 2.5 | 0 | 40 | 360 | 0 | 2 | 3 | 1 high-fat meat |
| Deli Thin Cut Ham | 2 oz | 80 | 2.5 | 25 | 1 | 0 | 30 | 700 | 0 | 5 | 9 | 1 lean meat |
| Deli Thin Cut Turkey Breast | 2 oz | 60 | 1.5 | 15 | 0 | 0 | 30 | 540 | 0 | 3 | 9 | 1 lean meat |
| Extra Lean Cooked Ham | 1 oz | 40 | 1 | 10 | 0 | 0 | 20 | 420 | 0 | 1 | 5 | 1 lean meat |
| Extra Lean Honey Cured Ham | 1 oz | 45 | 1.5 | 15 | 0 | 0 | 20 | 450 | 0 | 3 | 5 | 1 lean meat |
| Oven Roasted Turkey | 1 oz | 35 | 0.5 | 5 | 0 | 0 | 15 | 350 | 0 | 2 | 5 | 1 lean meat |

PROCESSED MEAT, BREAKFAST MEAT, LUNCH MEAT

| | Serving | Calories | Fat (g) | Cal. from Fat | Sat. Fat (g) | Trans Fat (g) | Chol. (mg) | Sod. (mg) | Carb. (g) | Fiber (g) | Prot. (g) | Servings/Exchanges |
|---|---|---|---|---|---|---|---|---|---|---|---|---|
| Thick Sliced Bologna | 2 oz | 180 | 15 | 140 | 5 | 0 | 60 | 620 | 0 | 4 | 5 | 1 high-fat meat, 1 fat |
| Turkey Bologna | 1 oz | 60 | 4.5 | 40 | 1.5 | 0 | 25 | 370 | 0 | 3 | 3 | 1 med-fat meat |
| ***Buddig*** | | | | | | | | | | | | |
| Beef | 2 oz | 90 | 5 | 45 | 2 | 0 | 40 | 790 | 0 | 1 | 10 | 1 med-fat meat |
| Chicken | 2 oz | 90 | 5 | 45 | 1.5 | 0 | 30 | 530 | 0 | 2 | 10 | 1 med-fat meat |
| Corned Beef | 2 oz | 90 | 5 | 45 | 2 | 0 | 40 | 760 | 0 | 1 | 10 | 1 med-fat meat |
| Ham | 2 oz | 90 | 5 | 45 | 2 | 0 | 35 | 760 | 0 | 1 | 10 | 1 med-fat meat |
| Honey Ham | 2 oz | 90 | 5 | 45 | 2 | 0 | 35 | 590 | 0 | 2 | 10 | 1 med-fat meat |
| Honey Turkey | 2 oz | 100 | 5 | 45 | 2 | 0 | 30 | 600 | 0 | 3 | 9 | 1 med-fat meat |
| Pastrami | 2 oz | 90 | 5 | 45 | 2 | 0 | 40 | 790 | 0 | 1 | 10 | 1 med-fat meat |
| Turkey | 2 oz | 90 | 5 | 45 | 2 | 0 | 30 | 600 | 0 | 2 | 10 | 1 med-fat meat |
| ***Deli Cuts*** | | | | | | | | | | | | |
| Honey Ham | 2 oz | 80 | 2.5 | 25 | 1 | 0 | 20 | 460 | 0 | 3 | 10 | 1 lean meat |
| Honey-Roasted Turkey | 2 oz | 80 | 2.5 | 25 | 1 | 0 | 20 | 460 | 0 | 4 | 9 | 1 lean meat |

| | | | | | | | | | | | | |
|---|---|---|---|---|---|---|---|---|---|---|---|---|
| Oven-Roasted Turkey | 2 oz | 70 | 2.5 | 25 | 1 | 0 | 20 | 460 | 0 | 2 | 10 | 1 lean meat |
| ***Butterball*** | | | | | | | | | | | | |
| All Natural Oven Roasted Turkey Breast | 2 oz | 60 | 1 | 10 | 0 | 0 | 35 | 280 | 0 | 0 | 13 | 2 lean meat |
| Extra Thin Sliced Oven Roasted Turkey Breast | 2 oz | 70 | 1.5 | 15 | 0.5 | 0 | 25 | 580 | 0 | 3 | 10 | 1 lean meat |
| Extra Thin Sliced Rotisserie Flavored Turkey Breast | 2 oz | 50 | 0.5 | 5 | 0 | 0 | 20 | 510 | 0 | 1 | 11 | 2 lean meat |
| Thin Sliced Honey Turkey Breast | 2 oz | 70 | 1 | 10 | 0 | 0 | 25 | 550 | 0 | 4 | 10 | 1 lean meat |
| Thin Sliced Oven Roasted Chicken Breast | 2 oz | 50 | 0.5 | 5 | 0 | 0 | 25 | 480 | 0 | 1 | 11 | 2 lean meat |
| Thin Sliced Oven Roasted Turkey Breast | 2 oz | 70 | 1.5 | 10 | 0.5 | 0 | 2 | 570 | 0 | 3 | 10 | 1 lean meat |

PROCESSED MEAT, BREAKFAST MEAT, LUNCH MEAT

| | Serving | Calories | Fat (g) | Cal. from Fat | Sat. Fat (g) | Trans Fat (g) | Chol. (mg) | Sod. (mg) | Carb. (g) | Fiber (g) | Prot. (g) | Servings/Exchanges |
|---|---|---|---|---|---|---|---|---|---|---|---|---|
| Thin Sliced Smoked Turkey Breast | 2 oz | 70 | 1.5 | 10 | 0.5 | 0 | 25 | 560 | 0 | 4 | 7 | 1 lean meat |
| ***Deep Fried Lunchmeat*** | | | | | | | | | | | | |
| Extra Thin Sliced Original Deep Fried Turkey Lunchmeat | 2 oz | 60 | 1.5 | 15 | 0 | 0 | 25 | 510 | 0 | 3 | 9 | 1 lean meat |
| Thick Sliced Original Deep Fried Turkey Lunchmeat | 1 oz | 30 | 0.5 | 5 | 0 | 0 | 15 | 260 | 0 | 1 | 5 | 1 lean meat |
| ***Deli Premium*** | | | | | | | | | | | | |
| Honey Roasted & Smoked Turkey Breast | 2 oz | 50 | 0 | 10 | 0 | 0 | 25 | 400 | 0 | 2 | 9 | 1 lean meat |
| Oven Roasted Chicken Breast | 2 oz | 60 | 0 | 10 | 0 | 0 | 25 | 440 | 0 | 1 | 11 | 2 lean meat |

| | | | | | | | | | | | | |
|---|---|---|---|---|---|---|---|---|---|---|---|---|
| Oven Roasted Turkey Breast | 2 oz | 50 | 0.5 | 5 | 0 | 0 | 40 | 440 | 0 | 0 | 12 | 2 lean meat |
| ***Celebrity*** | | | | | | | | | | | | |
| Black Forest Smoked Ham 99% Fat Free | 1 oz | 25 | 0 | 0 | 0 | 0 | 15 | 180 | 0 | <1 | 5 | 1 lean meat |
| Ham 99% Fat Free | 1 oz | 20 | 0 | 0 | 0 | 0 | 15 | 180 | 0 | 0 | 5 | 1 lean meat |
| Columbus Salame | | | | | | | | | | | | |
| Choice Roast Beef | 2 oz | 90 | 3 | 25 | 1 | 0 | 40 | 310 | 1 | 0 | 13 | 2 lean meat |
| Italian Style Salame | 1 oz | 110 | 9 | 80 | 4 | 0 | 10 | 420 | 0 | 0 | 6 | 1 high-fat meat |
| Maple Honey Turkey | 2 oz | 70 | 1 | 10 | 0 | 0 | 20 | 340 | 3 | 0 | 13 | 2 lean meat |
| Pan Roasted Turkey Breast | 2 oz | 50 | 0.5 | 5 | 0 | 0 | 25 | 480 | 0 | 0 | 12 | 2 lean meat |
| Peppered Salami | 1 oz | 110 | 9 | 80 | 4 | 0 | 10 | 420 | 0 | 0 | 6 | 1 high-fat meat |
| ***Farmer John Sliced Deli Meats*** | | | | | | | | | | | | |
| Bologna | 2 oz | 160 | 14 | 130 | 4.5 | 0.5 | 25 | 520 | 0 | 2 | 6 | 1 high-fat meat, 1 fat |
| Cotto Salami | 2 oz | 140 | 11 | 100 | 4 | 0 | 45 | 470 | 0 | 3 | 7 | 1 high-fat meat |

PROCESSED MEAT, BREAKFAST MEAT, LUNCH MEAT

| | Serving | Calories | Fat (g) | Cal. from Fat | Sat. Fat (g) | Trans Fat (g) | Chol. (mg) | Sod. (mg) | Carb. (g) | Fiber (g) | Prot. (g) | Servings/Exchanges |
|---|---|---|---|---|---|---|---|---|---|---|---|---|
| Ham Roll | 2 oz | 60 | 1.5 | 15 | 1 | 0 | 25 | 450 | 0 | 1 | 10 | 1 lean meat |
| Head Cheese | 1.4 oz | 100 | 7 | 60 | 4 | 0 | 30 | 400 | 0 | 0 | 8 | 1 med-fat meat |
| Mission Loaf | 2 oz | 60 | 1.5 | 15 | 1 | 0 | 25 | 450 | 0 | 1 | 10 | 1 lean meat |
| Oven Roasted Turkey Breast | 1 oz | 25 | 0 | 0 | 0 | 0 | 10 | 270 | 0 | 1 | 5 | 1 lean meat |
| ***Foster Farms*** | | | | | | | | | | | | |
| Mesquite Smoked Turkey Breast | 2 oz | 60 | 1.5 | 10 | 0 | 0 | 10 | 520 | 0 | 2 | 9 | 1 lean meat |
| Oven Roasted Turkey Breast | 2 oz | 60 | 2 | 20 | 0.5 | 0 | 15 | 440 | 0 | 1 | 9 | 1 lean meat |
| ***Hebrew National*** | | | | | | | | | | | | |
| Beef Bologna | 1 oz | 80 | 8 | 70 | 3.5 | 0 | 15 | 240 | 0 | 0 | 3 | 1 high-fat meat |
| Beef Salami | 2 oz | 150 | 13 | 120 | 6 | 0 | 35 | 420 | 0 | 0 | 8 | 1 high-fat meat, 1 fat |
| Corned Beef | 2 oz | 80 | 3.5 | 20 | 1.5 | 0 | 35 | 520 | 0 | 1 | 13 | 2 lean meat |

| | | | | | | | | | | | | |
|---|---|---|---|---|---|---|---|---|---|---|---|---|
| Lean Beef Salami | 2 oz | 90 | 5 | 50 | 3 | 0 | 25 | 480 | 0 | 1 | 9 | 1 med-fat meat |
| Pastrami | 2 oz | 80 | 3 | 25 | 1 | 0 | 30 | 520 | 0 | 1 | 11 | 2 lean meat |
| ***Hebrew National Franks*** | | | | | | | | | | | | |
| 97% Fat Free Beef Franks | 1 | 40 | 1 | 10 | 0 | 0 | 10 | 520 | 3 | 0 | 6 | 1 lean meat |
| Beef Franks | 1 | 150 | 14 | 130 | 6 | 0.5 | 25 | 460 | 1 | 0 | 6 | 1 high-fat meat, 1 fat |
| Jumbo Beef Franks | 1 | 270 | 25 | 230 | 10 | 0 | 45 | 810 | 2 | 0 | 10 | 1 high-fat meat, 3 fat |
| Reduced Fat Beef Franks | 1 | 110 | 9 | 80 | 3.5 | 0 | 20 | 490 | 2 | 0 | 5 | 1 high-fat meat |
| ***Hillshire Farm Deli Select*** | | | | | | | | | | | | |
| Baked Ham | 2 oz | 60 | 1.5 | 15 | 0.5 | 0 | 30 | 730 | 0 | 1 | 9 | 1 lean meat |
| Brown Sugar Baked Ham | 2 oz | 60 | 1.5 | 15 | 0.5 | 0 | 25 | 600 | 0 | 2 | 10 | 1 lean meat |
| Honey Ham | 2 oz | 70 | 1.5 | 15 | 0.5 | 0 | 30 | 720 | 0 | 3 | 9 | 1 lean meat |
| Honey Roasted Turkey Breast | 2 oz | 50 | 0.5 | 5 | 0 | 0 | 25 | 580 | 0 | 2 | 9 | 1 lean meat |

PROCESSED MEAT, BREAKFAST MEAT, LUNCH MEAT

| | Serving | Calories | Fat (g) | Cal. from Fat | Sat. Fat (g) | Trans Fat (g) | Chol. (mg) | Sod. (mg) | Carb. (g) | Fiber (g) | Prot. (g) | Servings/Exchanges |
|---|---|---|---|---|---|---|---|---|---|---|---|---|
| Oven Roasted Chicken Breast | 2 oz | 60 | 0.5 | 5 | 0 | 0 | 25 | 620 | 0 | 2 | 11 | 2 lean meat |
| Oven Roasted Turkey Breast | 2 oz | 50 | 0.5 | 5 | 0 | 0 | 25 | 610 | 0 | 1 | 10 | 1 lean meat |
| Pastrami | 2 oz | 60 | 1 | 10 | 0.5 | 0 | 30 | 600 | 0 | 0 | 11 | 2 lean meat |
| Roast Beef | 2 oz | 60 | 1 | 10 | 0.5 | 0 | 25 | 670 | 0 | 1 | 11 | 2 lean meat |
| Smoked Chicken Breast | 2 oz | 60 | 1 | 10 | 0 | 0 | 25 | 730 | 0 | 2 | 10 | 1 lean meat |
| Smoked Ham | 2 oz | 60 | 1.5 | 15 | 0.5 | 0 | 25 | 600 | 0 | 1 | 10 | 1 lean meat |
| Smoked Turkey Breast | 2 oz | 50 | 0.5 | 5 | 0 | 0 | 20 | 590 | 0 | 3 | 9 | 1 lean meat |
| Hillshire Farm Hearty Slices | | | | | | | | | | | | |
| Honey Ham | 1 oz | 30 | 0.5 | 5 | 0 | 0 | 10 | 260 | 0 | <1 | 5 | 1 lean meat |
| Honey Roasted Turkey | 1 oz | 25 | 0 | 0 | 0 | 0 | 10 | 260 | 0 | 1 | 6 | 1 lean meat |
| Oven Roasted Chicken | 1 oz | 25 | 0 | 0 | 0 | 0 | 15 | 280 | 0 | <1 | 5 | 1 lean meat |

| | | | | | | | | | | | | |
|---|---|---|---|---|---|---|---|---|---|---|---|---|
| Hillshire Farm Ultra Thin | | | | | | | | | | | | |
| Hard Salami | 1 oz | 110 | 10 | 90 | 4 | 0 | 30 | 500 | 0 | 0 | 6 | 1 high-fat meat |
| Honey Ham | 2 oz | 60 | 1.5 | 15 | 0.5 | 0 | 25 | 500 | 0 | 2 | 10 | 1 lean meat |
| Oven Roasted Turkey Breast | 2 oz | 50 | 0.5 | 5 | 0 | 0 | 20 | 620 | 0 | 2 | 9 | 1 lean meat |
| Roast Beef | 2 oz | 60 | 3 | 25 | 1 | 0 | 25 | 450 | 0 | 0 | 9 | 1 med-fat meat |
| Smoked Ham | 2 oz | 60 | 1.5 | 15 | 0.5 | 0 | 30 | 620 | 0 | 1 | 9 | 1 lean meat |
| ***Hormel Natural Choice*** | | | | | | | | | | | | |
| Deli Roast Beef | 2 oz | 70 | 2.5 | 25 | 1 | 0 | 25 | 500 | 0 | 0 | 11 | 2 lean meat |
| Honey Deli Ham 97% Fat Free | 2 oz | 70 | 1.5 | 15 | 0.5 | 0 | 25 | 520 | 0 | 3 | 10 | 1 lean meat |
| ***Land O'Frost*** | | | | | | | | | | | | |
| ***DeliShaved*** | | | | | | | | | | | | |
| Chicken | 2 oz | 90 | 6 | 50 | 1.5 | 0 | 30 | 760 | 0 | 0 | 10 | 1 med-fat meat |
| Honey Ham | 2 oz | 80 | 5 | 45 | 2 | 0 | 30 | 540 | 0 | 4 | 10 | 1 med-fat meat |
| Oven Roasted Turkey | 2 oz | 90 | 6 | 50 | 1.5 | 0 | 35 | 540 | 0 | 0 | 9 | 1 med-fat meat |

PROCESSED MEAT, BREAKFAST MEAT, LUNCH MEAT

| | Serving | Calories | Fat (g) | Cal. from Fat | Sat. Fat (g) | Trans Fat (g) | Chol. (mg) | Sod. (mg) | Carb. (g) | Fiber (g) | Prot. (g) | Servings/Exchanges |
|---|---|---|---|---|---|---|---|---|---|---|---|---|
| Smoked Turkey | 2 oz | 90 | 6 | 50 | 2 | 0 | 40 | 740 | 0 | 0 | 9 | 1 med-fat meat |
| ***Premium*** | | | | | | | | | | | | |
| Chicken Breast | 2 oz | 80 | 5 | 45 | 1 | 0 | 35 | 650 | 0 | 2 | 7 | 1 med-fat meat |
| Honey Ham | 1.8 oz | 70 | 3 | 25 | 1 | 0 | 25 | 530 | 0 | 2 | 9 | 1 lean meat |
| Smoked Ham | 1.8 oz | 60 | 3 | 25 | 1 | 0 | 25 | 560 | 0 | 1 | 9 | 1 lean meat |
| ***Select*** | | | | | | | | | | | | |
| Honey Smoked White Turkey | 3 oz | 110 | 4.5 | 40 | 1 | 0 | 35 | 1080 | 0 | 6 | 12 | 1 med-fat meat |
| Oven Roasted White Turkey | 1.9 oz | 70 | 3.5 | 35 | 1 | 0 | 25 | 630 | 0 | 1 | 8 | 1 med-fat meat |
| Smoked Ham | 3 oz | 100 | 5 | 45 | 1.5 | 0 | 45 | 1060 | 0 | 1 | 14 | 2 lean meat |
| Taste Escapes | | | | | | | | | | | | |
| Hickory Smoked Black Pepper Ham | 2 oz | 70 | 2.5 | 20 | 1 | 0 | 30 | 690 | 0 | 2 | 10 | 1 lean meat |

| | | | | | | | | | | | | |
|---|---|---|---|---|---|---|---|---|---|---|---|---|
| Hickory Smoked Maple Ham | 2 oz | 70 | 2 | 15 | 0.5 | 0 | 30 | 640 | 0 | 3 | 10 | 1 lean meat |
| Peppered Beef | 2 oz | 70 | 2 | 20 | 1 | 0 | 20 | 680 | 0 | 2 | 10 | 1 lean meat |
| ***Traditional*** | | | | | | | | | | | | |
| Chicken | 2 oz | 90 | 5 | 45 | 1.5 | 0 | 35 | 800 | 0 | 0 | 9 | 1 med-fat meat |
| Ham | 2 oz | 90 | 5 | 45 | 2 | 0 | 30 | 690 | 0 | 1 | 9 | 1 med-fat meat |
| Honey Ham | 2 oz | 90 | 4.5 | 40 | 1.5 | 0 | 30 | 610 | 0 | 3 | 9 | 1 med-fat meat |
| Honey Turkey | 2 oz | 90 | 5 | 45 | 1.5 | 0 | 35 | 780 | 3 | 0 | 9 | 1 med-fat meat |
| Turkey | 2 oz | 90 | 6 | 50 | 2 | 0 | 40 | 790 | 0 | 0 | 9 | 1 med-fat meat |
| ***Oscar Mayer*** | | | | | | | | | | | | |
| Baked Ham | 2.25 oz | 60 | 2 | 20 | 1 | 0 | 30 | 760 | 0 | 1 | 10 | 1 lean meat |
| Beef Bologna | 1 oz | 90 | 8 | 70 | 3.5 | 0 | 20 | 310 | 0 | 1 | 3 | 1 high-fat meat |
| Beef Cotto Salami | 1 oz | 60 | 4.5 | 40 | 2 | 0 | 20 | 360 | 0 | 1 | 4 | 1 med-fat meat |
| Beef Salami, Deli Thin | 1.8 oz | 150 | 13 | 120 | 6 | 1 | 40 | 640 | 0 | 1 | 8 | 1 high-fat meat |
| Boiled Ham | 2.25 oz | 60 | 2 | 20 | 1 | 0 | 30 | 820 | 0 | 1 | 10 | 1 lean meat |
| Bologna | 1 oz | 90 | 8 | 80 | 3 | 0 | 30 | 300 | 0 | 1 | 3 | 1 high-fat meat |

PROCESSED MEAT, BREAKFAST MEAT, LUNCH MEAT

| | Serving | Calories | Fat (g) | Cal. from Fat | Sat. Fat (g) | Trans Fat (g) | Chol. (mg) | Sod. (mg) | Carb. (g) | Fiber (g) | Prot. (g) | Servings/Exchanges |
|---|---|---|---|---|---|---|---|---|---|---|---|---|
| Bologna, 98% Fat Free | 1 oz | 25 | 0 | 0.5 | 0 | 0 | 10 | 240 | 0 | 3 | 3 | 1 lean meat |
| Braunschweiger Liver Sausage | 2 oz | 190 | 17 | 155 | 6 | 0 | 90 | 630 | 0 | 1 | 8 | 1 high-fat meat, 1 fat |
| Chopped Ham | 1 oz | 50 | 3 | 30 | 1.5 | 0 | 15 | 340 | 0 | 1 | 4 | 1 lean meat |
| Cotto Salami | 1 oz | 70 | 6 | 50 | 2 | 0 | 25 | 280 | 0 | 1 | 4 | 1 med-fat meat |
| Fat Free Bologna | 1 oz | 20 | 0 | 0 | 0 | 0 | 10 | 250 | 0 | 2 | 3 | 1 lean meat |
| Ham & Cheese Loaf | 1 oz | 60 | 4.5 | 40 | 2.5 | 0 | 20 | 350 | 0 | 1 | 4 | 1 med-fat meat |
| Hard Salami | 1 oz | 100 | 8 | 70 | 3 | 0 | 25 | 510 | 0 | 1 | 7 | 1 high-fat meat |
| Honey Ham | 2.25 oz | 70 | 2 | 20 | 1 | 0 | 30 | 770 | 0 | 2 | 11 | 2 lean meat |
| Honey Ham, 98% Fat Free | 2.25 oz | 70 | 2 | 20 | 1 | 0 | 30 | 770 | 0 | 2 | 11 | 2 lean meat |
| Light Beef Bologna | 1 oz | 60 | 4 | 35 | 1.5 | 0 | 15 | 310 | 0 | 2 | 3 | 1 med-fat meat |
| Liver Cheese | 1.5 oz | 120 | 10 | 90 | 3.5 | 0 | 80 | 420 | 0 | 1 | 6 | 1 high-fat meat |
| Olive Loaf | 1 oz | 70 | 6 | 55 | 2 | 0 | 20 | 360 | 0 | 2 | 3 | 1 med-fat meat |

| | | | | | | | | | | | | |
|---|---|---|---|---|---|---|---|---|---|---|---|---|
| Oven Roasted White Turkey | 1 oz | 25 | 1 | 10 | 0 | 0 | 10 | 340 | 0 | 1 | 6 | 1 lean meat |
| Pickle & Pimiento Loaf | 1 oz | 80 | 6 | 55 | 2 | 0 | 20 | 360 | 0 | 2 | 3 | 1 med-fat meat |
| Sandwich Spread | 2 oz | 130 | 9 | 80 | 4 | 0 | 25 | 460 | 0 | 9 | 4 | 1 high-fat meat |
| Turkey Bologna | 1 oz | 50 | 4 | 35 | 1 | 0 | 20 | 270 | 0 | 1 | 3 | 1 med-fat meat |
| Turkey Bologna, 50% Less Fat | 1 oz | 50 | 4 | 35 | 1 | 0 | 20 | 270 | 0 | 1 | 3 | 1 med-fat meat |
| Turkey Cotto Salami | 1 oz | 45 | 3 | 25 | 1 | 0 | 20 | 310 | 0 | 0 | 4 | 1 lean meat |
| Turkey Cotto Salami, 50% Less Fat | 1 oz | 45 | 3 | 25 | 1 | 0 | 20 | 310 | 0 | 0 | 4 | 1 lean meat |
| Turkey Ham | 1 oz | 35 | 1.5 | 10 | 0 | 0 | 20 | 350 | 0 | 1 | 5 | 1 lean meat |
| Turkey, Smoked, White, 95% Fat Free | 1 oz | 30 | 1 | 10 | 0 | 0 | 10 | 320 | 0 | 1 | 4 | 1 lean meat |
| Turkey, White, Smoked | 1 oz | 30 | 1 | 10 | 0 | 0 | 10 | 320 | 0 | 1 | 4 | 1 lean meat |
| ***Deli Fresh Meats*** | | | | | | | | | | | | |
| Brown Sugar Ham, Shaved | 1.8 oz | 60 | 1.5 | 10 | 0 | 0 | 25 | 740 | 0 | 3 | 9 | 1 lean meat |

PROCESSED MEAT, BREAKFAST MEAT, LUNCH MEAT

| | Serving | Calories | Fat (g) | Cal. from Fat | Sat. Fat (g) | Trans Fat (g) | Chol. (mg) | Sod. (mg) | Carb. (g) | Fiber (g) | Prot. (g) | Servings/Exchanges |
|---|---|---|---|---|---|---|---|---|---|---|---|---|
| Chicken Breast, Rotisserie Style, Shaved | 1.8 oz | 50 | 1 | 10 | 0 | 0 | 25 | 480 | 0 | 2 | 9 | 1 lean meat |
| Honey Ham-Shaved | 1.8 oz | 50 | 1 | 10 | 0.5 | 0 | 25 | 650 | 0 | 2 | 9 | 1 lean meat |
| Roast Beef Slow Roasted, Shaved | 1.8 oz | 60 | 2.5 | 20 | 1 | 0 | 30 | 520 | 0 | 0 | 10 | 1 lean meat |
| Smoked Ham, Shaved | 1.8 oz | 45 | 1 | 10 | 0 | 0 | 25 | 640 | 0 | 0 | 9 | 1 lean meat |
| Smoked Turkey Breast | 2.25 oz | 60 | 0.5 | 5 | 0 | 0 | 25 | 760 | 0 | 0 | 13 | 2 lean meat |
| ***Oscar Mayer Hot Dogs*** | | | | | | | | | | | | |
| Jumbo Beef Franks | 1 | 300 | 27 | 240 | 11 | 1.5 | 55 | 1090 | 2 | 0 | 10 | 1 high-fat meat, 3 fat |
| Jumbo Wieners | 1 | 290 | 27 | 240 | 10 | 0 | 60 | 930 | 2 | 0 | 10 | 1 high-fat meat, 3 fat |
| Quarter Pound Beef Franks | 1 | 370 | 34 | 310 | 14 | 1.5 | 70 | 1370 | 3 | 0 | 13 | 2 high-fat meat, 3 fat |
| Regular Beef Franks | 1 | 180 | 17 | 150 | 7 | 1 | 35 | 680 | 1 | 0 | 7 | 1 high-fat meat, 1 fat |

| | | | | | | | | | | | | |
|---|---|---|---|---|---|---|---|---|---|---|---|---|
| Turkey Franks | 1 | 100 | 8 | 70 | 2.5 | 0 | 30 | 510 | 2 | 0 | 5 | 1 high-fat meat |
| Wieners | 1 | 140 | 13 | 120 | 5 | 0 | 30 | 460 | <1 | 0 | 5 | 1 high-fat meat, 1 fat |
| ***Trader Joe's*** | | | | | | | | | | | | |
| Black Forest Ham | 2 oz | 70 | 1 | 10 | 0 | 0 | 35 | 730 | 0 | 2 | 12 | 1 lean meat |
| Oven Roasted Turkey Breast | 2 oz | 50 | 0 | 0 | 0 | 0 | 25 | 630 | 0 | 2 | 11 | 2 lean meat |
| Pastami | 2 oz | 80 | 2 | 15 | 0.5 | 0 | 25 | 270 | 0 | <1 | 13 | 2 lean meat |
| Roast Beef | 2 oz | 80 | 2 | 20 | 0.5 | 0 | 30 | 460 | 0 | 0 | 15 | 2 lean meat |
| Smoked Turkey Breast | 2 oz | 50 | 0 | 0 | 0 | 0 | 25 | 630 | 0 | 2 | 11 | 2 lean meat |
| **CANNED MEAT** | | | | | | | | | | | | |
| **Fish/Seafood** | | | | | | | | | | | | |
| Anchovies in Oil, Canned, Drained | 5 | 42 | 2 | 18 | <1 | 0 | 17 | 734 | 0 | 0 | 8 | 1 lean meat |
| Clams, Canned, Drained Solids | 1 oz | 42 | <1 | 5 | <1 | 0 | 19 | 32 | 1 | 0 | 7 | 1 lean meat |
| Clams, Smoked, Canned in Oil, Small | 5 | 88 | 6 | 54 | 1 | 0 | 19 | 161 | 1 | 0 | 7 | 1 med-fat meat |

PROCESSED MEAT, BREAKFAST MEAT, LUNCH MEAT

| | Serving | Calories | Fat (g) | Cal. from Fat | Sat. Fat (g) | Trans Fat (g) | Chol. (mg) | Sod. (mg) | Carb. (g) | Fiber (g) | Prot. (g) | Servings/Exchanges |
|---|---|---|---|---|---|---|---|---|---|---|---|---|
| Crab, Canned, Drained Solids | 1 oz | 28 | <1 | 5 | <1 | 0 | 26 | 95 | 0 | 0 | 6 | 1 lean meat |
| Salmon, Canned in Water | 1 oz | 40 | 2 | 18 | <1 | 0 | 11 | 139 | 0 | 0 | 6 | 1 lean meat |
| Sardines, Oil-Packed, Drained | 2 | 50 | 3 | 27 | <1 | 0 | 34 | 121 | 0 | 0 | 6 | 1 lean meat |
| Shrimp, Canned, Drained Solids | 1 oz | 34 | <1 | 0 | <1 | 0 | 50 | 48 | <1 | 0 | 7 | 1 lean meat |
| Squid, Pickled | 1 oz | 26 | <1 | 0 | <1 | 0 | 64 | 397 | 1 | 0 | 4 | 1 lean meat |
| Tuna, Canned in Oil, Drained | 1 oz | 56 | 2 | 9 | <1 | 0 | 5 | 100 | 0 | 0 | 8 | 1 lean meat |
| Tuna, Canned, Water Packed, Solids Only | 1 oz | 33 | <1 | 0 | <1 | 0 | 9 | 96 | 0 | 0 | 7 | 1 lean meat |
| **Beef** | | | | | | | | | | | | |
| Liver Pate, Canned | 2 Tbsp | 52 | 3 | 27 | 1 | 0 | 66 | 100 | 2 | 0 | 4 | 1 lean meat |

| | | | | | | | | | | | | |
|---|---|---|---|---|---|---|---|---|---|---|---|---|
| Pickled Beef Trip | 1 oz | 18 | <1 | 0 | <1 | 0 | 19 | 13 | 0 | 0 | 3 | 1 lean meat |
| **Pork** | | | | | | | | | | | | |
| Ham, Canned | 1 oz | 48 | 2 | 18 | <1 | 0 | 12 | 304 | <1 | 0 | 6 | 1 lean meat |
| Sausage, Vienna, Canned | 1 oz | 79 | 7 | 63 | 3 | 0 | 15 | 270 | <1 | 0 | 3 | 1 high-fat meat |
| **Canned Fish** | | | | | | | | | | | | |
| ***Bumble Bee*** | | | | | | | | | | | | |
| Blueback Salmon | 2.2 oz | 110 | 7 | 60 | 1.5 | 0 | 40 | 270 | 0 | 0 | 13 | 2 lean meat |
| Chunk Light Tuna in Oil | 2 oz | 70 | 3 | 25 | 0.5 | 0 | 25 | 180 | 0 | 0 | 13 | 2 lean meat |
| Chunk Light Tuna in Water | 2 oz | 50 | 0.5 | 5 | 0 | 0 | 3 | 180 | 0 | 0 | 13 | 2 lean meat |
| Chunk White Albacore Tuna, Very Low Sodium, in Water | 2 oz | 60 | 1 | 10 | 0 | 0 | 25 | 35 | 0 | 0 | 15 | 2 lean meat |
| Fancy Whole Baby Clams | 2 oz | 50 | 1 | 10 | 0.5 | 0 | 40 | 270 | 2 | 0 | 9 | 1 lean meat |

PROCESSED MEAT, BREAKFAST MEAT, LUNCH MEAT

| | Serving | Calories | Fat (g) | Cal. from Fat | Sat. Fat (g) | Trans Fat (g) | Chol. (mg) | Sod. (mg) | Carb. (g) | Fiber (g) | Prot. (g) | Servings/Exchanges |
|---|---|---|---|---|---|---|---|---|---|---|---|---|
| Jumbo Shrimp | 2 oz | 40 | 0 | 0 | 0 | 0 | 115 | 430 | 0 | 0 | 10 | 1 lean meat |
| Keta Salmon | 2.2 oz | 90 | 4 | 35 | 1 | 0 | 40 | 270 | 0 | 0 | 13 | 2 lean meat |
| Medium Red Salmon (Alaska Coho) | 2.2 oz | 90 | 5 | 45 | 1 | 0 | 40 | 270 | 0 | 0 | 12 | 2 lean meat |
| Medium Shrimp | 2 oz | 40 | 0 | 0 | 0 | 0 | 115 | 430 | 0 | 0 | 10 | 1 lean meat |
| Minced Clams | 2 oz | 25 | 0 | 0 | 0 | 0 | 10 | 320 | 2 | 0 | 4 | 1 lean meat |
| Pink Crabmeat | 2 oz | 35 | 0.5 | 5 | 0 | 0 | 50 | 300 | 0 | 0 | 7 | 1 lean meat |
| Pink Salmon | 2.2 oz | 90 | 5 | 45 | 1 | 0 | 40 | 270 | 0 | 0 | 12 | 2 lean meat |
| Premium Light Tuna in Water Pouch | 2 oz | 60 | 0.5 | 5 | 0 | 0 | 30 | 180 | 0 | 0 | 13 | 2 lean meat |
| Prime Fillet Albacore Steak Entrées, Mesquite Grilled | 4 oz | 150 | 1.5 | 10 | 0 | 0 | 40 | 370 | 0 | 0 | 35 | 5 lean meat |
| Prime Fillet Atlantic Salmon | 2 oz | 80 | 3 | 30 | 1.5 | 0 | 10 | 170 | 0 | 0 | 12 | 2 lean meat |

| | | | | | | | | | | | | |
|---|---|---|---|---|---|---|---|---|---|---|---|---|
| Prime Fillet Salmon Steaks | 4 oz | 160 | 3 | 25 | 0.5 | 0 | 45 | 690 | 8 | 0 | 24 | 3 lean meat |
| Prime Fillet Solid Light Tuna, Tonno in Oil | 2 oz | 110 | 5 | 50 | 1 | 0 | 30 | 220 | 0 | 0 | 15 | 2 lean meat |
| Prime Fillet Solid White Albacore in Water | 2 oz | 70 | 1 | 10 | 0 | 0 | 25 | 180 | 0 | 0 | 16 | 2 lean meat |
| Red Salmon (Sockeye) | 2.2 oz | 110 | 7 | 60 | 1.5 | 0 | 40 | 270 | 0 | 0 | 13 | 2 lean meat |
| Sardines in Oil | 2.7-oz can | 130 | 9 | 80 | 2 | 0 | 35 | 340 | 0 | 0 | 13 | 2 med-fat meat |
| Sardines in Water | 2.7-oz can | 120 | 7 | 70 | 2 | 0 | 35 | 340 | 0 | 0 | 13 | 2 lean meat |
| Sensations Easy Peel Bowls, Spicy Thai Chili | 3 oz | 110 | 3 | 30 | 0.5 | 0 | 25 | 350 | 2 | 0 | 18 | 2 lean meat |
| Sensations Easy Peel Tuna Bowls, Lemon & Cracked Pepper | 3 oz | 110 | 4 | 35 | 1 | 0 | 25 | 300 | 2 | 0 | 16 | 2 lean meat |

| | Serving | Calories | Fat (g) | Cal. from Fat | Sat. Fat (g) | Trans Fat (g) | Chol. (mg) | Sod. (mg) | Carb. (g) | Fiber (g) | Prot. (g) | Servings/Exchanges |
|---|---|---|---|---|---|---|---|---|---|---|---|---|
| Skinless Boneless Pink Salmon | 2 oz | 70 | 1.5 | 10 | 0 | 0 | 30 | 240 | 0 | 0 | 12 | 2 lean meat |
| Small Shrimp | 2 oz | 40 | 0 | 0 | 0 | 0 | 115 | 430 | 0 | 0 | 10 | 1 lean meat |
| Smoked Clams | 2 oz | 130 | 8 | 80 | 2 | 0 | 40 | 460 | 1 | 0 | 11 | 2 med-fat meat |
| Smoked Oysters | 2 oz | 120 | 7 | 60 | 1.5 | 0 | 35 | 210 | 6 | 0 | 10 | 1 med-fat meat |
| Smoked Salmon Fillets in Oil | 3 oz | 150 | 9 | 80 | 2 | 0 | 55 | 400 | 0 | 0 | 16 | 2 med-fat meat |
| Solid White Albacore Tuna in Oil | 2 oz | 80 | 3 | 25 | 0.5 | 0 | 25 | 180 | 0 | 0 | 14 | 2 lean meat |
| Solid White Albacore Tuna in Water | 2 oz | 60 | 1 | 10 | 0 | 0 | 25 | 180 | 0 | 0 | 13 | 2 lean meat |
| White Crabmeat | 2 oz | 40 | 1 | 10 | 0 | 0 | 50 | 300 | 0 | 0 | 8 | 1 lean meat |
| Whole Oysters | 2 oz | 70 | 3 | 30 | 0.5 | 0 | 45 | 140 | 3 | 0 | 7 | 1 lean meat |

***Chicken of the Sea***

| | | | | | | | | | | | | |
|---|---|---|---|---|---|---|---|---|---|---|---|---|
| Chunk Light Tuna in Oil | 2 oz | 100 | 6 | 50 | 1 | 0 | 25 | 250 | 0 | 0 | 10 | 1 med-fat meat |
| Chunk Light Tuna in Water | 2 oz | 50 | 0.5 | 50 | 0 | 0 | 25 | 250 | 0 | 0 | 11 | 2 lean meat |
| Chunk Light Tuna in Water Low Sodium | 2 oz | 50 | 0.5 | 50 | 0 | 0 | 25 | 90 | 0 | 0 | 11 | 2 lean meat |
| Chunk Light Tuna, 50% Less Sodium | 2 oz | 50 | 0.5 | 5 | 0 | 0 | 25 | 125 | 0 | 0 | 11 | 2 lean meat |
| Chunk White Albacore Low Sodium | 3 oz | 80 | 1 | 10 | 0 | 0 | 35 | 50 | 0 | 0 | 18 | 3 lean meat |
| Chunk White Albacore Tuna | 2 oz | 50 | 1 | 10 | 0 | 0 | 25 | 250 | 0 | 0 | 11 | 2 lean meat |
| Fancy Crabmeat | 2 oz | 40 | 0 | 0 | 0 | 0 | 50 | 400 | 2 | 0 | 7 | 1 lean meat |
| Genova Skinless Boneless Salmon in Water | 2 oz | 60 | 2 | 20 | 1 | 0 | 20 | 280 | 0 | 0 | 10 | 1 lean meat |
| Genova Solid White Albacore Tuna in Oil | 2 oz | 110 | 6 | 50 | 1 | 0 | 25 | 250 | 0 | 0 | 13 | 2 lean meat |

PROCESSED MEAT, BREAKFAST MEAT, LUNCH MEAT

| | Serving | Calories | Fat (g) | Cal. from Fat | Sat. Fat (g) | Trans Fat (g) | Chol. (mg) | Sod. (mg) | Carb. (g) | Fiber (g) | Prot. (g) | Servings/Exchanges |
|---|---|---|---|---|---|---|---|---|---|---|---|---|
| Genova Tonno Tuna in Olive Oil | 2 oz | 120 | 8 | 70 | 2 | 0 | 25 | 250 | 0 | 0 | 13 | 2 med-fat meat |
| Medium or Small Shrimp | 2 oz | 45 | 0.5 | 5 | 0 | 0 | 145 | 400 | 1 | 0 | 10 | 1 lean meat |
| Minced Clams | 1/4 cup | 30 | 0 | 0 | 0 | 0 | 12 | 370 | 2 | 0 | 5 | 1 lean meat |
| Pink Crabmeat | 2 oz | 30 | 0 | 0 | 0 | 0 | 50 | 400 | 0 | 0 | 7 | 1 lean meat |
| Sardines in Water | 3.75-oz can | 100 | 4 | 40 | 2 | 0 | 45 | 430 | 2 | 0 | 13 | 2 lean meat |
| Skinless & Boneless Pink Salmon | 2 oz | 60 | 2 | 20 | 0.5 | 0 | 20 | 280 | 0 | 0 | 10 | 1 lean meat |
| Smoked Oysters in Oil | 3.75 oz | 170 | 8 | 70 | 2 | 0 | 45 | 280 | 8 | 0 | 10 | 1 high-fat meat |
| Smoked Oysters in Water | 3.75 oz | 120 | 3 | 30 | 1 | 0 | 55 | 400 | 10 | 0 | 12 | 2 lean meat |
| Smoked Sardines in Oil | 3.75-oz can | 190 | 14 | 130 | 6 | 0 | 45 | 430 | 2 | 0 | 12 | 2 med-fat meat, 1 fat |

| | | | | | | | | | | | | |
|---|---|---|---|---|---|---|---|---|---|---|---|---|
| Solid White Albacore Tuna in Oil | 2 oz | 90 | 4 | 40 | 0 | 0 | 25 | 250 | 0 | 0 | 13 | 2 lean meat |
| Solid White Albacore Tuna in Water | 2 oz | 80 | 4 | 40 | 0 | 0 | 25 | 250 | 0 | 0 | 11 | 2 lean meat |
| Traditional Pink Salmon | 1/4 cup | 90 | 5 | 45 | 1 | 0 | 40 | 270 | 0 | 0 | 12 | 2 lean meat |
| Very Low Sodium Chunk White Albacore Tuna | 2 oz | 50 | 0.5 | 5 | 0 | 0 | 25 | 35 | 0 | 0 | 12 | 2 lean meat |
| Whole Baby Clams | 1/4 cup | 30 | 0 | 0 | 0 | 0 | 10 | 290 | 1 | 0 | 6 | 1 lean meat |
| Whole Oysters | 2 oz | 80 | 3 | 30 | 1 | 0 | 35 | 220 | 6 | 0 | 7 | 1 lean meat |
| ***Starkist*** | | | | | | | | | | | | |
| Chunk Light Tuna in Water | 2 oz | 50 | 1 | 0 | 0 | 0 | 25 | 180 | <1 | <1 | 11 | 2 lean meat |
| Hickory Smoked Tuna Creations | 2 oz | 80 | 2.5 | 0 | 0 | 0 | 30 | NA | <1 | 0 | 14 | 2 lean meat |
| Low Sodium Albacore | 2 oz | 50 | 0.5 | 0 | 0 | 0 | 20 | 125 | 0 | 0 | 12 | 2 lean meat |

PROCESSED MEAT, BREAKFAST MEAT, LUNCH MEAT

| | Serving | Calories | Fat (g) | Cal. from Fat | Sat. Fat (g) | Trans Fat (g) | Chol. (mg) | Sod. (mg) | Carb. (g) | Fiber (g) | Prot. (g) | Servings/Exchanges |
|---|---|---|---|---|---|---|---|---|---|---|---|---|
| Low Sodium Chunk Light Tuna | 2 oz | 50 | 0.5 | 0 | 0 | 0 | 20 | 125 | 0 | 0 | 12 | 2 lean meat |
| Solid White Albacore Tuna in Water | 2 oz | 70 | 2 | 0 | 0.5 | 0 | 25 | 200 | 0 | 0 | 13 | 2 lean meat |
| **Canned Chicken** | | | | | | | | | | | | |
| ***Swanson*** | | | | | | | | | | | | |
| Premium White Chunk Chicken Breast in Water | 2 oz | 50 | 1 | 10 | 0 | 0 | 25 | 260 | 1 | 0 | 9 | 1 lean meat |
| ***Tyson*** | | | | | | | | | | | | |
| Premium Chunk Chicken | 2 oz | 60 | 2 | 20 | 0 | 0 | 30 | 200 | 0 | 0 | 10 | 1 lean meat |
| Premium Chunk Chicken Pouch (97% Fat Free) | 2 oz | 70 | 1 | 15 | 0 | 0 | 45 | 210 | 0 | 0 | 14 | 2 lean meat |

| | Serving | Calories | Fat (g) | Cal. from Fat | Sat. Fat (g) | Trans Fat (g) | Chol. (mg) | Sod. (mg) | Carb. (g) | Fiber (g) | Prot. (g) | Servings/Exchanges |
|---|---|---|---|---|---|---|---|---|---|---|---|---|
| **RICE, RICE MIXES** | | | | | | | | | | | | |
| Brown Rice, Long Grain, Cooked | 1/2 cup | 108 | <1 | 0 | <1 | 0 | 0 | 5 | 22 | 2 | 3 | 1 1/2 starch |
| Brown Rice, Medium Grain, Cooked | 1/2 cup | 109 | <1 | 0 | <1 | 0 | 0 | 1 | 23 | 2 | 2 | 1 1/2 starch |
| White Rice, Glutinous, Cooked | 1/2 cup | 85 | <1 | 0 | 0 | 0 | 0 | 5 | 19 | <1 | 2 | 1 starch |
| White Rice, Long Grain, Cooked | 1/2 cup | 103 | <1 | 0 | <1 | 0 | 0 | 1 | 22 | <1 | 2 | 2 starch |
| White Rice, Long Grain, Instant, Cooked | 1/2 cup | 97 | <1 | 0 | <1 | 0 | 0 | 4 | 21 | <1 | 2 | 1 starch |
| White Rice, Long Grain, Parboiled, Cooked | 1/2 cup | 97 | <1 | 0 | <1 | 0 | 0 | 2 | 21 | <1 | 2 | 1/2 starch |
| White Rice, Medium Grain, Cooked | 1/2 cup | 121 | <1 | 0 | <1 | 0 | 0 | 0 | 27 | <1 | 2 | 2 starch |

RICE, RICE MIXES

| | Serving | Calories | Fat (g) | Cal. from Fat | Sat. Fat (g) | Trans Fat (g) | Chol. (mg) | Sod. (mg) | Carb. (g) | Fiber (g) | Prot. (g) | Servings/Exchanges |
|---|---|---|---|---|---|---|---|---|---|---|---|---|
| White Rice, Short Grain, Cooked | 1/2 cup | 121 | <1 | 0 | <1 | 0 | 0 | 0 | 27 | <1 | 2 | 2 starch |
| Wild Rice, Cooked | 1/2 cup | 83 | <1 | 0 | <1 | 0 | 0 | 3 | 18 | 2 | 3 | 1 starch |
| **Brands** | | | | | | | | | | | | |
| ***Knorr/Lipton*** | | | | | | | | | | | | |
| Cheddar Broccoli | 1 cup | 260 | 6 | 55 | 1 | 0 | <5 | 900 | 47 | 2 | 6 | 3 starch, 1 fat |
| Chicken Fried Rice | 1 cup | 270 | 8 | 75 | 1 | 0 | <5 | 750 | 46 | 2 | 6 | 3 starch, 2 fat |
| Spanish Rice | 1 cup | 290 | 7 | 65 | 1 | 0 | 0 | 860 | 50 | 2 | 6 | 3 starch, 1 fat |
| ***Mahatma*** | | | | | | | | | | | | |
| Authenic Spanish Rice | 2/3 cup | 180 | 0 | 5 | 0 | 0 | 0 | 650 | 42 | 1 | 4 | 3 starch |
| Brown Rice | 3/4 cup | 150 | 1 | 10 | 0 | 0 | 0 | 0 | 32 | 1 | 3 | 2 starch |
| Classic Pilaf | 2/3 cup | 190 | 0.5 | 5 | 0 | 0 | 0 | 790 | 43 | 1 | 5 | 3 starch |
| Gold Rice, Parboiled | 1 cup | 160 | 0 | 0 | 0 | 0 | 0 | 0 | 37 | 1 | 3 | 2 1/2 starch |
| Thai Jasmine Rice | 3/4 cup | 160 | 0 | 0 | 0 | 0 | 0 | 0 | 36 | 0 | 3 | 2 1/2 starch |

| | | | | | | | | | | | | |
|---|---|---|---|---|---|---|---|---|---|---|---|---|
| ***Minute Rice*** | | | | | | | | | | | | |
| Boil-In-Bag Rice | 1 cup | 180 | 0 | 0 | 0 | 0 | 0 | 10 | 42 | <1 | 4 | 3 starch |
| Brown Rice, Instant | 2/3 cup | 150 | 1.5 | 15 | 0 | 0 | 0 | 10 | 34 | 2 | 3 | 2 starch |
| White Rice, Instant | 1 cup | 200 | 0 | 0 | 0 | 0 | 0 | 5 | 45 | <1 | 5 | 3 starch |
| ***Near East*** | | | | | | | | | | | | |
| ***Long Grain & Wild Rice*** | | | | | | | | | | | | |
| Garlic & Herb | 1 cup | 220 | 4 | 35 | 2 | 0 | 10 | 720 | 43 | 2 | 5 | 3 starch, 1 fat |
| Original | 1 cup | 220 | 4 | 35 | 2 | 0 | 10 | 830 | 43 | 2 | 5 | 3 starch, 1 fat |
| ***Rice Pilaf*** | | | | | | | | | | | | |
| Garlic & Herb | 1 cup | 220 | 4 | 30 | 0.5 | 0 | 0 | 680 | 44 | 1 | 5 | 3 starch, 1 fat |
| Original | 1 cup | 220 | 4 | 30 | 2 | 0 | 10 | 820 | 44 | 1 | 5 | 3 starch, 1 fat |
| Roasted Chicken & Garlic | 1 cup | 220 | 3 | 25 | 1.5 | 0 | 5 | 600 | 44 | 2 | 5 | 3 starch, 1 fat |
| Spanish Rice | 1 cup | 310 | 8 | 70 | 5 | 0 | 20 | 1090 | 54 | 2 | 5 | 3 1/2 starch, 2 fat |
| Sundried Tomato & Basil | 1 cup | 290 | 7 | 60 | 1 | 0 | 0 | 1030 | 54 | 2 | 6 | 3 1/2 starch, 1 fat |

| | Serving | Calories | Fat (g) | Cal. from Fat | Sat. Fat (g) | Trans Fat (g) | Chol. (mg) | Sod. (mg) | Carb. (g) | Fiber (g) | Prot. (g) | Servings/Exchanges |
|---|---|---|---|---|---|---|---|---|---|---|---|---|
| Toasted Almond | 1 cup | 230 | 6 | 50 | 0 | 0 | 10 | 670 | 40 | 2 | 5 | 2 1/2 starch, 1 fat |
| Wild Mushroom & Herb | 1 cup | 220 | 4 | 30 | 2 | 0 | 10 | 570 | 43 | 1 | 5 | 3 starch, 1 fat |
| ***Rice-A-Roni*** | | | | | | | | | | | | |
| Beef | 1 cup | 310 | 9 | 80 | 1.5 | 1.5 | 0 | 1100 | 51 | 2 | 7 | 3 1/2 starch, 2 fat |
| Chicken & Garlic | 1 cup | 260 | 8 | 70 | 1.5 | 1.5 | 0 | 820 | 41 | 1 | 5 | 2 1/2 starch, 2 fat |
| Chicken & Broccoli | 1 cup | 220 | 5 | 45 | 1 | 1 | 0 | 1020 | 40 | 2 | 6 | 2 1/2 starch, 1 fat |
| Country Cheddar | 1 cup | 370 | 17 | 150 | 5 | 2 | 10 | 1080 | 49 | 2 | 6 | 3 starch, 3 fat |
| Creamy Four Cheese | 1 cup | 280 | 12 | 110 | 4 | 1.5 | 5 | 810 | 37 | 1 | 6 | 2 1/2 starch, 2 fat |
| Long Grain & Wild Rice | 1 cup | 240 | 6 | 50 | 1 | 1 | 0 | 910 | 42 | 2 | 5 | 3 starch, 1 fat |
| Mexican Style | 1 cup | 250 | 8 | 70 | 1.5 | 1 | 0 | 820 | 40 | 2 | 6 | 2 1/2 starch, 2 fat |
| Parmesan Chicken | 1 cup | 370 | 15 | 140 | 4.5 | 2 | 5 | 1360 | 51 | 3 | 8 | 3 1/2 starch, 3 fat |
| Spanish | 1 cup | 260 | 7 | 60 | 1.5 | 1 | 0 | 1340 | 44 | 2 | 6 | 3 starch, 1 fat |
| ***Rice-A-Roni Savory Whole Grain Blends*** | | | | | | | | | | | | |
| Chicken Herb Classico | 1 cup | 260 | 8 | 70 | 1 | 0 | 0 | 760 | 41 | 4 | 6 | 2 1/2 starch, 2 fat |

| | | | | | | | | | | | | |
|---|---|---|---|---|---|---|---|---|---|---|---|---|
| Roasted Garlic Italiano | 1 cup | 270 | 9 | 80 | 1.5 | 0 | 0 | 760 | 41 | 3 | 6 | 2 1/2 starch, 2 fat |
| Spanish | 1 cup | 250 | 8 | 60 | 1 | 0 | 0 | 760 | 42 | 3 | 5 | 3 starch, 2 fat |
| ***Uncle Ben's*** | | | | | | | | | | | | |
| ***Country Inn Rice Dishes*** | | | | | | | | | | | | |
| Broccoli Rice Au Gratin | 1 cup | 200 | 2 | 20 | 1 | 0 | 5 | 790 | 43 | 1 | 4 | 3 starch |
| Chicken & Broccoli | 1 cup | 190 | 1 | 10 | 0 | 0 | 0 | 910 | 42 | 1 | 5 | 3 starch |
| Chicken & Vegetable | 1 cup | 200 | 1.5 | 15 | 0.5 | 0 | 0 | 720 | 41 | 1 | 5 | 2 1/2 starch |
| Chicken & Wild Rice | 1 cup | 200 | 1 | 5 | 0.5 | 0 | 0 | 800 | 42 | 1 | 5 | 3 starch |
| Chicken Flavored | 1 cup | 200 | 1 | 10 | 0 | 0 | 0 | 940 | 41 | 1 | 6 | 2 1/2 starch |
| Mexican Fiesta | 1 cup | 200 | 1 | 5 | 0 | 0 | 0 | 680 | 42 | 1 | 5 | 3 starch |
| Oriental Fried Rice | 1 cup | 200 | 1 | 20 | 0 | 0 | 0 | 580 | 42 | 1 | 6 | 3 starch |
| Rice Pilaf | 1 cup | 200 | 0.5 | 5 | 0 | 0 | 0 | 640 | 43 | 1 | 5 | 3 starch |
| ***Long Grain & Wild Rice*** | | | | | | | | | | | | |
| Butter & Herb | 1 cup | 190 | 1 | 10 | 0 | 0 | 0 | 810 | 40 | 1 | 5 | 2 1/2 starch |
| Fast Cook Recipe | 1 cup | 190 | 0.5 | 5 | 0 | 0 | 0 | 680 | 41 | 1 | 5 | 2 1/2 starch |
| Original Recipe | 1 cup | 200 | 0 | 0 | 0 | 0 | 0 | 670 | 44 | 1 | 6 | 3 starch |

| | Serving | Calories | Fat (g) | Cal. from Fat | Sat. Fat (g) | Trans Fat (g) | Chol. (mg) | Sod. (mg) | Carb. (g) | Fiber (g) | Prot. (g) | Servings/Exchanges |
|---|---|---|---|---|---|---|---|---|---|---|---|---|
| Roasted Garlic & Olive Oil | 1 cup | 180 | 1 | 10 | 0 | 0 | 0 | 590 | 39 | 3 | 5 | 2 1/2 starch |
| Vegetable Pilaf | 1 cup | 180 | 1 | 10 | 0 | 0 | 0 | 610 | 40 | 3 | 5 | 2 1/2 starch |
| Whole Grain & Wild Rice with Mushroom | 1 cup | 200 | 1.5 | 10 | 1.5 | 0 | 0 | 570 | 42 | 3 | 6 | 3 starch |
| ***Ready Rice*** | | | | | | | | | | | | |
| Long Grain & Wild | 1 cup | 220 | 3 | 25 | 0 | 0 | 0 | 900 | 43 | 2 | 5 | 3 starch, 1 fat |
| Original Long Grain | 1 cup | 200 | 2.5 | 25 | 0 | 0 | 0 | 10 | 40 | 1 | 4 | 2 1/2 starch, 1 fat |
| Rice Pilaf | 1 cup | 220 | 3.5 | 35 | 0.5 | 0 | 0 | 970 | 42 | 2 | 6 | 2 1/2 starch, 1 fat |
| Roasted Chicken | 1 cup | 220 | 3.5 | 30 | 0 | 0 | 0 | 1020 | 41 | 2 | 5 | 2 1/2 starch |
| Spanish Style | 1 cup | 200 | 2.5 | 30 | 0 | 0 | 0 | 680 | 41 | 3 | 4 | 2 1/2 starch, 1 fat |
| Teriyaki Style | 1 cup | 220 | 3 | 25 | 0 | 0 | 5 | 870 | 42 | 3 | 6 | 3 starch, 1 fat |
| ***Ready Whole Grain Medley*** | | | | | | | | | | | | |
| Brown & Wild | 1 cup | 220 | 3.5 | 30 | 0 | 0 | 0 | 730 | 42 | 3 | 6 | 3 starch, 1 fat |

| | | | | | | | | | | | | |
|---|---|---|---|---|---|---|---|---|---|---|---|---|
| Santa Fe | 1 cup | 220 | 3 | 25 | 0 | 0 | 0 | 700 | 42 | 5 | 7 | 3 starch, 1 fat |
| Vegetable Harvest | 1 cup | 220 | 3 | 25 | 0 | 0 | 0 | 780 | 44 | 5 | 5 | 3 starch, 1 fat |
| ***White Rice*** | | | | | | | | | | | | |
| Boil-In-Bag | 1 cup | 190 | 0.5 | 5 | 0 | 0 | 0 | 0 | 44 | 1 | 4 | 3 starch |
| Instant | 1 cup | 190 | 0.5 | 5 | 0 | 0 | 0 | 15 | 43 | 1 | 3 | 3 starch |
| Original Converted Rice | 1 cup | 170 | 0 | 0 | 0 | 0 | 0 | 0 | 37 | 0 | 4 | 2 1/2starch |
| ***Whole Grain Brown Rice*** | | | | | | | | | | | | |
| Fast & Natural Instant Brown Rice | 1 cup | 170 | 1 | 10 | 0 | 0 | 0 | 20 | 36 | 2 | 4 | 2 1/2 starch |
| Natural Whole Grain Brown Rice | 1 cup | 170 | 1.5 | 10 | 0 | 0 | 0 | 0 | 35 | 2 | 5 | 2 starch |

| | Serving | Calories | Fat. (g) | Cal. from Fat | Sat. Fat (g) | Trans Fat (g) | Chol. (mg) | Sod. (mg) | Carb. (g) | Fiber (g) | Prot. (g) | Servings/Exchanges |
|---|---|---|---|---|---|---|---|---|---|---|---|---|
| **SALAD DRESSING** | | | | | | | | | | | | |
| Mayonnaise | 1 tsp | 33 | 4 | 35 | <1 | 0 | 2 | 26 | 0 | 0 | 0 | 1 fat |
| Mayonnaise, Fat-Free | 1 Tbsp | 13 | <1 | 0 | 0 | 0 | 1 | 126 | 2 | 0 | 0 | free |
| Mayonnaise, Light/ Reduced Fat | 1 Tbsp | 45 | 5 | 45 | <1 | 0 | 4 | 120 | 1 | 0 | 0 | 1 fat |
| Oil & Vinegar | 2 Tbsp | 144 | 16 | 145 | 3 | 0 | 0 | <1 | <1 | 0 | 0 | 3 fat |
| Salad Dressing, Fat-Free | 1 Tbsp | 20 | 0 | 0 | 0 | 0 | 0 | 145 | 5 | 0 | 0 | free |
| Salad Dressing, Reduced Fat, Cream Based | 2 Tbsp | 70 | 4 | 35 | <1 | 0 | 0 | 241 | 8 | 0 | 0 | 1/2 carb, 1 fat |
| Salad Dressing, Regular | 1 Tbsp | 69 | 7 | 65 | <1 | 0 | 0 | 125 | 2 | 0 | 0 | 1 fat |
| **Brands** | | | | | | | | | | | | |
| ***Bernstein's*** | | | | | | | | | | | | |
| Balsamic Italian | 2 Tbsp | 110 | 11 | 100 | 0.5 | 0 | 0 | 270 | 2 | 0 | 0 | 2 fat |

| | | | | | | | | | | | | |
|---|---|---|---|---|---|---|---|---|---|---|---|---|
| Basil Parmesan | 2 Tbsp | 100 | 10 | 90 | 1 | 0 | 5 | 400 | 2 | 0 | 1 | 2 fat |
| Cheese & Garlic Italian | 2 Tbsp | 110 | 11 | 100 | 1 | 0 | 0 | 340 | 2 | 0 | 1 | 2 fat |
| Cheese Fantastico | 2 Tbsp | 100 | 10 | 90 | 1 | 0 | 5 | 400 | 2 | 0 | 1 | 2 fat |
| Creamy Caesar | 2 Tbsp | 120 | 13 | 115 | 1 | 0 | 15 | 200 | 1 | 0 | 0 | 3 fat |
| Herb Garden French | 2 Tbsp | 130 | 12 | 110 | 1 | 0 | 0 | 260 | 6 | 0 | 0 | 1/2 carb, 2 fat |
| Light Fantastic Cheese Fantastico | 2 Tbsp | 25 | 1.5 | 15 | 0.5 | 0 | 0 | 370 | 2 | 0 | 1 | free |
| Light Fantastic Parmesan Garlic Ranch | 2 Tbsp | 50 | 2.5 | 25 | 0.5 | 0 | 5 | 330 | 6 | 0 | 1 | 1/2 carb, 1 fat |
| ***Best Foods*** | | | | | | | | | | | | |
| Canola Cholesterol Free Mayonnaise | 1 Tbsp | 45 | 4.5 | 40 | 0 | 0 | 0 | 90 | <1 | 0 | 0 | 1 fat |
| Light Mayonnaise | 1 Tbsp | 35 | 3.5 | 30 | 0 | 0 | <5 | 120 | 1 | 0 | 0 | 1 fat |
| Low Fat Mayonnaise Dressing | 1 Tbsp | 15 | 1 | 10 | 0 | 0 | 0 | 130 | 2 | 0 | 0 | free |

| | Serving | Calories | Fat (g) | Cal. from Fat | Sat. Fat (g) | Trans Fat (g) | Chol. (mg) | Sod. (mg) | Carb. (g) | Fiber (g) | Prot. (g) | Servings/Exchanges |
|---|---|---|---|---|---|---|---|---|---|---|---|---|
| Mayonnaise Dressing with Olive Oil | 1 Tbsp | 50 | 5 | 45 | 0.5 | 0 | 5 | 120 | <1 | 0 | 0 | 1 fat |
| Real Mayonnaise | 1 Tbsp | 90 | 10 | 90 | 1.5 | 0 | 5 | 85 | 0 | 0 | 0 | 2 fat |
| ***Cardini's*** | | | | | | | | | | | | |
| Balsamic Vinaigrette | 2 Tbsp | 100 | 8 | 80 | 1.5 | 0 | 0 | 250 | 5 | 0 | 0 | 2 fat |
| Fat Free Caesar | 2 Tbsp | 40 | 0 | 0 | 0 | 0 | 0 | 510 | 9 | 0 | 0 | 1/2 carb |
| Honey Mustard | 2 Tbsp | 140 | 13 | 120 | 2 | 0 | 0 | 220 | 5 | 0 | 0 | 3 fat |
| Italian | 2 Tbsp | 100 | 8 | 70 | 1 | 0 | 0 | 310 | 7 | 0 | 0 | 1/2 carb, 3 fat |
| Light Caesar | 2 Tbsp | 60 | 5 | 45 | 1 | 0 | 0 | 450 | 2 | 0 | 1 | 1 fat |
| Original Caesar | 2 Tbsp | 160 | 17 | 150 | 2.5 | 0 | 30 | 240 | 10 | 0 | 1 | 1/2 carb, 3 fat |
| Pear Vinaigrette | 2 Tbsp | 100 | 9 | 80 | 1.5 | 0 | 0 | 150 | 6 | 0 | 0 | 1/2 carb, 2 fat |
| Roasted Asian Sesame | 2 Tbsp | 120 | 10 | 90 | 1.5 | 0 | 0 | 360 | 7 | 0 | 0 | 1/2 carb, 2 fat |
| ***Dorothy Lynch*** | | | | | | | | | | | | |
| Fat Free Dressing | 2 Tbsp | 60 | 0 | 0 | 0 | 0 | 0 | 160 | 14 | 0 | 0 | 1 carb |

| | | | | | | | | | | | | |
|---|---|---|---|---|---|---|---|---|---|---|---|---|
| Home Style Dressing | 2 Tbsp | 110 | 6 | 55 | 1 | 0 | 0 | 170 | 12 | 0 | 0 | 1 carb, 1 fat |
| ***Girard's*** | | | | | | | | | | | | |
| Balsamic Basil | 2 Tbsp | 90 | 9 | 80 | 1.5 | 0 | 0 | 330 | 3 | 0 | 0 | 2 fat |
| Blue Cheese Vinaigrette | 2 Tbsp | 100 | 10 | 90 | 2 | 0 | 5 | 500 | 3 | 0 | 1 | 2 fat |
| Caesar | 2 Tbsp | 140 | 15 | 130 | 2.5 | 0 | 10 | 350 | 1 | 0 | 1 | 3 fat |
| Chinese Chicken Salad | 2 Tbsp | 120 | 11 | 100 | 1.5 | 0 | 0 | 350 | 6 | 0 | 0 | 1/2 carb, 2 fat |
| Greek Feta Vinaigrette | 2 Tbsp | 100 | 11 | 100 | 1.5 | 0 | 0 | 300 | 2 | 0 | 0 | 2 fat |
| Light Caesar | 2 Tbsp | 90 | 8 | 70 | 1.5 | 0 | 10 | 370 | 5 | 0 | 1 | 2 fat |
| Romano Cheese | 2 Tbsp | 130 | 13 | 120 | 2 | 0 | 0 | 500 | 2 | 0 | 1 | 3 fat |
| Spinach Salad | 2 Tbsp | 70 | 2 | 15 | 0 | 0 | 0 | 250 | 14 | 0 | 1 | 1 carb |
| ***Girard's Fat Free*** | | | | | | | | | | | | |
| Balsamic Vinaigrette | 2 Tbsp | 25 | 0 | 0 | 0 | 0 | 0 | 390 | 6 | 0 | 0 | 1/2 carb |
| Raspberry | 2 Tbsp | 60 | 0 | 0 | 0 | 0 | 0 | 210 | 14 | 0 | 0 | 1 carb |
| Fat Free Caesar | 2 Tbsp | 40 | 0 | 0 | 0 | 0 | 0 | 510 | 9 | 0 | 0 | 1/2 carb |
| ***Hidden Valley*** | | | | | | | | | | | | |
| Buttermilk Ranch Light | 2 Tbsp | 70 | 5 | 50 | 1 | 0 | 5 | 310 | 3 | 0 | 1 | 1 fat |

| | Serving | Calories | Fat (g) | Cal. from Fat | Sat. Fat (g) | Trans Fat (g) | Chol. (mg) | Sod. (mg) | Carb. (g) | Fiber (g) | Prot. (g) | Servings/Exchanges |
|---|---|---|---|---|---|---|---|---|---|---|---|---|
| Coleslaw Dressing | 2 Tbsp | 150 | 15 | 130 | 2.5 | 0 | 15 | 170 | 5 | 0 | 0 | 3 fat |
| Old-Fashioned Buttermilk Ranch | 2 Tbsp | 140 | 14 | 130 | 2 | 0 | 10 | 340 | 2 | 0 | 0 | 3 fat |
| Original Ranch | 2 Tbsp | 140 | 14 | 130 | 2.5 | 0 | 10 | 260 | 2 | 0 | 1 | 3 fat |
| Original Ranch Fat Free | 2 Tbsp | 30 | 0 | 0 | 0 | 0 | 0 | 310 | 6 | 0 | 0 | 1/2 carb |
| Original Ranch Light | 2 Tbsp | 80 | 7 | 70 | 1 | 0 | 5 | 290 | 3 | 0 | 1 | 1 fat |
| ***Ken's Steak House*** | | | | | | | | | | | | |
| Buttermilk Ranch | 2 Tbsp | 180 | 20 | 180 | 3 | 0 | 5 | 280 | 1 | 0 | 0 | 4 fat |
| Country French | 2 Tbsp | 130 | 12 | 110 | 1.5 | 0 | 0 | 150 | 9 | 0 | 0 | 1/2 carb, 2 fat |
| Lite Caesar | 2 Tbsp | 70 | 6 | 60 | 1 | 0 | 0 | 620 | 3 | 0 | 1 | 1 fat |
| Lite Country French | 2 Tbsp | 100 | 6 | 50 | 1 | 0 | 0 | 230 | 11 | 0 | 0 | 1 carb, 1 fat |
| Lite Olive Oil Vinaigrette | 2 Tbsp | 60 | 6 | 50 | 1 | 0 | 0 | 240 | 3 | 0 | 0 | 1 fat |
| ***Kraft*** | | | | | | | | | | | | |
| Catalina | 2 Tbsp | 130 | 11 | 100 | 1.5 | 0 | 0 | 380 | 7 | 0 | 0 | 1/2 carb, 2 fat |

| | | | | | | | | | | | | |
|---|---|---|---|---|---|---|---|---|---|---|---|---|
| Classic Caesar | 2 Tbsp | 130 | 12 | 110 | 2.5 | 0 | 15 | 380 | 2 | 0 | 2 | 2 fat |
| Honey Dijon Vinaigrette | 2 Tbsp | 90 | 7 | 60 | 0.5 | 0 | 0 | 340 | 6 | 0 | <1 | 1/2 carb, 1 fat |
| Ranch | 2 Tbsp | 120 | 12 | 110 | 2 | 0 | 5 | 370 | 3 | 0 | 0 | 2 fat |
| Roka Blue Cheese | 2 Tbsp | 120 | 13 | 120 | 2 | 0 | 5 | 380 | 1 | 0 | 0 | 3 fat |
| Thousand Island | 2 Tbsp | 110 | 10 | 90 | 1.5 | 0 | 0 | 330 | 5 | 0 | 0 | 2 fat |
| Three Cheese Ranch | 2 Tbsp | 120 | 12 | 110 | 2 | 0 | 0 | 360 | 3 | 0 | 0 | 2 fat |
| Zesty Italian | 2 Tbsp | 70 | 6 | 50 | 1 | 0 | 0 | 370 | 3 | 0 | 0 | 1 fat |
| ***Kraft Free (Fat Free)*** | | | | | | | | | | | | |
| Catalina | 2 Tbsp | 50 | 0 | 0 | 0 | 0 | 0 | 350 | 11 | 0 | 0 | 1 carb |
| French | 2 Tbsp | 45 | 0 | 0 | 0 | 0 | 0 | 290 | 11 | 0 | 0 | 1 carb |
| Honey Dijon | 2 Tbsp | 50 | 0 | 0 | 0 | 0 | 0 | 330 | 12 | 0 | 0 | 1 carb |
| Ranch | 2 Tbsp | 50 | 0 | 0 | 0 | 0 | 0 | 330 | 11 | 0 | 0 | 1 carb |
| ***Kraft Light*** | | | | | | | | | | | | |
| Caesar | 2 Tbsp | 60 | 4.5 | 40 | 1 | 0 | 10 | 320 | 3 | 0 | 0 | 1 fat |
| Ranch | 2 Tbsp | 80 | 6 | 60 | 1 | 0 | 10 | 440 | 7 | 0 | 0 | 1/2 carb, 1 fat |
| Red Wine Vinaigrette | 2 Tbsp | 45 | 4 | 35 | 0 | 0 | 0 | 310 | 3 | 0 | 0 | 1 fat |

| | Serving | Calories | Fat (g) | Cal. from Fat | Sat. Fat (g) | Trans Fat (g) | Chol. (mg) | Sod. (mg) | Carb. (g) | Fiber (g) | Prot. (g) | Servings/Exchanges |
|---|---|---|---|---|---|---|---|---|---|---|---|---|
| Thousand Island | 2 Tbsp | 60 | 3 | 20 | 0 | 0 | 10 | 340 | 11 | 0 | 0 | 1 carb |
| Three Cheese Ranch | 2 Tbsp | 70 | 8 | 70 | 1.5 | 0 | 0 | 450 | 2 | 0 | 0 | 2 fat |
| ***Kraft Miracle Whip, Mayonnaise*** | | | | | | | | | | | | |
| Mayonnaise | 1 Tbsp | 90 | 10 | 90 | 1.5 | 0 | 5 | 70 | 0 | 0 | 0 | 2 fat |
| Mayonnaise, Fat Free | 1 Tbsp | 10 | 0 | 0 | 0 | 0 | 0 | 120 | 2 | 0 | 0 | free |
| Mayonnaise, Light | 1 Tbsp | 45 | 4 | 35 | 0.5 | 0 | 5 | 95 | 2 | 0 | 0 | 1 fat |
| Mayonnaise, Reduced Fat with Olive Oil | 1 Tbsp | 45 | 4 | 35 | 0 | 0 | 0 | 95 | 2 | 0 | 0 | 1 fat |
| Miracle Whip | 1 Tbsp | 40 | 3.5 | 35 | 0.5 | 0 | 5 | 105 | 2 | 0 | 0 | 1 fat |
| Miracle Whip, Fat Free | 1 Tbsp | 15 | 0 | 0 | 0 | 0 | 0 | 125 | 3 | 0 | 0 | free |
| Miracle Whip, Light | 1 Tbsp | 25 | 1.5 | 15 | 0 | 0 | 5 | 140 | 3 | 0 | 0 | free |
| ***Litehouse*** | | | | | | | | | | | | |
| Big Bleu | 2 Tbsp | 160 | 17 | 150 | 2 | 0 | 15 | 230 | 1 | 0 | 1 | 3 fat |
| Coleslaw | 2 Tbsp | 100 | 8 | 70 | 0.5 | 0 | 5 | 120 | 8 | 0 | 0 | 1/2 carb, 2 fat |

| | | | | | | | | | | | | |
|---|---|---|---|---|---|---|---|---|---|---|---|---|
| Creamy Asian | 2 Tbsp | 130 | 13 | 110 | 1 | 0 | 10 | 170 | 4 | 0 | 0 | 3 fat |
| Creamy Cilantro | 2 Tbsp | 110 | 10 | 90 | 1 | 0 | 10 | 230 | 3 | 0 | 1 | 2 fat |
| Lite Bleu Cheese | 2 Tbsp | 70 | 6 | 60 | 0.5 | 0 | 5 | 240 | 2 | 0 | 1 | 1 fat |
| Lite Ranch | 2 Tbsp | 60 | 6 | 50 | 0.5 | 0 | 10 | 230 | 3 | 0 | 1 | 1 fat |
| Original Bleu Cheese | 2 Tbsp | 150 | 16 | 140 | 1.5 | 0 | 15 | 220 | 1 | 0 | 1 | 3 fat |
| Parmesan Caesar | 2 Tbsp | 100 | 10 | 90 | 1 | 0 | 5 | 220 | 3 | 0 | 1 | 2 fat |
| Ranch | 2 Tbsp | 120 | 12 | 110 | 1 | 0 | 10 | 220 | 2 | 0 | 1 | 2 fat |
| Sesame Ginger, Fat Free | 2 Tbsp | 35 | 0 | 0 | 0 | 0 | 0 | 230 | 8 | 0 | 0 | 1/2 carb |
| Spinach Salad | 2 Tbsp | 50 | 0 | 0 | 0 | 0 | 0 | 260 | 11 | 0 | 1 | 1 carb |
| Sweet & Sour | 2 Tbsp | 70 | 3.5 | 30 | 0 | 0 | 5 | 240 | 9 | 0 | 0 | 1/2 carb, 1 fat |
| Tangy Orange Citrus, Fat Free | 2 Tbsp | 50 | 0 | 0 | 0 | 0 | 0 | 190 | 13 | 0 | 0 | 1 carb |
| Thai Peanut | 2 Tbsp | 60 | 3 | 30 | 0 | 0 | 0 | 280 | 6 | 1 | 1 | 1/2 carb, 1 fat |
| ***Maple Grove Farms of Vermont*** | | | | | | | | | | | | |
| Fat Free Balsamic Vinaigrette | 2 Tbsp | 5 | 0 | 0 | 0 | 0 | 0 | 160 | 1 | 0 | 0 | free |

| | Serving | Calories | Fat (g) | Cal. from Fat | Sat. Fat (g) | Trans Fat (g) | Chol. (mg) | Sod. (mg) | Carb. (g) | Fiber (g) | Prot. (g) | Servings/Exchanges |
|---|---|---|---|---|---|---|---|---|---|---|---|---|
| Fat Free Cranberry Balsamic | 2 Tbsp | 20 | 0 | 0 | 0 | 0 | 0 | 180 | 7 | 0 | 0 | 1/2 carb |
| Fat Free Honey Dijon | 2 Tbsp | 40 | 0 | 0 | 0 | 0 | 0 | 200 | 10 | <1 | 0 | 1 carb |
| Honey Mustard | 2 Tbsp | 100 | 8 | 70 | 0.5 | 0 | 0 | 260 | 8 | 0 | <1 | 1/2 carb, 2 fat |
| Light Caesar | 2 Tbsp | 60 | 4.5 | 40 | 1 | 0 | 5 | 270 | 4 | 0 | 0 | 1 fat |
| Light Romano | 2 Tbsp | 40 | 3.5 | 30 | 0 | 0 | 0 | 260 | 1 | 0 | <1 | 1 fat |
| Parmesan & Cracked Pepper | 2 Tbsp | 120 | 11 | 100 | 1 | 0 | 0 | 360 | 3 | 0 | <1 | 2 fat |
| ***Marie's*** | | | | | | | | | | | | |
| Balsamic Vinaigrette | 2 Tbsp | 50 | 4.5 | 40 | 0.5 | 0 | 0 | 220 | 3 | 0 | 0 | 1 fat |
| Caesar | 2 Tbsp | 170 | 19 | 170 | 3.5 | 0 | 15 | 170 | 1 | 0 | 1 | 4 fat |
| Chunky Blue Cheese | 2 Tbsp | 160 | 17 | 150 | 3.5 | 0 | 15 | 170 | 0 | 0 | 1 | 3 fat |
| Coleslaw | 2 Tbsp | 150 | 13 | 120 | 2 | 0 | 10 | 170 | 8 | 0 | 0 | 1/2 carb, 3 fat |
| Creamy Ranch | 2 Tbsp | 170 | 19 | 170 | 3 | 0 | 15 | 150 | 1 | 0 | 1 | 4 fat |

| | | | | | | | | | | | | |
|---|---|---|---|---|---|---|---|---|---|---|---|---|
| Italian Vinaigrette | 2 Tbsp | 80 | 8 | 70 | 1.5 | 0 | 0 | 350 | 3 | 0 | 0 | 2 fat |
| Lite Chunky Blue Cheese | 2 Tbsp | 80 | 6 | 60 | 1.5 | 0 | 5 | 280 | 7 | 4 | 1 | 1/2 carb, 1 fat |
| Lite Creamy Ranch | 2 Tbsp | 90 | 6 | 60 | 1 | 0 | 5 | 240 | 6 | 0 | 1 | 1/2 carb, 1 fat |
| Poppy Seed | 2 Tbsp | 150 | 13 | 120 | 2 | 0 | 10 | 170 | 8 | 0 | 0 | 1/2 carb, 3 fat |
| Premium Spinach Salad | 2 Tbsp | 70 | 1.5 | 15 | 0 | 0 | 0 | 330 | 13 | 0 | 1 | 1 carb |
| Raspberry Vinaigrette | 2 Tbsp | 40 | 0.5 | 5 | 0 | 0 | 0 | 60 | 8 | 0 | 0 | 1/2 carb |
| Red Wine Vinaigrette | 2 Tbsp | 60 | 4.5 | 40 | 0.5 | 0 | 0 | 210 | 6 | 0 | 0 | 1/2 carb, 1 fat |
| Thousand Island | 2 Tbsp | 150 | 15 | 140 | 2.5 | 0 | 15 | 210 | 4 | 0 | 0 | 3 fat |
| Yogurt Feta Cheese | 2 Tbsp | 70 | 7 | 60 | 1.5 | 0 | 15 | 190 | 2 | 0 | 1 | 1 fat |
| ***Newman's Own*** | | | | | | | | | | | | |
| Balsamic Vinaigrette | 2 Tbsp | 90 | 9 | 80 | 1 | 0 | 0 | 350 | 3 | 0 | 0 | 2 fat |
| Caesar | 2 Tbsp | 150 | 16 | 140 | 1.5 | 0 | 0 | 420 | 1 | 0 | 1 | 3 fat |
| Family Recipe Italian | 2 Tbsp | 120 | 13 | 120 | 1 | 0 | 0 | 400 | 1 | 0 | 1 | 3 fat |
| Olive Oil & Vinegar | 2 Tbsp | 150 | 16 | 150 | 2.5 | 0 | 0 | 150 | 1 | 0 | 0 | 3 fat |
| Ranch | 2 Tbsp | 140 | 15 | 130 | 2 | 0 | 10 | 250 | 2 | 0 | 0 | 3 fat |

SALAD DRESSING

| | Serving | Calories | Fat (g) | Cal. from Fat | Sat. Fat (g) | Trans Fat (g) | Chol. (mg) | Sod. (mg) | Carb. (g) | Fiber (g) | Prot. (g) | Servings/Exchanges |
|---|---|---|---|---|---|---|---|---|---|---|---|---|
| ***Newman's Own Lighten Up*** | | | | | | | | | | | | |
| Balsamic Vinaigrette | 2 Tbsp | 45 | 4 | 40 | 0.5 | 0 | 0 | 470 | 2 | 0 | 0 | 1 fat |
| Caesar | 2 Tbsp | 70 | 6 | 50 | 1 | 0 | 5 | 520 | 3 | 0 | 1 | 1 fat |
| Honey Mustard | 2 Tbsp | 70 | 4 | 35 | 0.5 | 0 | 0 | 290 | 7 | 0 | 0 | 1 fat |
| Italian | 2 Tbsp | 60 | 6 | 50 | 1 | 0 | 0 | 260 | 0 | 0 | 0 | 1 fat |
| Raspberry & Walnut | 2 Tbsp | 70 | 5 | 45 | 0.5 | 0 | 0 | 120 | 7 | 0 | 0 | 1/2 carb, 1 fat |
| ***Rao's Homemade*** | | | | | | | | | | | | |
| 8 Star Balsamic | 2 Tbsp | 140 | 14 | 130 | 1.5 | 0 | 0 | 240 | 2 | 0 | 0 | 3 fat |
| Caesar Salad | 2 Tbsp | 80 | 8 | 70 | 1 | 0 | 0 | 310 | 2 | 0 | 1 | 2 fat |
| Italian Herb | 2 Tbsp | 80 | 8 | 70 | 0.5 | 0 | 0 | 370 | 2 | 0 | 0 | 2 fat |
| Roasted Garlic Vinaigrette | 2 Tbsp | 140 | 16 | 140 | 1.5 | 0 | 0 | 180 | 1 | 0 | 0 | 3 fat |
| ***Seven Seas*** | | | | | | | | | | | | |
| Creamy Italian | 2 Tbsp | 110 | 12 | 110 | 2 | 0 | 0 | 510 | 2 | 0 | 0 | 2 fat |

| | | | | | | | | | | | | |
|---|---|---|---|---|---|---|---|---|---|---|---|---|
| Green Goddess | 2 Tbsp | 130 | 13 | 120 | 2 | 0 | 0 | 260 | 2 | 0 | 0 | 3 fat |
| Red Wine Vinaigrette | 2 Tbsp | 90 | 9 | 80 | 1 | 0 | 0 | 470 | 2 | 0 | 0 | 2 fat |
| Viva Italian Fat Free | 2 Tbsp | 15 | 0 | 0 | 0 | 0 | 0 | 480 | 2 | 0 | 0 | free |
| Viva Italian Reduced Fat | 2 Tbsp | 45 | 4 | 35 | 0.5 | 0 | 0 | 370 | 2 | 0 | 0 | 1 fat |
| Viva Robust Italian | 2 Tbsp | 90 | 9 | 80 | 0.5 | 0 | 0 | 380 | 2 | 0 | 0 | 2 fat |
| ***South Beach*** | | | | | | | | | | | | |
| Italian with Extra Virgin Olive Oil | 2 Tbsp | 50 | 4.5 | 40 | 0 | 0 | 0 | 300 | 3 | 0 | 0 | 1 fat |
| Ranch | 2 Tbsp | 70 | 7 | 60 | 1 | 0 | 0 | 300 | 2 | 0 | 1 | 1 fat |
| ***Trader Joe's*** | | | | | | | | | | | | |
| Balsamic Vinaigrette | 2 Tbsp | 80 | 6 | 60 | 0 | 0 | 0 | 60 | 5 | 0 | 0 | 1 fat |
| Fat Free Balsamic Vinaigrette | 2 Tbsp | 25 | 0 | 0 | 0 | 0 | 0 | 170 | 6 | 0 | 0 | 1/2 carb |
| Goddess | 2 Tbsp | 130 | 13 | 120 | 1 | 0 | 0 | 320 | 1 | 0 | 1 | 3 fat |
| Organic Red Wine & Olive Oil Vinaigrette | 2 Tbsp | 140 | 15 | 140 | 2 | 0 | 0 | 190 | 0 | 0 | 0 | 3 fat |

| | Serving | Calories | Fat (g) | Cal. from Fat | Sat. Fat (g) | Trans Fat (g) | Chol. (mg) | Sod. (mg) | Carb. (g) | Fiber (g) | Prot. (g) | Servings/Exchanges |
|---|---|---|---|---|---|---|---|---|---|---|---|---|
| Raspberry Vinaigrette | 2 Tbsp | 35 | 1.5 | 15 | 0 | 0 | 0 | 75 | 5 | 0 | 0 | 1 fat |
| Romano Caesar | 2 Tbsp | 180 | 20 | 180 | 1.5 | 0 | 1 | 150 | <1 | 0 | <1 | 4 fat |
| Sesame Soy Ginger Vinaigrette | 2 Tbsp | 35 | 0 | 0 | 0 | 0 | 0 | 230 | 9 | 0 | 0 | 1/2 carb |
| Sweet Poppyseed | 2 Tbsp | 90 | 5 | 45 | 0.5 | 0 | 0 | 45 | 11 | 0 | 0 | 1 carb, 1 fat |
| Tuscan Italian | 2 Tbsp | 80 | 7 | 60 | 0.5 | 0 | 0 | 240 | 5 | 0 | 0 | 1 fat |
| ***Vidalia*** | | | | | | | | | | | | |
| Creamy Vidalia | 2 Tbsp | 60 | 4.5 | 40 | 0 | 0 | 0 | 160 | 7 | 0 | 0 | 1/2 carb, 1 fat |
| Honey Mustard | 2 Tbsp | 60 | 3.5 | 35 | 3.5 | 0 | 0 | 95 | 6 | 0 | 0 | 1/2 carb, 1 fat |
| Raspberry Vinaigrette | 2 Tbsp | 35 | 0 | 0 | 0 | 0 | 0 | 25 | 9 | 0 | 0 | 1/2 carb |
| Sun Dried Tomato | 2 Tbsp | 90 | 8 | 70 | 1 | 0 | 0 | 330 | 4 | 0 | 0 | 2 fat |
| ***Wish-Bone*** | | | | | | | | | | | | |
| Blue Cheese with Gorgonzola | 2 Tbsp | 140 | 15 | 140 | 2.5 | 0 | <5 | 300 | 1 | 0 | 0 | 3 fat |

| | | | | | | | | | | |
|---|---|---|---|---|---|---|---|---|---|---|
| Chunky Blue Cheese | 2 Tbsp | 150 | 15 | 140 | 2.5 | 0 | 5 | 260 | 2 | 0 | 0 | 3 fat |
| Creamy Caesar | 2 Tbsp | 170 | 18 | 160 | 3 | 0 | 10 | 300 | 1 | 0 | <1 | 4 fat |
| Creamy Italian | 2 Tbsp | 110 | 10 | 90 | 1.5 | 0 | 0 | 240 | 4 | 0 | <1 | 2 fat |
| Deluxe French | 2 Tbsp | 120 | 11 | 100 | 1.5 | 0 | 0 | 170 | 5 | 0 | <1 | 2 fat |
| Fat Free Western | 2 Tbsp | 50 | 0 | 0 | 0 | 0 | 0 | 280 | 12 | 0 | 0 | 1 carb |
| House Italian | 2 Tbsp | 100 | 10 | 90 | 1.5 | 0 | 5 | 260 | 3 | 0 | 0 | 2 fat |
| Italian | 2 Tbsp | 80 | 7 | 60 | 1 | 0 | 0 | 510 | 3 | 0 | 0 | 2 fat |
| Olive Oil Vinaigrette | 2 Tbsp | 60 | 5 | 45 | 0.5 | 0 | 0 | 250 | 4 | 0 | 0 | 1 fat |
| Ranch | 2 Tbsp | 120 | 13 | 120 | 2 | 0 | 5 | 250 | 2 | 0 | 0 | 3 fat |
| Raspberry Hazelnut Vinaigrette | 2 Tbsp | 80 | 5 | 45 | 0.5 | 0 | 0 | 260 | 9 | 0 | 0 | 1/2 carb, 1 fat |
| Red Wine Vinaigrette | 2 Tbsp | 80 | 5 | 45 | 1 | 0 | 0 | 240 | 9 | 0 | 0 | 1/2 carb, 1 fat |
| Russian | 2 Tbsp | 120 | 6 | 50 | 1 | 0 | 0 | 360 | 14 | 0 | 0 | 1 carb, 1 fat |
| Sweet & Spicy French | 2 Tbsp | 130 | 12 | 110 | 1.5 | 0 | 0 | 330 | 6 | 0 | 0 | 1/2 carb, 2 fat |
| Thousand Island | 2 Tbsp | 130 | 12 | 110 | 2 | 0 | 10 | 300 | 6 | 0 | 0 | 1/2 carb, 2 fat |
| Western | 2 Tbsp | 160 | 12 | 110 | 1.5 | 0 | 0 | 230 | 11 | 0 | 0 | 1 carb, 2 fat |

| | Serving | Calories | Fat (g) | Cal. from Fat | Sat. Fat (g) | Trans Fat (g) | Chol. (mg) | Sod. (mg) | Carb. (g) | Fiber (g) | Prot. (g) | Servings/Exchanges |
|---|---|---|---|---|---|---|---|---|---|---|---|---|
| ***Wish-Bone Fat Free*** | | | | | | | | | | | | |
| Chunky Blue Cheese | 2 Tbsp | 35 | 0 | 0 | 0 | 0 | 0 | 270 | 7 | <1 | <1 | 1/2 carb |
| Italian | 2 Tbsp | 20 | 0 | 0 | 0 | 0 | 0 | 350 | 4 | 0 | 0 | free |
| Ranch | 2 Tbsp | 30 | 0 | 0 | 0 | 0 | 0 | 280 | 7 | <1 | 0 | 1/2 carb |
| Red Wine Vinaigrette | 2 Tbsp | 30 | 0 | 0 | 0 | 0 | 0 | 230 | 7 | 0 | 0 | 1/2 carb |

| | Serving | Calories | Fat (g) | Cal. from Fat | Sat. Fat (g) | Trans Fat (g) | Chol. (mg) | Sod. (mg) | Carb. (g) | Fiber (g) | Prot. (g) | Servings/Exchanges |
|---|---|---|---|---|---|---|---|---|---|---|---|---|
| **SAUCES, GRAVIES, CONDIMENTS, RELISHES** | | | | | | | | | | | | |
| Apple Butter | 2 Tbsp | 65 | <1 | 0 | <1 | 0 | 0 | 0 | 17 | <1 | <1 | 1 carb |
| Catsup/Ketchup | 1 Tbsp | 16 | <1 | 0 | <1 | 0 | 0 | 182 | 4 | <1 | <1 | free |
| Catsup/Ketchup, Low Sodium | 1 Tbsp | 16 | <1 | 0 | <1 | 0 | 0 | 3 | 4 | <1 | <1 | free |
| Chutney | 1 Tbsp | 26 | <1 | 0 | <1 | 0 | 0 | 38 | 7 | <1 | <1 | 1/2 carb |
| Gravy, Au Jus, Canned | 1/2 cup | 19 | <1 | 0 | <1 | NA | 0 | 60 | 3 | 0 | 1 | free |
| Gravy, Beef, Canned | 1/2 cup | 62 | 3 | 27 | 1 | NA | 4 | 652 | 6 | <1 | 4 | 1/2 carb, 1 fat |
| Gravy, Beef, Homemade | 1/2 cup | 89 | 5 | 45 | 2 | 0 | 3 | 767 | 7 | <1 | 4 | 1/2 carb, 1 fat |
| Gravy, Brown, Dry Mix with Water | 1/2 cup | 38 | <1 | 0 | <1 | 0 | 1 | 538 | 7 | <1 | 1 | 1/2 carb |
| Gravy, Chicken Giblet, Homemade | 1/2 cup | 97 | 5 | 45 | 1 | 0 | 55 | 683 | 6 | <1 | 6 | 1/2 carb, 1 fat |
| Gravy, Chicken, Canned | 1/2 cup | 94 | 7 | 63 | 2 | NA | 2 | 687 | 7 | <1 | 2 | 1/2 carb, 1 fat |

SAUCES, GRAVIES, CONDIMENTS, RELISHES

| | Serving | Calories | Fat (g) | Cal. from Fat | Sat. Fat (g) | Trans Fat (g) | Chol. (mg) | Sod. (mg) | Carb. (g) | Fiber (g) | Prot. (g) | Servings/Exchanges |
|---|---|---|---|---|---|---|---|---|---|---|---|---|
| Gravy, Mushroom, Canned | 1/2 cup | 60 | 6 | 54 | <1 | NA | 0 | 678 | 7 | <1 | 2 | 1/2 carb, 1 fat |
| Gravy, Sausage | 1/2 cup | 206 | 16 | 144 | 6 | NA | 33 | 408 | 8 | <1 | 8 | 1/2 carb, 3 fat |
| Gravy, Turkey, Canned | 1/2 cup | 61 | 3 | 27 | <1 | NA | 2 | 687 | 6 | <1 | 3 | 1/2 starch, 1 fat |
| Guacamole with Tomatoes | 1 Tbsp | 17 | 2 | 17 | <1 | 0 | 0 | 27 | 1 | <1 | <1 | free |
| Honey | 1 Tbsp | 64 | 0 | 0 | 0 | 0 | 0 | <1 | 17 | <1 | <1 | 1 carb |
| Horseradish, Prepared | 1 Tbsp | 7 | <1 | 0 | <1 | 0 | 0 | 47 | 2 | <1 | <1 | free |
| Jam, Cherry/Strawberry | 1 Tbsp | 54 | <1 | 0 | 0 | 0 | 0 | 2 | 14 | <1 | <1 | 1 carb |
| Jam/Marmalade, Artifically Sweetened | 1 Tbsp | 2 | <1 | 0 | <1 | 0 | 0 | 0 | 11 | <1 | <1 | free |
| Jam/Marmalade, Reduced Sugar | 1 Tbsp | 36 | <1 | 0 | <1 | 0 | 0 | 5 | 9 | <1 | <1 | 1/2 carb |
| Jam/Preserves | 1 Tbsp | 48 | <1 | 0 | <1 | 0 | 0 | 8 | 13 | <1 | <1 | 1 carb |

| | | | | | | | | | | | | |
|---|---|---|---|---|---|---|---|---|---|---|---|---|
| Jelly | 1 Tbsp | 52 | <1 | 0 | <1 | 0 | 0 | 7 | 14 | <1 | <1 | 1 carb |
| Jelly, Blackberry | 1 Tbsp | 50 | 0 | 0 | 0 | 0 | 0 | 10 | 13 | 0 | 0 | 1 carb |
| Jelly, Dietetic | 1 Tbsp | 6 | 0 | 0 | 0 | 0 | 0 | <1 | 11 | <1 | <1 | free |
| Jelly, Reduced Sugar | 1 Tbsp | 34 | <1 | 0 | <1 | 0 | 0 | <1 | 9 | <1 | <1 | 1/2 carb |
| Marmalade, Orange | 1 Tbsp | 49 | 0 | 0 | 0 | 0 | 0 | 11 | 13 | <1 | <1 | 1 carb |
| Mustard, Dijon | 1 Tbsp | 19 | 1 | 9 | <1 | 0 | 0 | 379 | 2 | <1 | <1 | free |
| Mustard, Honey | 1 Tbsp | 50 | 3 | 27 | <1 | 0 | 0 | 91 | 7 | <1 | <1 | 1/2 carb |
| Mustard, Prepared | 1 Tbsp | 12 | <1 | 0 | <1 | 0 | 0 | 196 | 1 | <1 | <1 | free |
| Olives, Green, Pitted | 10 | 45 | 5 | 45 | <1 | 0 | 0 | 936 | <1 | <1 | <1 | 1 fat |
| Olives, Small Ripe | 10 | 37 | 3 | 27 | <1 | 0 | 0 | 279 | 2 | 1 | <1 | 1 fat |
| Olives, Stuffed Green | 10 | 41 | 5 | 41 | <1 | 0 | 0 | 827 | <1 | <1 | <1 | 1 fat |
| Peppers, Pickled Hot Jalapeño | 2 | 8 | <1 | 0 | <1 | 0 | 0 | 121 | 2 | <1 | <1 | free |
| Pickle Slices, Dill | 10 | 11 | <1 | 0 | <1 | 0 | 0 | 769 | 3 | <1 | <1 | free |
| Pickle Slices, Dill, Low Sodium | 10 | 11 | <1 | 0 | <1 | 0 | 0 | 11 | 3 | <1 | <1 | free |

SAUCES, GRAVIES, CONDIMENTS, RELISHES

| | Serving | Calories | Fat (g) | Cal. from Fat | Sat. Fat (g) | Trans Fat (g) | Chol. (mg) | Sod. (mg) | Carb. (g) | Fiber (g) | Prot. (g) | Servings/Exchanges |
|---|---|---|---|---|---|---|---|---|---|---|---|---|
| Pickle Slices, Fresh Pack | 4 | 22 | <1 | 0 | 0 | 0 | 0 | 202 | 5 | <1 | <1 | free |
| Pickle Slices, Sour | 10 | 8 | <1 | 0 | <1 | 0 | 0 | 846 | 2 | <1 | <1 | free |
| Pickle, Dill | 1 | 12 | <1 | 0 | <1 | 0 | 0 | 833 | 3 | <1 | <1 | free |
| Pickle, Dill, Low Sodium | 1 | 12 | <1 | 0 | <1 | 0 | 0 | 12 | 3 | <1 | <1 | free |
| Pickle, Sour | 1 | 4 | <1 | 0 | <1 | 0 | 0 | 423 | <1 | <1 | <1 | free |
| Pickle, Sweet | 1 medium | 41 | <1 | 0 | <1 | 0 | 0 | 329 | 11 | <1 | <1 | 1/2 carb |
| Relish, Hot Dog | 1 Tbsp | 14 | <1 | 0 | <1 | 0 | 0 | 167 | 4 | <1 | <1 | free |
| Relish, Sweet Pickle | 1 Tbsp | 20 | <1 | 0 | <1 | 0 | 0 | 124 | 5 | <1 | <1 | free |
| Sauce, Bearnaise, Homemade | 1/2 cup | 321 | 34 | 306 | 20 | 0 | 237 | 444 | 1 | <1 | 2 | 7 fat |
| Sauce, Black Bean | 1/2 cup | 129 | 6 | 54 | 1 | 0 | 0 | 1322 | 14 | 2 | 3 | 1 starch, 1 fat |
| Sauce, Cheese | 1/2 cup | 221 | 16 | 144 | 10 | 0 | 36 | 515 | 9 | <1 | 10 | 1/2 carb, 1 med-fat meat, 2 fat |

| | | | | | | | | | | | | |
|---|---|---|---|---|---|---|---|---|---|---|---|---|
| Sauce, Curry | 1/2 cup | 74 | 6 | 54 | 1 | 0 | 0 | 392 | 3 | <1 | 3 | 1 fat |
| Sauce, Hollandaise, Dry Mix & Water | 1/2 cup | 119 | 10 | 90 | 6 | 0 | 26 | 783 | 7 | <1 | 2 | 1/2 carb, 2 fat |
| Sauce, Hot Chili/Red Pepper | 2 Tbsp | 7 | <1 | 0 | <1 | 0 | 0 | 8 | 1 | <1 | <1 | free |
| Sauce, Hot Green Chili | 1 Tbsp | 6 | <1 | 0 | 0 | 0 | 0 | 4 | 2 | <1 | <1 | free |
| Sauce, Salsa/Mexican, Homemade | 1/2 cup | 23 | <1 | 0 | <1 | 0 | 0 | 468 | 5 | 1 | <1 | 1 vegetable |
| Sauce, Soy | 1 Tbsp | 10 | <1 | 0 | <1 | 0 | 0 | 1028 | 2 | 0 | <1 | free |
| Sauce, Spanish-Style Tomato | 1/2 cup | 40 | <1 | 0 | <1 | 0 | 0 | 576 | 9 | 2 | 2 | 1/2 carb |
| Sauce, Tartar | 1 Tbsp | 74 | 8 | 72 | 2 | 0 | 7 | 99 | <1 | <1 | <1 | 2 fat |
| Sauce, Teriyaki | 1 Tbsp | 15 | 0 | 0 | 0 | 0 | 0 | 690 | 3 | <1 | 1 | free |
| Sauce, White, Homemade | 1/2 cup | 178 | 14 | 126 | 4 | 0 | 14 | 185 | 10 | <1 | 4 | 1/2 starch, 3 fat |
| Sauce, Worcestershire | 1 Tbsp | 11 | 0 | 0 | 0 | 0 | 0 | 167 | 3 | 0 | 0 | free |

SAUCES, GRAVIES, CONDIMENTS, RELISHES

| | Serving | Calories | Fat (g) | Cal. from Fat | Sat. Fat (g) | Trans Fat (g) | Chol. (mg) | Sod. (mg) | Carb. (g) | Fiber (g) | Prot. (g) | Servings/Exchanges |
|---|---|---|---|---|---|---|---|---|---|---|---|---|
| Syrup, Maple | 1 Tbsp | 52 | <1 | 0 | 0 | 0 | 0 | 2 | 13 | 0 | 0 | 1 carb |
| Syrup, Pancake | 1 Tbsp | 57 | 0 | 0 | 0 | 0 | 0 | 17 | 15 | 0 | 0 | 1 carb |
| **Brands** | | | | | | | | | | | | |
| ***A1 Steakhouse*** | | | | | | | | | | | | |
| Marinade, Carb Well | 1 Tbsp | 5 | 0 | 0 | 0 | 0 | 0 | 230 | 1 | 0 | 0 | free |
| Marinade, Chicago Steakhouse | 1 Tbsp | 20 | 1 | 10 | 0 | 0 | 0 | 270 | 3 | 0 | 0 | free |
| Marinade, Ginger Teriyaki | 1 Tbsp | 25 | 0 | 0 | 0 | 0 | 0 | 490 | 5 | 0 | 0 | free |
| Marinade, Jamaican Jerk | 1 Tbsp | 25 | 0.5 | 5 | 0 | 0 | 0 | 190 | 5 | 0 | 0 | free |
| Marinade, New Orleans Cajun | 1 Tbsp | 25 | 0 | 0 | 0 | 0 | 0 | 180 | 5 | 0 | 0 | free |
| Marinade, Texas Mesquite | 1 Tbsp | 15 | 0 | 0 | 0 | 0 | 0 | 400 | 4 | 0 | 0 | free |

| | | | | | | | | | | | | |
|---|---|---|---|---|---|---|---|---|---|---|---|---|
| Steak Sauce | 1 Tbsp | 15 | 0 | 0 | 0 | 0 | 0 | 280 | 3 | 0 | 0 | free |
| ***Aunt Jemima*** | | | | | | | | | | | | |
| Butter Lite Syrup | 1/4 cup | 100 | 0 | 0 | 0 | 0 | 0 | 210 | 26 | 1 | 0 | 2 carb |
| Butter Rich Syrup | 1/4 cup | 210 | 0 | 0 | 0 | 0 | 0 | 210 | 53 | 0 | 0 | 3 1/2 carb |
| Country Rich Lite Syrup | 1/4 cup | 100 | 0 | 0 | 0 | 0 | 0 | 180 | 26 | 1 | 0 | 2 carb |
| Country Rich Syrup | 1/4 cup | 210 | 0 | 0 | 0 | 0 | 0 | 120 | 53 | 0 | 0 | 3 1/2 carb |
| Lite Syrup | 1/4 cup | 100 | 0 | 0 | 0 | 0 | 0 | 190 | 26 | 0 | 0 | 2 carb |
| Original Syrup | 1/4 cup | 210 | 0 | 0 | 0 | 0 | 0 | 120 | 52 | 0 | 0 | 3 1/2 carb |
| ***Betty Crocker*** | | | | | | | | | | | | |
| Bac-Os Bits or Chips | 1 1/2 Tbsp | 30 | 1.5 | 10 | 0 | 0 | 0 | 120 | 2 | 0 | 3 | 1 fat |
| ***Braswell's*** | | | | | | | | | | | | |
| Pear Preserves | 1 Tbsp | 30 | 0 | 0 | 0 | 0 | 0 | 0 | 7 | 0 | 0 | 1/2 carb |
| Red Pepper Jelly | 1 Tbsp | 35 | 0 | 0 | 0 | 0 | 0 | 0 | 9 | 0 | 0 | 1/2 carb |
| ***Campbell's*** | | | | | | | | | | | | |
| Gravy, Beef | 1/4 cup | 25 | 3 | 25 | 1 | 0 | 5 | 270 | 3 | 0 | 1 | 1 fat |

SAUCES, GRAVIES, CONDIMENTS, RELISHES

| | Serving | Calories | Fat (g) | Cal. from Fat | Sat. Fat (g) | Trans Fat (g) | Chol. (mg) | Sod. (mg) | Carb. (g) | Fiber (g) | Prot. (g) | Servings/Exchanges |
|---|---|---|---|---|---|---|---|---|---|---|---|---|
| Gravy, Chicken | 1/4 cup | 40 | 3 | 25 | 1 | 0 | 5 | 260 | 3 | 0 | 0 | 1 fat |
| Gravy, Country Style Cream Gravy | 1/4 cup | 45 | 3 | 25 | 1 | 0 | 5 | 190 | 3 | 0 | 1 | 1 fat |
| Gravy, Cream Style Sausage Gravy | 1/4 cup | 70 | 5 | 45 | 1.5 | 0 | 5 | 270 | 4 | 0 | 2 | 1 fat |
| Gravy, Turkey | 1/4 cup | 25 | 1 | 10 | 0.5 | 0 | 0 | 270 | 3 | 0 | 1 | free |
| ***Cary's*** | | | | | | | | | | | | |
| Syrup, Maple | 1/4 cup | 210 | 0 | 0 | 0 | 0 | 0 | 5 | 53 | 0 | 0 | 3 1/2 carb |
| Syrup, Sugar Free | 1/4 cup | 30 | 0 | 0 | 0 | 0 | 0 | 115 | 12 | 0 | 0 | 1 carb |
| ***Claussen*** | | | | | | | | | | | | |
| Pickle Relish, Sweet | 1 Tbsp | 14 | <1 | 0 | <1 | 0 | 0 | 90 | 3 | NA | <1 | free |
| Pickles, Bread 'n Butter | 1 oz | 20 | 0 | 0 | 0 | 0 | 0 | 180 | 4 | 0 | 0 | free |
| Pickles, Kosher Dill, Halves | 1 | 5 | 0 | 0 | 0 | 0 | 0 | 270 | 1 | 0 | 0 | free |

| | | | | | | | | | | | | |
|---|---|---|---|---|---|---|---|---|---|---|---|---|
| Pickles, Kosher Dill Mini Dills | 1 | 5 | 0 | 0 | 0 | 0 | 0 | 290 | <1 | <1 | <1 | free |
| Pickles, Kosher Dill Sandwich Slices | 1 | 5 | 0 | 0 | 0 | 0 | 0 | 420 | 1 | 0 | 0 | free |
| Pickles, Kosher Dill Spears | 1 | 5 | 0 | 0 | 0 | 0 | 0 | 312 | <1 | 0 | 0 | free |
| ***Dynasty*** | | | | | | | | | | | | |
| Bead Molasses | 1 Tbsp | 60 | 0 | 0 | 0 | 0 | 0 | 45 | 16 | 0 | 0 | 1 carb |
| Chinese Brown Gravy Sauce | 1 Tbsp | 60 | 0 | 0 | 0 | 0 | 0 | 65 | 14 | 0 | 0 | 1 carb |
| Hoisin Sauce | 2 Tbsp | 50 | 1 | 10 | 0 | 0 | 0 | 410 | 9 | 0 | 0 | 1/2 carb |
| Hot Chili Oil | 1 tsp | 40 | 4 | 40 | 0.5 | 0 | 0 | 0 | 0 | 0 | 0 | 1 fat |
| Spicy Hot Kung Pao Sauce | 2 Tbsp | 45 | 1.5 | 15 | 0 | 0 | 0 | 590 | 7 | 0 | 1 | 1/2 carb |
| ***Emeril's*** | | | | | | | | | | | | |
| BAM! B-Q Sauce, Kicked Up | 2 Tbsp | 40 | 0 | 0 | 0 | 0 | 0 | 360 | 11 | 0 | 0 | 1 carb |

| | Serving | Calories | Fat (g) | Cal. from Fat | Sat. Fat (g) | Trans Fat (g) | Chol. (mg) | Sod. (mg) | Carb. (g) | Fiber (g) | Prot. (g) | Servings/Exchanges |
|---|---|---|---|---|---|---|---|---|---|---|---|---|
| BAM! B-Q Sauce, Sweet | 2 Tbsp | 45 | 0 | 0 | 0 | 0 | 0 | 390 | 12 | 0 | 0 | 1 carb |
| Dijon Mustard | 1 Tbsp | 5 | 0 | 0 | 0 | 0 | 0 | 120 | 1 | 0 | 0 | free |
| ***Famous Dave's*** | | | | | | | | | | | | |
| BBQ Sauce, Devil's Spit | 2 Tbsp | 50 | 0 | 0 | 0 | 0 | 0 | 350 | 12 | <1 | 0 | 1 carb |
| BBQ Sauce, Rich & Sassy | 2 Tbsp | 60 | 0 | 0 | 0 | 0 | 0 | 350 | 15 | <1 | 0 | 1 carb |
| BBQ Sauce, Sweet & Zesty | 2 Tbsp | 70 | 0 | 0 | 0 | 0 | 0 | 320 | 17 | 0 | 0 | 1 carb |
| ***Fifty50*** | | | | | | | | | | | | |
| Sugar Free, Low Calorie, Strawberry Spread | 1 Tbsp | 5 | 0 | 0 | 0 | 0 | 0 | 25 | 3 | 0 | 0 | free |
| ***Franco-American*** | | | | | | | | | | | | |
| Gravy, Slow Roast Beef | 1/4 cup | 25 | 0.5 | 5 | 0 | 0 | 5 | 310 | 3 | 0 | 1 | free |

| | | | | | | | | | | | | |
|---|---|---|---|---|---|---|---|---|---|---|---|---|
| Gravy, Slow Roast Chicken | 1/4 cup | 20 | 0.5 | 5 | 0 | 0 | <5 | 240 | 3 | 0 | 1 | free |
| Gravy, Slow Roast Turkey | 1/4 cup | 25 | 0 | 0 | 0 | 0 | <5 | 320 | 4 | 0 | 1 | free |
| ***Grey Poupon*** | | | | | | | | | | | | |
| Country Dijon Mustard | 1 tsp | 5 | 0 | 0 | 0 | 0 | 0 | 120 | 0 | 0 | 0 | free |
| ***Heinz*** | | | | | | | | | | | | |
| 57 Sauce | 1 Tbsp | 20 | 0 | 0 | 0 | 0 | 0 | 190 | 4 | 0 | 0 | free |
| Chili Sauce | 1 Tbsp | 20 | 0 | 0 | 0 | 0 | 0 | 230 | 5 | 0 | 0 | free |
| Cocktail Sauce | 1/4 cup | 60 | 0 | 0 | 0 | 0 | 0 | 690 | 15 | 0 | 1 | 1 carb |
| Gravy, Home Style Classic Chicken | 1/4 cup | 30 | 2 | 20 | 0.5 | 0 | <5 | 250 | 3 | 0 | 0 | 1 fat |
| Gravy, Home Style Rich Mushroom | 1/4 cup | 20 | 0.5 | 5 | 0 | 0 | 0 | 320 | 3 | 0 | <1 | free |
| Gravy, Home Style Roasted Turkey | 1/4 cup | 25 | 1 | 0 | 0 | 0 | <5 | 290 | 3 | 0 | 1 | free |

SAUCES, GRAVIES, CONDIMENTS, RELISHES

| | Serving | Calories | Fat (g) | Cal. from Fat | Sat. Fat (g) | Trans Fat (g) | Chol. (mg) | Sod. (mg) | Carb. (g) | Fiber (g) | Prot. (g) | Servings/Exchanges |
|---|---|---|---|---|---|---|---|---|---|---|---|---|
| Gravy, Home Style Savory Beef | 1/4 cup | 30 | 1 | 10 | 0.5 | 0 | <5 | 390 | 4 | 0 | 1 | 1 fat |
| Worcestershire Sauce | 1 tsp | 0 | 0 | 0 | 0 | 0 | 0 | 60 | 0 | 0 | 0 | free |
| ***Hormel*** | | | | | | | | | | | | |
| Real Bacon Bits | 1 Tbsp | 25 | 1.5 | 15 | 1 | 0 | 5 | 240 | 0 | 0 | 3 | 1 fat |
| Real Bacon Pieces | 1 Tbsp | 25 | 1.5 | 15 | 0.5 | 0 | 5 | 200 | 0 | 0 | 3 | 1 fat |
| ***Hunt's*** | | | | | | | | | | | | |
| BBQ Sauce, Hickory & Brown Sugar | 2 Tbsp | 70 | 0 | 0 | 0 | 0 | 0 | 390 | 18 | <1 | 0 | 1 carb |
| BBQ Sauce, Honey Hickory | 2 Tbsp | 50 | 0 | 0 | 0 | 0 | 0 | 420 | 13 | <1 | 0 | 1 carb |
| BBQ Sauce, Original | 2 Tbsp | 60 | 0 | 0 | 0 | 0 | 0 | 280 | 15 | <1 | 0 | 1 carb |
| ***Jack Daniels*** | | | | | | | | | | | | |
| Barbecue Sauce, Hickory Brown Sugar | 2 Tbsp | 50 | 0 | 0 | 0 | 0 | 0 | 290 | 13 | 0 | 0 | 1 carb |

| | | | | | | | | | | | | |
|---|---|---|---|---|---|---|---|---|---|---|---|---|
| Barbecue Sauce, Honey Smokehouse | 2 Tbsp | 50 | 0 | 0 | 0 | 0 | 0 | 290 | 12 | 0 | 0 | 1 carb |
| Steak Sauce, Original | 1 Tbsp | 50 | 0 | 0 | 0 | 0 | 0 | 290 | 12 | 0 | 0 | 1 carb |
| ***Karo*** | | | | | | | | | | | | |
| Dark Corn Syrup | 2 Tbsp | 120 | 0 | 0 | 0 | 0 | 0 | 45 | 31 | 0 | 0 | 2 carb |
| Light Corn Syrup | 2 Tbsp | 120 | 0 | 0 | 0 | 0 | 0 | 35 | 30 | 0 | 0 | 2 carb |
| Lite Syrup | 2 Tbsp | 80 | 0 | 0 | 0 | 0 | 0 | 80 | 20 | 0 | 0 | 1 carb |
| Pancake Syrup | 4 Tbsp | 240 | 0 | 0 | 0 | 0 | 0 | 85 | 63 | 0 | 0 | 4 carb |
| ***KC Masterpiece*** | | | | | | | | | | | | |
| Barbecue Sauce, Hickory Brown Sugar | 2 Tbsp | 60 | 0 | 0 | 0 | 0 | 0 | 320 | 15 | 0 | 0 | 1 carb |
| Barbecue Sauce, Mesquite | 2 Tbsp | 60 | 0 | 0 | 0 | 0 | 0 | 260 | 14 | 0 | 0 | 1 carb |
| Barbecue Sauce, Original | 2 Tbsp | 60 | 0 | 0 | 0 | 0 | 0 | 240 | 15 | 0 | 0 | 1 carb |
| Marinade, Caribbean Jerk | 1 Tbsp | 25 | 0 | 0 | 0 | 0 | 0 | 320 | 6 | 0 | 0 | 1/2 carb |

SAUCES, GRAVIES, CONDIMENTS, RELISHES

| | Serving | Calories | Fat (g) | Cal. from Fat | Sat. Fat (g) | Trans Fat (g) | Chol. (mg) | Sod. (mg) | Carb. (g) | Fiber (g) | Prot. (g) | Servings/Exchanges |
|---|---|---|---|---|---|---|---|---|---|---|---|---|
| Marinade, Garlic & Herb | 1 Tbsp | 30 | 1 | 10 | 0 | 0 | 0 | 220 | 5 | 0 | 0 | 1/2 carb |
| Marinade, Honey Teriyaki | 1 Tbsp | 40 | 0.5 | 5 | 0 | 0 | 0 | 360 | 9 | 0 | <1 | 1/2 carb |
| Marinade, Lemon Pepper | 1 Tbsp | 40 | 1.5 | 15 | 0 | 0 | 0 | 310 | 7 | 0 | 0 | 1/2 carb |
| Marinade, Roasted Garlic Balsamic | 1 Tbsp | 15 | 0 | 0 | 0 | 0 | 0 | 220 | 4 | 0 | 0 | free |
| ***Kitchen Bouquet*** | | | | | | | | | | | | |
| Browning & Seasoning Sauce | 1 tsp | 15 | 0 | 0 | 0 | 0 | 0 | 10 | 3 | 0 | 0 | free |
| ***Knott's Berry Farm*** | | | | | | | | | | | | |
| Apple Cinnamon Jelly | 1 Tbsp | 50 | 0 | 0 | 0 | 0 | 0 | 0 | 13 | 0 | 0 | 1 carb |
| Apricot Preserves | 1 Tbsp | 50 | 0 | 0 | 0 | 0 | 0 | 0 | 13 | 0 | 0 | 1 carb |
| Bing Cherry Preserves | 1 Tbsp | 50 | 0 | 0 | 0 | 0 | 0 | 0 | 13 | 0 | 0 | 1 carb |

| | | | | | | | | | | | | |
|---|---|---|---|---|---|---|---|---|---|---|---|---|
| Boysenberry Light Preserves | 1 Tbsp | 20 | 0 | 0 | 0 | 0 | 0 | 0 | 5 | 0 | 0 | free |
| Boysenberry Preserves | 1 Tbsp | 50 | 0 | 0 | 0 | 0 | 0 | 0 | 13 | 0 | 0 | 1 carb |
| California Plum Jam | 1 Tbsp | 50 | 0 | 0 | 0 | 0 | 0 | 0 | 13 | 0 | 0 | 1 carb |
| Jalapeño Jelly | 1 Tbsp | 50 | 0 | 0 | 0 | 0 | 0 | 0 | 13 | 0 | 0 | 1 carb |
| Mint Flavored Apple Jelly | 1 Tbsp | 50 | 0 | 0 | 0 | 0 | 0 | 0 | 13 | 0 | 0 | 1 carb |
| Red Currant Jelly | 1 Tbsp | 50 | 0 | 0 | 0 | 0 | 0 | 10 | 13 | 0 | 0 | 1 carb |
| Seedless Blackberry Jam | 1 Tbsp | 50 | 0 | 0 | 0 | 0 | 0 | 0 | 13 | 0 | 0 | 1 carb |
| Seedless Red Raspberry Jam | 1 Tbsp | 50 | 0 | 0 | 0 | 0 | 0 | 0 | 13 | 0 | 0 | 1 carb |
| Strawberry Preserves | 1 Tbsp | 50 | 0 | 0 | 0 | 0 | 0 | 0 | 13 | 0 | 0 | 1 carb |
| ***Kraft*** | | | | | | | | | | | | |
| Barbecue Sauce, Hickory Smoke | 2 Tbsp | 60 | 0 | 0 | 0 | 0 | 0 | 430 | 13 | 0 | 0 | 1 carb |
| Barbecue Sauce, Honey | 2 Tbsp | 50 | 0 | 0 | 0 | 0 | 0 | 360 | 13 | 0 | 0 | 1 carb |

SAUCES, GRAVIES, CONDIMENTS, RELISHES

| | Serving | Calories | Fat (g) | Cal. from Fat | Sat. Fat (g) | Trans Fat (g) | Chol. (mg) | Sod. (mg) | Carb. (g) | Fiber (g) | Prot. (g) | Servings/Exchanges |
|---|---|---|---|---|---|---|---|---|---|---|---|---|
| Barbecue Sauce, Honey Hickory Smoke | 2 Tbsp | 70 | 0 | 0 | 0 | 0 | 0 | 460 | 16 | 0 | 0 | 1 carb |
| Barbecue Sauce, Honey Roasted Garlic | 2 Tbsp | 50 | 0 | 0 | 0 | 0 | 0 | 350 | 12 | 0 | 0 | 1 carb |
| Barbecue Sauce, Light Original | 2 Tbsp | 20 | 0 | 0 | 0 | 0 | 0 | 340 | 5 | 0 | 0 | free |
| Barbecue Sauce, Mesquite Smoke | 2 Tbsp | 50 | 0 | 0 | 0 | 0 | 0 | 450 | 12 | 0 | 0 | 1 carb |
| Barbecue Sauce, Original | 2 Tbsp | 50 | 0 | 0 | 0 | 0 | 0 | 440 | 12 | 0 | 0 | 1 carb |
| Sauce, Cocktail | 1/4 cup | 60 | 0.5 | 5 | 0 | 0 | 0 | 880 | 11 | 1 | 1 | 1 carb |
| Sauce, Coleslaw Maker | 1/4 cup | 110 | 9 | 80 | 1.5 | 10 | 0 | 230 | 7 | 0 | 0 | 1/2 carb, 2 fat |
| Sauce, Horseradish | 1 tsp | 15 | 1.5 | 15 | 0 | 0 | 0 | 40 | 1 | 0 | 0 | free |
| Sauce, Sweet & Sour | 2 Tbsp | 60 | 0 | 0 | 0 | 0 | 0 | 130 | 13 | 0 | 0 | 1 carb |
| Sauce, Tartar | 2 Tbsp | 60 | 4.5 | 40 | 0.5 | 0 | 5 | 230 | 4 | 0 | 0 | 1 fat |

| | | | | | | | | | | | | |
|---|---|---|---|---|---|---|---|---|---|---|---|---|
| Sauce, Tartar, Fat Free | 2 Tbsp | 25 | 0 | 0 | 0 | 0 | 0 | 200 | 5 | 0 | 0 | free |
| Sauce, Tartar, Lemon & Herb | 2 Tbsp | 150 | 16 | 140 | 2.5 | 0 | 15 | 170 | 1 | 0 | 0 | 3 fat |
| ***La Choy*** | | | | | | | | | | | | |
| Marinade & Sauce, Teriyaki | 1 Tbsp | 40 | 0 | 0 | 0 | 0 | 0 | 570 | 10 | 0 | <1 | 1/2 carb |
| Sauce, Soy | 1 Tbsp | 10 | 0 | 0 | 0 | 0 | 0 | 1160 | 1 | 0 | 1 | free |
| Sauce, Soy, Lite | 1 Tbsp | 15 | 0 | 0 | 0 | 0 | 0 | 550 | 2 | 0 | 1 | free |
| Sauce, Sweet & Sour | 1 Tbsp | 60 | 0 | 0 | 0 | 0 | 0 | 110 | 14 | 0 | 0 | 1 carb |
| ***La Victoria*** | | | | | | | | | | | | |
| Enchilada Sauce, Green | 1/4 cup | 15 | 0 | 0 | 0 | 0 | 0 | 310 | 3 | 0 | 0 | free |
| Enchilada Sauce, Red | 1/4 cup | 15 | 2 | 10 | 0 | 0 | 0 | 310 | 2 | 0 | 0 | free |
| Taco Sauce, Green | 1 Tbsp | 0 | 0 | 0 | 0 | 0 | 0 | 70 | <1 | 0 | 0 | free |
| Taco Sauce, Red | 1 Tbsp | 5 | 0 | 0 | 0 | 0 | 0 | 90 | 1 | 0 | 0 | free |
| ***Las Palmas*** | | | | | | | | | | | | |
| Enchilada Sauce, Green | 1/4 cup | 25 | 1.5 | 15 | 0 | 0 | 0 | 340 | 1 | 0 | 0 | free |

| | Serving | Calories | Fat (g) | Cal. from Fat | Sat. Fat (g) | Trans Fat (g) | Chol. (mg) | Sod. (mg) | Carb. (g) | Fiber (g) | Prot. (g) | Servings/Exchanges |
|---|---|---|---|---|---|---|---|---|---|---|---|---|
| Enchilada Sauce, Original Style | 1/4 cup | 15 | 0.5 | 5 | 0 | 0 | 0 | 330 | 2 | 1 | 0 | free |
| Sauce, Red Chile | 1/4 cup | 15 | 0 | 0 | 0 | 0 | 0 | 330 | 2 | 1 | 0 | free |
| ***Lawry's*** | | | | | | | | | | | | |
| Marinade, Baja Chipotle | 1 Tbsp | 15 | 0 | 0 | 0 | 0 | 0 | 390 | 4 | 0 | 0 | free |
| Marinade, Herb & Garlic | 1 Tbsp | 10 | 0 | 0 | 0 | 0 | 0 | 420 | 2 | 0 | 0 | free |
| Marinade, Lemon Pepper | 1 Tbsp | 10 | 0 | 0 | 0 | 0 | 0 | 390 | 2 | 0 | 0 | free |
| Marinade, Mesquite | 1 Tbsp | 5 | 0 | 0 | 0 | 0 | 0 | 350 | 1 | 0 | 0 | free |
| Marinade, Sesame Ginger | 1 Tbsp | 30 | 0 | 0 | 0 | 0 | 0 | 580 | 7 | 0 | 0 | 1/2 carb |
| Marinade, Tequila Lime | 1 Tbsp | 15 | 0 | 0 | 0 | 0 | 0 | 490 | 4 | 0 | 0 | free |
| Marinade, Teriyaki | 1 Tbsp | 20 | 0 | 0 | 0 | 0 | 0 | 560 | 5 | 0 | 0 | free |
| ***Log Cabin*** | | | | | | | | | | | | |
| Original Syrup | 1/4 cup | 210 | 0 | 0 | 0 | 0 | 0 | 105 | 52 | 0 | 0 | 3 1/2 carb |

| | | | | | | | | | | | | |
|---|---|---|---|---|---|---|---|---|---|---|---|---|
| Sugar Free Syrup | 1/4 cup | 30 | 0 | 0 | 0 | 0 | 0 | 110 | 11 | 0 | 0 | 1 carb |
| ***Maple Grove Farms Cozy Cottage*** | | | | | | | | | | | | |
| Blueberry Syrup | 1/4 cup | 210 | 0 | 0 | 0 | 0 | 0 | 120 | 52 | 0 | 0 | 3 1/2 carb |
| Maple Syrup | 1/4 cup | 200 | 0 | 0 | 0 | 0 | 0 | 5 | 53 | 0 | 0 | 3 1/2 carb |
| ***McCormick*** | | | | | | | | | | | | |
| Bac'n Pieces, Bits | 1 Tbsp | 30 | 1 | 10 | 0 | 0 | 0 | 180 | 2 | 0 | 3 | 1 fat |
| Salad Toppins | 1 1/3 Tbsp | 35 | 1.5 | 15 | 0 | 0 | 0 | 70 | 3 | 0 | 2 | 1 fat |
| ***Mezzetta*** | | | | | | | | | | | | |
| Cocktail Onions | 8 pieces | 5 | 0 | 0 | 0 | 0 | 0 | 300 | 1 | 0 | 0 | free |
| Garlic Olives | 1 | 10 | 1 | 10 | 0 | 0 | 0 | 140 | 0 | 0 | 0 | free |
| Grape Leaves | 1 leaf | 5 | 0 | 0 | 0 | 0 | 0 | 100 | 1 | 0 | 0 | free |
| Jalapeño Stuffed Olives | 1 | 10 | 1 | 10 | 0 | 0 | 0 | 140 | 1 | 0 | 0 | free |
| Martini Olives | 1 | 10 | 1 | 10 | 0 | 0 | 0 | 170 | 1 | 0 | 0 | free |
| Roasted Bell Peppers | 1 1/2 Tbsp | 10 | 0 | 0 | 0 | 0 | 0 | 110 | 1 | 0 | 0 | free |

| | Serving | Calories | Fat (g) | Cal. from Fat | Sat. Fat (g) | Trans Fat (g) | Chol. (mg) | Sod. (mg) | Carb. (g) | Fiber (g) | Prot. (g) | Servings/Exchanges |
|---|---|---|---|---|---|---|---|---|---|---|---|---|
| Sliced Jalapeño Peppers | 1/4 cup | 5 | 0 | 0 | 0 | 0 | 0 | 380 | 1 | 0 | 0 | free |
| Spanish Queen Olives | 1 | 10 | 1 | 10 | 0 | 0 | 0 | 170 | 1 | 1 | 0 | free |
| Sweet Banana Peppers | 3 | 10 | 0 | 0 | 0 | 0 | 0 | 320 | 1 | 0 | 0 | free |
| Sweet Cherry Peppers Relish | 3 pieces | 15 | 0.5 | 5 | 0 | 0 | 0 | 340 | 2 | 1 | 1 | free |
| ***Mrs. Butterworth's*** | | | | | | | | | | | | |
| Original Syrup | 1/4 cup | 210 | 0 | 0 | 0 | 0 | 0 | 115 | 53 | 0 | 0 | 3 1/2 carb |
| ***Mrs. Dash*** | | | | | | | | | | | | |
| 10 Minute Marinade, Lemon Herb Peppercorn | 1 Tbsp | 25 | 2 | 20 | 0 | 0 | 0 | 0 | 2 | 0 | 0 | free |
| 10 Minute Marinade, Mesquite Grille | 1 Tbsp | 25 | 1.5 | 15 | 0 | 0 | 0 | 0 | 2 | 0 | 0 | free |

| | | | | | | | | | | | | |
|---|---|---|---|---|---|---|---|---|---|---|---|---|
| 10 Minute Marinade, Southwest Chipotle | 1 Tbsp | 20 | 1.5 | 15 | 0 | 0 | 0 | 0 | 2 | 0 | 0 | free |
| 10 Minute Marinade, Zesty Garlic Herb | 1 Tbsp | 25 | 2 | 20 | 0 | 0 | 0 | 0 | 3 | 0 | 0 | free |
| ***Musselman's*** | | | | | | | | | | | | |
| Apple Butter | 1 Tbsp | 30 | 0 | 0 | 0 | 0 | 0 | 0 | 8 | 0 | 0 | 1/2 carb |
| ***Old El Paso*** | | | | | | | | | | | | |
| Enchilada Sauce, Green Chile Mild | 1/4 cup | 25 | 1.5 | 15 | 0 | 0 | 0 | 280 | 4 | 0 | 0 | free |
| Enchilada Sauce, Mild | 1/4 cup | 20 | 0 | 0 | 0 | 0 | 0 | 360 | 3 | 0 | 0 | free |
| Taco Sauce, Hot | 1 Tbsp | 5 | 0 | 0 | 0 | 0 | 0 | 90 | 1 | 0 | 0 | free |
| Taco Sauce, Medium | 1 Tbsp | 5 | 0 | 0 | 0 | 0 | 0 | 90 | 1 | 0 | 0 | free |
| Taco Sauce, Mild | 1 Tbsp | 5 | 0 | 0 | 0 | 0 | 0 | 90 | 1 | 0 | 0 | free |
| ***Ortega*** | | | | | | | | | | | | |
| Enchilada Sauce | 1/4 cup | 10 | 0.5 | 5 | 0 | 0 | 0 | 340 | 4 | <1 | <1 | free |
| Sauce Picante, Mild | 1/4 cup | 10 | 0 | 0 | 0 | 0 | 0 | 220 | 2 | 0 | 1 | free |

SAUCES, GRAVIES, CONDIMENTS, RELISHES

| | Serving | Calories | Fat (g) | Cal. from Fat | Sat. Fat (g) | Trans Fat (g) | Chol. (mg) | Sod. (mg) | Carb. (g) | Fiber (g) | Prot. (g) | Servings/Exchanges |
|---|---|---|---|---|---|---|---|---|---|---|---|---|
| Taco Sauce, Original | 1 Tbsp | 10 | 0 | 0 | 0 | 0 | 0 | 60 | 1 | 0 | 0 | free |
| ***Oscar Mayer*** | | | | | | | | | | | | |
| Bacon Bits | 1 Tbsp | 25 | 1.5 | 15 | 0.5 | 0 | 5 | 170 | 0 | 0 | 2 | free |
| ***Polaner*** | | | | | | | | | | | | |
| All Fruit Strawberry Spread | 1 Tbsp | 40 | 0 | 0 | 0 | 0 | 0 | 0 | 10 | 0 | 0 | 1/2 carb |
| Strawberry Preserves | 1 Tbsp | 50 | 0 | 0 | 0 | 0 | 0 | 0 | 13 | 0 | 0 | 1 carb |
| Sugar Free Strawberry Preserves | 1 Tbsp | 10 | 0 | 0 | 0 | 0 | 0 | 0 | 5 | 0 | 0 | free |
| ***Progresso*** | | | | | | | | | | | | |
| Artichoke Hearts, Marinated | 2 pieces | 60 | 5 | 45 | 1 | 0.5 | 0 | 110 | 2 | 0 | 0 | 1 fat |
| Sauce, Lobster | 1/2 cup | 100 | 7 | 60 | 1 | 0 | 5 | 430 | 6 | 2 | 3 | 1/2 carb, 1 fat |
| Sauce, Red Clam with Tomato & Basil | 1/2 cup | 60 | 1 | 10 | 0 | 0 | 10 | 350 | 8 | 1 | 4 | 1 carb |

| | | | | | | | | | | | | |
|---|---|---|---|---|---|---|---|---|---|---|---|---|
| Sauce, White Clam, Deluxe | 1/2 cup | 150 | 10 | 90 | 1.5 | 0 | 20 | 710 | 5 | 0 | 9 | 1 med-fat meat, 1 fat |
| ***Regina*** | | | | | | | | | | | | |
| Cooking Wine, Red | 1/4 cup | 20 | 1 | 9 | 0 | 0 | 0 | 365 | 1 | 0 | 1 | free |
| Cooking Wine, Sherry | 1/4 cup | 20 | 0 | 0 | 0 | 0 | 0 | 70 | 5 | 0 | 1 | free |
| Vinegar, Red Wine | 1 oz | 4 | 0 | 0 | 0 | 0 | 0 | 0 | 0 | 0 | 0 | free |
| Vinegar, White Wine | 1 oz | 4 | 0 | 0 | 0 | 0 | 0 | 0 | 1 | 0 | 0 | free |
| ***Smucker's*** | | | | | | | | | | | | |
| Apricot Preserves | 1 Tbsp | 50 | 0 | 0 | 0 | 0 | 0 | 0 | 13 | 0 | 0 | 1 carb |
| Apricot-Pineapple Preserves | 1 Tbsp | 50 | 0 | 0 | 0 | 0 | 0 | 0 | 13 | 0 | 0 | 1 carb |
| Blueberry Syrup | 1/4 cup | 210 | 0 | 0 | 0 | 0 | 0 | 0 | 52 | 0 | 0 | 3 1/2 carb |
| Boysenberry Preserves | 1 Tbsp | 50 | 0 | 0 | 0 | 0 | 0 | 0 | 13 | 0 | 0 | 1 carb |
| Boysenberry Syrup | 1/4 cup | 210 | 0 | 0 | 0 | 0 | 0 | 0 | 52 | 0 | 0 | 3 1/2 carb |
| Cider Apple Butter | 1 Tbsp | 45 | 0 | 0 | 0 | 0 | 0 | 10 | 11 | 0 | 0 | 1 carb |
| Concord Grape Jam | 1 Tbsp | 50 | 0 | 0 | 0 | 0 | 0 | 0 | 13 | 0 | 0 | 1 carb |

| | Serving | Calories | Fat (g) | Cal. from Fat | Sat. Fat (g) | Trans Fat (g) | Chol. (mg) | Sod. (mg) | Carb. (g) | Fiber (g) | Prot. (g) | Servings/Exchanges |
|---|---|---|---|---|---|---|---|---|---|---|---|---|
| Currant Jelly | 1 Tbsp | 50 | 0 | 0 | 0 | 0 | 0 | 0 | 13 | 0 | 0 | 1 carb |
| Low Sugar Apricot | 1 Tbsp | 25 | 0 | 0 | 0 | 0 | 0 | 0 | 6 | 0 | 0 | 1/2 carb |
| Low Sugar Apricot Preserves | 1 Tbsp | 25 | 0 | 0 | 0 | 0 | 0 | 0 | 6 | 0 | 0 | 1/2 carb |
| Low Sugar Concord Grape Jelly | 1 Tbsp | 25 | 0 | 0 | 0 | 0 | 0 | 0 | 6 | 0 | 0 | 1/2 carb |
| Low Sugar Strawberry Preserves | 1 Tbsp | 25 | 0 | 0 | 0 | 0 | 0 | 0 | 6 | 0 | 0 | 1/2 carb |
| Red Raspberry Preserves | 1 Tbsp | 50 | 0 | 0 | 0 | 0 | 0 | 0 | 13 | 0 | 0 | 1 carb |
| Reduced Sugar Sweet Orange Marmalade | 1 Tbsp | 25 | 0 | 0 | 0 | 0 | 0 | 0 | 6 | 0 | 0 | 1/2 carb |
| Seedless Strawberry Jam | 1 Tbsp | 50 | 0 | 0 | 0 | 0 | 0 | 0 | 13 | 0 | 0 | 1 carb |

| | | | | | | | | | | | | |
|---|---|---|---|---|---|---|---|---|---|---|---|---|
| Simply Fruit Spreadable Fruit, Strawberry | 1 Tbsp | 40 | 0 | 0 | 0 | 0 | 0 | 0 | 10 | 0 | 0 | 1/2 carb |
| Squeeze Grape Jelly | 1 Tbsp | 50 | 0 | 0 | 0 | 0 | 0 | 5 | 13 | 0 | 0 | 1 carb |
| Squeeze Strawberry Fruit Spread | 1 Tbsp | 50 | 0 | 0 | 0 | 0 | 0 | 0 | 13 | 0 | 0 | 1 carb |
| Strawberry Preserves | 1 Tbsp | 50 | 0 | 0 | 0 | 0 | 0 | 0 | 13 | 0 | 0 | 1 carb |
| Sugar Free Blackberry with Splenda | 1 Tbsp | 10 | 0 | 0 | 0 | 0 | 0 | 0 | 5 | 0 | 0 | free |
| Sugar Free Strawberry with Nutra Sweet | 1 Tbsp | 10 | 0 | 0 | 0 | 0 | 0 | 0 | 5 | 0 | 0 | free |
| Sweet Orange Marmalade Preserves | 1 Tbsp | 50 | 0 | 0 | 0 | 0 | 0 | 0 | 13 | 0 | 0 | 1 carb |
| ***Tabasco*** | | | | | | | | | | | | |
| Sauce, Green Pepper | 1 tsp | 0 | 0 | 0 | 0 | 0 | 0 | 150 | 0 | 0 | 0 | free |
| Sauce, Pepper | 1 tsp | 0 | 0 | 0 | 0 | 0 | 0 | 35 | 0 | 0 | 0 | free |
| ***Trappey's Red Devil*** | | | | | | | | | | | | |
| Cayenne Pepper Sauce | 1 tsp | 0 | 0 | 0 | 0 | 0 | 0 | 150 | 0 | 0 | 0 | free |

| | Serving | Calories | Fat (g) | Cal. from Fat | Sat. Fat (g) | Trans Fat (g) | Chol. (mg) | Sod. (mg) | Carb. (g) | Fiber (g) | Prot. (g) | Servings/Exchanges |
|---|---|---|---|---|---|---|---|---|---|---|---|---|
| ***Vermont*** | | | | | | | | | | | | |
| Sugar Free Low Calorie Syrup | 1/4 cup | 25 | 0 | 0 | 0 | 0 | 0 | 110 | 7 | 0 | 0 | 1/2 carb |
| ***Vlasic*** | | | | | | | | | | | | |
| Sweet Gherkins | 1 oz | 35 | 0 | 0 | 0 | 0 | 0 | 170 | 9 | 0 | 0 | 1/2 carb |
| Sweet Relish | 1 Tbsp | 15 | 0 | 0 | 0 | 0 | 0 | 140 | 4 | 0 | 0 | free |
| ***Welch's*** | | | | | | | | | | | | |
| Concord Grape Jam | 1 Tbsp | 50 | 0 | 0 | 0 | 0 | 0 | 10 | 13 | 0 | 0 | 1 carb |
| Concord Grape Jelly | 1 Tbsp | 50 | 0 | 0 | 0 | 0 | 0 | 10 | 13 | 0 | 0 | 1 carb |
| Squeezable Concord Grape Jelly | 1 Tbsp | 50 | 0 | 0 | 0 | 0 | 0 | 10 | 13 | 0 | 0 | 1 carb |
| Squeezable Strawberry Spread | 1 Tbsp | 50 | 0 | 0 | 0 | 0 | 0 | 10 | 13 | 0 | 0 | 1 carb |
| Strawberry Spread | 1 Tbsp | 50 | 0 | 0 | 0 | 0 | 0 | 10 | 13 | 0 | 0 | 1 carb |

| | Serving | Calories | Fat (g) | Cal. from Fat | Sat. Fat (g) | Trans Fat (g) | Chol. (mg) | Sod. (mg) | Carb. (g) | Fiber (g) | Prot. (g) | Servings/Exchanges |
|---|---|---|---|---|---|---|---|---|---|---|---|---|
| **SNACKS, CRACKERS, CHIPS, POPCORN, SNACK BARS** | | | | | | | | | | | | |
| Chips, Bagel | 5 | 298 | 7 | 63 | 1 | 0 | 0 | 419 | 52 | 6 | 6 | 3 1/2 starch, 1 fat |
| Chips, Potato | 3/4 oz | 114 | 7 | 65 | 2 | 0 | 0 | 171 | 11 | <1 | 2 | 1 starch, 1 fat |
| Chips, Potato, Baked | 3/4 oz | 82 | 1 | 10 | 0 | 0 | 0 | 112 | 17 | 1.5 | 2 | 1 starch |
| Chips, Potato, Fat Free | 3/4 oz | 56 | 0 | 0 | 0 | 0 | 0 | 150 | 14 | <1 | 2 | 1 starch |
| Crackers, Animal | 8 | 89 | 3 | 25 | 0.5 | 0 | 0 | 79 | 15 | 0 | 1 | 1 starch |
| Crackers, Graham | 3 squares | 99 | 2 | 20 | <1 | 0 | 0 | 142 | 18 | <1 | 2 | 1 starch |
| Crackers, Matzoh, Plain | 3/4 oz | 83 | <1 | 0 | <1 | 0 | 0 | 0 | 18 | <1 | 2 | 1 starch |
| Crackers, Oyster | 20 | 86 | 2 | 20 | <1 | 0 | 0 | 214 | 14 | <1 | 2 | 1 starch |
| Crackers, Round Butter Type | 6 | 90 | 5 | 45 | 0.5 | 0 | 0 | 152 | 11 | <1 | 1 | 1 starch, 1 fat |
| Crackers, Saltines | 6 | 77 | 2 | 20 | <1 | 0 | 0 | 193 | 13 | 0.5 | 2 | 1 starch |
| Crackers, Whole Wheat, Baked | 5 | 89 | 3.5 | 30 | <1 | 0 | 0 | 132 | 14 | 2 | 2 | 1 starch, 1 fat |

SNACKS, CRACKERS, CHIPS, POPCORN

| | Serving | Calories | Fat (g) | Cal. from Fat | Sat. Fat (g) | Trans Fat (g) | Chol. (mg) | Sod. (mg) | Carb. (g) | Fiber (g) | Prot. (g) | Servings/Exchanges |
|---|---|---|---|---|---|---|---|---|---|---|---|---|
| Crackers, Whole Wheat, Reduced Fat | 5 | 80 | 2 | 20 | <1 | 0 | 0 | 110 | 15 | 2.5 | 2 | 1 starch |
| Crispbread | 2 slices | 73 | <1 | 0 | 0 | 0 | 0 | 53 | 16 | 3 | 2 | 1 starch |
| Granola Bar | 1 | 134 | 6 | 55 | 1 | 0 | 0 | 83 | 18 | 1.5 | 3 | 1 starch, 1 fat |
| Granola Bar, Chewy, Low Fat | 1 | 109 | 2 | 20 | 0.5 | 0 | 0 | 70 | 22 | 1 | 1 | 1 1/2 starch |
| Meal Replacement Bar, Small | 1 1/3 oz bar | 140 | 4 | 35 | 2 | 0 | 2 | 75 | 22 | 4 | 6 | 1 1/2 starch, 1 fat |
| Meal Replacement Bar, Medium | 2 oz bar | 202 | 5 | 45 | 3 | 0 | 2 | 130 | 27 | 2 | 12 | 2 carb, 1 med-fat meat |
| Melba Toast | 4 pieces | 78 | <1 | 0 | 0 | 0 | 0 | 166 | 15 | 1 | 2 | 1 starch |
| Oriental Snack Mix | 1 oz | 155 | 12 | 108 | 5 | 0 | 0 | 235 | 9 | 4 | 5 | 1/2 starch, 2 fat |
| Pita Chips | 3/4 oz | 86 | 3 | 25 | 1 | 0 | 0 | 246 | 12 | <1 | 2 | 1 starch, 1 fat |
| Popcorn, Microwave, 94% Fat Free | 3 cups | 65 | 1 | 10 | <1 | 0 | 0 | 155 | 14 | 2.5 | 2 | 1 starch |

| | | | | | | | | | | | | |
|---|---|---|---|---|---|---|---|---|---|---|---|---|
| Popcorn, Microwave, Butter | 3 cups | 96 | 6 | 55 | 3 | 0 | 0 | 216 | 11 | 2 | 2 | 1 starch, 1 fat |
| Popcorn, No Salt Added | 3 cup | 93 | 1 | 10 | 0 | 0 | 0 | 2 | 19 | 3.5 | 3 | 1 starch |
| Pretzels, Sticks or Rings | 3/4 oz | 80 | <1 | 0 | 0 | 0 | 0 | 360 | 17 | <1 | 2 | 1 starch |
| Rice Cakes | 2 | 70 | <1 | 0 | 0 | 0 | 0 | 59 | 15 | <1 | 2 | 1 starch |
| Sandwich Crackers, Cheese Filled | 3 | 100 | 4 | 35 | 1 | 0 | 0 | 294 | 13 | <1 | 2 | 1 starch, 1 fat |
| Sandwich Crackers, Peanut Butter | 3 | 102 | 5 | 45 | 1 | 0 | 0 | 198 | 12 | <1 | 2 | 1 starch, 1 fat |
| Tortilla Chips | 3/4 oz | 106 | 6 | 55 | 1 | 0 | 0 | 131 | 13 | <1 | 2 | 1 starch, 1 fat |
| Tortilla Chips, Fat Free | 3/4 oz | 82 | <1 | 0 | 0 | 0 | 0 | 111 | 18 | 3 | 2 | 1 starch |
| Trail Mix, Fruit Based | 1 oz | 115 | 5 | 45 | 2 | 0 | 0 | 3 | 19 | 2 | 2 | 1 starch, 1 fat |
| **Brands** | | | | | | | | | | | | |
| ***Act II Microwave Popcorn*** | | | | | | | | | | | | |
| 94% Fat Free Butter Popcorn | 3 Tbsp | 130 | 2.5 | 20 | 0.5 | 0 | 0 | 310 | 28 | 5 | 4 | 2 starch, 1 fat |

SNACKS, CRACKERS, CHIPS, POPCORN

| | Serving | Calories | Fat (g) | Cal. from Fat | Sat. Fat (g) | Trans Fat (g) | Chol. (mg) | Sod. (mg) | Carb. (g) | Fiber (g) | Prot. (g) | Servings/Exchanges |
|---|---|---|---|---|---|---|---|---|---|---|---|---|
| 94% Fat Free Kettle Corn | 3 Tbsp | 130 | 2.5 | 20 | 1 | 0 | 0 | 370 | 28 | 5 | 4 | 2 starch, 1 fat |
| Light Butter Popcorn | 2 Tbsp | 110 | 4.5 | 40 | 2 | 0 | 0 | 400 | 19 | 3 | 3 | 1 starch, 1 fat |
| Movie Theatre Pop 'n Serve Tub | 2 Tbsp | 160 | 10 | 90 | 2 | 4.5 | 0 | 300 | 18 | 3 | 3 | 1 starch, 2 fat |
| ***Austin*** | | | | | | | | | | | | |
| Cheese Crackers with Cheddar Cheese | 1 pkg | 190 | 10 | 90 | 2.5 | 0 | 0 | 350 | 23 | <1 | 3 | 1 1/2 starch, 2 fat |
| Cheese Crackers with Peanut Butter | 1 pkg | 190 | 10 | 90 | 1.5 | 0 | 0 | 330 | 23 | 1 | 4 | 1 1/2 starch, 2 fat |
| Toasty Crackers with Peanut Butter | 1 pkg | 130 | 6 | 50 | 1 | 0 | 0 | 200 | 16 | <1 | 3 | 1 starch, 1 fat |
| ***Barbara's Bakery*** | | | | | | | | | | | | |
| Crunchy Organic Granola Bar, Oats & Honey | 2 bars | 190 | 8 | 70 | 1 | 0 | 0 | 60 | 27 | 3 | 4 | 2 carb, 2 fat |

| | | | | | | | | | | | | |
|---|---|---|---|---|---|---|---|---|---|---|---|---|
| Fruit & Yogurt Bar, Strawberry Apple | 1 bar | 150 | 3 | 25 | 0 | 0 | 0 | 125 | 28 | 1 | 3 | 2 carb, 1 fat |
| Nature's Choice Multigrain Cereal Bar, Apple Cinnamon | 1 bar | 140 | 2 | 20 | 0 | 0 | 0 | 80 | 28 | 1 | 2 | 2 carb |
| ***Betty Crocker*** | | | | | | | | | | | | |
| Fruit By The Foot | 1 roll | 80 | 1 | 10 | 0 | 0 | 0 | 45 | 17 | 0 | 0 | 1 carb |
| Fruit Gushers | 1 pouch | 90 | 1 | 10 | 0 | 0 | 0 | 45 | 20 | 0 | 0 | 1 carb |
| Fruit Roll-Ups | 1 | 50 | 1 | 5 | 0 | 0 | 0 | 55 | 12 | 0 | 0 | 1 carb |
| Fruit-Flavored Shapes, Batman | 1 pouch | 80 | 0 | 0 | 0 | 0 | 0 | 30 | 21 | 0 | 0 | 1 1/2 carb |
| ***Cracker Jack*** | | | | | | | | | | | | |
| Original | 1/2 cup | 120 | 2 | 15 | 0 | 0 | 0 | 70 | 23 | 1 | 2 | 1 1/2 carb |
| ***Entenmann's*** | | | | | | | | | | | | |
| Apple Cinnamon Cereal Bar | 1 bar | 140 | 3 | 25 | 1.5 | 0 | 0 | 105 | 28 | 1 | 1 | 2 carb, 1 fat |

| | Serving | Calories | Fat (g) | Cal. from Fat | Sat. Fat (g) | Trans Fat (g) | Chol. (mg) | Sod. (mg) | Carb. (g) | Fiber (g) | Prot. (g) | Servings/Exchanges |
|---|---|---|---|---|---|---|---|---|---|---|---|---|
| Chewy Chocolate Chip Cereal Bar | 1 bar | 150 | 6 | 50 | 2.53 | 0 | 5 | 110 | 25 | 2 | 2 | 1 1/2 carb, 1 fat |
| Strawberry Cereal Bar | 1 bar | 140 | 3 | 25 | 1.5 | 0 | 0 | 105 | 28 | 1 | 1 | 2 carb, 1 fat |
| ***Extend Bar*** | | | | | | | | | | | | |
| Peanut Butter Chocolate Delight | 1 bar | 150 | 3 | 30 | 1 | 0 | 0 | 180 | 21 | 5 | 11 | 1 1/2 carb, 1 lean meat |
| ***Franklin*** | | | | | | | | | | | | |
| Crunch 'n Munch, Buttery Toffee | 2/3 cup | 140 | 5 | 45 | 1.5 | 0 | <5 | 160 | 23 | 1 | 2 | 1 1/2 carb, 1 fat |
| Crunch 'n Munch, Caramel | 2/3 cup | 150 | 6 | 50 | 2.5 | 0 | 10 | 100 | 23 | <1 | 2 | 1 1/2 carb, 1 fat |
| ***Frito-Lay*** | | | | | | | | | | | | |
| Baken-ets Fried Pork Skins, Traditional | 8 | 90 | 6 | 55 | 2 | 0 | 15 | 550 | <1 | <1 | 7 | 1 med-fat meat |

| | | | | | | | | | | | | |
|---|---|---|---|---|---|---|---|---|---|---|---|---|
| Cheetos, Baked | 1 oz | 130 | 5 | 45 | 1 | 0 | 0 | 240 | 19 | 0 | 2 | 1 starch, 1 fat |
| Cheetos, Baked! 100 Calorie Mini Bites | 1 pkg | 100 | 4 | 35 | 0.5 | 0 | 0 | 180 | 14 | 0 | 2 | 1 starch, 1 fat |
| Cheetos, Crunchy | 1 oz | 160 | 10 | 90 | 2 | 0 | <5 | 290 | 15 | <1 | 2 | 1 starch, 2 fat |
| Cheetos, Flamin' Hot | 1 oz | 170 | 11 | 100 | 1.5 | 0 | 0 | 250 | 15 | <1 | 2 | 1 starch, 2 fat |
| Cheetos, Natural White Cheddar Puffs | 1 oz | 150 | 9 | 80 | 1.5 | 0 | 0 | 290 | 16 | <1 | 2 | 1 starch, 2 fat |
| Cheetos, Puffs | 1 oz | 160 | 10 | 90 | 1.5 | 0 | 0 | 370 | 15 | <1 | 2 | 1 starch, 2 fat |
| Chester's Butter Popcorn | 1 oz | 160 | 11 | 100 | 1.5 | 0 | 0 | 300 | 12 | <1 | 1 | 1 starch 2 fat |
| Chester's Cheddar Cheese Popcorn | 1 oz | 150 | 10 | 90 | 1.5 | 0 | 0 | 200 | 15 | 3 | 2 | 1 starch, 2 fat |
| Crackers, Peanut Butter on Toast | 1 pkg | 200 | 10 | 90 | 2.5 | 1 | 0 | 310 | 23 | 2 | 4 | 1 1/2 starch, 2 fat |
| Crackers, Peanut Butter Sandwich Crackers | 1 pkg | 190 | 9 | 80 | 2.5 | 1 | 0 | 370 | 23 | 2 | 5 | 1 1/2 starch, 2 fat |

SNACKS, CRACKERS, CHIPS, POPCORN

| | Serving | Calories | Fat (g) | Cal. from Fat | Sat. Fat (g) | Trans Fat (g) | Chol. (mg) | Sod. (mg) | Carb. (g) | Fiber (g) | Prot. (g) | Servings/Exchanges |
|---|---|---|---|---|---|---|---|---|---|---|---|---|
| Doritos, 100 Calorie Mini Bites, Nacho Cheese | 1 pkg | 100 | 6 | 60 | 1 | 0 | 0 | 140 | 12 | 0 | 2 | 1 starch, 1 fat |
| Doritos, Cooler Ranch | 1 oz | 150 | 8 | 70 | 1 | 0 | 0 | 180 | 18 | 2 | 2 | 1 starch, 2 fat |
| Doritos, Diablo | 1 oz | 150 | 8 | 70 | 1 | 0 | 0 | 310 | 17 | 2 | 2 | 1 starch, 2 fat |
| Doritos, Last Call Jalapeño Popper | 1 oz | 150 | 8 | 70 | 1.5 | 0 | 0 | 230 | 17 | 2 | 2 | 1 starch, 2 fat |
| Doritos, Nacho Cheese | 1 oz | 150 | 8 | 70 | 1.5 | 0 | 0 | 180 | 17 | 1 | 2 | 1 starch, 2 fat |
| Doritos, Reduced Fat Nacho Cheese | 1 pkg | 130 | 5 | 45 | 1 | 0 | 0 | 220 | 19 | 1 | 2 | 1 starch, 1 fat |
| Doritos, Reduced Fat, Cool Ranch | 1 pkg | 130 | 5 | 45 | 1 | 0 | 0 | 160 | 19 | 2 | 2 | 1 starch, 1 fat |
| Doritos, Salsa Verde | 1 oz | 140 | 7 | 70 | 1 | 0 | 0 | 210 | 19 | 1 | 2 | 1 starch, 1 fat |
| Doritos, Spicy Nacho | 1 oz | 140 | 7 | 60 | 1 | 0 | 0 | 210 | 18 | 1 | 2 | 1 starch, 1 fat |
| Doritos, Toasted Corn | 1 oz | 140 | 7 | 60 | 1 | 0 | 0 | 120 | 18 | 1 | 2 | 1 starch, 1 fat |

| | | | | | | | | | | | | |
|---|---|---|---|---|---|---|---|---|---|---|---|---|
| Fritos, BBQ | 1 oz | 150 | 10 | 90 | 1.5 | 0 | 0 | 280 | 16 | 1 | 2 | 1 starch, 2 fat |
| Fritos, Chili Cheese | 1 oz | 160 | 10 | 90 | 1.5 | 0 | 0 | 260 | 15 | 1 | 2 | 1 starch, 2 fat |
| Fritos, Flamin' Hot | 1 oz | 160 | 10 | 90 | 1.5 | 0 | 0 | 160 | 15 | 1 | 2 | 1 starch, 2 fat |
| Fritos, Flavor Twists, Honey BBQ | 1 oz | 160 | 10 | 90 | 1.5 | 0 | 0 | 210 | 16 | 1 | 2 | 1 starch, 2 fat |
| Fritos, Original | 1 oz | 160 | 10 | 90 | 1.5 | 0 | 0 | 170 | 15 | 1 | 2 | 1 starch, 2 fat |
| Fritos, Scoops | 1 oz | 160 | 10 | 90 | 1.5 | 0 | 0 | 110 | 16 | 1 | 2 | 1 starch, 2 fat |
| Funyuns Onion Flavored Rings | 1 oz | 140 | 7 | 60 | 1 | 0 | 0 | 270 | 18 | <1 | 2 | 1 starch, 1 fat |
| Lay's, Baked BBQ Potato Chips | 1 oz | 120 | 3 | 30 | 0.5 | 0 | 0 | 210 | 22 | 2 | 2 | 1 1/2 starch, 1 fat |
| Lay's, Baked Original Potato Chips | 1 oz | 120 | 2 | 15 | 0 | 0 | 0 | 180 | 23 | 2 | 2 | 1 1/2 starch |
| Lay's, Baked Sour Cream & Onion Potato Chips | 1 oz | 120 | 3 | 25 | 0.5 | 0 | 0 | 210 | 21 | 2 | 2 | 1 1/2 starch, 1 fat |

SNACKS, CRACKERS, CHIPS, POPCORN

| | Serving | Calories | Fat (g) | Cal. from Fat | Sat. Fat (g) | Trans Fat (g) | Chol. (mg) | Sod. (mg) | Carb. (g) | Fiber (g) | Prot. (g) | Servings/Exchanges |
|---|---|---|---|---|---|---|---|---|---|---|---|---|
| Lay's, BBQ Potato Chips | 1 oz | 150 | 10 | 90 | 1 | 0 | 0 | 200 | 15 | 1 | 2 | 1 starch, 2 fat |
| Lay's, Classic Potato Chips | 1 oz | 150 | 10 | 90 | 1 | 0 | 0 | 180 | 15 | 1 | 2 | 1 starch, 2 fat |
| Lay's, Kettle Cooked, Original | 1 oz | 150 | 8 | 80 | 1 | 0 | 0 | 110 | 18 | 1 | 2 | 1 starch, 2 fat |
| Lay's, Light Original | 1 oz | 75 | 0 | 0 | 0 | 0 | 0 | 200 | 17 | 1 | 2 | 1 starch |
| Lay's, Natural Sea Salt & Vinegar | 1 oz | 140 | 7 | 60 | 1 | 0 | 0 | 260 | 17 | 1 | 2 | 1 starch, 1 fat |
| Lay's, Salt & Vinegar Potato Chips | 1 oz | 150 | 10 | 90 | 1 | 0 | 0 | 380 | 15 | 1 | 2 | 1 starch, 2 fat |
| Lay's, Stax, Original Potato Crisps | 1 oz | 150 | 9 | 80 | 1 | 0 | 0 | 160 | 16 | 1 | 2 | 1 starch, 2 fat |
| Lay's, Wavy Au Gratin Potato Chips | 1 oz | 150 | 10 | 90 | 1.5 | 0 | <5 | 200 | 14 | 1 | 2 | 1 starch, 2 fat |

| | | | | | | | | | | | | |
|---|---|---|---|---|---|---|---|---|---|---|---|---|
| Lay's, Wavy Original Potato Chips | 1 oz | 150 | 10 | 90 | 1 | 0 | 0 | 180 | 15 | 1 | 2 | 1 starch, 2 fat |
| Lay's, Wavy Ranch Potato Chips | 1 oz | 150 | 10 | 80 | 1.5 | 0 | 0 | 200 | 16 | 1 | 2 | 1 starch, 2 fat |
| Munchies, Flamin' Hot Snack Mix | 3/4 cup | 140 | 7 | 60 | 1 | 0 | 0 | 200 | 18 | 1 | 2 | 1 starch, 1 fat |
| Munchos Potato Crisps | 1 oz | 160 | 10 | 90 | 1.5 | 0 | 0 | 230 | 16 | 1 | 1 | 1 starch, 2 fat |
| Rold Gold, Cheddar Cheese Tiny Twists Pretzels | 1 oz | 110 | 1 | 10 | 0 | 0 | 0 | 370 | 22 | 1 | 3 | 1 1/2 starch |
| Rold Gold, Classic Style Tiny Twists Pretzels | 1 oz | 110 | 1 | 10 | 0 | 0 | 0 | 450 | 23 | 1 | 3 | 1 1/2 starch |
| Rold Gold, Fat Free Tiny Twists Pretzels | 1 oz | 100 | 0 | 0 | 0 | 0 | 0 | 420 | 23 | 1 | 3 | 1 1/2 starch |
| Rold Gold, Honey Mustard Tiny Twists Pretzels | 1 oz | 110 | 1 | 10 | 0 | 0 | 0 | 430 | 23 | 1 | 3 | 1 1/2 starch |

SNACKS, CRACKERS, CHIPS, POPCORN

| | Serving | Calories | Fat (g) | Cal. from Fat | Sat. Fat (g) | Trans Fat (g) | Chol. (mg) | Sod. (mg) | Carb. (g) | Fiber (g) | Prot. (g) | Servings/Exchanges |
|---|---|---|---|---|---|---|---|---|---|---|---|---|
| Rold Gold, Pretzel Sticks | 1 oz | 100 | 0 | 0 | 0 | 0 | 0 | 580 | 23 | 1 | 2 | 1 1/2 starch |
| Ruffles, Authentic Barbecue Flavored | 1 oz | 150 | 10 | 90 | 1 | 0 | 0 | 190 | 16 | 1 | 2 | 1 starch, 2 fat |
| Ruffles, Baked, Cheddar & Sour Cream | 1 oz | 120 | 3.5 | 30 | 0.5 | 0 | 0 | 270 | 21 | 2 | 2 | 1 1/2 starch, 1 fat |
| Ruffles, Baked, Original | 1 oz | 120 | 3 | 30 | 0 | 0 | 0 | 200 | 21 | 2 | 2 | 1 1/2 starch, 1 fat |
| Ruffles, Cheddar & Sour Cream | 1 oz | 160 | 11 | 90 | 1.5 | 0 | 0 | 230 | 14 | 1 | 2 | 1 starch, 2 fat |
| Ruffles, Light Original | 1 oz | 70 | 0 | 0 | 0 | 0 | 0 | 190 | 17 | 1 | 2 | 1 starch |
| Ruffles, Original | 1oz | 160 | 10 | 90 | 1 | 0 | 0 | 160 | 14 | 1 | 2 | 1 starch, 2 fat |
| Ruffles, Sour Cream & Onion | 1 oz | 160 | 11 | 90 | 1.5 | 0 | 0 | 190 | 14 | 1 | 2 | 1 starch, 2 fat |
| Santitas White Corn Tortilla Chips | 1 oz | 130 | 6 | 50 | 1 | 0 | 0 | 110 | 19 | 1 | 2 | 1 starch, 1 fat |

| | | | | | | | | | | | | |
|---|---|---|---|---|---|---|---|---|---|---|---|---|
| Santitas Yellow Corn Tortilla Chips | 1 oz | 140 | 6 | 50 | 1 | 0 | 0 | 110 | 19 | 2 | 2 | 1 starch, 1 fat |
| Smartfood White Cheddar Cheese Popcorn | 1 pkg | 100 | 6 | 60 | 1.5 | 0 | <5 | 180 | 9 | 1 | 2 | 1/2 starch, 1 fat |
| Smartfood White Cheddar Cheese Popcorn, Reduced Fat | 3 cups | 140 | 6 | 50 | 1.5 | 0 | <5 | 280 | 19 | 3 | 4 | 1 starch, 1 fat |
| Sunchips, French Onion | 1 oz | 140 | 6 | 60 | 1 | 0 | 0 | 130 | 18 | 2 | 2 | 1 starch, 1 fat |
| Sunchips, Harvest Cheddar | 1 oz | 140 | 6 | 50 | 1 | 0 | 0 | 160 | 19 | 2 | 2 | 1 starch, 1 fat |
| Sunchips, Original | 1 oz | 140 | 6 | 50 | 1 | 0 | 0 | 120 | 19 | 2 | 2 | 1 starch, 1 fat |
| Tostitos, Baked Scoops | 1 oz | 120 | 3 | 25 | 0.5 | 0 | 0 | 125 | 22 | 2 | 1 | 1 1/2 starch, 1 fat |
| Tostitos, Bite Size Rounds | 1 oz | 140 | 8 | 70 | 1 | 0 | 0 | 110 | 18 | 1 | 2 | 1 starch, 2 fat |
| Tostitos, Crispy Rounds | 1 oz | 140 | 7 | 70 | 1 | 0 | 0 | 120 | 18 | 1 | 2 | 1 starch, 1 fat |

SNACKS, CRACKERS, CHIPS, POPCORN

| | Serving | Calories | Fat (g) | Cal. from Fat | Sat. Fat (g) | Trans Fat (g) | Chol. (mg) | Sod. (mg) | Carb. (g) | Fiber (g) | Prot. (g) | Servings/Exchanges |
|---|---|---|---|---|---|---|---|---|---|---|---|---|
| Tostitos, Restaurant Style | 1 oz | 140 | 7 | 60 | 1 | 0 | 0 | 115 | 19 | 2 | 2 | 1 starch, 1 fat |
| Tostitos, Restaurant Style, Hint of Lime | 1 oz | 150 | 8 | 70 | 1 | 0 | 0 | 160 | 18 | 1 | 2 | 1 starch, 2 fat |
| ***Gardetto's*** | | | | | | | | | | | | |
| Snack Mix, Original | 1/2 cup | 150 | 6 | 60 | 1 | 1 | 0 | 270 | 20 | 1 | 3 | 1 starch, 1 fat |
| Snack Mix, Reduced Fat Original | 1/2 cup | 130 | 4 | 35 | 1 | 0.5 | 0 | 330 | 20 | 1 | 3 | 1 starch, 1 fat |
| ***General Mills*** | | | | | | | | | | | | |
| Bugles, Original | 1 1/3 cup | 160 | 9 | 80 | 8 | 0 | 0 | 310 | 18 | <1 | 1 | 1 starch, 2 fat |
| Cheerios Snack Mix, Cheddar | 2/3 cup | 120 | 3 | 30 | 0.5 | 0 | 0 | 310 | 21 | 1 | 3 | 1 1/2 carb, 1 fat |
| Cheerios Snack Mix, Original | 2/3 cup | 130 | 3.5 | 30 | 0.5 | 0 | 0 | 290 | 22 | 1 | 3 | 1 1/2 carb, 1 fat |

| | | | | | | | | | | | | |
|---|---|---|---|---|---|---|---|---|---|---|---|---|
| Chex Mix Bar, Chocolate Chunk | 1 bar | 140 | 3 | 30 | 0 | 0 | 0 | 135 | 26 | 2 | 2 | 2 carb, 1 fat |
| Chex Mix Select, Chocolate Turtle | 1/2 cup | 130 | 4.5 | 40 | 2 | 0 | <5 | 130 | 20 | <1 | 2 | 1 starch, 1 fat |
| Chex Mix Sweet 'n Salty, Trail Mix | 1/2 cup | 140 | 5 | 45 | 1.5 | 0 | 0 | 140 | 23 | 1 | 2 | 1 1/2 starch, 1 fat |
| Chex Mix, Bold Party Blend | 1/2 cup | 120 | 4.5 | 40 | 1 | 0.5 | 0 | 260 | 18 | <1 | 2 | 1 starch, 1 fat |
| Chex Mix, Cheddar | 1/2 cup | 120 | 3.5 | 30 | 0.5 | 0 | 0 | 210 | 20 | 1 | 2 | 1 starch, 1 fat |
| Chex Mix, Peanut Lovers | 1/2 cup | 140 | 5 | 50 | 1 | 0 | 0 | 270 | 20 | 1 | 3 | 1 starch, 1 fat |
| Chex Mix, Traditional | 1/2 cup | 110 | 3 | 30 | 0.5 | 0 | 0 | 240 | 19 | <1 | 2 | 1 starch, 1 fat |
| Fiber One Chewy Bar, Oats & Caramel | 1 bar | 140 | 3.5 | 30 | 1.5 | 0 | 0 | 105 | 30 | 9 | 2 | 2 carb, 1 fat |
| Fiber One Chewy Bar, Oats & Peanut Butter | 1 bar | 150 | 4.5 | 40 | 2 | 0 | 0 | 105 | 28 | 9 | 3 | 2 carb, 1 fat |

SNACKS, CRACKERS, CHIPS, POPCORN

| | Serving | Calories | Fat (g) | Cal. from Fat | Sat. Fat (g) | Trans Fat (g) | Chol. (mg) | Sod. (mg) | Carb. (g) | Fiber (g) | Prot. (g) | Servings/Exchanges |
|---|---|---|---|---|---|---|---|---|---|---|---|---|
| ***Health Valley Organic*** | | | | | | | | | | | | |
| Cereal Bar, Strawberry Cobbler | 1 bar | 130 | 2.5 | 20 | 0 | 0 | 0 | 85 | 26 | 1 | 2 | 2 carb, 1 fat |
| Crackers, Sesame | 4 | 70 | 3 | 30 | 0 | 0 | 0 | 200 | 10 | <1 | 1 | 1/2 starch, 1 fat |
| Crackers, Stoned Wheat | 4 | 70 | 3 | 30 | 0 | 0 | 0 | 170 | 10 | <1 | 1 | 1/2 starch, 1 fat |
| Graham Crackers, Amaranth Bran | 6 | 120 | 3 | 25 | 0 | 0 | 0 | 80 | 22 | 3 | 3 | 1 1/2 starch, 1 fat |
| Graham Crackers, Oat Bran | 6 | 120 | 3 | 25 | 0 | 0 | 0 | 80 | 22 | 3 | 3 | 1 1/2 carb, 1 fat |
| Granola Bar, Chocolate Chewy | 1 bar | 110 | 2 | 20 | 1 | 0 | 0 | 10 | 22 | <1 | 1 | 1 1/2 carb |
| ***Jolly Time*** | | | | | | | | | | | | |
| Blast O Butter Popcorn | 3 1/2 cups | 150 | 12 | 110 | 3 | 4 | 0 | 340 | 19 | 9 | 3 | 1 starch, 2 fat |

| | | | | | | | | | | | | |
|---|---|---|---|---|---|---|---|---|---|---|---|---|
| Healthy Pop Popcorn, 94% Fat Free | 5 cups | 90 | 2 | 20 | 0 | 0 | 0 | 210 | 23 | 9 | 3 | 1 1/2 starch |
| Mallow Magic Popcorn | 2 1/2 cups | 170 | 12 | 110 | 2 | 3 | 0 | 170 | 16 | 3 | 1 | 1 starch, 2 fat |
| The Big Cheez Popcorn | 3 1/2 cups | 160 | 11 | 100 | 2.5 | 4 | 0 | 340 | 17 | 6 | 2 | 1 starch, 2 fat |
| ***Kashi*** | | | | | | | | | | | | |
| TLC Fruit & Grain Bar, Dark Chocolate Coconut | 1 bar | 120 | 3.5 | 30 | 1.5 | 0 | 0 | 50 | 21 | 4 | 4 | 1 1/2 carb, 1 fat |
| TLC Fruit & Grain Bar, Raspberry Chocolate | 1 bar | 120 | 3 | 30 | 0.5 | 0 | 0 | 50 | 21 | 4 | 4 | 1 1/2 carb, 1 fat |
| ***Kay's Naturals*** | | | | | | | | | | | | |
| Better Balance Pretzel Sticks, Jalapeño Honey Mustard | 1 oz | 120 | 6 | 60 | 1.5 | 0 | 0 | 150 | 9 | 2 | 10 | 1/2 carb, 1 med-fat meat |
| Better Balance Pretzel Sticks, Wasabi | 1 oz | 120 | 6 | 60 | 1.5 | 0 | 0 | 200 | 9 | 2 | 10 | 1/2 carb, 1 med-fat meat |

SNACKS, CRACKERS, CHIPS, POPCORN

| | Serving | Calories | Fat (g) | Cal. from Fat | Sat. Fat (g) | Trans Fat (g) | Chol. (mg) | Sod. (mg) | Carb. (g) | Fiber (g) | Prot. (g) | Servings/Exchanges |
|---|---|---|---|---|---|---|---|---|---|---|---|---|
| ***Keebler*** | | | | | | | | | | | | |
| Crackers, Club, Multi-Grain | 4 | 70 | 3 | 25 | 0 | 0 | 0 | 120 | 9 | <1 | 1 | 1/2 starch, 1 fat |
| Crackers, Club, Original | 4 | 70 | 3 | 25 | 0.5 | 0 | 0 | 125 | 9 | <1 | <1 | 1/2 starch, 1 fat |
| Crackers, Club, Reduced Fat | 5 | 70 | 2 | 20 | 0 | 0 | 0 | 150 | 12 | <1 | 1 | 1 starch |
| Crackers, Graham, Cinnamon | 8 | 130 | 3.5 | 35 | 1 | 0 | 0 | 140 | 23 | 1 | 2 | 1 1/2 starch, 1 fat |
| Crackers, Graham, Cinnamon, Low-Fat | 8 | 110 | 1.5 | 15 | 0 | 0 | 0 | 140 | 23 | 1 | 2 | 1 1/2 starch |
| Crackers, Graham, Original | 8 | 120 | 1 | 30 | 1 | 0 | 0 | 160 | 22 | 1 | 2 | 1 1/2 starch |
| Crackers, Honey Graham | 8 | 140 | 4 | 35 | 1 | 0 | 0 | 150 | 23 | <1 | 2 | 1 1/2 starch, 1 fat |

| | | | | | | | | | | | | |
|---|---|---|---|---|---|---|---|---|---|---|---|---|
| Crackers, Honey Graham, Bug Bites | 13 | 130 | 4 | 35 | 1.5 | 0 | 0 | 125 | 22 | <1 | 2 | 1 1/2 starch, 1 fat |
| Crackers, Krispy Soup & Oyster | 16 | 60 | 1.5 | 15 | 0 | 0 | 0 | 230 | 11 | <1 | 1 | 1 starch |
| Crackers, Toasteds, Buttercrisps | 5 | 80 | 4 | 35 | 0.5 | 0 | 0 | 150 | 10 | <1 | <1 | 1/2 starch, 1 fat |
| Crackers, Toasteds, Onion | 5 | 80 | 3 | 35 | 0.5 | 0 | 0 | 150 | 10 | <1 | <1 | 1/2 starch, 1 fat |
| Crackers, Toasteds, Sesame | 5 | 80 | 4 | 35 | 0.5 | 0 | 0 | 140 | 10 | <1 | 1 | 1/2 starch, 1 fat |
| Crackers, Toasteds, Wheat | 5 | 80 | 3.5 | 30 | 0.5 | 0 | 0 | 150 | 10 | <1 | 1 | 1/2 starch, 1 fat |
| Crackers, Town House Original | 5 | 80 | 4.5 | 40 | 1 | 0 | 0 | 130 | 10 | <1 | <1 | 1/2 starch, 1 fat |
| Crackers, Town House, Reduced Fat | 6 | 60 | 1.5 | 15 | 0 | 0 | 0 | 160 | 11 | <1 | 1 | 1 starch |
| Crackers, Wheatables, Original Golden Wheat | 17 | 140 | 6 | 50 | 1.5 | 0 | 0 | 340 | 20 | 1 | 2 | 1 starch, 1 fat |

SNACKS, CRACKERS, CHIPS, POPCORN

| | Serving | Calories | Fat (g) | Cal. from Fat | Sat. Fat (g) | Trans Fat (g) | Chol. (mg) | Sod. (mg) | Carb. (g) | Fiber (g) | Prot. (g) | Servings/Exchanges |
|---|---|---|---|---|---|---|---|---|---|---|---|---|
| Crackers, Wheatables, Reduced Fat | 19 | 140 | 4 | 35 | 1 | 0 | 0 | 320 | 22 | 1 | 2 | 1 1/2 starch, 1 fat |
| Crackers, Zesta Saltines, Original | 5 | 60 | 1.5 | 15 | 0 | 0 | 0 | 150 | 11 | <1 | 1 | 1 starch |
| Crackers, Zesta Saltines, Whole Wheat | 5 | 60 | 1.5 | 15 | 0 | 0 | 0 | 230 | 11 | <1 | 1 | 1 starch |
| ***Kellogg's*** | | | | | | | | | | | | |
| FiberPlus Antioidants Bar, Chocolate Chip | 1 bar | 120 | 4 | 40 | 2 | 0 | 0 | 55 | 26 | 9 | 2 | 2 carb, 1 fat |
| Nutri-Grain Cereal Bars (All Varieties) | 1 bar | 130 | 3 | 30 | 0.5 | 0 | 0 | 120 | 24 | 2 | 2 | 1 1/2 carb, 1 fat |
| Nutri-Grain Yogurt Bar, Strawberry | 1 bar | 140 | 3.5 | 30 | 0.5 | 0 | 0 | 110 | 25 | 2 | 2 | 1 1/2 carb, 1 fat |
| Rice Krispies Treats, Original | 1 | 90 | 2.5 | 20 | 1 | 0 | 0 | 105 | 17 | 0 | 1 | 1 starch, 1 fat |

| | | | | | | | | | | | | |
|---|---|---|---|---|---|---|---|---|---|---|---|---|
| Special K Bars | 1 bar | 90 | 1.5 | 15 | 1 | 0 | 0 | 95 | 18 | <1 | 1 | 1 carb |
| ***Kraft/Nabisco*** | | | | | | | | | | | | |
| Barnum's Animal Crackers | 10 | 120 | 4 | 35 | <1 | 0 | 0 | 140 | 22 | 0 | 0 | 1 1/2 starch, 1 fat |
| Better Cheddars, Baked Snack Crackers | 22 | 160 | 8 | 70 | 1.5 | 0 | 5 | 360 | 18 | <1 | 3 | 1 starch, 2 fat |
| Chicken-In-A-Biskit Crackers | 12 | 160 | 8 | 70 | 1.5 | 0 | 0 | 310 | 19 | 1 | 2 | 1 starch, 2 fat |
| Handi-Snacks, Premium Breadsticks 'n Cheez | 1 pkg | 110 | 4.5 | 40 | 1 | 0 | 5 | 350 | 14 | 0 | 3 | 1 starch, 1 fat |
| Handi-Snacks, Ritz Crackers 'n Cheez | 1 pkg | 100 | 6 | 50 | 1.5 | 0 | <5 | 330 | 11 | 0 | 2 | 1 starch, 1 fat |
| Honey Maid Grahams, Cinnamon | 8 | 130 | 2.5 | 25 | 0.5 | 0 | 0 | 170 | 25 | 1 | 2 | 1 1/2 starch, 1 fat |
| Honey Maid Grahams, Cinnamon, Low Fat | 8 | 120 | 1.5 | 15 | 0 | 0 | 0 | 180 | 26 | 1 | 2 | 2 starch |
| Honey Maid Grahams, Honey | 8 | 130 | 3 | 25 | 0.5 | 0 | 0 | 190 | 24 | 1 | 2 | 1 1/2 starch, 1 fat |

SNACKS, CRACKERS, CHIPS, POPCORN

| | Serving | Calories | Fat (g) | Cal. from Fat | Sat. Fat (g) | Trans Fat (g) | Chol. (mg) | Sod. (mg) | Carb. (g) | Fiber (g) | Prot. (g) | Servings/Exchanges |
|---|---|---|---|---|---|---|---|---|---|---|---|---|
| Honey Maid Grahams, Honey, Low Fat | 8 | 120 | 2 | 15 | 0 | 0 | 0 | 190 | 25 | 1 | 2 | 1 1/2 starch |
| Premium Saltine Crackers | 5 | 60 | 1.5 | 10 | 0 | 0 | 0 | 190 | 11 | 0 | 1 | 1 starch |
| Premium Saltine Crackers, Hint of Salt | 5 | 60 | 1.5 | 10 | 0 | 0 | 0 | 30 | 12 | 0 | 1 | 1 starch |
| Ritz Bits, Cheese | 13 | 150 | 9 | 80 | 3 | 0 | 0 | 250 | 17 | 0 | 2 | 1 starch, 2 fat |
| Ritz Bits, Peanut Butter | 12 | 140 | 8 | 70 | 1.5 | 0 | 0 | 240 | 16 | 1 | 3 | 1 starch, 2 fat |
| Ritz Crackers | 5 | 80 | 4.5 | 40 | 1 | 0 | 10 | 135 | 10 | 0 | 1 | 1 starch, 1 fat |
| Ritz Crackers, Hint of Salt | 5 | 80 | 4 | 35 | 1 | 0 | 0 | 35 | 10 | 0 | 1 | 1/2 starch, 1 fat |
| Ritz Crackers, Reduced Fat | 5 | 70 | 2 | 20 | 0 | 0 | 0 | 160 | 11 | 0 | 1 | 1 starch |
| Ritz Crackers, Whole Wheat | 5 | 70 | 2.5 | 25 | 0.5 | 0 | 0 | 120 | 11 | <1 | 1 | 1 starch, 1 fat |

| | | | | | | | | | | | | |
|---|---|---|---|---|---|---|---|---|---|---|---|---|
| Sociables | 5 | 70 | 3.5 | 30 | 0.5 | 0 | 0 | 140 | 9 | 0 | 1 | 1/2 starch, 1 fat |
| Triscuit Thin Crisps, Parmesan Garlic | 15 | 140 | 5 | 40 | 1 | 0 | 0 | 180 | 22 | 3 | 3 | 1 1/2 starch, 1 fat |
| Triscuits | 6 | 120 | 4.5 | 40 | 1 | 0 | 0 | 180 | 19 | 3 | 3 | 1 starch, 1 fat |
| Triscuits, Reduced Fat | 7 | 120 | 3 | 25 | 0.5 | 0 | 0 | 160 | 21 | 3 | 3 | 1 1/2 starch, 1 fat |
| Vegetable Thins, Baked Snack Crackers | 21 | 150 | 7 | 60 | 2 | 0 | 0 | 320 | 19 | 1 | 2 | 1 starch, 1 fat |
| Wheat Thins Toasted Chips, Multi-Grain | 14 | 120 | 4 | 35 | 0.5 | 0 | 0 | 240 | 20 | 1 | 2 | 1 starch, 1 fat |
| Wheat Thins, Multi-Grain | 15 | 140 | 4.5 | 40 | 0.5 | 0 | 0 | 230 | 22 | 2 | 2 | 1 1/2 starch, 1 fat |
| Wheat Thins, Original | 16 | 140 | 5 | 45 | 1 | 0 | 0 | 230 | 22 | 2 | 2 | 1 1/2 starch, 1 fat |
| Wheat Thins, Reduced Fat | 16 | 130 | 3.5 | 35 | 0.5 | 0 | 0 | 260 | 21 | 1 | 2 | 1 1/2 starch, 1 fat, |
| ***Orville Redenbacher's Gourmet Popping Corn*** | | | | | | | | | | | | |
| Butter | 4 1/2 cups | 170 | 12 | 110 | 6 | 0 | 0 | 260 | 17 | 3 | 2 | 1 starch, 2 fat |

SNACKS, CRACKERS, CHIPS, POPCORN

| | Serving | Calories | Fat (g) | Cal. from Fat | Sat. Fat (g) | Trans Fat (g) | Chol. (mg) | Sod. (mg) | Carb. (g) | Fiber (g) | Prot. (g) | Servings/Exchanges |
|---|---|---|---|---|---|---|---|---|---|---|---|---|
| Kettle Korn | 5 cups | 170 | 13 | 110 | 7 | 0 | <5 | 130 | 16 | 3 | 2 | 1 starch, 3 fat |
| Light Butter | 5 1/2 cups | 120 | 5 | 45 | 2.5 | 0 | 0 | 190 | 19 | 4 | 3 | 1 starch, 1 fat |
| Movie Theatre Butter | 4 1/2 cups | 170 | 12 | 110 | 6 | 0 | 0 | 360 | 16 | 3 | 2 | 1 starch, 2 fat |
| Smart Pop! 94% Fat Free Butter | 6 1/2 cups | 110 | 2 | 20 | 0.5 | 0 | 0 | 220 | 24 | 4 | 3 | 1 1/2 starch |
| Tender White | 3 1/2 cups | 170 | 12 | 110 | 6 | 0 | 0 | 250 | 15 | 2 | 3 | 1 starch, 2 fat |
| Ultimate Butter | 5 cups | 170 | 12 | 110 | 6 | 0 | 0 | 380 | 16 | 3 | 2 | 1 starch, 2 fat |
| ***Pepperidge Farm*** | | | | | | | | | | | | |
| Crackers, Cheese Crisps, Four Cheese | 20 | 140 | 6 | 55 | 1 | 0 | <5 | 270 | 19 | 1 | 3 | 1 starch, 1 fat |
| Crackers, Golden Butter | 4 | 70 | 2.5 | 25 | 1 | 0 | <5 | 100 | 11 | 0 | 1 | 1 starch, 1 fat |

| | | | | | | | | | | | | |
|---|---|---|---|---|---|---|---|---|---|---|---|---|
| Crackers, Harvest Wheat | 3 | 80 | 3.5 | 30 | 0.5 | 0 | 0 | 125 | 11 | <1 | 1 | 1 starch, 1 fat |
| Goldfish Crackers, Chocolate Grahams | 50 | 130 | 4 | 35 | 1 | 0 | 0 | 125 | 22 | 2 | 2 | 1 1/2 starch, 1 fat |
| Goldfish Crackers, Honey Graham | 50 | 140 | 4.5 | 40 | 1 | 0 | 0 | 150 | 23 | 1 | 2 | 1 1/2 starch, 1 fat |
| Goldfish Crackers, Original | 55 | 140 | 5 | 45 | 1 | 0 | <5 | 250 | 20 | <1 | 4 | 1 starch, 1 fat |
| Goldfish Crackers, Parmesan | 60 | 130 | 4 | 35 | 1 | 0 | 0 | 280 | 20 | <1 | 4 | 1 starch, 1 fat |
| Goldfish Crackers, Pizza Flavor | 55 | 140 | 5 | 45 | 1 | 0 | 0 | 230 | 20 | <1 | 3 | 1 starch, 1 fat |
| Goldfish Crackers, Pretzel | 43 | 130 | 2.5 | 25 | 0.5 | 0 | 0 | 430 | 24 | <1 | 3 | 1 1/2 starch, 1 fat |
| Goldfish Crackers, Whole Grain | 55 | 140 | 5 | 45 | 1 | 0 | <5 | 250 | 19 | 2 | 4 | 1 starch, 1 fat |

SNACKS, CRACKERS, CHIPS, POPCORN

| | Serving | Calories | Fat (g) | Cal. from Fat | Sat. Fat (g) | Trans Fat (g) | Chol. (mg) | Sod. (mg) | Carb. (g) | Fiber (g) | Prot. (g) | Servings/Exchanges |
|---|---|---|---|---|---|---|---|---|---|---|---|---|
| Snack Sticks, Toasted Sesame | 12 | 140 | 5 | 45 | 1 | 0 | 0 | 290 | 20 | 2 | 4 | 1 starch, 1 fat |
| ***Planters*** | | | | | | | | | | | | |
| Double Peanut Bar | 1 | 220 | 13 | 110 | 3 | 0 | 0 | 160 | 22 | 3 | 7 | 1 1/2 carb, 3 fat |
| Fiddle Faddle | 3/4 cup | 150 | 7 | 63 | 3 | 0 | 10 | 180 | 20 | 1 | 2 | 1 carb, 1 fat |
| Fiddle Faddle, Fat-Free | 1 cup | 110 | 0 | 0 | 0 | 0 | 0 | 210 | 28 | 0 | 2 | 2 carb |
| ***Poore Brothers*** | | | | | | | | | | | | |
| Chips, Original | 1 oz | 140 | 9 | 80 | 2.5 | 0 | 0 | 180 | 15 | 1 | 2 | 1 starch, 2 fat |
| Chips, Salt & Vinegar | 1 oz | 150 | 9 | 80 | 2.5 | 0 | 0 | 470 | 15 | 1 | 2 | 1 starch, 2 fat |
| ***Pop-Secret Microwave Popcorn*** | | | | | | | | | | | | |
| 94% Fat Free Butter | 6 cups | 120 | 2 | 20 | 0.5 | 0 | 0 | 400 | 26 | 4 | 4 | 2 starch |
| Butter | 4 cups | 180 | 11 | 100 | 2.5 | 5 | 0 | 330 | 17 | 3 | 3 | 1 starch, 2 fat |
| Homestyle | 4 cups | 180 | 11 | 100 | 1.5 | 5 | 0 | 410 | 18 | 3 | 3 | 1 starch, 2 fat |
| Kettle Corn | 4 cups | 180 | 13 | 120 | 3 | 6 | 0 | 150 | 15 | 3 | 2 | 1 starch, 3 fat |

| | | | | | | | | | | | | |
|---|---|---|---|---|---|---|---|---|---|---|---|---|
| Movie Theater Butter | 4 cups | 180 | 12 | 100 | 2.5 | 5 | 0 | 300 | 18 | 3 | 2 | 1 starch, 2 fat |
| ***Power Bar*** | | | | | | | | | | | | |
| Performance Energy Bar, Chocolate | 1 | 240 | 3 | 30 | 1 | 0 | 0 | 200 | 45 | 3 | 8 | 3 carb, 1 fat |
| Performance Energy Bar, Vanilla Crisp | 1 | 240 | 3.5 | 35 | 0.5 | 0 | 0 | 200 | 45 | 1 | 8 | 3 carb, 1 fat |
| ***Pringles*** | | | | | | | | | | | | |
| Chips, Original | 1 oz | 150 | 9 | 90 | 2.5 | 0 | 0 | 150 | 15 | 1 | 1 | 1 starch, 2 fat |
| Chips, Original, Light | 1 oz | 70 | 0 | 0 | 0 | 0 | 0 | 160 | 15 | 0 | 1 | 1 starch |
| Chips, Sour Cream & Onion | 1 oz | 150 | 9 | 80 | 2.5 | 0 | 0 | 170 | 15 | 1 | 1 | 1 starch, 2 fat |
| Chips, Sour Cream & Onion, Light | 1 oz | 70 | 0 | 0 | 0 | 0 | 0 | 190 | 15 | 1 | 2 | 1 starch |
| ***Quaker*** | | | | | | | | | | | | |
| Cheesy Nacho Tortillaz | 1 oz | 130 | 5 | 45 | 0.5 | 0 | 0 | 230 | 20 | 1 | 2 | 1 carb, 1 fat |
| Chewy 25% Less Sugar Bar, Baked Apple | 1 bar | 100 | 3.5 | 30 | 1 | 0 | 0 | 75 | 17 | 3 | 1 | 1 carb, 1 fat |

SNACKS, CRACKERS, CHIPS, POPCORN

| | Serving | Calories | Fat (g) | Cal. from Fat | Sat. Fat (g) | Trans Fat (g) | Chol. (mg) | Sod. (mg) | Carb. (g) | Fiber (g) | Prot. (g) | Servings/Exchanges |
|---|---|---|---|---|---|---|---|---|---|---|---|---|
| Chewy Granola Bar, Chocolate Chip | 1 bar | 100 | 3 | 20 | 0.5 | 0 | 15 | 80 | 19 | 1 | 1 | 1 carb |
| Fiber & Omega-3 Bar, Peanut Butter Chocolate | 1 bar | 150 | 5 | 45 | 2 | 0 | 0 | 35 | 25 | 9 | 3 | 1 1/2 carb, 1 fat |
| Granola Bites | 1 bag | 90 | 3.5 | 30 | 2 | 0 | 0 | 30 | 14 | 2 | 2 | 1 carb, 1 fat |
| Mini Rice Cakes, Apple Cinnamon | 8 | 60 | 0 | 0 | 0 | 0 | 0 | 50 | 15 | 0 | 1 | 1 carb |
| Mini Rice Cakes, Caramel Corn | 7 | 60 | 0 | 0 | 0 | 0 | 0 | 150 | 13 | 0 | 1 | 1 carb |
| Rice Cakes, Apple Cinnamon | 1 | 50 | 0 | 0 | 0 | 0 | 0 | 0 | 11 | 0 | 1 | 1 carb |
| Rice Cakes, Butter Popped Corn | 1 | 35 | 0 | 0 | 0 | 0 | 0 | 45 | 8 | 0 | 1 | 1/2 carb |
| Rice Cakes, Caramel Corn | 1 | 50 | 0 | 0 | 0 | 0 | 0 | 30 | 11 | 0 | 1 | 1 carb |

| | | | | | | | | | | | | |
|---|---|---|---|---|---|---|---|---|---|---|---|---|
| Rice Cakes, Peanut Butter Chocolate Chip | 1 | 60 | 1 | 10 | 0 | 0 | 0 | 70 | 12 | 0 | 1 | 1 carb |
| Rice Cakes, Salt Free | 1 | 35 | 0 | 0 | 0 | 0 | 0 | 0 | 7 | 0 | 1 | 1 carb |
| ***Ross*** | | | | | | | | | | | | |
| Chewy Glucerna Meal Bar, Oatmeal Raisin | 1 bar | 220 | 6 | 50 | 3.5 | 0 | <5 | 105 | 35 | 2 | 10 | 2 carb, 1 med-fat meat |
| ***Ry Krisp*** | | | | | | | | | | | | |
| Crackers, Seasoned, Fat Free | 2 | 60 | 1 | 10 | 0 | 0 | 0 | 80 | 11 | 3 | 1 | 1 starch |
| Crackers, Sesame Rye | 2 | 60 | 1.5 | 15 | 0 | 0 | 0 | 80 | 10 | 3 | 1 | 1/2 starch |
| ***Snyder's of Hanover*** | | | | | | | | | | | | |
| Butter Snaps | 24 | 120 | 1 | 10 | 0 | 0 | 0 | 270 | 25 | 1 | 3 | 1 1/2 starch |
| Honey Mustard & Onion Nibblers | 13 | 130 | 3 | 25 | 1.5 | 0 | 0 | 95 | 23 | <1 | 3 | 1 1/2 starch, 1 fat |
| Hot Buffalo Wing Pieces | 1/3 cup | 140 | 7 | 60 | 3 | 0 | 0 | 380 | 17 | <1 | 2 | 1 starch, 1 fat |
| Mini Pretzels | 20 | 110 | 0 | 0 | 0 | 0 | 0 | 250 | 25 | <1 | 3 | 1 1/2 starch |
| Rods | 3 | 120 | 1 | 10 | 0 | 0 | 0 | 290 | 24 | 1 | 3 | 1 1/2 starch |

SNACKS, CRACKERS, CHIPS, POPCORN

| | Serving | Calories | Fat (g) | Cal. from Fat | Sat. Fat (g) | Trans Fat (g) | Chol. (mg) | Sod. (mg) | Carb. (g) | Fiber (g) | Prot. (g) | Servings/Exchanges |
|---|---|---|---|---|---|---|---|---|---|---|---|---|
| ***South Beach Living*** | | | | | | | | | | | | |
| High Protein Cereal Bar, Peanut Butter | 1 | 140 | 5 | 50 | 2 | 0 | 0 | 160 | 15 | 3 | 10 | 1 carb, 1 med-fat meat |
| ***Stacy's*** | | | | | | | | | | | | |
| Pita Chips, Multigrain | 1 oz | 140 | 5 | 50 | 0.5 | 0 | 0 | 270 | 19 | 2 | 3 | 1 starch, 1 fat |
| Pita Chips, Simply Naked | 1 oz | 130 | 5 | 45 | 0.5 | 0 | 0 | 270 | 19 | 1 | 3 | 1 starch, 1 fat |
| ***Sunshine*** | | | | | | | | | | | | |
| Cheez-It, Original | 27 | 150 | 8 | 70 | 3 | 0 | 0 | 250 | 17 | <1 | 3 | 1 starch, 2 fat |
| Cheez-It, Party Mix | 1/2 cup | 130 | 4.5 | 40 | 1 | 0 | 0 | 370 | 20 | 1 | 3 | 1 starch, 1 fat |
| Cheez-It, Reduced Fat | 29 | 130 | 4.5 | 45 | 1 | 0 | 0 | 320 | 20 | <1 | 4 | 1 starch, 1 fat |
| Cheez-It, White Cheddar | 25 | 130 | 4 | 35 | 1 | 0 | 0 | 240 | 22 | <1 | 3 | 1 1/2 starch, 1 fat |
| Krispy Saltine Crackers | 5 | 60 | 1.5 | 15 | 0 | 0 | 0 | 150 | 11 | <1 | 1 | 1 starch |
| Krispy Saltine Crackers, Wheat | 5 | 60 | 1.5 | 15 | 0 | 0 | 0 | 230 | 11 | <1 | 1 | 1 starch |

# SOUPS, STEW, CHILI

| | Serving | Calories | Fat (g) | Cal. from Fat | Sat. Fat (g) | Trans Fat (g) | Chol. (mg) | Sod. (mg) | Carb. (g) | Fiber (g) | Prot. (g) | Servings/Exchanges |
|---|---|---|---|---|---|---|---|---|---|---|---|---|
| **READY-TO-SERVE CANNED SOUP** | | | | | | | | | | | | |
| **Brands** | | | | | | | | | | | | |
| ***Campbell's Chunky*** | | | | | | | | | | | | |
| Baked Potato with Cheddar & Bacon Bits | 1 cup | 190 | 9 | 80 | 3 | 0 | 10 | 790 | 23 | 3 | 5 | 1 1/2 carb, 2 fat |
| Beef & Dumplings with Hearty Vegetables | 1 cup | 130 | 2 | 20 | 0.5 | 0 | 25 | 800 | 20 | 2 | 8 | 1 carb, 1 lean meat |
| Beef with Country Vegetables | 1 cup | 130 | 3 | 25 | 1 | 0 | 15 | 920 | 18 | 4 | 8 | 1 carb, 1 lean meat |
| Beef with White & Wild Rice | 1 cup | 140 | 1.5 | 15 | 0.5 | 0 | 10 | 890 | 24 | 2 | 8 | 1 1/2 carb, 1 lean meat |
| Chicken & Dumplings | 1 cup | 180 | 8 | 70 | 2 | 0 | 30 | 890 | 19 | 3 | 8 | 1 carb, 1 med-fat meat, 1 fat |

SOUPS, STEW, CHILI

| | Serving | Calories | Fat (g) | Cal. from Fat | Sat. Fat (g) | Trans Fat (g) | Chol. (mg) | Sod. (mg) | Carb. (g) | Fiber (g) | Prot. (g) | Servings/Exchanges |
|---|---|---|---|---|---|---|---|---|---|---|---|---|
| Chicken Broccoli Cheese & Potato | 1 cup | 210 | 11 | 100 | 4 | 0 | 20 | 880 | 20 | 3 | 7 | 1 carb, 1 med-fat meat, 1 fat |
| Classic Chicken Noodle | 1 cup | 120 | 3 | 25 | 1 | 0 | 25 | 790 | 14 | 2 | 8 | 1 carb, 1 lean meat |
| Grilled Chicken & Sausage Gumbo | 1 cup | 140 | 3 | 25 | 1.5 | 0 | 20 | 850 | 21 | 2 | 7 | 1 1/2 carb, 1 lean meat |
| Hearty Bean 'N' Ham | 1 cup | 180 | 2 | 20 | 0.5 | 0 | 10 | 780 | 30 | 5 | 11 | 2 carb, 1 lean meat |
| Hearty Chicken & Vegetable | 1 cup | 110 | 2 | 20 | 0.5 | 0 | 15 | 710 | 17 | 3 | 6 | 1 carb, 1 lean meat |
| Manhattan Clam Chowder | 1 cup | 130 | 3.5 | 30 | 1 | 0 | 5 | 830 | 19 | 3 | 5 | 1 carb, 1 fat |
| New England Clam Chowder | 1 cup | 230 | 13 | 115 | 2 | 0 | 10 | 890 | 20 | 3 | 7 | 1 carb, 1 med-fat meat, 2 fat |
| Old Fashioned Vegetable Beef | 1 cup | 120 | 2.5 | 20 | 1 | 0 | 15 | 890 | 17 | 4 | 8 | 1 carb, 1 lean meat |
| Roasted Beef Tips with Vegetables | 1 cup | 130 | 1.5 | 15 | 0.5 | 0 | 15 | 800 | 20 | 2 | 8 | 1 carb, 1 lean meat |

| | | | | | | | | | | | | |
|---|---|---|---|---|---|---|---|---|---|---|---|---|
| Salisbury Steak Mushrooms & Onions | 1 cup | 140 | 4.5 | 40 | 2.5 | 0 | 15 | 800 | 19 | 2 | 7 | 1 carb, 1 med-fat meat |
| Sirloin Burger with Country Vegetables | 1 cup | 130 | 2.5 | 20 | 1 | 0 | 15 | 800 | 18 | 4 | 10 | 1 carb, 1 lean meat |
| Split Pea & Ham | 1 cup | 190 | 2.5 | 20 | 1 | 0 | 10 | 780 | 30 | 5 | 12 | 2 carb, 1 lean meat |
| Steak & Potato | 1 cup | 120 | 2 | 20 | 0.5 | 0 | 15 | 920 | 18 | 3 | 8 | 1 carb, 1 lean meat |
| ***Campbell's Chunky Fully Loaded*** | | | | | | | | | | | | |
| Creamy Chicken Alfredo | 1 cup | 230 | 12 | 110 | 5 | 0 | 30 | 780 | 18 | 2 | 12 | 1 carb, 1 med-fat meat, 1 fat |
| Rigatoni & Meatball | 1 cup | 210 | 7 | 65 | 3 | 0 | 20 | 800 | 25 | 8 | 11 | 1 1/2 carb, 1 med-fat meat |
| Turkey Pot Pie | 1 cup | 200 | 8 | 70 | 1.5 | 0 | 35 | 800 | 21 | 4 | 11 | 1 1/2 carb, 1 med-fat meat, 1 fat |
| Campbell's Chunky Healthy Request | 1 cup | 140 | 3.5 | 32 | 1.5 | 0 | 10 | 730 | 24 | 2 | 3 | 1 1/2 carb, 1 fat |
| Chicken Corn Chowder | 1 cup | 140 | 3 | 25 | 1 | 0 | 10 | 410 | 22 | 2 | 7 | 1 1/2 carb, 1 lean meat |
| Chicken Noodle | 1 cup | 120 | 2.5 | 20 | 1 | 0 | 10 | 410 | 17 | 2 | 8 | 1 carb, 1 lean meat |

| | Serving | Calories | Fat (g) | Cal. from Fat | Sat. Fat (g) | Trans Fat (g) | Chol. (mg) | Sod. (mg) | Carb. (g) | Fiber (g) | Prot. (g) | Servings/Exchanges |
|---|---|---|---|---|---|---|---|---|---|---|---|---|
| New England Clam Chowder | 1 cup | 130 | 3 | 25 | 1 | 0 | 10 | 410 | 20 | 2 | 5 | 1 carb, 1 fat |
| Old Fashioned Vegetable Beef | 1 cup | 120 | 2 | 20 | 1 | 0 | 10 | 410 | 19 | 3 | 7 | 1 carb, 1 lean meat |
| Sirloin Burger | 1 cup | 130 | 2 | 20 | 1 | 0 | 15 | 410 | 19 | 3 | 9 | 1 carb, 1 lean meat |
| Vegetable | 1 cup | 120 | 1 | 10 | 0.5 | 0 | 0 | 410 | 24 | 4 | 4 | 1 1/2 carb |
| ***Campbell's Low Sodium*** | | | | | | | | | | | | |
| Chicken Broth | 1 can | 25 | 0.5 | 5 | 0.5 | 0 | 5 | 140 | 1 | 0 | 4 | free |
| Chicken with Noodles | 1 can | 160 | 4.5 | 40 | 1.5 | 0 | 30 | 140 | 17 | 2 | 12 | 1 carb, 1 med-fat meat |
| Chunky Vegetable Beef | 1 can | 170 | 4.5 | 40 | 1.5 | 0 | 30 | 50 | 18 | 6 | 14 | 1 carb, 2 lean meat |
| Cream of Mushroom | 1 can | 160 | 8 | 70 | 2.5 | 0 | 10 | 60 | 19 | 3 | 4 | 1 carb, 2 fat |
| Split Pea | 1 can | 240 | 4 | 35 | 1.5 | 0 | 5 | 30 | 38 | 6 | 12 | 2 1/2 carb, 1 med-fat meat |
| Tomato with Tomato Pieces | 1 can | 150 | 4 | 45 | 1.5 | 0 | 10 | 90 | 25 | 4 | 4 | 1 1/2 carb, 1 fat |

| | | | | | | | | | | | | |
|---|---|---|---|---|---|---|---|---|---|---|---|---|
| ***Campbell's Select Harvest*** | | | | | | | | | | | | |
| Light Italian-Style Vegetable | 1 cup | 50 | 0 | 0 | 0 | 0 | 0 | 480 | 14 | 4 | 3 | 1 carb |
| Light Minestrone with Whole Grain Pasta | 1 cup | 80 | 0.5 | 0 | 0 | 0 | 0 | 480 | 14 | 4 | 4 | 1 carb |
| Light Roasted Chicken with Italian Herbs | 1 cup | 80 | 2.5 | 25 | 0.5 | 0 | 10 | 480 | 8 | 3 | 6 | 1/2 carb, 1 lean meat |
| Light Vegetable & Pasta | 1 cup | 60 | 0 | 0 | 0 | 0 | 0 | 480 | 13 | 4 | 3 | 1 carb |
| ***Health Valley Organic (Fat Free)*** | | | | | | | | | | | | |
| Black Bean, No Added Salt | 1 cup | 130 | 1 | 10 | 0 | 0 | 0 | 25 | 25 | 5 | 7 | 1 1/2 carb |
| Chicken Noodle | 1 cup | 80 | 2 | 20 | 0 | 0 | 10 | 480 | 11 | 1 | 4 | 1 carb, 1 lean meat |
| Italian Minestrone, 40% Less Sodium | 1 cup | 110 | 0 | 0 | 0 | 0 | 0 | 470 | 26 | 7 | 6 | 2 carb |
| Lentil, No Added Salt | 1 cup | 100 | 1 | 10 | 0 | 0 | 0 | 25 | 21 | 8 | 8 | 1 1/2 carb |
| Minestrone, No Added Salt | 1 cup | 70 | 0 | 0 | 0 | 0 | 0 | 45 | 17 | 3 | 3 | 1 carb |

| | Serving | Calories | Fat (g) | Cal. from Fat | Sat. Fat (g) | Trans Fat (g) | Chol. (mg) | Sod. (mg) | Carb. (g) | Fiber (g) | Prot. (g) | Servings/Exchanges |
|---|---|---|---|---|---|---|---|---|---|---|---|---|
| Split Pea, No Added Salt | 1 cup | 110 | 0 | 0 | 0 | 0 | 0 | 115 | 23 | 8 | 10 | 1 1/2 carb, 1 very lean meat |
| Tomato Vegetable, 40% Less Sodium | 1 cup | 70 | 0 | 0 | 0 | 0 | 0 | 470 | 17 | 5 | 3 | 1 carb |
| Tomato, No Added Salt | 1 cup | 80 | 0 | 0 | 0 | 0 | 0 | 35 | 18 | 1 | 3 | 1 carb |
| Vegetable Barley, 40% Less Sodium | 1 cup | 80 | 0 | 0 | 0 | 0 | 0 | 480 | 19 | 4 | 3 | 1 carb |
| Vegetable, No Added Salt | 1 cup | 90 | 0 | 0 | 0 | 0 | 0 | 70 | 16 | 4 | 3 | 1 carb |
| ***Healthy Choice*** | | | | | | | | | | | | |
| Bean & Ham | 1 cup | 180 | 2 | 20 | 1 | 0 | 5 | 480 | 29 | 10 | 11 | 2 carb, 1 lean meat |
| Chicken & Dumplings | 1 cup | 140 | 2.5 | 20 | 0.5 | 0 | 20 | 480 | 21 | 3 | 9 | 1 1/2 carb, 1 lean meat |
| Chicken with Rice | 1 cup | 110 | 1.5 | 15 | 0 | 0 | 10 | 480 | 17 | 3 | 7 | 1 carb, 1 lean meat |
| Country Vegetable | 1 cup | 110 | 1 | 10 | 0 | 0 | 0 | 480 | 19 | 4 | 5 | 1 carb |
| Fiesta Chicken | 1 cup | 120 | 2 | 20 | 0.5 | 0 | 15 | 480 | 20 | 3 | 6 | 1 carb, 1 lean meat |

| | | | | | | | | | | | | |
|---|---|---|---|---|---|---|---|---|---|---|---|---|
| Garden Vegetable | 1 cup | 120 | 0.5 | 5 | 0 | 0 | 5 | 480 | 24 | 4 | 5 | 1 1/2 carb |
| Hearty Chicken | 1 cup | 130 | 2 | 15 | 0.5 | 0 | 20 | 480 | 20 | 3 | 9 | 1 carb, 1 lean meat |
| New England Clam Chowder | 1 cup | 110 | 1 | 10 | 0.5 | 0 | 10 | 480 | 19 | 2 | 5 | 1 carb |
| Old Fashioned Chicken Noodle | 1 cup | 100 | 1.5 | 15 | 0 | 0 | 15 | 480 | 13 | 2 | 9 | 1 carb, 1 lean meat |
| Split Pea & Ham | 1 cup | 170 | 2 | 15 | 0.5 | 0 | 5 | 480 | 22 | 3 | 9 | 1 1/2 carb, 1 lean meat |
| Vegetable Beef | 1 cup | 130 | 1 | 10 | 0 | 0 | 15 | 480 | 22 | 4 | 9 | 1 1/2 carb, l lean meat |
| Zesty Gumbo | 1 cup | 100 | 2 | 15 | 0.5 | 0 | 20 | 480 | 16 | 4 | 6 | 1 carb |
| ***Progresso (99% Fat Free)*** | | | | | | | | | | | | |
| Beef Barley | 1 cup | 120 | 1.5 | 15 | 0.5 | 0 | 10 | 720 | 20 | 4 | 7 | 1 carb, 1 lean meat |
| Chicken Noodle | 1 cup | 90 | 2 | 20 | 0.5 | 0 | 20 | 670 | 12 | 1 | 6 | 1 carb, 1 lean meat |
| Lentil | 1 cup | 140 | 1.5 | 15 | 0 | 0 | 0 | 500 | 25 | 3 | 8 | 1 1/2 carb, 1 lean meat |
| Minestrone | 1 cup | 100 | 1 | 10 | 0 | 0 | 0 | 600 | 19 | 5 | 5 | 1 carb |
| New England Clam Chowder | 1 cup | 110 | 1.5 | 15 | 0 | 0 | 5 | 810 | 21 | 2 | 4 | 1 1/2 carb |

SOUPS, STEW, CHILI

| | Serving | Calories | Fat (g) | Cal. from Fat | Sat. Fat (g) | Trans Fat (g) | Chol. (mg) | Sod. (mg) | Carb. (g) | Fiber (g) | Prot. (g) | Servings/Exchanges |
|---|---|---|---|---|---|---|---|---|---|---|---|---|
| ***Progresso*** | | | | | | | | | | | | |
| Beef & Vegetable | 1 cup | 120 | 2 | 15 | 1 | 0 | 15 | 690 | 18 | 2 | 8 | 1 carb, 1 lean meat |
| Chickarina w/Meatballs | 1 cup | 130 | 5 | 45 | 2 | 0 | 20 | 690 | 14 | 1 | 8 | 1 carb, 1 med-fat meat |
| Chicken & Wild Rice | 1 cup | 100 | 1.5 | 15 | 0.5 | 0 | 15 | 650 | 15 | 1 | 6 | 1 carb, 1 lean meat |
| Chicken Noodle | 1 cup | 100 | 2.5 | 20 | 0.5 | 0 | 20 | 690 | 12 | 1 | 7 | 1 carb, 1 lean meat |
| Creamy Mushroom | 1 cup | 120 | 8 | 70 | 2 | 0 | 5 | 890 | 9 | 1 | 2 | 1/2 carb, 2 fat |
| Creamy Tomato Basil | 1 cup | 130 | 4 | 35 | 1 | 0 | 5 | 690 | 26 | 7 | 3 | 2 carb, 1 fat |
| French Onion | 1 cup | 50 | 1 | 10 | 0 | 0 | 0 | 690 | 9 | 1 | 2 | 1/2 carb |
| Green Split Pea | 1 cup | 160 | 2 | 20 | 0.5 | 0 | 0 | 690 | 28 | 4 | 9 | 2 carb, 1 lean meat |
| Hearty Black Bean | 1 cup | 160 | 1 | 10 | 0.5 | 0 | <5 | 690 | 29 | 8 | 8 | 2 carb |
| Hearty Penne in Chicken Broth | 1 cup | 80 | 1 | 10 | 0 | 0 | 0 | 710 | 14 | 1 | 3 | 1 carb |
| Hearty Tomato | 1 cup | 110 | 0.5 | 5 | 0 | 0 | 0 | 690 | 24 | 3 | 3 | 1 1/2 carb |
| Lentil | 1 cup | 160 | 2 | 20 | 0.5 | 0 | 0 | 810 | 30 | 5 | 9 | 2 carb, 1 lean meat |

| | | | | | | | | | | | | |
|---|---|---|---|---|---|---|---|---|---|---|---|---|
| Macaroni & Bean | 1 cup | 160 | 3.5 | 30 | 1 | 0 | 0 | 690 | 25 | 6 | 8 | 1 1/2 carb, 1 lean meat |
| Manhattan Clam Chowder | 1 cup | 100 | 2 | 20 | 0 | 0 | 5 | 690 | 17 | 2 | 3 | 1 carb |
| Minestrone | 1 cup | 100 | 2 | 20 | 0.5 | 0 | 0 | 690 | 20 | 4 | 4 | 1 carb |
| Potato Broccoli & Cheese Chowder | 1 cup | 210 | 12 | 110 | 3.5 | 0 | 15 | 860 | 20 | 2 | 5 | 1 carb, 2 fat |
| Roasted Chicken Rotini | 1 cup | 80 | 2 | 15 | 0.5 | 0 | 10 | 670 | 10 | <1 | 5 | 1/2 carb, 1 lean meat |
| Southwestern Style Corn Chowder | 1 cup | 120 | 2 | 15 | 0.5 | 0 | 10 | 740 | 18 | 2 | 6 | 1 carb, 1 lean meat |
| Split Pea with Ham | 1 cup | 140 | 1 | 10 | 0 | 0 | 5 | 690 | 24 | 4 | 9 | 1 1/2 carb, 1 lean meat |
| Tomato Basil | 1 cup | 150 | 3 | 30 | 0.5 | 0 | 0 | 680 | 29 | 2 | 3 | 2 carb, 1 fat |
| Tomato Rotini | 1 cup | 130 | 0.5 | 5 | 0 | 0 | 0 | 690 | 28 | 4 | 4 | 2 carb |
| Turkey Noodle | 1 cup | 80 | 1 | 10 | 0 | 0 | 15 | 690 | 12 | 1 | 5 | 1 carb, 1 lean meat |
| Vegetable | 1 cup | 80 | 0 | 0 | 0 | 0 | 0 | 660 | 15 | 3 | 5 | 1 carb |
| Vegetarian Vegetable with Barley | 1 cup | 80 | 0 | 0 | 0 | 0 | 0 | 670 | 18 | 3 | 3 | 1 carb |

| | Serving | Calories | Fat (g) | Cal. from Fat | Sat. Fat (g) | Trans Fat (g) | Chol. (mg) | Sod. (mg) | Carb. (g) | Fiber (g) | Prot. (g) | Servings/Exchanges |
|---|---|---|---|---|---|---|---|---|---|---|---|---|
| **CONDENSED CANNED SOUP** | | | | | | | | | | | | |
| **Brands** | | | | | | | | | | | | |
| ***Campbell's Condensed*** | | | | | | | | | | | | |
| Bean with Bacon | 1/2 cup | 160 | 3 | 30 | 1.5 | 0 | 5 | 860 | 25 | 8 | 8 | 1 1/2 carb, 1 lean meat |
| Beef Broth | 1/2 cup | 10 | 0 | 0 | 0 | 0 | 0 | 860 | 1 | 0 | 2 | free |
| Beef Consommé | 1/2 cup | 20 | 0 | 0 | 0 | 0 | 0 | 810 | 1 | 0 | 4 | free |
| Beef Noodle | 1/2 cup | 70 | 2 | 20 | 0.5 | 0 | 10 | 820 | 8 | <1 | 4 | 1/2 carb, 1 lean meat |
| Beefy Mushroom | 1/2 cup | 50 | 2 | 20 | 0.5 | 0 | 5 | 890 | 6 | 0 | 3 | 1/2 carb |
| Broccoli Cheese | 1/2 cup | 100 | 4.5 | 40 | 2 | 0 | 5 | 820 | 12 | 0 | 2 | 1 carb, 1 fat |
| Chicken & Dumplings | 1/2 cup | 70 | 2.5 | 20 | 1 | 0 | 10 | 760 | 10 | 1 | 3 | 1/2 carb, 1 fat |
| Chicken & Stars | 1/2 cup | 70 | 2 | 20 | 0.5 | 0 | 5 | 480 | 11 | 1 | 3 | 1 carb |
| Chicken Alphabet | 1/2 cup | 70 | 1.5 | 20 | 0.5 | 0 | 5 | 480 | 12 | 1 | 3 | 1 carb |
| Chicken Broth | 1/2 cup | 20 | 1 | 10 | 0 | 0 | <5 | 770 | 1 | 0 | 1 | free |
| Chicken Gumbo | 1/2 cup | 70 | 1 | 10 | 0.5 | 0 | 5 | 870 | 12 | 1 | 2 | 1 carb |

| | | | | | | | | | | | | |
|---|---|---|---|---|---|---|---|---|---|---|---|---|
| Chicken Noodle | 1/2 cup | 60 | 2 | 20 | 0.5 | 0 | 15 | 890 | 8 | 1 | 3 | 1/2 carb |
| Chicken Won Ton | 1/2 cup | 60 | 1 | 10 | 0.5 | 0 | 10 | 870 | 8 | 0 | 4 | 1/2 carb |
| Cream of Asparagus | 1/2 cup | 110 | 9 | 80 | 2 | 0 | 5 | 830 | 9 | 3 | 2 | 1/2 carb, 2 fat |
| Cream of Broccoli | 1/2 cup | 90 | 3.5 | 30 | 1 | 0 | 5 | 750 | 12 | 1 | 2 | 1 carb, 1 fat |
| Cream of Celery | 1/2 cup | 90 | 6 | 55 | 0.5 | 0 | 5 | 860 | 9 | 3 | 1 | 1/2 carb, 1 fat |
| Cream of Chicken | 1/2 cup | 120 | 8 | 70 | 2.5 | 0 | 10 | 870 | 10 | 2 | 3 | 1/2 carb, 2 fat |
| Cream of Mushroom | 1/2 cup | 100 | 7 | 65 | 1.5 | 0 | 5 | 870 | 9 | 2 | 1 | 1/2 carb, 1 fat |
| French Onion | 1/2 cup | 45 | 1.5 | 15 | 1 | 0 | <5 | 900 | 6 | 1 | 2 | 1/2 carb |
| Golden Mushroom | 1/2 cup | 80 | 3.5 | 30 | 1 | 0 | 5 | 890 | 10 | 1 | 2 | 1/2 carb, 1 fat |
| Green Pea | 1/2 cup | 180 | 3 | 25 | 1 | 0 | 0 | 870 | 28 | 4 | 9 | 2 carb, 1 lean meat |
| Lentil | 1/2 cup | 140 | 1 | 10 | 0.5 | 0 | 0 | 800 | 24 | 6 | 9 | 1 1/2 carb, 1 lean meat |
| Manhattan Clam Chowder | 1/2 cup | 60 | 0.5 | 5 | 0.5 | 0 | 0 | 880 | 12 | 2 | 2 | 1 carb |
| Minestrone | 1/2 cup | 90 | 1 | 10 | 0.5 | 0 | 5 | 960 | 17 | 3 | 4 | 1 carb |
| New England Clam Chowder | 1/2 cup | 90 | 2.5 | 20 | 0.5 | 0 | 5 | 880 | 13 | 1 | 4 | 1 carb, 1 fat |

| | Serving | Calories | Fat (g) | Cal. from Fat | Sat. Fat (g) | Trans Fat (g) | Chol. (mg) | Sod. (mg) | Carb. (g) | Fiber (g) | Prot. (g) | Servings/Exchanges |
|---|---|---|---|---|---|---|---|---|---|---|---|---|
| Pepper Pot | 1/2 cup | 90 | 4 | 35 | 1.5 | 0 | 25 | 980 | 9 | 1 | 5 | 1/2 carb, 1 fat |
| Split Pea with Ham & Bacon | 1/2 cup | 180 | 3.5 | 30 | 2 | 0 | 5 | 850 | 27 | 5 | 10 | 2 carb, 1 med-fat meat |
| Tomato | 1/2 cup | 90 | 0 | 0 | 0 | 0 | 0 | 480 | 20 | 1 | 2 | 1 carb |
| Tomato Bisque | 1/2 cup | 130 | 3.5 | 30 | 1.5 | 0 | 5 | 880 | 23 | 1 | 2 | 1 1/2 carb, 1 fat |
| Vegetable | 1/2 cup | 100 | 0.5 | 5 | 0.5 | 0 | 5 | 890 | 20 | 3 | 4 | 1 carb |
| ***Campbell's Condensed Light*** | | | | | | | | | | | | |
| Chicken Gumbo | 1/2 cup | 70 | 1 | 10 | 0.5 | 0 | 5 | 870 | 12 | 1 | 2 | 1 carb |
| Italian-Style Wedding | 1/2 cup | 80 | 2 | 20 | 1 | 0 | 5 | 790 | 12 | 2 | 4 | 1 carb |
| ***Campbell's Healthy Request Condensed*** | | | | | | | | | | | | |
| Chicken Noodle | 1/2 cup | 60 | 2 | 20 | 0.5 | 0 | 10 | 410 | 8 | 1 | 3 | 1/2 carb |
| Chicken Rice | 1/2 cup | 70 | 1.5 | 15 | 0.5 | 0 | 5 | 410 | 13 | 1 | 2 | 1 carb |
| Cream of Celery | 1/2 cup | 70 | 2 | 20 | 0.5 | 0 | <5 | 410 | 12 | 1 | 1 | 1 carb |
| Cream of Chicken | 1/2 cup | 80 | 2.5 | 20 | 1 | 0 | 5 | 410 | 12 | 1 | 2 | 1 carb |

| | | | | | | | | | | | | |
|---|---|---|---|---|---|---|---|---|---|---|---|---|
| Cream of Mushroom | 1/2 cup | 70 | 2 | 20 | 0.5 | 0 | 5 | 410 | 10 | 1 | 2 | 1/2 carb, 1 fat |
| Homestyle Chicken Noodle | 1/2 cup | 70 | 2 | 20 | 0.5 | 0 | 10 | 410 | 10 | 1 | 3 | 1/2 carb, 1 fat |
| Minestrone | 1/2 cup | 80 | 0.5 | 5 | 0 | 0 | 0 | 410 | 15 | 3 | 3 | 1 carb |
| Tomato | 1/2 cup | 90 | 1.5 | 15 | 0.5 | 0 | 0 | 410 | 17 | 1 | 2 | 1 carb |
| Vegetable | 1/2 cup | 100 | 1 | 9 | 10 | 0 | 0 | 410 | 20 | 3 | 4 | 1 carb |
| **READY-TO-SERVE SINGLE-SERVING CANNED SOUP** | | | | | | | | | | | | |
| **Brands** | | | | | | | | | | | | |
| ***Campbell's Soup at Hand*** | | | | | | | | | | | | |
| Chicken & Stars | 1 Container | 70 | 2 | 20 | 0.5 | 0 | 5 | 960 | 10 | 1 | 3 | 1 carb |
| Classic Tomato | 1 Container | 120 | 0.5 | 5 | 0 | 0 | 0 | 890 | 25 | 2 | 3 | 1 1/2 carb |
| Cream of Broccoli | 1 Container | 150 | 7 | 65 | 2 | 0 | 5 | 890 | 17 | 7 | 3 | 1 carb, 1 fat |
| Creamy Chicken | 1 Container | 150 | 8 | 70 | 2.5 | 0 | 10 | 880 | 9 | 2 | 3 | 1/2 carb, 2 fat |

| | Serving | Calories | Fat (g) | Cal. from Fat | Sat. Fat (g) | Trans Fat (g) | Chol. (mg) | Sod. (mg) | Carb. (g) | Fiber (g) | Prot. (g) | Servings/Exchanges |
|---|---|---|---|---|---|---|---|---|---|---|---|---|
| Creamy Tomato | 1 Container | 180 | 4 | 35 | 1 | 0 | 5 | 940 | 32 | 2 | 4 | 2 carb, 1 fat |
| Creamy Tomato Parmesan Bisque | 1 Container | 220 | 7 | 65 | 2 | 0 | 10 | 810 | 35 | 2 | 5 | 2 carb, 1 fat |
| New England Clam Chowder | 1 Container | 160 | 10 | 90 | 2 | 0 | 5 | 890 | 13 | 5 | 4 | 1 carb, 2 fat |
| Vegetable Beef | 1 Container | 70 | 1 | 10 | 0.5 | 0 | 5 | 930 | 11 | 1 | 3 | 1 carb |
| Vegetable with Mini Round Noodles | 1 Container | 100 | 0.5 | 5 | 0 | 0 | 5 | 650 | 21 | 1 | 2 | 1 1/2 carb |
| ***Campbell's Microwavable Classic Bowls*** | | | | | | | | | | | | |
| Chicken Noodle | 1 cup | 70 | 2 | 20 | 0.5 | 0 | 15 | 870 | 10 | <1 | 4 | 1/2 carb, 1 lean meat |
| Tomato | 1 cup | 110 | 0 | 0 | 0 | 0 | 0 | 790 | 24 | 3 | 3 | 1 1/2 carb |
| Vegetable Beef | 1 cup | 80 | 0.5 | 5 | 0.5 | 0 | 10 | 880 | 15 | 3 | 5 | 1 carb |

| | | | | | | | | | | | | |
|---|---|---|---|---|---|---|---|---|---|---|---|---|
| ***Healthy Choice Microwavable Bowls*** | | | | | | | | | | | | |
| Beef Pot Roast | 1 cup | 110 | 1 | 10 | 0 | 0 | 0 | 480 | 18 | 5 | 7 | 1 carb, 1 lean meat |
| Chicken with Rice | 1 cup | 90 | 1.5 | 15 | 0.5 | 0 | 15 | 440 | 13 | 2 | 6 | 1 carb, 1 lean meat |
| Country Vegetable | 1 cup | 100 | 0.5 | 5 | 0 | 0 | 0 | 480 | 21 | 5 | 4 | 1 1/2 carb |
| ***Knorr Ready to Serve*** | | | | | | | | | | | | |
| Broccoli with Boursin Cheese | 1 cup | 140 | 9 | 80 | 5 | 0 | 15 | 810 | 12 | 1 | 2 | 1 carb, 2 fat |
| Classic Tomato with Real Cream | 1 cup | 140 | 3 | 25 | 1.5 | 0 | 0 | 650 | 25 | 3 | 3 | 1 1/2 carb, 1 fat |
| Red Soup | 1 cup | 120 | 2.5 | 25 | 0.5 | 0 | 0 | 650 | 20 | 3 | 3 | 1 carb, 1 fat |
| Rustic Vegetable & Potato | 1 cup | 80 | 1.5 | 15 | 1 | 0 | 5 | 730 | 14 | 2 | 2 | 1 carb |
| **MULTI-SERVE SOUP MIX** | | | | | | | | | | | | |
| **Brands** | | | | | | | | | | | | |
| ***Bear Creek*** | | | | | | | | | | | | |
| Creamy Potato | 1 cup | 150 | 3.5 | 35 | 2 | 0 | 0 | 860 | 27 | 0 | 2 | 2 carb, 1 fat |

| | Serving | Calories | Fat (g) | Cal. from Fat | Sat. Fat (g) | Trans Fat (g) | Chol. (mg) | Sod. (mg) | Carb. (g) | Fiber (g) | Prot. (g) | Servings/Exchanges |
|---|---|---|---|---|---|---|---|---|---|---|---|---|
| Minestrone | 1 cup | 110 | 0 | 0 | 0 | 0 | 0 | 870 | 23 | 2 | 4 | 1 1/2 carb |
| Tortilla | 1 cup | 90 | 0.5 | 5 | 0 | 0 | 0 | 830 | 22 | 5 | 3 | 1 1/2 carb |
| Vegetable Beef | 1 cup | 115 | 0.5 | 5 | 0 | 0 | 0 | 740 | 25 | 3 | 5 | 1 1/2 carb |
| ***Fantastic Foods Simmer Soups*** | | | | | | | | | | | | |
| Blarneystone Creamy Potato | 1 cup | 110 | 2 | 15 | 1 | 0 | 5 | 760 | 28 | 3 | 9 | 2 carb |
| Dutch Split Pea | 1 cup | 120 | 1 | 10 | 1 | 0 | 0 | 590 | 21 | 5 | 8 | 1 1/2 carb |
| Vegetarian Chicken Noodle | 1 cup | 90 | 1 | 10 | 0 | 0 | 0 | 700 | 14 | 1 | 7 | 1 carb, 1 lean meat |
| **SINGLE-SERVING SOUP MIX** | | | | | | | | | | | | |
| **Brands** | | | | | | | | | | | | |
| ***Health Valley (Fat Free Soup Cups)*** | | | | | | | | | | | | |
| Chicken Flavored Noodles w/Vegetable | 1/2 cup | 110 | 0 | 0 | 0 | 0 | 0 | 390 | 24 | 3 | 5 | 1 1/2 carb |

| | | | | | | | | | | | | |
|---|---|---|---|---|---|---|---|---|---|---|---|---|
| Creamy Potato with Broccoli | 1/3 cup | 80 | 0 | 0 | 0 | 0 | 0 | 390 | 17 | 3 | 4 | 1 carb |
| Lentil with Couscous | 1/3 cup | 130 | 0 | 0 | 0 | 0 | 0 | 310 | 28 | 5 | 7 | 2 carb |
| Spicy Black Bean with Couscous | 1/3 cup | 130 | 0 | 0 | 0 | 0 | 0 | 290 | 29 | 5 | 6 | 2 carb |
| ***Lipton Cup-a-Soup*** | | | | | | | | | | | | |
| Chicken Noodle | 1 envelope | 45 | 1 | 10 | 0 | 0 | 10 | 540 | 8 | 0 | 2 | 1/2 carb |
| ***Maruchan Noodle Cups*** | | | | | | | | | | | | |
| Chicken | 1 container | 290 | 12 | 110 | 6 | 0 | 0 | 1200 | 38 | 2 | 7 | 2 1/2 carb, 2 fat |
| ***Maruchan Ramen Noodle Soup*** | | | | | | | | | | | | |
| Chicken | 1/2 pkg | 190 | 7 | 70 | 3.5 | 0 | 0 | 830 | 26 | 1 | 5 | 2 carb, 1 fat |
| ***Nissin Noodle Cup*** | | | | | | | | | | | | |
| Chicken | 1 container | 300 | 13 | 120 | 7 | 0 | <5 | 1060 | 38 | 2 | 6 | 2 1/2 carb, 3 fat |

| | Serving | Calories | Fat (g) | Cal. from Fat | Sat. Fat (g) | Trans Fat (g) | Chol. (mg) | Sod. (mg) | Carb. (g) | Fiber (g) | Prot. (g) | Servings/Exchanges |
|---|---|---|---|---|---|---|---|---|---|---|---|---|
| ***Nissin Top Ramen Noodle Soup*** | | | | | | | | | | | | |
| Chicken | 1/2 pkg | 190 | 7 | 60 | 3.5 | 0 | 0 | 910 | 26 | 2 | 5 | 2 carb, 1 fat |
| **CHILI & STEW** | | | | | | | | | | | | |
| **Brands** | | | | | | | | | | | | |
| ***Amy's Organic*** | | | | | | | | | | | | |
| Black Bean Chili | 1 cup | 200 | 3 | 30 | 0 | 0 | 0 | 680 | 31 | 13 | 13 | 2 carb, 1 lean meat |
| Medium Chili | 1 cup | 280 | 9 | 80 | 1 | 0 | 0 | 680 | 35 | 7 | 15 | 2 carb, 2 med-fat meat |
| Medium Chili with Vegetables | 1 cup | 190 | 6 | 50 | 0.5 | 0 | 0 | 590 | 29 | 8 | 7 | 2 carb, 1 fat |
| Southwestern Black Bean Chili | 1 cup | 240 | 4 | 35 | 0.5 | 0 | 0 | 680 | 40 | 10 | 12 | 2 1/2 carb, 1 med-fat meat |
| Spicy Chili | 1 cup | 250 | 9 | 80 | 1 | 0 | 0 | 340 | 30 | 7 | 13 | 2 carb, 1 med-fat meat, 1 fat |
| ***Campbell's*** | | | | | | | | | | | | |

| | | | | | | | | | | | | |
|---|---|---|---|---|---|---|---|---|---|---|---|---|
| Chunky Hot & Spicy Beef & Bean Chili | 1 cup | 230 | 8 | 70 | 3.5 | 0.5 | 30 | 870 | 25 | 8 | 15 | 1 1/2 carb, 2 med-fat meat |
| Chunky Grilled Steak Chili with Beans | 1 cup | 200 | 3 | 25 | 1 | 0 | 15 | 870 | 27 | 7 | 16 | 2 carb, 1 lean meat |
| Chunky Hold the Beans Chili | 1 cup | 240 | 10 | 90 | 4 | 0.5 | 35 | 770 | 20 | 5 | 18 | 1 carb, 2 med-fat meat |
| Chunky Roadhouse Beef & Bean Chili | 1 cup | 230 | 8 | 70 | 3.5 | 0.5 | 30 | 870 | 25 | 8 | 15 | 1 1/2 carb, 2 med-fat meat |
| ***Dennison's*** | | | | | | | | | | | | |
| Chunky Chili Con Carne with Beans | 1 cup | 300 | 10 | 90 | 4.5 | 0.5 | 40 | 1020 | 32 | 9 | 20 | 2 carb, 2 med-fat meat |
| Hot Chili Con Carne with Beans | 1 cup | 350 | 14 | 130 | 6 | 1 | 40 | 930 | 36 | 11 | 21 | 2 1/2 carb, 2 med-fat meat, 1 fat |
| Original Chili Con Carne with Beans | 1 cup | 360 | 14 | 130 | 6 | 1 | 40 | 1030 | 38 | 11 | 20 | 2 1/2 carb, 2 med-fat meat, 1 fat |
| ***Dinty Moore*** | | | | | | | | | | | | |
| Beef Stew | 1 cup | 210 | 10 | 90 | 4 | 0 | 30 | 970 | 19 | 1 | 11 | 1 carb, 1 med-fat meat, 1 fat |

| | Serving | Calories | Fat (g) | Cal. from Fat | Sat. Fat (g) | Trans Fat (g) | Chol. (mg) | Sod. (mg) | Carb. (g) | Fiber (g) | Prot. (g) | Servings/Exchanges |
|---|---|---|---|---|---|---|---|---|---|---|---|---|
| ***Health Valley Chunky Chili*** | | | | | | | | | | | | |
| Vegetarian, Mild | 1 cup | 150 | 1 | 0 | 0 | 0 | 0 | 480 | 31 | 10 | 9 | 2 carb, 1 lean meat |
| Vegetarian, Mild, Black Bean Mole | 1 cup | 150 | 1 | 0 | 0 | 0 | 0 | 480 | 32 | 8 | 10 | 2 carb, 1 lean meat |
| Vegetarian, Mild, No Salt Added | 1 cup | 150 | 1 | 0 | 0 | 0 | 0 | 75 | 31 | 10 | 9 | 2 carb, 1 lean meat |
| Vegetarian, Mild, Three Bean Chipotle | 1 cup | 150 | 1 | 0 | 0 | 0 | 0 | 480 | 32 | 10 | 10 | 2 carb, 1 lean meat |
| Vegetarian, Spicy | 1 cup | 150 | 1 | 0 | 0 | 0 | 0 | 480 | 31 | 10 | 9 | 2 carb, 1 lean meat |
| Vegetarian, Spicy, Black Bean Mango | 1 cup | 150 | 1 | 0 | 0 | 0 | 0 | 480 | 32 | 8 | 10 | 2 carb, 1 lean meat |
| ***Hormel Chili*** | | | | | | | | | | | | |
| Chili No Beans | 1 cup | 220 | 9 | 80 | 4 | 0 | 40 | 970 | 18 | 3 | 16 | 1 carb, 2 med-fat meat |
| Chili with Beans | 1 cup | 260 | 7 | 60 | 3 | 0 | 30 | 1200 | 33 | 7 | 16 | 2 carb, 1 med-fat meat |

| | | | | | | | | | | | | |
|---|---|---|---|---|---|---|---|---|---|---|---|---|
| Chunky Chili No Beans | 1 cup | 210 | 8 | 70 | 3.5 | 0 | 40 | 1130 | 19 | 4 | 16 | 1 carb, 2 med-fat meat |
| Chunky Chili with Beans | 1 cup | 260 | 7 | 60 | 3 | 0 | 30 | 1160 | 32 | 7 | 17 | 2 carb, 2 lean meat |
| Hot Chili No Beans | 1 cup | 220 | 9 | 80 | 4 | 0 | 40 | 970 | 18 | 3 | 16 | 1 carb, 2 med-fat meat |
| Hot Chili with Beans | 1 cup | 260 | 7 | 60 | 3 | 0 | 30 | 1190 | 33 | 7 | 16 | 2 carb, 1 med-fat meat |
| Less Sodium Chili with Beans | 1 cup | 260 | 7 | 60 | 3 | 0 | 30 | 880 | 33 | 7 | 16 | 2 carb, 1 med-fat meat |
| Turkey Chili with Beans, 98% Fat Free | 1 cup | 210 | 3 | 25 | 1 | 0 | 45 | 1250 | 28 | 6 | 17 | 2 carb, 2 lean meat |
| ***Hormel Chili Master*** | | | | | | | | | | | | |
| Chipotle Chicken Chili with Beans | 1 cup | 240 | 7 | 65 | 2 | 0 | 50 | 970 | 28 | 7 | 17 | 2 carb, 2 lean meat |
| Roasted Tomato Chili with Beans | 1 cup | 210 | 6 | 55 | 2 | 0 | 25 | 990 | 25 | 7 | 14 | 2 carb, 2 lean meat |
| White Chicken Chili with Beans | 1 cup | 220 | 8 | 70 | 4 | 0 | 50 | 990 | 17 | 4 | 19 | 1 1/2 carb, 2 med-fat meat |

| | Serving | Calories | Fat (g) | Cal. from Fat | Sat. Fat (g) | Trans Fat (g) | Chol. (mg) | Sod. (mg) | Carb. (g) | Fiber (g) | Prot. (g) | Servings/Exchanges |
|---|---|---|---|---|---|---|---|---|---|---|---|---|
| ***Shelton's*** | | | | | | | | | | | | |
| Mild Turkey Chili | 1 cup | 220 | 2.5 | 20 | 0.5 | 0 | 50 | 1060 | 29 | 6 | 21 | 2 carb, 2 lean meat |
| Spicy Turkey Chili | 1 cup | 220 | 2.5 | 20 | 0.5 | 0 | 50 | 1060 | 29 | 6 | 21 | 2 carb, 2 lean meat |
| ***Stagg Chili*** | | | | | | | | | | | | |
| Chunkero Chili with Beans | 1 cup | 320 | 16 | 140 | 6 | 0.5 | 40 | 850 | 28 | 6 | 16 | 2 carb, 1 med-fat meat, 2 fat |
| Classic Chili with Beans | 1 cup | 330 | 17 | 150 | 7 | 0.05 | 45 | 810 | 27 | 6 | 16 | 2 carb, 1 med-fat meat, 2 fat |
| Country Brand Chili with Beans | 1 cup | 330 | 17 | 150 | 7 | 1 | 35 | 1140 | 28 | 6 | 15 | 2 carb, 1 med-fat meat, 2 fat |
| Dynamite Hot Chili with Beans | 1 cup | 340 | 17 | 150 | 7 | 1 | 40 | 800 | 30 | 8 | 17 | 2 carb, 2 med-fat meat, 1 fat |
| Fiesta Grille Chili with Beans | 1 cup | 250 | 10 | 90 | 4 | 0 | 40 | 950 | 25 | 6 | 15 | 1 1/2 carb, 2 med-fat meat |

| | | | | | | | | | | | | |
|---|---|---|---|---|---|---|---|---|---|---|---|---|
| Laredo Chili with Beans | 1 cup | 310 | 17 | 150 | 7 | 1 | 40 | 1100 | 25 | 7 | 15 | 1 1/2 carb, 2 med-fat meat, 1 fat |
| Ranch House Chicken Chili | 1 cup | 240 | 8 | 70 | 2 | 0 | 55 | 780 | 26 | 7 | 17 | 2 carb, 2 med-fat meat |
| Silverado Beef Chili with Beans | 1 cup | 250 | 7 | 60 | 3 | 0 | 30 | 860 | 30 | 6 | 17 | 2 carb, 2 lean meat |
| Steak House Chili No Beans | 1 cup | 320 | 22 | 200 | 10 | 1 | 65 | 1080 | 14 | 2 | 17 | 1 carb, 2 med-fat meat, 2 fat |
| Turkey Ranchero Chili with Beans | 1 cup | 240 | 3 | 25 | 1 | 0 | 35 | 880 | 31 | 6 | 22 | 2 carb, 2 lean meat |
| Vegetable Garden Four-Bean Chili | 1 cup | 200 | 1 | 10 | 0 | 0 | 0 | 890 | 37 | 8 | 10 | 2 1/2 carb, 1 lean meat |
| ***Trader Joe's*** | | | | | | | | | | | | |
| 99% Fat Free Beef Chili with Beans | 1 cup | 230 | 3 | 25 | 1 | 0 | 40 | 880 | 33 | 6 | 18 | 2 carb, 2 lean meat |
| Chicken Chili with Beans | 1 cup | 290 | 9 | 80 | 3 | 0 | 50 | 810 | 32 | 6 | 19 | 2 carb, 2 med-fat meat |

| | Serving | Calories | Fat (g) | Cal. from Fat | Sat. Fat (g) | Trans Fat (g) | Chol. (mg) | Sod. (mg) | Carb. (g) | Fiber (g) | Prot. (g) | Servings/Exchanges |
|---|---|---|---|---|---|---|---|---|---|---|---|---|
| Organic Vegetarian Chili | 1 cup | 190 | 6 | 60 | 0.5 | 0 | 0 | 590 | 26 | 7 | 8 | 2 carb, 1 fat |
| Turkey Chili with Beans | 1 cup | 230 | 3 | 25 | 1 | 0 | 40 | 800 | 30 | 7 | 21 | 2 carb, 2 lean meat |
| ***Wolf Brand*** | | | | | | | | | | | | |
| Chili Hot Dog Sauce | 2 Tbsp | 30 | 1 | 10 | 0 | 0 | 0 | 140 | 4 | 1 | 1 | 1/2 carb |
| Chili No Beans | 1 cup | 410 | 28 | 250 | 12 | 1.5 | 55 | 1020 | 20 | 7 | 23 | 1 carb, 3 med-fat meat, 3 fat |

## SWEET BREADS, MUFFINS, PASTRIES, DONUTS

| | Serving | Calories | Fat (g) | Cal. from Fat | Sat. Fat (g) | Trans Fat (g) | Chol. (mg) | Sod. (mg) | Carb. (g) | Fiber (g) | Prot. (g) | Servings/Exchanges |
|---|---|---|---|---|---|---|---|---|---|---|---|---|
| Baklava | 22-inch piece | 333 | 23 | 207 | 9 | NA | 36 | 291 | 29 | 2 | 5 | 2 carb, 4 fat |
| Bread, Banana | 1 slice | 178 | 5 | 45 | 2 | NA | 34 | 170 | 31 | 1 | 3 | 2 carb, 1 fat |
| Bread, Date Nut | 1 slice | 217 | 10 | 90 | 2 | NA | 28 | 140 | 30 | <1 | 3 | 2 carb, 2 fat |
| Bread, Fruit, No Nuts | 1 slice | 150 | 6 | 54 | 2 | NA | 22 | 109 | 23 | <1 | 2 | 1 1/2 carb, 1 fat |
| Cream Puff with Custard Filling | 1 | 335 | 20 | 180 | 5 | NA | 174 | 375 | 30 | <1 | 9 | 2 carb, 4 fat |
| Crepe/French Pancake | 1 | 239 | 13 | 117 | 4 | NA | 163 | 274 | 22 | <1 | 9 | 1 1/2 carb, 3 fat |
| Croissant, Cheese | 1 medium | 236 | 12 | 108 | 6 | NA | 37 | 316 | 27 | 2 | 5 | 2 carb, 2 fat |
| Danish Pastry, Cinnamon | 1, 4 inches | 262 | 15 | 135 | 4 | NA | 14 | 241 | 29 | <1 | 5 | 2 carb, 3 fat |
| Danish Pastry, Fruit-Filled | 1, 4 inches | 263 | 13 | 115 | 3.5 | NA | 81 | 251 | 34 | 1 | 4 | 2 carb, 3 fat |

## SWEET BREADS, MUFFINS, PASTRIES, DONUTS

| | Serving | Calories | Fat (g) | Cal. from Fat | Sat. Fat (g) | Trans Fat (g) | Chol. (mg) | Sod. (mg) | Carb. (g) | Fiber (g) | Prot. (g) | Servings/Exchanges |
|---|---|---|---|---|---|---|---|---|---|---|---|---|
| Donut Cake | 1 | 196 | 11 | 100 | 3 | NA | 4 | 262 | 21 | <1 | 3 | 1 1/2 carb, 2 fat |
| Donut, Cake, Sugared/Glazed | 1 | 192 | 10 | 90 | 2 | NA | 14 | 181 | 23 | <1 | 2 | 1 1/2 carb, 2 fat |
| Donut, Cake, with Chocolate Icing | 1 | 194 | 11 | 100 | 6 | NA | 8 | 178 | 22 | <1 | 2 | 1 1/2 carb, 2 fat |
| Donut, Custard-Filled with Icing | 1 | 261 | 13 | 117 | 6 | NA | 21 | 125 | 34 | 1 | 3 | 2 carb, 3 fat |
| Donut, Yeast, Crème Filled | 1 | 307 | 21 | 189 | 6 | NA | 20 | 263 | 26 | <1 | 5 | 2 carb, 4 fat |
| Donut, Yeast, Glazed | 1 | 239 | 12 | 110 | 3 | NA | 18 | 232 | 30 | 1 | 4 | 2 carb, 2 fat |
| Donut, Yeast, Jelly Filled | 1 | 289 | 16 | 144 | 4 | NA | 22 | 190 | 33 | <1 | 5 | 1 1/2 carb, 2 fat |
| Eclair, Chocolate with Custard Filling | 1 | 262 | 16 | 144 | 4 | NA | 127 | 337 | 24 | <1 | 6 | 1 1/2 carb, 3 fat |
| Muffin | 1 small | 133 | 5 | 45 | 1 | NA | 18 | 210 | 19 | 1 | 3 | 1 carb, 1 fat |

| | | | | | | | | | | | | |
|---|---|---|---|---|---|---|---|---|---|---|---|---|
| Muffin, Cheese | 1 small | 184 | 8 | 72 | 3 | NA | 30 | 274 | 23 | <1 | 5 | 1 1/2 carb, 2 fat |
| Muffin, Chocolate Chip | 1 small | 190 | 9 | 81 | 3 | NA | 25 | 186 | 27 | 1 | 4 | 2 carb, 2 fat |
| Muffin, Cranberry Nut | 1 small | 164 | 5 | 45 | 2 | NA | 39 | 326 | 25 | <1 | 4 | 1 1/2 carb, 1 fat |
| Muffin, Oat Bran | 1 small | 175 | 8 | 70 | 1 | NA | 0 | 444 | 55 | 5 | 8 | 3 1/2 carb, 2 fat |
| Muffin, Pumpkin with Raisins & Nuts | 1 small | 181 | 4 | 36 | <1 | NA | 26 | 154 | 34 | 1 | 3 | 2 carb, 1 fat |
| Muffin, Wheat Bran | 1 small | 161 | 7 | 63 | 2 | NA | 19 | 335 | 24 | 2 | 4 | 1 1/2 carb, 1 fat |
| Muffin, Whole Wheat | 1 small | 142 | 6 | 54 | 2 | NA | 21 | 283 | 20 | 3 | 4 | 1 carb, 1 fat |
| Muffin, Zucchini with Nuts | 1 small | 210 | 11 | 99 | 2 | NA | 37 | 169 | 26 | <1 | 3 | 2 carb, 2 fat |
| Pannetone or Italian Sweetbread | 1 slice | 86 | 2 | 18 | 1 | NA | 19 | 96 | 15 | <1 | 2 | 1 carb |
| Sweet Roll | 1 roll | 264 | 12 | 110 | 2 | NA | 47 | 272 | 36 | 2 | 4 | 2 1/2 carb, 2 fat |
| Sweet Roll, Cheese | 1 roll | 238 | 12 | 108 | 4 | NA | 40 | 236 | 29 | <1 | 5 | 2 carb, 2 fat |
| Sweet Roll, Cinnamon Raisin | 1 roll | 223 | 10 | 90 | 2 | NA | 40 | 230 | 31 | 1 | 4 | 2 carb, 2 fat |

SWEET BREADS, MUFFINS, PASTRIES, DONUTS

| | Serving | Calories | Fat (g) | Cal. from Fat | Sat. Fat (g) | Trans Fat (g) | Chol. (mg) | Sod. (mg) | Carb. (g) | Fiber (g) | Prot. (g) | Servings/Exchanges |
|---|---|---|---|---|---|---|---|---|---|---|---|---|
| Sweet Roll, Cinnamon with Raisins & Nuts | 1 | 196 | 7 | 63 | 2 | NA | 13 | 185 | 30 | 1 | 4 | 2 carb, 1 fat |
| **Brands** | | | | | | | | | | | | |
| ***Betty Crocker*** | | | | | | | | | | | | |
| Muffin Mix, Apple Streusel | 1 | 230 | 8 | 70 | 2 | 0 | 35 | 280 | 37 | <1 | 3 | 2 1/2 carb, 2 fat |
| Muffin Mix, Banana Nut | 1 | 210 | 9 | 80 | 2 | 0 | 35 | 250 | 27 | <1 | 2 | 2 carb, 2 fat |
| Muffin Mix, Lemon Poppy Seed | 1 | 200 | 8 | 70 | 1.5 | 0 | 35 | 230 | 30 | 0 | 3 | 2 carb, 2 fat |
| Muffin Mix, Wild Blueberry | 1 | 180 | 7 | 60 | 1.5 | 0 | 35 | 230 | 27 | <1 | 3 | 2 carb, 1 fat |
| Quick Bread Mix, Banana | 1 slice | 170 | 7 | 60 | 1.5 | 0 | 35 | 210 | 25 | 0 | 3 | 1 1/2 carb, 1 fat |
| Quick Bread Mix, Cinnamon Streusel | 1 slice | 180 | 7 | 60 | 1.5 | 0 | 30 | 160 | 28 | 0 | 2 | 2 carb, 1 fat |

| | | | | | | | | | | | | |
|---|---|---|---|---|---|---|---|---|---|---|---|---|
| Quick Bread Mix, Cranberry Orange | 1 slice | 180 | 6 | 60 | 1.5 | 0 | 35 | 180 | 29 | <1 | 3 | 2 carb, 1 fat |
| ***Duncan Hines*** | | | | | | | | | | | | |
| Muffin Mix, Blueberry Streusel, Whole Grain | 1 | 210 | 8 | 70 | 1.5 | 0 | 35 | 230 | 32 | 3 | 3 | 2 carb, 2 fat |
| Muffin Mix, Chocolate Chip, Whole Grain | 1 | 190 | 7 | 60 | 2 | 0 | 35 | 290 | 32 | 3 | 3 | 2 carb, 1 fat |
| Muffin Mix, Cinnamon Swirl, Whole Grain | 1 | 220 | 8 | 70 | 1.5 | 0 | 35 | 230 | 34 | 3 | 3 | 2 carb, 2 fat |
| ***Eggo Bake Shop (Frozen)*** | | | | | | | | | | | | |
| Mini Muffin Tops, Blueberry | 1 | 140 | 5 | 45 | 1.5 | 0 | 15 | 280 | 21 | 0 | 2 | 1 1/2 carb, 1 fat |
| Swirlz, Strawberry | 1 | 150 | 3 | 30 | 1 | 0 | 10 | 270 | 28 | <1 | 3 | 2 carb, 1 fat |
| Twists, Apple | 1 | 190 | 7 | 60 | 3.5 | 0 | 15 | 220 | 29 | <1 | 3 | 2 carb, 1 fat |
| ***Entenmann's*** | | | | | | | | | | | | |
| Apple Puffs | 1 | 290 | 14 | 130 | 7 | 0 | 0 | 260 | 39 | 1 | 3 | 2 1/2 carb, 3 fat |

SWEET BREADS, MUFFINS, PASTRIES, DONUTS

| | Serving | Calories | Fat (g) | Cal. from Fat | Sat. Fat (g) | Trans Fat (g) | Chol. (mg) | Sod. (mg) | Carb. (g) | Fiber (g) | Prot. (g) | Servings/Exchanges |
|---|---|---|---|---|---|---|---|---|---|---|---|---|
| Cheese Topped Buns | 1 | 320 | 15 | 140 | 6 | 0 | 55 | 320 | 40 | 1 | 6 | 2 1/2 carb, 3 fat |
| Cherry Cheese Danish | 1/9 | 200 | 9 | 80 | 3.5 | 0 | 25 | 170 | 25 | <1 | 3 | 1 1/2 carb, 2 fat |
| Cinnamon Swirl Rolls | 1 | 320 | 14 | 130 | 5 | 0 | 45 | 280 | 44 | 2 | 5 | 3 carb, 3 fat |
| Coffee Cake, Crumb | 1/10 | 260 | 13 | 120 | 4 | 0 | 15 | 210 | 34 | 1 | 3 | 2 carb, 3 fat |
| Danish Pastry Twist, Raspberry | 1/8 | 220 | 11 | 100 | 4.5 | 0 | 15 | 170 | 29 | <1 | 3 | 2 carb, 2 fat |
| Danish, Cheese Crumb | 1/9 | 200 | 10 | 90 | 4 | 0 | 35 | 190 | 35 | <1 | 3 | 2 carb, 2 fat |
| Donuts, Frosted Devil Food | 1 | 310 | 18 | 160 | 12 | 0 | 10 | 170 | 36 | 2 | 3 | 2 1/2 carb, 4 fat |
| Donuts, Frosted Popettes | 4 | 320 | 23 | 210 | 14 | 0 | 10 | 180 | 28 | 1 | 2 | 2 carb, 5 fat |
| Donuts, Glazed Crullers | 2 | 210 | 12 | 210 | 6 | 0 | 10 | 140 | 25 | 0 | 1 | 1 1/2 carb, 2 fat |
| Donuts, Glazed Popems | 4 | 220 | 10 | 90 | 5 | 0 | 0 | 170 | 30 | 0 | 2 | 2 carb, 2 fat |
| Donuts, Rich Frosted | 1 | 300 | 20 | 180 | 13 | 0 | 10 | 190 | 30 | 1 | 2 | 2 carb, 4 fat |

| | | | | | | | | | | | | |
|---|---|---|---|---|---|---|---|---|---|---|---|---|
| Eclair | 1 | 260 | 9 | 80 | 2.5 | 0 | 65 | 190 | 46 | 3 | 3 | 3 carb, 2 fat |
| Little Bites Banana Chocolate Chip Muffins | 1 pkg | 180 | 8 | 70 | 2 | 0 | 20 | 125 | 25 | <1 | 2 | 1 1/2 carb, 2 fat |
| Little Bites Blueberry Muffins | 1 pkg | 180 | 8 | 70 | 1.5 | 0 | 25 | 190 | 25 | 0 | 2 | 1 1/2 carb, 2 fat |
| Pecan Danish Ring | 1/8 | 240 | 15 | 140 | 3.5 | 0 | 20 | 150 | 24 | 1 | 3 | 1 1/2 carb, 3 fat |
| ***Hostess*** | | | | | | | | | | | | |
| Donettes, Frosted | 4 | 270 | 17 | 150 | 11 | 0 | 15 | 210 | 29 | 1 | 2 | 2 carb, 3 fat |
| Donettes, Powdered | 4 | 230 | 11 | 100 | 5 | 0 | 20 | 230 | 31 | <1 | 2 | 2 carb, 2 fat |
| Donuts, Powdered | 1 | 190 | 9 | 80 | 4 | 0 | 10 | 230 | 25 | 0 | 2 | 1 1/2 carb, 2 fat |
| Mini Muffins, Banana Walnut | 1 pkg | 260 | 16 | 150 | 2.5 | 0 | 30 | 140 | 27 | <1 | 3 | 2 carb, 3 fat |
| Mini Muffins, Blueberry | 1 pkg | 260 | 14 | 120 | 2.5 | 0 | 40 | 170 | 30 | <1 | 3 | 2 carb, 3 fat |
| ***Jiffy*** | | | | | | | | | | | | |
| Muffin Mix, Apple Cinnamon | 1/4 cup | 180 | 5 | 60 | 2 | 0 | <5 | 320 | 26 | 0 | 2 | 2 carb, 1 fat |

SWEET BREADS, MUFFINS, PASTRIES, DONUTS

| | Serving | Calories | Fat (g) | Cal. from Fat | Sat. Fat (g) | Trans Fat (g) | Chol. (mg) | Sod. (mg) | Carb. (g) | Fiber (g) | Prot. (g) | Servings/Exchanges |
|---|---|---|---|---|---|---|---|---|---|---|---|---|
| Muffin Mix, Banana Nut | 1/4 cup | 170 | 4.5 | 50 | 2 | 0 | <5 | 310 | 25 | <1 | 2 | 1 1/2 carb, 1 fat |
| Muffin Mix, Blueberry | 1/4 cup | 180 | 5 | 60 | 2 | 0 | <5 | 320 | 26 | 0 | 2 | 2 carb, 1 fat |
| ***Kellogg's*** | | | | | | | | | | | | |
| Pop-Tarts Pastry, Blueberry | 1 | 210 | 5 | 50 | 2 | 0 | 0 | 180 | 37 | <1 | 2 | 2 1/2 carb, 1 fat |
| Pop-Tarts Pastry, Brown Sugar Cinnamon | 1 | 210 | 8 | 70 | 2.5 | 0 | 0 | 190 | 34 | 1 | 2 | 2 carb, 2 fat |
| Pop-Tarts Pastry, Cherry, Frosted | 1 | 200 | 5 | 45 | 1.5 | 0 | 0 | 160 | 38 | <1 | 2 | 2 1/2 carb, 1 fat |
| Pop-Tarts Pastry, Chocolate Chip Cookie Dough | 1 | 200 | 5 | 45 | 2 | 0 | 0 | 190 | 35 | <1 | 2 | 2 carb, 1 fat |
| Pop-Tarts Pastry, Chocolate Fudge, Frosted | 1 | 200 | 5 | 45 | 1.5 | 0 | 0 | 230 | 37 | 1 | 3 | 2 1/2 carb, 1 fat |

| | | | | | | | | | | | | |
|---|---|---|---|---|---|---|---|---|---|---|---|---|
| Pop-Tarts Pastry, Raspberry, Frosted | 1 | 200 | 5 | 45 | 1.5 | 0 | 0 | 160 | 38 | <1 | 2 | 2 1/2 carb, 1 fat |
| Pop-Tarts Pastry, S'mores, Frosted | 1 | 200 | 6 | 45 | 1.5 | 0 | 0 | 210 | 36 | <1 | 3 | 2 1/2 carb, 1 fat |
| Pop-Tarts Pastry, Strawberry, Frosted | 1 | 200 | 5 | 45 | 1.5 | 0 | 0 | 170 | 38 | 1 | 2 | 2 1/2 carb, 1 fat |
| Pop-Tarts Pastry, Whole Grain, 20% Fiber, Strawberry | 1 | 190 | 5 | 45 | 1.5 | 0 | 0 | 150 | 35 | 5 | 2 | 2 carb, 1 fat |
| ***Kraft Bagel-fuls*** | | | | | | | | | | | | |
| Blueberry, Bagel with Cream Cheese | 1 | 190 | 4.5 | 40 | 2.5 | 0 | 10 | 190 | 30 | 2 | 6 | 2 carb, 1 fat |
| Original, Plain Bagel with Cream Cheese | 1 | 200 | 5 | 50 | 3 | 0 | 15 | 200 | 31 | 2 | 6 | 2 carb, 1 fat |
| Strawberry & Cream Cheese Bagel | 1 | 190 | 3 | 30 | 1.5 | 0 | 5 | 180 | 34 | 2 | 6 | 2 carb, 1 fat |

SWEET BREADS, MUFFINS, PASTRIES, DONUTS

| | Serving | Calories | Fat (g) | Cal. from Fat | Sat. Fat (g) | Trans Fat (g) | Chol. (mg) | Sod. (mg) | Carb. (g) | Fiber (g) | Prot. (g) | Servings/Exchanges |
|---|---|---|---|---|---|---|---|---|---|---|---|---|
| ***Little Debbie*** | | | | | | | | | | | | |
| Coffee Cake, Apple Streusel | 1 | 190 | 5 | 45 | 1.5 | 0 | 10 | 160 | 35 | 0 | 2 | 2 carb, 1 fat |
| Donut Stick | 1 | 230 | 14 | 130 | 7 | 0 | 10 | 160 | 25 | 0 | 2 | 1 1/2 carb, 3 fat |
| Honey Bun | 1 | 220 | 12 | 110 | 6 | 0 | <5 | 170 | 26 | <1 | 3 | 2 carb, 2 fat |
| Mini Frosted Donuts | 4 | 290 | 17 | 150 | 10 | 0 | 15 | 230 | 32 | 1 | 3 | 2 carb, 3 fat |
| Mini Powdered Donuts | 4 | 210 | 10 | 90 | 5 | 0 | 15 | 220 | 29 | 0 | 2 | 2 carb, 2 fat |
| Muffin, Banana Nut | 1 | 210 | 9 | 80 | 1.5 | 0 | 10 | 170 | 30 | <1 | 3 | 2 carb, 2 fat |
| Muffin, Blueberry | 1 | 190 | 8 | 70 | 1.5 | 0 | 10 | 140 | 27 | 1 | 3 | 2 carb, 2 fat |
| Muffin, Chocolate Chip | 1 | 210 | 9 | 80 | 2 | 0 | 20 | 170 | 28 | 1 | 3 | 2 carb, 2 fat |
| Pecan Spinwheel | 1 | 100 | 4 | 35 | 1 | 0 | <5 | 75 | 16 | <1 | 1 | 1 carb, 1 fat |
| ***Pepperidge Farm Puff Pastry*** | | | | | | | | | | | | |
| Apple Turnover | 1 | 270 | 15 | 135 | 8 | 0 | 0 | 230 | 31 | 1 | 4 | 2 carb, 3 fat |
| Cherry Turnover | 1 | 270 | 15 | 135 | 8 | 0 | 0 | 230 | 31 | 1 | 4 | 2 carb, 3 fat |

| | | | | | | | | | | | | |
|---|---|---|---|---|---|---|---|---|---|---|---|---|
| Raspberry Turnover | 1 | 280 | 15 | 135 | 8 | 0 | 0 | 230 | 34 | 2 | 4 | 2 carb, 3 fat |
| ***Pillsbury (Refrigerated)*** | | | | | | | | | | | | |
| Cinnamon Rolls with Icing | 1 | 140 | 5 | 45 | 1.5 | 2 | 0 | 340 | 23 | <1 | 2 | 1 1/2 carb, 1 fat |
| Cinnamon Rolls with Icing, Reduced Fat | 1 | 130 | 3.5 | 30 | 2.5 | 0 | 0 | 340 | 24 | <1 | 2 | 1 1/2 carb, 1 fat |
| Flaky Supreme Cinnamon Rolls with Icing | 1 | 370 | 19 | 170 | 5 | 5 | 0 | 650 | 48 | 1 | 4 | 3 carb, 4 fat |
| Flaky Twists with Icing | 1 | 180 | 9 | 80 | 2.5 | 0 | 0 | 310 | 22 | <1 | 2 | 1 1/2 carb, 2 fat |
| Orange Sweet Rolls with Icing | 1 | 160 | 6 | 50 | 1.5 | 1.5 | 0 | 350 | 26 | <1 | 2 | 2 carb, 1 fat |
| Toaster Strudel Frozen Pastries, Apple | 1 | 190 | 8 | 80 | 3.5 | 1 | 5 | 180 | 26 | <1 | 3 | 2 carb, 2 fat |
| Toaster Strudel Frozen Pastries, Strawberry | 1 | 190 | 8 | 80 | 3.5 | 1 | 5 | 180 | 26 | <1 | 3 | 2 carb, 2 fat |

# VEGETABLES, VEGETABLE JUICES

| | Serving | Calories | Fat (g) | Cal. from Fat | Sat. Fat (g) | Trans Fat (g) | Chol. (mg) | Sod. (mg) | Carb. (g) | Fiber (g) | Prot. (g) | Servings/Exchanges |
|---|---|---|---|---|---|---|---|---|---|---|---|---|
| Alfalfa Sprouts | 1 cup | 10 | <1 | 0 | 0 | 0 | 0 | 2 | 1 | <1 | 1 | free |
| Artichoke Hearts, Canned, Drained | 1/2 cup | 30 | 0 | 0 | 0 | 0 | 0 | 240 | 6 | 1 | 2 | 1 vegetable |
| Artichokes, Cooked | 1/2 | 30 | <1 | 0 | 0 | 0 | 0 | 57 | 7 | <1 | 3 | 1 vegetable |
| Arugula, Raw | 1 cup | 5 | 0 | 0 | 0 | 0 | 0 | 6 | <1 | 0 | <1 | free |
| Asparagus, Canned, Drained | 1/2 cup | 23 | <1 | 0 | 0 | 0 | 0 | 347 | 3 | 2 | 3 | 1 vegetable |
| Asparagus, Frozen, Cooked | 1/2 cup | 25 | <1 | 0 | 0 | 0 | 0 | 4 | 4 | 1 | 3 | 1 vegetable |
| Aspargus, Fresh, Cooked | 4 spears | 14 | 0 | 0 | 0 | 0 | 0 | 7 | 3 | 1 | 2 | free |
| Baby Corn, Canned | 1/2 cup | 20 | 0 | 0 | 0 | 0 | 0 | 10 | 5 | 2 | 1 | 1 vegetable |
| Bamboo Shoots, Canned | 1/2 cup | 12 | 0 | 0 | 0 | 0 | 0 | 5 | 2 | <1 | 1 | free |

| | | | | | | | | | | | | |
|---|---|---|---|---|---|---|---|---|---|---|---|---|
| Bamboo Shoots, Sliced, Raw | 1 cup | 41 | <1 | 0 | <1 | 0 | 0 | 6 | 8 | 3 | 4 | 1 vegetable |
| Bean Sprouts, Fresh, Cooked | 1/2 cup | 13 | 0 | 0 | 0 | 0 | 0 | 6 | 3 | <1 | 1 | free |
| Beans, Green, Canned | 1/2 cup | 14 | 0 | 0 | 0 | 0 | 0 | 178 | 3 | 1 | <1 | 1 vegetable |
| Beans, Green, Fresh, Cooked | 1/2 cup | 22 | 0 | 0 | 0 | 0 | 0 | 1 | 5 | 2 | 1 | 1 vegetable |
| Beans, Green, Frozen | 1/2 cup | 19 | 0 | 0 | 0 | 0 | 0 | 1 | 4 | 2 | <1 | 1 vegetable |
| Beets, Canned | 1/2 cup | 26 | 0 | 0 | 0 | 0 | 0 | 165 | 6 | 1 | <1 | 1 vegetable |
| Beets, Harvard, Diced | 1/2 cup | 136 | 4 | 36 | <1 | 0 | 0 | 287 | 25 | 2 | <1 | 1 carb, 1 vegetable, 1 fat |
| Beets, Pickled | 1/2 cup | 74 | <1 | 0 | <1 | 0 | 0 | 301 | 19 | 1 | <1 | 1 carb, 1 vegetable |
| Bitter Melon Gourd, Cooked | 1/2 cup | 12 | 0 | 0 | 0 | 0 | 0 | 4 | 3 | 1 | <1 | 1 vegetable |
| Bok Choy | 1 cup | 9 | 0 | 0 | 0 | 0 | 0 | 46 | 2 | <1 | 1 | free |
| Broccoli, Fresh, Cooked | 1/2 cup | 22 | 0 | 0 | 0 | 0 | 0 | 20 | 4 | 2 | 2 | 1 vegetable |

## VEGETABLES, VEGETABLE JUICES

| | Serving | Calories | Fat (g) | Cal. from Fat | Sat. Fat (g) | Trans Fat (g) | Chol. (mg) | Sod. (mg) | Carb. (g) | Fiber (g) | Prot. (g) | Servings/Exchanges |
|---|---|---|---|---|---|---|---|---|---|---|---|---|
| Broccoli, Frozen, Cooked | 1/2 cup | 26 | 0 | 0 | 0 | 0 | 0 | 22 | 5 | 3 | 3 | 1 vegetable |
| Brussels Sprouts, Frozen, Cooked | 1/2 cup | 33 | 0 | 0 | 0 | 0 | 0 | 18 | 7 | 3 | 3 | 1 vegetable |
| Cabbage, Fresh, Cooked | 1/2 cup | 17 | 0 | 0 | 0 | 0 | 0 | 6 | 3 | 2 | <1 | 1 vegetable |
| Cabbage, Green, Raw | 1 cup | 18 | 0 | 0 | 0 | 0 | 0 | 13 | 4 | 2 | 1 | 1 vegetable |
| Cabbage, Red, Cooked | 1/2 cup | 16 | 0 | 0 | <1 | 0 | 0 | 6 | 4 | 2 | <1 | 1 vegetable |
| Carrot Juice, Canned | 1/2 cup | 47 | <1 | 0 | <1 | 0 | 0 | 34 | 11 | <1 | 1 | 2 vegetable |
| Carrots, Canned | 1/2 cup | 36 | 0 | 0 | 0 | 0 | 0 | 344 | 8 | 2 | 1 | 1 vegetable |
| Carrots, Fresh, Cooked | 1/2 cup | 35 | 0 | 0 | 0 | 0 | 0 | 51 | 8 | 3 | <1 | 1 vegetable |
| Carrots, Raw | 1 cup | 50 | 0 | 0 | 0 | 0 | 0 | 84 | 12 | 4 | 1 | 2 vegetable |
| Cassava, Cooked | 1/3 cup | 70 | 0 | 0 | 0 | 0 | 0 | 7 | 17 | <1 | <1 | 1 starch |
| Cassava, Raw | 1/4 cup | 83 | 0 | 0 | 0 | 0 | 0 | 7 | 20 | 1 | 1 | 1 starch |
| Cauliflower, Fresh, Raw | 1 cup | 25 | 0 | 0 | 0 | 0 | 0 | 30 | 5 | 3 | 2 | 1 vegetable |

| | | | | | | | | | | | | |
|---|---|---|---|---|---|---|---|---|---|---|---|---|
| Cauliflower, Frozen, Cooked | 1/2 cup | 17 | 0 | 0 | 0 | 0 | 0 | 16 | 3 | 2 | 1 | 1 vegetable |
| Celery, Fresh, Cooked | 1/2 cup | 14 | 0 | 0 | 0 | 0 | 0 | 68 | 3 | 1 | <1 | 1 vegetable |
| Celery, Fresh, Raw | 1 cup | 17 | 0 | 0 | 0 | 0 | 0 | 99 | 4 | 2 | <1 | 1 vegetable |
| Chard, Swiss, Fresh, Cooked | 1/2 cup | 18 | 0 | 0 | 0 | 0 | 0 | 158 | 4 | 2 | 2 | 1 vegetable |
| Chayote Squash, Cooked | 1/2 cup | 19 | 0 | 0 | 0 | 0 | 0 | 1 | 4 | 2 | <1 | 1 vegetable |
| Coleslaw Mix | 1/2 cup | 17 | 0 | 0 | 0 | 0 | 0 | 15 | 3 | 2 | 0 | 1 vegetable |
| Collard Greens, Fresh, Cooked | 1/2 cup | 26 | 0 | 0 | 0 | 0 | 0 | 15 | 6 | 3 | 1 | 1 vegetable |
| Corn on the Cob, Cooked | 1/2 large ear | 66 | <1 | 0 | 0 | 0 | 0 | 3 | 16 | 2 | 2 | 1 starch |
| Corn, Canned | 1/2 cup | 66 | <1 | 0 | 0 | 0 | 0 | 175 | 15 | 2 | 2 | 1 starch |
| Corn, Frozen, Cooked | 1/2 cup | 66 | <1 | 0 | 0 | 0 | 0 | 4 | 16 | 2 | 2 | 1 starch |
| Cucumber, Raw | 1 cup | 16 | 0 | 0 | 0 | 0 | 0 | 2 | 4 | <1 | <1 | 1 vegetable |

## VEGETABLES, VEGETABLE JUICES

| | Serving | Calories | Fat (g) | Cal. from Fat | Sat. Fat (g) | Trans Fat (g) | Chol. (mg) | Sod. (mg) | Carb. (g) | Fiber (g) | Prot. (g) | Servings/Exchanges |
|---|---|---|---|---|---|---|---|---|---|---|---|---|
| Eggplant, Fresh, Cooked | 1/2 cup | 17 | 0 | 0 | 0 | 0 | 0 | 0 | 4 | 1 | <1 | 1 vegetable |
| Endive/Escarole, Raw | 1 cup | 9 | 0 | 0 | 0 | 0 | 0 | 11 | 2 | 2 | <1 | 1 vegetable |
| Green Onions, Raw | 1 cup | 32 | 0 | 0 | 0 | 0 | 0 | 16 | 7 | 3 | 2 | 1 vegetable |
| Heart of Palm, Canned | 1/2 cup | 20 | 0.5 | 5 | 0 | 0 | 0 | 311 | 3 | 2 | 2 | 1 vegetable |
| Hominy, Yellow, Canned | 1/2 cup | 90 | 1 | 10 | 0 | 0 | 0 | 157 | 18 | 3 | 2 | 1 starch |
| Jicama | 1/2 cup | 30 | 0 | 0 | 0 | 0 | 0 | 3 | 7 | 3 | <1 | 1 vegetable |
| Kale, Fresh, Cooked | 1/2 cup | 18 | 0 | 0 | 0 | 0 | 0 | 15 | 4 | 1 | 1 | 1 vegetable |
| Kohlrabi, Cooked | 1/2 cup | 24 | 0 | 0 | 0 | 0 | 0 | 17 | 6 | <1 | 2 | 1 vegetable |
| Leeks, Cooked | 1/2 cup | 16 | 0 | 0 | 0 | 0 | 0 | 5 | 4 | <1 | <1 | 1 vegetable |
| Lettuce, Butterhead, Raw | 1 cup | 7 | 0 | 0 | 0 | 0 | 0 | 3 | 1 | 0 | 0 | 1 vegetable |
| Lettuce, Iceberg, Raw | 1 cup | 7 | <1 | 0 | 0 | 0 | 0 | 5 | 1 | <1 | <1 | 1 vegetable |
| Lettuce, Romaine, Chopped | 1 cup | 9 | <1 | 0 | <1 | 0 | 0 | 5 | 1 | 1 | <1 | free |

| | | | | | | | | | | | | |
|---|---|---|---|---|---|---|---|---|---|---|---|---|
| Lettuce, Romaine, Raw | 1 cup | 9 | <1 | 0 | 0 | 0 | 0 | 5 | 1 | 1 | <1 | 1 vegetable |
| Lima Beans, Frozen, Cooked | 1/2 cup | 94 | 0 | 0 | 0 | 0 | 0 | 26 | 18 | 5 | 6 | 1 starch |
| Luffa, Cooked | 1/2 cup | 20 | 0 | 0 | 0 | 0 | 0 | 12 | 4 | 2 | 2 | 1 vegetable |
| Mixed Vegetables with Corn, Frozen, Cooked | 1 cup | 80 | 0 | 0 | 0 | 0 | 0 | 80 | 18 | 4 | 4 | 1 starch |
| Mixed Vegetables with Pasta, Frozen, Cooked | 1 cup | 80 | 0 | 0 | 0 | 0 | 0 | 39 | 15 | 5 | 3 | 1 starch |
| Mixed Vegetables, No Corn, Peas, or Pasta | 1/2 cup | 20 | 0 | 0 | 0 | 0 | 0 | 15 | 3 | 1 | 1 | 1 vegetable |
| Mung Bean Sprouts, Cooked | 1/2 cup | 13 | 0 | 0 | 0 | 0 | 0 | 6 | 3 | <1 | 1 | 1 vegetable |
| Mushrooms, Canned | 1/2 cup | 20 | 0 | 0 | 0 | 0 | 0 | 332 | 4 | 2 | 1 | 1 vegetable |
| Mushrooms, Fresh | 1 cup | 15 | 0 | 0 | 0 | 0 | 0 | 4 | 2 | <1 | 2 | free |
| Mustard Greens, Fresh, Cooked | 1/2 cup | 10 | 0 | 0 | 0 | 0 | 0 | 11 | 2 | 1 | 2 | 1 vegetable |

VEGETABLES, VEGETABLE JUICES

| | Serving | Calories | Fat (g) | Cal. from Fat | Sat. Fat (g) | Trans Fat (g) | Chol. (mg) | Sod. (mg) | Carb. (g) | Fiber (g) | Prot. (g) | Servings/Exchanges |
|---|---|---|---|---|---|---|---|---|---|---|---|---|
| Okra, Frozen, Cooked | 1/2 cup | 34 | 0 | 0 | 0 | 0 | 0 | 3 | 5 | 3 | 2 | 1 vegetable |
| Onions, Fresh, Cooked | 1/2 cup | 46 | 0 | 0 | 0 | 0 | 0 | 3 | 11 | 2 | 1 | 2 vegetable |
| Onions, Fresh, Raw | 1 cup | 67 | 0 | 0 | 0 | 0 | 0 | 5 | 16 | 2 | 2 | 3 vegetable |
| Oriental Radish, Fresh | 1 cup | 21 | 0 | 0 | 0 | 0 | 0 | 24 | 5 | 2 | <1 | 1 vegetable |
| Parsnips, Fresh, Cooked | 1/2 cup | 63 | 0 | 0 | 0 | 0 | 0 | 8 | 15 | 3 | 1 | 1 starch |
| Pea Pods, Fresh, Cooked | 1/2 cup | 34 | 0 | 0 | 0 | 0 | 0 | 3 | 6 | 2 | 3 | 1 vegetable |
| Pea Pods, Raw | 1 cup | 61 | 0 | 0 | 0 | 0 | 0 | 6 | 11 | 4 | 4 | 2 vegetable |
| Peas, Green, Canned | 1/2 cup | 59 | 0 | 0 | 0 | 0 | 0 | 214 | 11 | 4 | 4 | 1 starch |
| Peas, Green, Fresh, Cooked | 1/2 cup | 67 | 0 | 0 | 0 | 0 | 0 | 2 | 13 | 4 | 4 | 1 starch |
| Peas, Green, Frozen, Cooked | 1/2 cup | 62 | 0 | 0 | 0 | 0 | 0 | 70 | 11 | 4 | 4 | 1 starch |
| Peas, Sugar Snap, Frozen, Uncooked | 1/2 cup | 30 | 0 | 0 | 0 | 0 | 0 | 3 | 5 | 2 | 2 | 1 vegetable |

| | | | | | | | | | | | | |
|---|---|---|---|---|---|---|---|---|---|---|---|---|
| Peppers, Green, Fresh | 1 cup | 18 | 0 | 0 | 0 | 0 | 0 | 3 | 4 | 2 | <1 | 1 vegetable |
| Peppers, Hot Green Chili, Canned | 1/2 cup | 25 | 0 | 0 | 0 | 0 | 0 | 565 | 3 | 3 | 0 | 1 vegetable |
| Peppers, Red, Fresh, Cooked | 1/2 cup | 19 | 0 | 0 | 0 | 0 | 0 | 1 | 5 | <1 | <1 | 1 vegetable |
| Plantains, Cooked | 1/3 cup | 59 | 0 | 0 | 0 | 0 | 0 | 3 | 16 | 1 | <1 | 1 starch |
| Potatoes, Baked with Skin | 3 oz | 79 | 0 | 0 | 0 | 0 | 0 | 9 | 18 | 2 | 2 | 1 starch |
| Potatoes, French Fried, Frozen, Baked | 1 cup | 98 | 3 | 25 | 0.5 | 0 | 0 | 18 | 16 | 2 | 2 | 1 starch, 1 fat |
| Potatoes, Fresh, Mashed, with Milk | 1/2 cup | 85 | <1 | 0 | 0 | 0 | 0 | 250 | 19 | 2 | 2 | 1 starch |
| Potatoes, White, Cooked, Peeled | 3 oz | 73 | 0 | 0 | 0 | 0 | 0 | 4 | 17 | 2 | 2 | 1 starch |
| Pumpkin, canned | 1 cup | 83 | 0 | 0 | 0 | 0 | 0 | 12 | 20 | 7 | 3 | 1 starch |
| Radicchio, Raw | 1 cup | 9 | 0 | 0 | 0 | 0 | 0 | 9 | 2 | 0 | 0 | 1 vegetable |

## VEGETABLES, VEGETABLE JUICES

| | Serving | Calories | Fat (g) | Cal. from Fat | Sat. Fat (g) | Trans Fat (g) | Chol. (mg) | Sod. (mg) | Carb. (g) | Fiber (g) | Prot. (g) | Servings/Exchanges |
|---|---|---|---|---|---|---|---|---|---|---|---|---|
| Radishes | 1 cup | 20 | 0 | 0 | 0 | 0 | 0 | 28 | 4 | 2 | <1 | 1 vegetable |
| Rutabagas, Fresh, Cooked | 1/2 cup | 33 | 0 | 0 | 0 | 0 | 0 | 17 | 7 | 2 | 1 | 1 vegetable |
| Sauerkraut, Canned | 1/2 cup | 23 | 0 | 0 | 0 | 0 | 0 | 471 | 5 | 3 | 1 | 1 vegetable |
| Soybean Sprouts, Cooked | 1/2 cup | 38 | 2 | 20 | 0 | 0 | 0 | 5 | 3 | <1 | 4 | 1 vegetable |
| Spinach, Canned | 1/2 cup | 25 | 0 | 0 | 0 | 0 | 0 | 29 | 4 | 3 | 3 | 1 vegetable |
| Spinach, Frozen, Cooked | 1/2 cup | 13 | 0 | 0 | 0 | 0 | 0 | 92 | 5 | 4 | 4 | 1 vegetable |
| Spinach, Raw | 1 cup | 12 | 0 | 0 | 0 | 0 | 0 | 44 | 2 | 3 | 2 | 1 vegetable |
| Squash, Summer, Fresh, Cooked | 1/2 cup | 18 | 0 | 0 | 0 | 0 | 0 | 1 | 4 | 1 | <1 | 1 vegetable |
| Squash, Summer, Raw | 1 cup | 18 | 0 | 0 | 0 | 0 | 0 | 2 | 4 | 3 | 1 | 1 vegetable |
| Squash, Winter, Cooked | 1 cup | 39 | <1 | 0 | 0 | 0 | 0 | 1 | 9 | 3 | <1 | 1/2 starch |

| | | | | | | | | | | | | |
|---|---|---|---|---|---|---|---|---|---|---|---|---|
| Succotash, Frozen, Cooked | 1/2 cup | 79 | <1 | 0 | 0 | 0 | 0 | 38 | 17 | 4 | 4 | 1 starch |
| Tomato Juice | 1/2 cup | 21 | 0 | 0 | 0 | 0 | 0 | 440 | 5 | <1 | <1 | 1 vegetable |
| Tomato Paste, Canned | 1/2 cup | 110 | 1 | 9 | <1 | 0 | 0 | 1034 | 25 | 6 | 5 | 1 starch, 1 vegetable |
| Tomato Sauce | 1/2 cup | 37 | 0 | 0 | 0 | 0 | 0 | 738 | 9 | 2 | 2 | 1 vegetable |
| Tomatoes, Canned | 1/2 cup | 24 | 0 | 0 | 0 | 0 | 0 | 250 | 6 | 1 | 1 | 1 vegetable |
| Tomatoes, Raw | 1 cup | 32 | 0 | 0 | 0 | 0 | 0 | 9 | 7 | 2 | 2 | 1 vegetable |
| Tossed Green Salad | 3/4 cup | 19 | 0 | 0 | <1 | 0 | 0 | 11 | 4 | 1 | <1 | 1 vegetable |
| Turnip Greens, Fresh, Cooked | 1/2 cup | 14 | 0 | 0 | 0 | 0 | 0 | 21 | 3 | 3 | <1 | 1 vegetable |
| Turnips, Fresh, Cooked | 1/2 cup | 17 | 0 | 0 | 0 | 0 | 0 | 12 | 4 | 2 | <1 | 1 vegetable |
| Vegetable Juice | 1/2 cup | 25 | 0 | 0 | 0 | 0 | 0 | 310 | 6 | <1 | <1 | 1 vegetable |
| Vegetable Juice Cocktail | 1/2 cup | 23 | 0 | 0 | <1 | 0 | 0 | 442 | 6 | 1 | <1 | 1 vegetable |
| Water Chestnuts, Canned | 1/2 cup | 40 | 0 | 0 | 0 | 0 | 0 | 18 | 9 | 3 | <1 | 1 vegetable |
| Watercress, Raw | 1 cup | 4 | 0 | 0 | 0 | 0 | 0 | 14 | <1 | <1 | <1 | 1 vegetable |

VEGETABLES, VEGETABLE JUICES

| | Serving | Calories | Fat (g) | Cal. from Fat | Sat. Fat (g) | Trans Fat (g) | Chol. (mg) | Sod. (mg) | Carb. (g) | Fiber (g) | Prot. (g) | Servings/Exchanges |
|---|---|---|---|---|---|---|---|---|---|---|---|---|
| Yams, Cooked | 1/2 cup | 79 | 0 | 0 | 0 | 0 | 0 | 5 | 19 | 3 | 1 | 1 starch |
| Yard-Long Beans, Fresh, Cooked | 1/2 cup | 24 | 0 | 0 | 0 | 0 | 0 | 2 | 5 | 2 | 1 | 1 vegetable |
| Zucchini, Fresh, Cooked | 1/2 cup | 14 | 0 | 0 | 0 | 0 | 0 | 3 | 4 | 1 | <1 | 1 vegetable |
| Zucchini, Raw | 1 cup | 18 | 0 | 0 | 0 | 0 | 0 | 11 | 4 | 1 | 1 | 1 vegetable |
| **Brands** | | | | | | | | | | | | |
| ***Betty Crocker*** | | | | | | | | | | | | |
| Mashed Potatoes, Four Cheese | 1/2 cup | 170 | 7 | 30 | 2 | 0 | 5 | 490 | 22 | 1 | 4 | 1 1/2 starch, 1 fat |
| Mashed Potatoes, Roasted Garlic | 1/2 cup | 120 | 3.5 | 30 | 1 | 0.5 | 0 | 520 | 21 | 1 | 2 | 1 1/2 starch, 1 fat |
| Potatoes, Au Gratin | 1/2 cup | 150 | 5 | 50 | 1.5 | 1 | <5 | 660 | 24 | 1 | 3 | 1 1/2 starch, 1 fat |
| Potatoes, Cheddar & Bacon | 2/3 cup | 140 | 5 | 45 | 1 | 1 | 0 | 690 | 23 | 1 | 3 | 1 1/2 starch, 1 fat |

| | | | | | | | | | | | | |
|---|---|---|---|---|---|---|---|---|---|---|---|---|
| Potatoes, Cheesy Scalloped | 1/2 cup | 140 | 5 | 45 | 1 | 1 | 0 | 690 | 22 | 2 | 2 | 1 1/2 starch, 1 fat |
| Potatoes, Deluxe Loaded Au Gratin | 2/3 cup | 140 | 4 | 35 | 1 | 0 | 0 | 660 | 24 | 1 | 3 | 1 1/2 starch, 1 fat |
| Potatoes, Julienne | 2/3 cup | 140 | 5 | 45 | 1.5 | 1 | <5 | 670 | 21 | 1 | 1 | 1 1/2 starch, 1 fat |
| Potatoes, Loaded Au Gratin | 2/3 cup | 140 | 4 | 35 | 2 | 0 | 5 | 660 | 24 | 1 | 3 | 1 1/2 starch, 1 fat |
| Potatoes, Scalloped | 1/2 cup | 130 | 3 | 30 | 1 | 0 | <5 | 660 | 23 | 1 | 2 | 1 1/2 starch, 1 fat |
| Potatoes, Skillet Hash Browns | 1/2 cup | 120 | 4 | 35 | 1 | 0.5 | 0 | 440 | 18 | 2 | 2 | 1 starch, 1 fat |
| Potatoes, Sour Cream 'n Chive | 2/3 cup | 120 | 3 | 30 | 1 | 0 | <5 | 760 | 22 | 1 | 2 | 1 1/2 starch, 1 fat |
| Potatoes, Three Cheese | 2/3 cup | 120 | 3 | 25 | 1 | 0 | 0 | 630 | 23 | 1 | 2 | 1 1/2 starch, 1 fat |
| ***Birds Eye*** | | | | | | | | | | | | |
| Asian Vegetable in Sesame Ginger Sauce | 1 cup | 60 | 1 | 10 | 0 | 0 | 0 | 630 | 12 | 2 | 2 | 2 vegetable |

VEGETABLES, VEGETABLE JUICES

| | Serving | Calories | Fat (g) | Cal. from Fat | Sat. Fat (g) | Trans Fat (g) | Chol. (mg) | Sod. (mg) | Carb. (g) | Fiber (g) | Prot. (g) | Servings/Exchanges |
|---|---|---|---|---|---|---|---|---|---|---|---|---|
| Asparagus Stir-Fry | 1 cup | 90 | 0 | 0 | 0 | 0 | 0 | 30 | 16 | 2 | 4 | 2 vegetable |
| Baby Corn & Vegetable Blend | 2/3 cup | 50 | 1 | 10 | 0 | 0 | 0 | 10 | 9 | 3 | 2 | 1 vegetable |
| Baby Sweet Peas & Pearl Onions | 2/3 cup | 60 | 0 | 0 | 0 | 0 | 0 | 0 | 12 | 3 | 4 | 1 starch |
| Broccoli & Cauliflower Mixture | 1 cup | 25 | 0 | 0 | 0 | 0 | 0 | 25 | 4 | 2 | 1 | 1 vegetable |
| Broccoli & Cheese Sauce | 1/2 cup | 90 | 5 | 45 | 3 | 0 | 5 | 490 | 8 | 1 | 3 | 1 vegetable, 1 fat |
| California Blend & Cheddar Cheese | 1/2 cup | 80 | 4 | 35 | 2 | 0 | 5 | 390 | 8 | 1 | 2 | 1 vegetable, 1 fat |
| Creamed Spinach | 1/2 cup | 90 | 4 | 35 | 2.5 | 0 | 10 | 500 | 9 | 4 | 3 | 1 vegetable, 1 fat |
| Green Beans & Lightly Toasted Almonds | 3/4 cup | 80 | 3.5 | 30 | 0 | 0 | 0 | 410 | 8 | 3 | 3 | 1 vegetable, 1 fat |

| | | | | | | | | | | | | |
|---|---|---|---|---|---|---|---|---|---|---|---|---|
| Peas & Pearl Onions in Lightly Seasoned Sauce | 2/3 cup | 90 | 0 | 0 | 0 | 0 | 0 | 510 | 17 | 4 | 5 | 1 starch |
| Roasted Potatoes & Broccoli | 2/3 cup | 100 | 3.5 | 35 | 2 | 0 | 0 | 470 | 15 | 1 | 2 | 1 starch, 1 fat |
| Sweet Corn & Butter Sauce | 1/2 cup | 110 | 1.5 | 15 | 0.5 | 0 | 0 | 190 | 21 | 1 | 2 | 1 1/2 starch |
| Szechuan Vegetable in Sesame Sauce | 1 cup | 60 | 1.5 | 15 | 0 | 0 | 0 | 460 | 9 | 2 | 1 | 1 vegetable |
| ***Campbell's*** | | | | | | | | | | | | |
| Tomato Juice | 8 oz | 50 | 0 | 0 | 0 | 0 | 0 | 680 | 10 | 2 | 2 | 2 vegetable |
| Tomato Juice, Low Sodium | 8 oz | 50 | 0 | 0 | 0 | 0 | 0 | 140 | 10 | 2 | 2 | 2 vegetable |
| V8 Calcium Enriched | 8 oz | 50 | 0 | 0 | 0 | 0 | 0 | 480 | 11 | 2 | 2 | 2 vegetable |
| V8 Diet Splash Berry Blend Juice Drink | 8 oz | 10 | 0 | 0 | 0 | 0 | 0 | 35 | 3 | 0 | 0 | free |

VEGETABLES, VEGETABLE JUICES

| | Serving | Calories | Fat (g) | Cal. from Fat | Sat. Fat (g) | Trans Fat (g) | Chol. (mg) | Sod. (mg) | Carb. (g) | Fiber (g) | Prot. (g) | Servings/Exchanges |
|---|---|---|---|---|---|---|---|---|---|---|---|---|
| V8 Diet Splash Tropical Blend Juice Drink | 8 oz | 10 | 0 | 0 | 0 | 0 | 0 | 35 | 3 | 0 | 0 | free |
| V8 High Fiber | 8 oz | 70 | 0 | 0 | 0 | 0 | 0 | 480 | 13 | 5 | 2 | 1 carb |
| V8 Low Sodium | 8 oz | 50 | 0 | 0 | 0 | 0 | 0 | 140 | 10 | 2 | 2 | 2 vegetable |
| V8 Spicy Hot | 8 oz | 50 | 0 | 0 | 0 | 0 | 0 | 480 | 10 | 2 | 2 | 2 vegetable |
| V8 Splash Strawberry Kiwi Juice Drink | 8 oz | 70 | 0 | 0 | 0 | 0 | 0 | 50 | 18 | 0 | 0 | 1 carb |
| V8 Vegetable Juice | 8 oz | 50 | 0 | 0 | 0 | 0 | 0 | 420 | 10 | 2 | 2 | 2 vegetable |
| ***Contadina*** | | | | | | | | | | | | |
| Tomato Paste | 2 Tbsp | 30 | 0 | 0 | 0 | 0 | 0 | 20 | 6 | 1 | 2 | 1 vegetable |
| Tomato Paste, Italian | 2 Tbsp | 35 | <1 | 0 | 0 | 0 | 0 | 290 | 7 | 1 | 1 | 1 vegetable |
| Tomato Sauce | 1/4 cup | 15 | 0 | 0 | 0 | 0 | 0 | 280 | 3 | <1 | <1 | 1 vegetable |
| Tomato Sauce with Italian Herbs | 1/4 cup | 15 | 0 | 0 | 0 | 0 | 0 | 320 | 4 | 1 | <1 | 1 vegetable |

| | | | | | | | | | | | | |
|---|---|---|---|---|---|---|---|---|---|---|---|---|
| Tomato Sauce, Extra Thick & Zesty | 1/4 cup | 20 | 0 | 0 | 0 | 0 | 0 | 340 | 3 | 1 | 1 | 1 vegetable |
| Tomatoes, Crushed | 1/4 cup | 20 | 0 | 0 | 0 | 0 | 0 | 150 | 3 | <1 | <1 | 1 vegetable |
| Tomatoes, Italian (Pear) | 1/2 cup | 25 | 0 | 0 | 0 | 0 | 0 | 220 | 4 | 1 | 1 | 1 vegetable |
| Tomatoes, Recipe Ready | 1/2 cup | 25 | <1 | 0 | 0 | 0 | 0 | 570 | 5 | 1 | 1 | 1 vegetable |
| Tomatoes, Stewed | 1/2 cup | 35 | 0 | 0 | 0 | 0 | 0 | 220 | 9 | 1 | 1 | 2 vegetable |
| Tomatoes, Stewed with Italian Herbs | 1/2 cup | 35 | 0 | 0 | 0 | 0 | 0 | 260 | 8 | 1 | 1 | 1 vegetable |
| Tomatoes, Whole Peeled | 1/2 cup | 25 | 0 | 0 | 0 | 0 | 0 | 218 | 4 | 1 | 1 | 1 vegetable |
| ***Green Giant*** | | | | | | | | | | | | |
| Alfredo Vegetables | 1/2 cup | 60 | 1.5 | 15 | 0 | 0 | 0 | 340 | 10 | 2 | 3 | 2 vegetable |
| Asparagus Cuts, No Sauce | 1/2 cup | 20 | 0 | 0 | 0 | 0 | 0 | 90 | 3 | <1 | 2 | 1 vegetable |
| Baby Brussels Sprouts & Butter Sauce | 1/2 cup | 60 | 1 | 10 | 0.5 | 0 | <5 | 320 | 9 | 3 | 3 | 2 vegetable |

| | Serving | Calories | Fat (g) | Cal. from Fat | Sat. Fat (g) | Trans Fat (g) | Chol. (mg) | Sod. (mg) | Carb. (g) | Fiber (g) | Prot. (g) | Servings/Exchanges |
|---|---|---|---|---|---|---|---|---|---|---|---|---|
| Baby Sweet Peas & Butter Sauce | 3/4 cup | 80 | 1.5 | 15 | 1 | 0 | <5 | 340 | 14 | 4 | 5 | 1 starch |
| Baby Sweet Peas, No Sauce | 1/2 cup | 60 | 0.5 | 5 | 0 | 0 | 0 | 190 | 13 | 4 | 4 | 1 starch |
| Baby Vegetable Medley | 3/4 cup | 40 | 1 | 10 | 0 | 0 | <5 | 250 | 9 | 2 | 1 | 2 vegetable |
| Broccoli & Carrots | 3/4 cup | 60 | 3 | 25 | 0 | 0 | 0 | 260 | 8 | 3 | 2 | 2 vegetable |
| Broccoli & Three Cheese Sauce | 1/2 cup | 45 | 1.5 | 15 | 0.5 | 0 | 0 | 420 | 7 | 2 | 3 | 1 vegetable |
| Broccoli Spears & Butter Sauce | 3 spears | 40 | 1.5 | 15 | 1 | 0 | <5 | 330 | 6 | 2 | 2 | 1 vegetable |
| Broccoli Spears, No Sauce | 3 spears | 25 | 0 | 0 | 0 | 0 | 0 | 120 | 4 | 2 | 2 | 1 vegetable |
| Cream Style Corn | 1/2 cup | 110 | 1 | 10 | 0 | 0 | 0 | 320 | 24 | 2 | 2 | 1 1/2 starch |
| Creamed Spinach | 1/2 cup | 70 | 2.5 | 25 | 1.5 | 0 | 0 | 510 | 9 | 1 | 3 | 1 vegetable, 1 fat |
| Cut Green Beans | 1/2 cup | 20 | 0 | 0 | 0 | 0 | 0 | 400 | 4 | 1 | 1 | 1 vegetable |

| | | | | | | | | | | | | |
|---|---|---|---|---|---|---|---|---|---|---|---|---|
| Cut Green Beans, 50% Less Sodium | 1/2 cup | 20 | 0 | 0 | 0 | 0 | 0 | 200 | 4 | 1 | 1 | 1 vegetable |
| Green Bean Casserole | 2/3 cup | 110 | 8 | 70 | 3 | 1 | 0 | 450 | 9 | 4 | 5 | 1 vegetable, 2 fat |
| Niblets Corn & Butter Sauce | 2/3 cup | 90 | 2 | 20 | 1 | 0 | <5 | 320 | 15 | 3 | 3 | 1 starch |
| Sugar Snap Peas, No Sauce | 1/2 cup | 45 | 0 | 0 | 0 | 0 | 0 | 95 | 10 | 2 | 2 | 1/2 starch |
| Sweet Niblets Corn, No Added Salt | 1/2 cup | 90 | 1 | 10 | 0 | 0 | 0 | 0 | 18 | 1 | 2 | 1 starch |
| Sweet Peas | 1/2 cup | 60 | 0 | 0 | 0 | 0 | 0 | 400 | 12 | 3 | 4 | 1 starch |
| Sweet Peas, 50% Less Sodium | 1/2 cup | 60 | 0 | 0 | 0 | 0 | 0 | 200 | 11 | 3 | 4 | 1 starch |
| Teriyaki Vegetables | 1 1/4 cup | 40 | 4 | 40 | 0 | 0 | 0 | 400 | 9 | 2 | 2 | 2 vegetable |
| ***Libby's*** | | | | | | | | | | | | |
| Bavarian Style Sauerkraut | 2 Tbsp | 10 | 0 | 0 | 0 | 0 | 0 | 200 | 3 | <1 | 0 | free |

| | Serving | Calories | Fat (g) | Cal. from Fat | Sat. Fat (g) | Trans Fat (g) | Chol. (mg) | Sod. (mg) | Carb. (g) | Fiber (g) | Prot. (g) | Servings/Exchanges |
|---|---|---|---|---|---|---|---|---|---|---|---|---|
| Pumpkin, Solid Pack, Canned | 1/2 cup | 40 | 0.5 | 5 | 0 | 0 | 0 | 5 | 9 | 5 | 2 | 2 vegetable |
| ***Ore-Ida*** | | | | | | | | | | | | |
| Country Style Fries | 3 oz | 130 | 4.5 | 40 | 1 | 0 | 0 | 300 | 20 | 2 | 2 | 1 starch, 1 fat |
| Country Style Hash Browns | 1 1/4 cup | 70 | 0 | 0 | 0 | 0 | 0 | 20 | 16 | 1 | 2 | 1 starch |
| Crispers | 3 oz | 220 | 13 | 120 | 3 | 0 | 0 | 390 | 23 | 2 | 2 | 1 1/2 starch, 3 fat |
| Crispy Crowns | 11 pieces | 170 | 10 | 90 | 2.5 | 0 | 0 | 490 | 21 | 2 | 2 | 1 1/2 starch, 2 fat |
| Extra Crispy Easy Fries | 3 oz | 180 | 8 | 70 | 1.5 | 0 | 0 | 400 | 25 | 2 | 2 | 1 1/2 starch, 2 fat |
| Extra Crispy Fast Food Fries | 3 oz | 160 | 6 | 60 | 1 | 0 | 0 | 440 | 23 | 2 | 2 | 1 1/2 starch, 1 fat |
| Extra Crispy Golden Crinkles | 3 oz | 170 | 7 | 60 | 1.5 | 0 | 0 | 410 | 24 | 2 | 2 | 1 1/2 starch, 1 fat |
| Extra Crispy Seasoned Crinkles | 3 oz | 150 | 6 | 60 | 1 | 0 | 0 | 450 | 22 | 2 | 2 | 1 1/2 starch, 1 fat |

| Golden Crinkles | 3 oz | 120 | 3.5 | 35 | 2 | 0 | 0 | 310 | 20 | 2 | 2 | 1 starch, 1 fat |
|---|---|---|---|---|---|---|---|---|---|---|---|---|
| Golden Fries | 3 oz | 130 | 3.5 | 20 | 2 | 0 | 0 | 310 | 21 | 2 | 2 | 1 1/2 starch, 1 fat |
| Potatoes O'Brien | 3/4 cup | 60 | 0 | 0 | 0 | 0 | 0 | 40 | 13 | 2 | 1 | 1 starch |
| Shoestrings | 3 oz | 140 | 5 | 45 | 2.5 | 0 | 0 | 320 | 22 | 2 | 2 | 1 1/2 starch, 1 fat |
| Southern Style Hash Browns | 2/3 cup | 70 | 0 | 0 | 0 | 0 | 0 | 30 | 16 | 2 | 2 | 1 starch |
| Steak Fries | 3 oz | 110 | 3 | 25 | 1.5 | 0 | 0 | 300 | 19 | 2 | 2 | 1 starch, 1 fat |
| Steam n' Mash Cut Red Potatoes | 3/4 cup | 70 | 0 | 0 | 0 | 0 | 0 | 270 | 15 | 1 | 2 | 1 starch |
| Steam n' Mash Cut Russet Potatoes | 3/4 cup | 80 | 0 | 0 | 0 | 0 | 0 | 260 | 17 | 2 | 2 | 1 starch |
| Steam n' Mash Cut Sweet Potatoes | 1 cup | 90 | 0 | 0 | 0 | 0 | 0 | 30 | 20 | 3 | 1 | 1 starch |
| Tater Tots | 9 pieces | 170 | 8 | 70 | 1.5 | 0 | 0 | 420 | 20 | 2 | 2 | 1 starch, 2 fat |
| Zesties | 3 oz | 150 | 5 | 45 | 1 | 0 | 0 | 320 | 22 | 2 | 2 | 1 1/2 starch, 1 fat |

## VEGETARIAN FOODS

| | Serving | Calories | Fat (g) | Cal. from Fat | Sat. Fat (g) | Trans Fat (g) | Chol. (mg) | Sod. (mg) | Carb. (g) | Fiber (g) | Prot. (g) | Servings/Exchanges |
|---|---|---|---|---|---|---|---|---|---|---|---|---|
| Bacon Strips, Soy Based | 3 strips | 68 | 3 | 25 | 0 | 0 | 0 | 428 | 2 | <1 | 9 | 1 lean meat |
| Breakfast Links, Soy Based | 1 link | 64 | 5 | 45 | <1 | 0 | 0 | 222 | 3 | <1 | 5 | 1 med-fat meat |
| Breakfast Patty, Meatless, Soy Based | 1 patty | 79 | 3 | 25 | 0.5 | 0 | 0 | 270 | 3 | 2 | 10 | 1 lean meat |
| Chicken Slices, Soy Based | 2 slices | 132 | 8 | 72 | 1 | 0 | 0 | 474 | 4 | 3 | 10 | 1 med-fat meat, 1 fat |
| Edamame | 1/2 cup | 95 | 4 | 35 | 0.5 | 0 | 0 | 5 | 8 | 4 | 8 | 1/2 carb, 1 med-fat meat |
| Falafel | 3 patties | 170 | 9 | 80 | 1 | 0 | 0 | 150 | 16 | 2 | 7 | 1 carb, 1 med-fat meat, 1 fat |
| Frankfurter/Hot Dog, Meatless, Soy Based | 1 | 70 | 2 | 20 | 0 | 0 | 0 | 280 | 6 | 1 | 8 | 1/2 carb, 1 lean meat |

| | | | | | | | | | | | | |
|---|---|---|---|---|---|---|---|---|---|---|---|---|
| Luncheon Meat, Soy Based | 1 slice | 188 | 11 | 100 | 2 | 0 | 0 | 576 | 6 | 3 | 17 | 1/2 carb, 2 med-fat meat |
| Meat Patties, Soy Based | 1 patty | 117 | 5 | 45 | 0.5 | 0 | 0 | 468 | 10 | 4 | 12 | 1/2 carb, 2 lean meat |
| Meatless Beef Crumbles, Soy Based | 2 oz | 60 | 0.5 | 5 | 0 | 0 | 0 | 270 | 6 | 3 | 13 | 1/2 carb, 2 lean meat |
| Meatless Sausage Crumbles, Soy Based | 2 oz | 60 | 0 | 0 | 0 | 0 | 0 | 490 | 8 | 2 | 7 | 1/2 carb, 1 lean meat |
| Meatless Burger, Vegetable & Starch Based | 1 patty | 130 | 3 | 25 | 1 | 0 | 15 | 290 | 12 | 4 | 13 | 1 carb, 1 lean meat |
| Miso | 1/2 cup | 274 | 8 | 70 | 1.5 | 0 | 0 | 5126 | 36 | 7 | 16 | 2 1/2 carb, 1 med-fat meat, 1 fat |
| Miso Sauce | 1/2 cup | 191 | 3 | 25 | <1 | 0 | 0 | 2008 | 36 | 3 | 7 | 2 1/2 carb, 1 fat |
| Nuggets, Breaded, Soy Based | 2 | 90 | 3.5 | 30 | 0.5 | 0 | 0 | 250 | 9 | 2 | 7 | 1/2 carb, 1 lean meat |
| Tempeh (Bean Cake) | 1/4 cup | 84 | 3 | 25 | 0 | 0 | 0 | 3 | 7 | 0 | 8 | 1/2 carb, 1 lean meat |
| Tofu Yogurt | 1 cup | 246 | 5 | 45 | <1 | 0 | 0 | 92 | 42 | <1 | 9 | 3 carb, 1 fat |

| | Serving | Calories | Fat (g) | Cal. from Fat | Sat. Fat (g) | Trans Fat (g) | Chol. (mg) | Sod. (mg) | Carb. (g) | Fiber (g) | Prot. (g) | Servings/Exchanges |
|---|---|---|---|---|---|---|---|---|---|---|---|---|
| Tofu, Firm, Raw | 1/2 cup | 80 | 5 | 45 | 1 | 0 | 0 | 14 | 2 | 1 | 9 | 1 med-fat meat |
| Tofu, Lite, Firm, Silken | 1/2 cup | 45 | 2 | 20 | 0 | 0 | 0 | 82 | 2 | 0 | 8 | 1 lean meat |
| **Brands** | | | | | | | | | | | | |
| ***Health Valley Organic*** | | | | | | | | | | | | |
| No Salt Added Spicy Vegetarian Chili | 1 cup | 150 | 1 | 10 | 0 | 0 | 0 | 75 | 31 | 10 | 9 | 2 starch, 1 lean meat |
| Vegetarian Black Bean Chili | 1 cup | 150 | 1 | 10 | 0 | 0 | 0 | 480 | 32 | 8 | 10 | 2 starch, 1 lean meat |
| Vegetarian Chili with Three Beans | 1 cup | 150 | 1 | 10 | 0 | 0 | 0 | 480 | 32 | 10 | 10 | 2 starch, 1 lean meat |
| ***Lightlife*** | | | | | | | | | | | | |
| Gimme Lean Beef | 2 oz | 70 | 0 | 0 | 0 | 0 | 0 | 350 | 10 | 2 | 7 | 1/2 carb, 1 lean meat |
| Gimme Lean Sausage | 2 oz | 60 | 0 | 0 | 0 | 0 | 0 | 310 | 7 | 3 | 7 | 1/2 carb, 1 lean meat |
| Honey BBQ Wings | 4 wings | 120 | 3 | 25 | 0 | 0 | 0 | 430 | 16 | 4 | 13 | 1 carb, 1 lean meat |

| | | | | | | | | | | | | |
|---|---|---|---|---|---|---|---|---|---|---|---|---|
| Light Burgers, Original | 1/3 cup | 120 | 1.5 | 15 | 0 | 0 | 0 | 500 | 12 | 3 | 16 | 1 carb, 2 lean meat |
| Light Burgers, Veggie | 1 | 140 | 4 | 35 | 0.5 | 0 | 0 | 370 | 16 | 4 | 10 | 1 carb, 1 med-fat meat |
| Organic Soy Tempeh | 4 oz | 230 | 8 | 70 | 1 | 0 | 0 | 10 | 16 | 12 | 22 | 1 carb, 3 lean meat |
| Smart Bacon | 2 slices | 20 | 1 | 10 | 0 | 0 | 0 | 140 | 0 | 0 | 2 | free |
| Smart BBQ | 1/4 cup | 70 | 0 | 0 | 0 | 0 | 0 | 380 | 13 | 1 | 6 | 1 carb, 1 lean meat |
| Smart Chili | 1 cup | 260 | 0.5 | 5 | 0 | 0 | 0 | 820 | 44 | 12 | 19 | 3 carb, 1 lean meat |
| Smart Deli Bologna | 4 slices | 70 | 0 | 0 | 0 | 0 | 0 | 490 | 4 | 1 | 14 | 2 lean meat |
| Smart Deli Turkey | 4 slices | 100 | 3.5 | 30 | 0.5 | 0 | 0 | 300 | 5 | 2 | 13 | 2 lean meat |
| Smart Dogs | 1 | 45 | 0 | 0 | 0 | 0 | 0 | 310 | 2 | <1 | 8 | 1 lean meat |
| Smart Dogs Jumbo | 1 | 80 | 1 | 5 | 0 | 0 | 0 | 560 | 3 | 2 | 15 | 2 lean meat |
| Smart Ground Original | 1/3 cup | 70 | 0 | 0 | 0 | 0 | 0 | 310 | 6 | 3 | 12 | 1/2 carb, 2 lean meat |
| Smart Links, Breakfast | 2 links | 100 | 3.5 | 30 | 0.5 | 0 | 0 | 580 | 8 | 4 | 10 | 1/2 carb, 1 lean meat |
| Smart Sausage, Chorizo Style | 1 link | 140 | 8 | 70 | 1 | 0 | 0 | 590 | 5 | <1 | 12 | 2 lean meat |
| Smart Sausage, Italian Style | 1 | 140 | 7 | 70 | 1 | 0 | 0 | 500 | 7 | 1 | 13 | 1/2 carb, 2 lean meat |

VEGETARIAN FOODS

| | Serving | Calories | Fat (g) | Cal. from Fat | Sat. Fat (g) | Trans Fat (g) | Chol. (mg) | Sod. (mg) | Carb. (g) | Fiber (g) | Prot. (g) | Servings/Exchanges |
|---|---|---|---|---|---|---|---|---|---|---|---|---|
| Smart Sausage, Smoked Style | 1 patty | 150 | 7 | 70 | 1 | 0 | 0 | 580 | 9 | 2 | 13 | 1/2 carb, 2 lean meat |
| Smart Strips, Chick'n | 3 oz | 80 | 0 | 0 | 0 | 0 | 0 | 520 | 6 | 4 | 14 | 1/2 carb, 2 lean meat |
| Tempehtations, Ginger Teriyaki | 3 oz | 160 | 5 | 45 | 1 | 0 | 0 | 560 | 18 | 5 | 11 | 1 carb, 1 med-fat meat |
| Tofu Pups | 1 | 60 | 2.5 | 20 | 0.5 | 0 | 0 | 300 | 2 | 1 | 8 | 1 lean meat |
| ***Morningstar Farms*** | | | | | | | | | | | | |
| Asian Veggie Patties | 1 patty | 100 | 4 | 35 | 0.5 | 0 | 0 | 490 | 10 | 2 | 7 | 1/2 carb, 1 lean meat |
| Breakfast Pattie, Organic Soy | 1 | 80 | 3 | 25 | 0.5 | 0 | 0 | 240 | 4 | 1 | 8 | 1 lean meat |
| Buffalo Wing Veggie Wings | 5 | 200 | 8 | 70 | 1 | 0 | 0 | 640 | 20 | 3 | 12 | 1 carb, 1 med-fat meat, 1 fat |
| Chik Patties Original | 1 | 140 | 5 | 45 | 0.5 | 0 | 0 | 590 | 16 | 2 | 8 | 1 carb, 1 med-fat meat |
| Chik'n Nuggets | 4 | 190 | 9 | 80 | 1.5 | 0 | 0 | 600 | 19 | 4 | 12 | 1 carb, 1 med-fat meat, 1 fat |

| | | | | | | | | | | | | |
|---|---|---|---|---|---|---|---|---|---|---|---|---|
| Classic Veggie Burgers, Organic Soy | 1 | 150 | 6 | 50 | 0.5 | 0 | 0 | 280 | 10 | 3 | 14 | 1/2 carb, 2 lean meat |
| Garden Veggie Patties Veggie Burgers | 1 | 110 | 3.5 | 30 | 0.5 | 0 | 0 | 350 | 9 | 3 | 10 | 1/2 carb, 1 lean meat |
| Grillers Chik'n Veggie Patties | 1 | 80 | 3 | 30 | 0 | 0 | 0 | 350 | 7 | 5 | 9 | 1/2 carb, 1 lean meat |
| Grillers Original | 1 burger | 130 | 6 | 50 | 1 | 0 | 0 | 260 | 5 | 2 | 15 | 2 lean meat |
| Grillers Prime Veggie Burgers | 1 | 170 | 9 | 80 | 1 | 0 | 0 | 360 | 4 | 2 | 17 | 2 lean meat |
| Hickory BBQ Riblets | 1 | 220 | 3.5 | 30 | 0 | 0 | 0 | 810 | 35 | 5 | 18 | 2 carb, 2 lean meat |
| Italian Herb Chik Patties | 1 | 170 | 5 | 45 | 0.5 | 0 | 0 | 480 | 22 | 2 | 10 | 1 1/2 carb, 1 med-fat meat |
| Maple Flavored Veggie Sausage Patties | 1 patty | 80 | 3 | 25 | 0.5 | 0 | 0 | 250 | 5 | <1 | 10 | 1 lean meat |
| Meal Starters Chik'n Strips | 12 | 140 | 3.5 | 30 | 0.5 | 0 | 0 | 510 | 6 | 1 | 23 | 1/2 carb, 3 lean meat |

| | Serving | Calories | Fat (g) | Cal. from Fat | Sat. Fat (g) | Trans Fat (g) | Chol. (mg) | Sod. (mg) | Carb. (g) | Fiber (g) | Prot. (g) | Servings/Exchanges |
|---|---|---|---|---|---|---|---|---|---|---|---|---|
| Meal Starters Grillers Recipe Crumbles | 2/3 cup | 80 | 2.5 | 20 | 0 | 0 | 0 | 230 | 5 | 3 | 10 | 1 lean meat |
| Meal Starters Sausage Style Recipe Crumbles | 2/3 cup | 90 | 2.5 | 25 | 0 | 0 | 0 | 420 | 5 | 3 | 11 | 2 lean meat |
| Original Chik'n Tenders | 2 | 190 | 7 | 60 | 1 | 0 | 0 | 580 | 20 | 3 | 12 | 1 carb, 1 med-fat meat |
| Spicy Black Bean Burger | 1 | 210 | 7 | 65 | 1 | 1 | 0 | 700 | 24 | 7 | 17 | 1 1/2 carb, 2 lean meat |
| Veggie Bacon Strips | 2 strips | 60 | 4.5 | 40 | 0.5 | 0 | 0 | 230 | 2 | 1 | 2 | 1 fat |
| Veggie Bites, Broccoli Cheddar Snacks | 3 pieces | 180 | 10 | 90 | 2.5 | 0 | 5 | 550 | 15 | 2 | 8 | 1 carb, 1 med-fat meat, 1 fat |
| Veggie Bites, Spinach Artichoke Snacks | 3 pieces | 190 | 10 | 90 | 2.5 | 0 | 0 | 570 | 16 | 2 | 9 | 1 carb, 1 med-fat meat, 1 fat |
| Veggie Cakes, Ginger Teriyaki | 1 patty | 110 | 1.5 | 15 | 0.5 | 0 | 0 | 320 | 19 | 2 | 5 | 1 carb, 1 lean meat |

| | | | | | | | | | | | | |
|---|---|---|---|---|---|---|---|---|---|---|---|---|
| Veggie Cakes, Southwestern Style | 1 patty | 130 | 3 | 30 | 1 | 0 | 5 | 340 | 21 | 2 | 6 | 1 1/2 carb, 1 lean meat |
| Veggie Italian Style Sausage | 1 link | 120 | 6 | 50 | 0.5 | 0 | 0 | 350 | 7 | 1 | 10 | 1/2 carb, 1 med-fat meat |
| Veggie Sausage Links | 2 links | 80 | 3 | 25 | 0.5 | 0 | 0 | 300 | 3 | 2 | 9 | 1 lean meat |
| ***Worthington/Loma Linda*** | | | | | | | | | | | | |
| Chic-ketts | 1 slice | 110 | 5 | 45 | 1 | 0 | 0 | 390 | 3 | 2 | 14 | 2 lean meat |
| Dinner Roast | 1 slice | 180 | 11 | 100 | 1.5 | 0 | 0 | 580 | 6 | 3 | 14 | 1/2 carb, 2 med-fat meat |
| Fried Chik'n with Gravy | 2 pieces | 130 | 6 | 50 | 1 | 0 | 0 | 430 | 9 | 3 | 9 | 1/2 carb, 1 med-fat meat |
| FriPats | 1 patty | 130 | 6 | 50 | 1 | 0 | 0 | 320 | 5 | 3 | 15 | 2 lean meat |
| Leanies Links | 1 link | 100 | 7 | 60 | 1 | 0 | 0 | 430 | 2 | 1 | 8 | 1 med-fat meat |
| Meatless Chicken Roll | 1 slice | 90 | 4.5 | 40 | 0.5 | 0 | 0 | 240 | 2 | 1 | 9 | 1 med-fat meat |
| Prosage Link | 2 links | 80 | 3 | 30 | 0.5 | 0 | 0 | 320 | 3 | 2 | 9 | 1 lean meat |
| Stakelets | 1 piece | 150 | 7 | 70 | 1 | 0 | 0 | 480 | 7 | 2 | 14 | 1/2 carb, 2 lean meat |

| | Serving | Calories | Fat (g) | Cal. from Fat | Sat. Fat (g) | Trans Fat (g) | Chol. (mg) | Sod. (mg) | Carb. (g) | Fiber (g) | Prot. (g) | Servings/Exchanges |
|---|---|---|---|---|---|---|---|---|---|---|---|---|
| Stripples | 2 strips | 60 | 4.5 | 40 | 0.5 | 0 | 0 | 220 | 2 | 1 | 2 | 1 fat |
| ***Yves Veggie Cuisine*** | | | | | | | | | | | | |
| Chicken Skewers | 1 | 100 | 1 | 10 | 0 | 0 | 0 | 450 | 7 | 4 | 15 | 1/2 carb, 2 lean meat |
| Classic Mac 'n' Soy Cheese | 1 bowl | 340 | 9 | 80 | 1.5 | 0 | 0 | 880 | 52 | 3 | 13 | 3 1/2 carb, 1 med-fat meat, 1 fat |
| Good Dog | 1 | 70 | 3.5 | 30 | 0 | 0 | 0 | 430 | 1 | 0 | 8 | 1 lean meat |
| Hot Dog | 1 | 50 | 0.5 | 5 | 0 | 0 | 0 | 400 | 2 | 0 | 10 | 1 lean meat |
| Meatless Breakfast Patties | 2 | 80 | 2 | 15 | 0 | 0 | 0 | 350 | 4 | 2 | 11 | 2 lean meat |
| Meatless Canadian Bacon | 3 slices | 80 | 0.5 | 5 | 0 | 0 | 0 | 400 | 2 | 0 | 17 | 2 lean meat |
| Meatless Chicken Burger | 1 | 100 | 3 | 25 | 0 | 0 | 0 | 420 | 5 | 2 | 15 | 2 lean meat |
| Meatless Chili | 1 bowl | 240 | 1 | 10 | 0 | 0 | 0 | 850 | 37 | 14 | 21 | 2 1/2 carb, 2 lean meat |

| | | | | | | | | | | | | |
|---|---|---|---|---|---|---|---|---|---|---|---|---|
| Meatless Deli Bologna Slices | 4 slices | 80 | 2.5 | 20 | 0 | 0 | 0 | 480 | 2 | 0 | 14 | 2 lean meat |
| Meatless Deli Turkey Slices | 4 slices | 100 | 1.5 | 15 | 0 | 0 | 0 | 340 | 5 | 0 | 15 | 2 lean meat |
| Meatless Ground Round Original | 1/3 cup | 60 | 0.5 | 5 | 0 | 0 | 0 | 270 | 5 | 2 | 10 | 1 lean meat |
| Meatless Ground Turkey | 1/3 cup | 60 | 1 | 10 | 0 | 0 | 0 | 330 | 4 | 2 | 14 | 2 lean meat |
| Meatless Ham Slices | 4 slices | 100 | 2 | 20 | 0 | 0 | 0 | 480 | 5 | 0 | 15 | 2 lean meat |
| Meatless Lasagna | 1 bowl | 300 | 3 | 25 | 0.5 | 0 | 0 | 650 | 51 | 4 | 17 | 3 1/2 carb, 2 lean meat |
| Tofu Dogs | 1 | 45 | 1 | 5 | 0 | 0 | 0 | 300 | 2 | 0 | 8 | 1 lean meat |
| Veggie Brat Classic | 1 | 160 | 5 | 50 | 0 | 0 | 0 | 840 | 1 | 1 | 19 | 3 lean meat |

# Index

## *G*



## *H*

## Q



## R



## S